Nutrition
and
Diet Therapy
Edition 2

Carroll A. Lutz, MA, RN
Associate Professor Emerita of Nursing
Jackson Community College
Jackson, Michigan

Karen Rutherford Przytulski, MS, RD
Director of Dietary
Doctors Hospital of Jackson
Registered Dietitian
Hospicc of Jackson
Jackson, Michigan

F. A. DAVIS COMPANY • Philadelphia

F. A. Davis Company
1915 Arch Street
Philadelphia, PA 19103

Copyright © 1997 by F. A. Davis Company

Printed in the United States of America

Last digit indicates print number: 10 9 8 7 6 5 4 3 2 1

Managing Editor, Nursing: Lisa Biello
Nursing Development Editor: Melanie Freely
Cover Design By: Louis Forgione
Cover Art By: Donna Dalton

As new scientific information becomes available through basic and clinical research, recommended treatments and drug therapies undergo changes. The author(s) and publisher have done everything possible to make this book accurate, up to date, and in accord with accepted standards at the time of publication. The authors, editors, and publisher are not responsible for errors or omissions or for consequences from application of the book, and make no warranty, expressed or implied, in regard to the contents of the book. Any practice described in this book should be applied by the reader in accordance with professional standards of care used in regard to the unique circumstances that may apply in each situation. The reader is advised always to check product information (package inserts) for changes and new information regarding dose and contraindications before administering any drug. Caution is especially urged when using new or infrequently ordered drugs.

Library of Congress Cataloging–in–Publication Data

Lutz, Carroll A.
    Nutrition and diet therapy / Carroll A. Lutz, Karen Rutherford
Przytulski.—2nd ed.
      p.   cm.
    Includes bibliographical references and index.
    ISBN 0–8036–0231–6 (pbk.)
    1. Dietetics. 2. Diet therapy. 3. Nutrition. I. Przytulski,
Karen Rutherford. II. Title.
    [DNLM: 1. Diet Therapy. 2. Nutrition. 3. Diet. WB 400 L975n
1997]
RM217.L88 1997
613.2—dc21
DNLM/DLC
for Library of Congress
                                        94–4030
                                        CIP

Paul—this one's for you.

Karen Rutherford Przytulski

To all my teachers, including family, friends, colleagues,
students, and editors, with appreciation for our ongoing and uplifting dialogue

Carroll A. Lutz

Preface

The second edition of *Nutrition and Diet Therapy* is designed to provide the beginning student with an understanding of the fundamentals of nutrition as it relates to the promotion and maintenance of optimal health. Practical applications and treatment of nutrition-related pathologies are stressed.

The second edition contains two new chapters: Individualizing Client Care (including cultural considerations) and Care of the Terminally Ill. In addition, the chapter on food management has been completely revised to include information on food safety and meal planning.

This book was written to meet the educational needs of nursing students, dietetic assistants, diet technicians, and others. Support materials for the nursing student include case studies with examples of care plans presented throughout the text and clinical analysis study questions. The goal of these support materials is to promote critical thinking. There is currently an information explosion related to the science of nutrition. As researchers discover new and more effective treatments for nutrition-related disorders and health maintenance, the ability to think critically becomes more important for professional growth and development. Students need to be able to know the facts and apply information in a clinical environment. This text has been developed to facilitate this process.

This text can be used to teach a complete course in nutrition or as a desk reference for practitioners. The student using this book needs no previous exposure to anatomy, physiology, or medical terminology. Subjects are fully supported by diagrams, illustrations, figures, or tables.

The content of *Nutrition and Diet Therapy, ed 2,* is organized into three units.

Unit One, **The Role of Nutrients in the Human Body,** covers basic information on nutrition as a science and how this information is applied through the nursing process. A thorough discussion of all the essential nutrients includes definitions and a description of functions, effects of excesses and deficiencies, and food sources. Information on the use of food in the body and how the body maintains energy balance completes the unit.

Unit Two, **Family and Community Nutrition,** provides an overview of topics such as nutrition in the life cycle, food management, and nutrient delivery.

Unit Three, **Clinical Nutrition,** focuses on the care of clients with pathologies caused by or that cause nutritional impairments. Pathological conditions include diabetes mellitus and hypoglycemia, cardiovascular disease, renal disease, gastrointestinal disease, cancer, and AIDS. Other topics discussed include food, nutrient, and drug interactions; weight control; nutrition during stress; and care of the client with a terminal illness.

Special features are used throughout the text to facilitate the teaching and learning process. All of the chapters include the following:

Study Aids—Chapter Review Questions and Clinical Analysis Questions that are similar to those on the NCLEX examination. Answers to the Study Aids questions are available in Appendix I.

Case Study with a proposed **Nursing Care Plan**—Allows the student to see how the nutrition principles described in the chapter are applied in a specific clinical situation.

Clinical Applications—Cover a variety of topics that emphasize application to clinical practice or curent use in the health care professions.

Clinical Calculations—Isolate and explain many of the mathematical calculations that are used in nutritional science.

This text also includes the following aids:

Glossary—Includes over 700 entries.

Teaching Aids—An **Instructor's Guide** that includes transparency masters, crossword puzzles, and classroom activities is available. Ideas for teaching the course as a stand alone or integrated into the curriculum are also presented.

Cybertest—An electronic testbank containing hundreds of questions arranged by chapter.

We believe that *Nutrition and Diet Therapy, ed 2,* provides the clinical information necessary for a fuller understanding of the relationship between the knowledge about nutrition and diet and its clinical application. This text balances direct explanations of the underlying science with the clinical responsibilities of the health care professional.

Acknowledgments

A project as massive as the writing of a textbook requires the assistance of many people. We would first like to thank all the organizations and publishers that gave permission for the use of their material. We would also like to thank Russell Tobe, J.D., D.O., B.S.E.E. for the many hours he spent reviewing selected portions of the manuscript. This textbook would have been much less without his unselfish devotion to this project.

Many of our peers contributed to this project. In particular we would like to thank The Jackson Community College Learning Resources Center staff, Cliff Taylor, Marion VanLoo, Joyce Bradley, and Wendy White. They were fantastically persistent in obtaining interlibrary loans. A special thanks to F. A. Davis staff: Bob Martone, Ruth DeGeorge, Melanie Freely, Herb Powell, and Peter Faber for their ongoing enthusiasm. We thank our students for their challenging questions and continuing inspiration. Lastly, we thank our husbands, Bob and Paul, for tolerating if not understanding our compulsion to write.

Consultants

Ellen J. Anderson, MS, RD
Research Dietitian Manager
Massachusetts General Hospital
Boston, MA

Carlene Bradham, MNSc
Adult Psychiatric Clinical Specialist
University of Arkansas
Little Rock, AR

Louise Brentin, BSN, MSN
Chair, Nursing Division
Delta College
University Center, MI

Patricia A. Eagan, BSN, MSN, RN, C
Instructor
Jefferson School of Nursing
Pine Bluff, AR

Bernardine Fitzloff, BSN, MSN
Academic Faculty
Concordia University
Oak Park, IL

Jean Foote, RN, C, MS
Associate Professor
Grand Canyon University
Phoenix, AZ

Karen Hauersperger, RD, LDN, MS, EdS
Instructor
Queens College
Charlotte, NC

Sue Heiber, RN, BSN, MNEd
Professor
Community College of Allegheny County
West Mifflin, PA

Theresa Isom, RN, BS, BSN, MS
Nursing Coordinator
Tennessee Technical Center
Memphis, TN

Starr Mitchell, RN, BSN, MSN
Chairman, Department of Nursing
Sandhills Community College
Pinehurst, NC

Lynn O'Reilly, BS, MS
Instructor
Endicott College
Beverly, MA

Gretchen Plotkin, MA, MS
Assistant Professor
SUNY Morrisville
Morrisville, NY

Margaret Skulnik, RN, BS, MS, CDE
Clinical Coordinator
Durham Technical Community College
Durham, NC

Nancy Spahr, BS, MS, MBA
Professor
New Hampshire Technical Institute
Concord, NH

Irene A. Farquhar Taylor, RN, BSN
Practical Nursing Program Coordinator
Bellingham Technical College
Bellingham, WA

Roselena Thorpe, RN, PhD
Professor/Department Chairperson
Community College Allegheny County
Pittsburgh, PA

Larry Tonzi, RN, MSN
Professor
North Maine Technical College
Presque Isle, ME

Contents

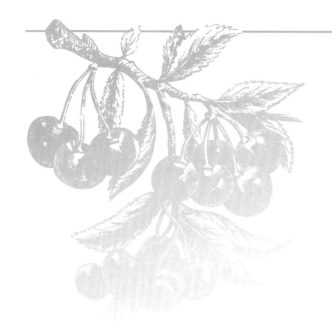

The Role of Nutrients in the Human Body

CHAPTER 1

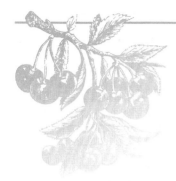

Evolution and the Science of Nutrition

LEARNING OBJECTIVES

After completing this chapter, the student should be able to:

1 Discuss the relationship between the biologic evolution of the human body and present nutritional concerns.
2 State the three functions of nutrients.
3 Identify the six classes of nutrients.
4 Discuss the effects of malnutrition on health and provide examples.
5 Describe the relationship between nutrition and health.

Food and health are now and always have been connected. In this chapter, we compare our ancestors' food habits and their effect on health with those of modern people. Our understanding of health concepts has changed considerably in the last 5 to 8 million years. This chapter examines past and present views about health and health care and how these views affect the role of health care professionals. In addition, the chapter discusses the concept of nutrition as a science and introduces some basic terminology.

Evolution of the Human Body and Emergence of Health Issues

Throughout history our ancestors survived on a number of different diets. What early humans ate in any particular geographic area depended on the climate, their hunting and gathering skills, the state of their food-processing technology, and what foods were available. The human body evolved the capability to subsist on a wide variety of foodstuffs of both plant and animal origin.

Effect of Agriculture

The emergence of agriculture led to population expansion. Individuals learned to work together to grow crops and began to live together in larger groups to protect the cultivated fields and harvested food stores, leading to the development of villages and towns. Food distribution systems evolved for the rationing of the harvest from one growing season to the next. This helped assure a food supply in the event of a poor harvest or natural disaster.

However, agriculture, especially single-crop agriculture, limited the variety of foods available to a given community. Today we understand that growth deficiencies can result from diets based on single-crop agriculture because no single food can furnish all the raw materials necessary for human growth and healthful maintenance. Variety, moderation, and balance in the diet are all necessary for health.

Adaptation to Feast and Famine Conditions

Seasonal and cyclical variations in food availability affected our ancestors. An example of a seasonal variation is the abundance of food during summer and fall compared with the scarcity of food late in winter. A **cyclical variation** refers to a recurring series of events such as a period of drought and famine followed by a period of plentiful rainfall.

Biologically, the human body adapted to these feast-or-famine conditions by developing the capacity to store energy as fat. While this adaptation enabled human beings to survive famine, individuals did not always receive optimal nourishment. The situation is much the same today. Famine still exists in many third world countries, and even in the developed countries there are population groups—notably, the poor, the young, and the elderly—that suffer from **malnutrition**.

Food Safety Issues

Frequently, we paint a picture of the so-called natural man or woman, imagining a time when healthy, happy people subsisted on unprocessed foods. Though free from pesticides and additives, the food our ancestors ate was not always safe. Meat, for example, was often rancid and contained parasites; fungal infestations contaminated not only stored grain but also grain in the fields; and heavy metals leached out of utensils into food, often with fatal effects. Notwithstanding these and other hazards, humans still managed to survive as a species.

Our Ancestors' View of Health

In the past, attitudes about **health** were often linked to following or not following the laws of a supernatural being. For example, the recurrent epidemics of bubonic plague that swept Europe during the Middle Ages were thought to be the result of witchcraft and the work of the devil. With the discovery of bacteria in the late 1880s and the subsequent discovery and use of antibiotics in the 1940s, many diseases were better understood and treatable. Until recent decades, the primary focus of health care was on curing an existing disease. Slowly, in part as a result of scientific progress, the thrust of health care delivery has shifted from curing an existing disease to preventing disease. The use of vaccines is one form of prevention. The consumption of substances in food, which can help to prevent certain diseases, is another example of prevention.

Current Attitudes toward Health and Health Care

Today many diseases are linked to lifestyle behaviors such as smoking, lack of adequate physical activity, and poor nutritional habits. Health care providers emphasize the relationship between lifestyle and risk of disease development. People are increasingly managing their health problems and making personal commitments to lead healthier lives. Nutrition is, in part, a preventive science—given sufficient resources, how and what one eats is a lifestyle choice.

The ability to detect disease early with the help of highly sophisticated technology is another major focus of health care delivery. Not only can it sometimes reduce suffering and mortality, but early disease detection also enables people to alter behaviors, including food habits, that can help to retard disease progression. Although early identification of disease frequently results in a cost saving to the client, educating and screening clients for disease is expensive to society. Can we afford to pay for disease detection and health education? The answer depends largely on the willingness of health care providers to educate clients during each client encounter.

The Emerging Role of the Health Care Professional

Changing attitudes about health have altered the role of the health care professional. No longer is the client totally reliant on the physician; his or her care is now in the hands of a number of allied health personnel. Indeed, a hospital client's health care team may include more than 15 members. The respective titles and responsibilities of the major members of the health care team are outlined below.

Physician

The physician is responsible for the diagnosis and treatment of the medical condition. He or she manages the medical care, orders laboratory tests, prescribes medications and diet, and explains the treatment plan to the client.

Registered Dietitian

The registered dietitian (RD), together with the physician, has the responsibility to meet the client's nutritional needs. This includes interpreting the physician's diet order in terms of the client's food habits and food choices, evaluating the client's response to the therapeutic diet, and providing nutrition education and counseling for clients.

Dietetic Technician

The dietetic technician (DT) assists the dietitian by taking nutrition histories and body measurements, reviewing records, and monitoring clients' food intake.

Registered Nurse

The registered nurse (RN) is responsible for the patient's daily health care, including his or her nutritional care. The RN communicates with the physician and the dietitian regarding the client's response to food, including intake and tolerance, provides nutrition education, if needed, and records information on the client's chart.

Licensed Practical Nurse

The licensed practical nurse (LPN), supervised by an RN, feeds clients, monitors food consumption, measures intake and output, and records data.

Other Health Care Personnel

Other health care personnel who may be involved in client care include the clinical pharmacist, the licensed social worker, the medical technologist, the nurse practitioner, and physical and occupational therapists. There now is a national trend toward client care technicians and associates who will be the bedside caregivers.

Client As the Focus of the Health Care Provider

The client is the focus of the health care team, and both the client and the family members should be involved in the care plan. Clients who participate in their own care are more likely to achieve the goals or objectives set.

Nutrition Is a Science

Stated simply, **nutrition** is the relationship of humans to food. Our study of nutrition will include a discussion of the following topics:

- The chemical content of food
- The use of food by the body
- The relationship of food to health
- The selection of food
- Techniques to change food behavior
- The diet as treatment for disease
- The relationship between medications and food intake

As this list shows, the science of nutrition encompasses ideas from many other sciences: biology, chemistry, economics, educational theory, medicine, pharmacology, physiology, psychology, and sociology. This connection with other disciplines suggests far-reaching implications of good nutrition.

Nutrients

The science of nutrition has historically been based on the nutrients found in food. **Nutrients** are chem-

---

Cyclical variation—A recurring series of events during a specified time period.

Health—A state of complete physical, mental, and social well-being, not just the absence of disease or infirmity.

Nutrition—The science of food and its relation to humans.

Nutrient—A chemical substance supplied by food that the body needs for growth, maintenance, and repair.

ical substances supplied by food that the body needs for growth, maintenance, and repair. Nutrients can be divided into six groups:

1. Carbohydrates (often abbreviated as CHO)
2. Fats (lipids)
3. Proteins
4. Minerals
5. Vitamins
6. Water

Each group will be discussed in a separate chapter.

Nutrients may be either essential or nonessential, depending on whether the body can or cannot manufacture them. When the body requires a nutrient for growth or maintenance but lacks the ability to manufacture it in amounts sufficient to meet bodily needs, the nutrient, called **essential** must be supplied by foods in the diet. Vitamin C, vitamin A, and calcium are just three examples of the more than 40 essential nutrients. However, if the nutrient is not needed in the diet because the body can make its own, the nutrient is called **nonessential.**

Functions of Nutrients

All nutrients perform one or more of the following functions: They serve as a source of energy or heat, support the growth and maintenance of tissue, and/or aid the regulation of basic body processes. These three life-sustaining functions collectively fall under the term **metabolism** which is the sum of all physical and chemical changes that take place in the body. Nutrients have specific metabolic functions and interact with one another to maintain the human organism.

Phytochemicals

Phytochemicals are nonnutrient food components or food chemicals that provide medical or health benefits, including the prevention or treatment of a disease. The relationship between chronic diseases such as heart disease, diabetes, high blood pressure, and cancer to phytochemicals is an area of active research. This research is so new that the definitions of nutrients and phytochemicals are blurred. According to the American Institute for Cancer Research, phytochemicals differ from vitamins and minerals in that they have no *known* nutritional value. Isothiocyanates, saponins, indols, isoflavones, and allyl sulfides are a few of the phytochemicals currently under study. This group of compounds will be discussed in subsequent chapters.

Source of Energy or Heat

Energy is defined in the physical sciences as the capacity to do work. Energy can take several forms: electric, thermal (heat), and mechanical. All food enters the body as potential chemical energy. The body processes the chemical energy stored in food and converts it into other energy forms. For example, chemical energy can be transformed into electric signals in nerves, which is changed to mechanical energy in muscles. Carbohydrates, fats, and proteins are the nutrients that supply energy, and for this reason they are referred to as the **energy nutrients.**

Growth and Maintenance of Tissues

Some nutrients provide the raw materials for building the body's structure and participate in the continued growth and maintenance of the necessary tissues. Water, proteins, fats, and minerals are the nutrient classes that contribute in a major way to building the body's structure.

Regulation of Body Processes

Some nutrients control or regulate the chemical processes in the body. For example, certain minerals and protein help regulate how water is distributed in the body. Vitamins participate in the series of reactions needed to generate energy. Even though vitamins themselves are not energy sources, if the body lacks a particular vitamin, the body will not be an efficient producer of energy.

Malnutrition

Too much or too little of a nutrient can interfere with health and well-being. There is a beneficial range of intake for any nutrient; to go below or above that range is incompatible with optimal health. Thus, **malnutrition** (poor nutrition) occurs when body cells receive too much or too little of one or more nutrients.

Undernutrition

Malnutrition includes **undernutrition** which is the result of a deficiency of one or more nutrients. Undernutrition can be related to:

- The inability to obtain foods that contain the essential nutrients
- Failure to consume essential nutrients
- The poor use of nutrients by the body

- Disease conditions that increase the body's need for nutrients
- A too-rapid excretion of nutrients from the body

Undernutrition occurs in many different circumstances. For example, stress caused by trauma, surgery, or burns is frequently a cause of malnutrition. Persons exposed to these severe and prolonged stressors may be malnourished even though consuming a "normal diet." Prolonged physical stress causes the body to break down internal protein stores, resulting in larger amounts of nutrients being lost in the urine. Mental and emotional stress has not been as clearly linked to malnutrition.

Although not widespread, undernutrition in the United States does exist. It generally occurs as a result of poverty, illness, neglect, poor dietary planning, environmental hazards, and prolonged hospitalization. Especially vulnerable groups are children, pregnant women, and the elderly. For example, malnourished children grow at a slower rate, are prone to infections, and are more likely to have mental and developmental problems.

Overnutrition

Malnutrition includes **overnutrition,** which is the excessive intake of nutrients. For example, when ingested in very high doses once or habitually, preformed vitamin A can cause headache, vomiting, bone abnormalities, and liver damage. Vitamin D toxicity can lead to the deposit of calcium in soft tissues, with consequent irreversible kidney and cardiovascular damage. Overnutrition is often associated with the use of self-prescribed over-the-counter vitamin and mineral supplements. Overnutrition is also associated with eating too much food and hence an excessive intake of many nutrients.

Nutrition and Health

Good nutrition is essential for good health. Nutrition is related to physical growth and development, body composition, and mental development. Research has shown that certain dietary substances can either protect persons from chronic diseases or predispose them toward chronic diseases. Medical treatment for many diseases includes diet therapy. Nutrition is thus both a preventive and therapeutic science.

Physical Growth and Development

Heredity determines much of the growth pattern and genetic potential of each individual. Malnutrition can delay or prevent an individual from achieving his or her genetic potential. For example, without calcium, phosphorus, and protein, bones cannot grow properly; children who are malnourished may never reach their genetic potential for height. Slowed growth may be one of the first clinically measurable indicators of inadequate dietary intake in children. Thus, diligent health care providers measure an infant's height and weight and plot them on growth charts on each visit. Examples of growth charts commonly used to plot the height and weight of infants and children can be found in Appendix D.

Body Composition

Nutrient intake can affect body composition, which in turn can affect health. The composition of the human body can be divided into four main substances (water, fat, ash, and protein) and one minor substance (carbohydrate) (see Fig. 1–1). One-half to three-quarters of the body is made up of water. A normally active woman has a body fat content of between 18 and 22 percent. A normally active man has a body fat content of between 15 and 19 percent. Body ash comprises about 6 percent of body weight. **Ash** is the leftover portion or residue that remains after something is burned, as in a charcoal fire. Body ash is the body's mineral content. For example, the human skeleton is partly composed of the minerals calcium and phosphorus.

About 15 percent of body weight consists of protein. The male body contains more protein than the female body. With age, the typical person's body composition becomes higher in fat and lower in protein. Protein is stored primarily in muscle tissue, organs, and certain body chemicals. When a person loses body protein, he or she is losing muscle tissue, organ mass, and/or the protein stored in body chemicals. Preservation of body protein and optimal health go hand in hand. Common sense dictates

---

Energy nutrients—The chemical substances in food that are able to supply fuel; refers collectively to carbohydrates, fat, and protein.

Malnutrition—Poor nutrition; results when the body's cells receive either an excess or a deficiency of one or more nutrients.

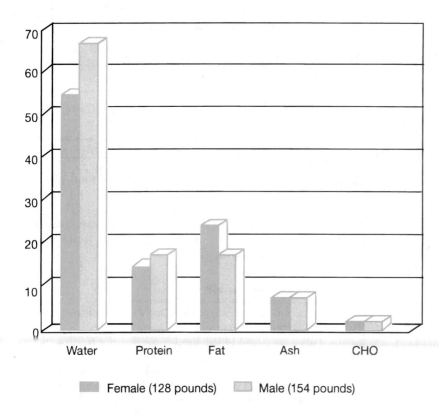

FIGURE 1–1 Approximate body composition of a sample 25-year-old man (154 lb) and woman (128 lb). Note that the typical woman has a higher percentage of body fat than does the typical man. The man has a higher percentage of lean body mass. The percentage of ash content is equal in both sexes. The human body has minimal carbohydrate content.

that a loss of structural body content (heart muscle, kidney, liver, blood proteins, etc.) is undesirable.

A person's body fat and protein content can be modified by food intake and/or exercise. For example, exercise increases body protein content by increasing muscle content. Eating too much food or the wrong kind of food increases the fat content of the body since fat is stored for future use.

Mental Development

The relationship between undernutrition and the development of a child's brain in structure, size, and function is being researched. It has been found that undernourished babies have smaller and fewer brain cells. However, the relationship between intelligence and the size and number of brain cells is not clear. There is some evidence that infants less than 6 months of age are particularly vulnerable to the effects of malnutrition on their mental development. Some nutritional deficiencies may cause permanent impairment of the central nervous system (CNS) in young infants.

Some conditions that affect the CNS may be reversible through diet. For example, nutrition plays an important role in the prevention and management of some forms of dementia. **Dementia** is defined as the impairment of intellectual function that is usually progressive and interferes with normal social and occupational activities. *Impairment* means any condition that causes one to deteriorate; *progressive* means to become more severe or to spread to other parts. Excessive alcohol intake or nutritional deficiencies may result in dementia. Correction of the deficiency or the removal of alcohol from the diet may improve intellectual function. Not all forms of dementia are directly related to poor nutrition. Alzheimer's disease may not be.

Diet As Therapy

A special or modified diet is often an important component of a client's total medical care. For example, diet is an important part of the treatment for clients with metabolic diseases such as diabetes and hypoglycemia. Special dietary measures are often required to maintain the lives of patients who have chronic heart, kidney, liver, and gastrointestinal diseases. These diets must also take into consideration the effects of medications on nutrients. Adjustments in the diet are also necessary for other situations, such as highly stressful or traumatic events. Persons suffering from severe burns, broken bones, or surgery may require dietary adjustment.

Although rare, some clients have a single-nutrient deficiency. Often, just adding foods to the diet that contain the missing nutrient is sufficient. The last section of this book is devoted to describing various diets for specific clinical situations.

Summary

Nutrition has been defined as the science of food and its relation to people. Our bodies and our attitudes about health and nutrition have evolved over millions of years. Health is a state of complete physical, mental, and social well-being, not just the absence of disease or infirmity. Nutrition is vital to optimal health. The principles of nutrition are applied by a team of health care members to promote health and treat many diseases. The science of nutrition is based on chemicals in foods called nutrients, which function (1) to provide fuel sources, (2) to support tissue growth and maintenance, and/or (3) to regulate body processes. A nutrient is called essential if the body requires it and is unable to manufacturer it in sufficient amounts to meet bodily needs. A balanced nutrient intake is vital for physical growth and development, optimal body composition, mental development, and the prevention of disease.

Study Aids

Chapter Review

1. In general, women's bodies contain more _____ and less _____ than men's bodies.
   a. Carbohydrate, protein
   b. Fat, water
   c. Protein, ash
   d. Water, fat

2. The human body adapted to feast or famine by developing the capacity to store excess:
   a. Fluid
   b. Carbohydrate
   c. Fat
   d. Protein

3. The following is *not* one of the traditional classes of nutrients:
   a. Phytochemicals
   b. Vitamins
   c. Minerals
   d. Proteins

4. The following is an energy nutrient:
   a. Water
   b. Carbohydrates
   c. Vitamins
   d. Minerals

5. Malnutrition always occurs as a result of:
   a. The consumption of a chemically designed diet
   b. A low income
   c. Infirmity
   d. Overnutrition

Clinical Analysis

1. Mrs. A believes she can cleanse her body of toxic compounds by abstaining from all food for 10 days. The nurse should:
   a. Tell Mrs. A she needs to drink extra fluids for this approach to succeed.
   b. Ignore Mrs. A.
   c. Agree with Mrs. A.
   d. Explain to Mrs. A the importance of variety, balance, and moderation in the diet.

2. Mr. and Mrs. J are members of a local fitness club and have recently had their body fat content analyzed. Mr. J is unhappy because his wife's body fat content (20 percent) is higher than his body fat content (15 percent). He asks for your opinion. An appropriate response would be:
   a. A normally active woman has a body fat content between 18 and 22 percent. He should not worry.
   b. A normally active woman has a body fat content of between 15 and 19 percent and his wife should work harder on her figure.
   c. A person's body fat content is not that important.
   d. If his wife would increase her protein intake, her body fat content would decrease.

3. Billie is a 3-month-old male who weighs 8 lb and is 19 1/2 in long. His mother asks you to evaluate

---

Dementia—Impairment of intellectual function that usually is progressive and interferes with normal social and occupational activities

his growth. (*Hint:* Use the growth chart in Appendix D for boys, birth to 36 months.) You should tell her:

a. Billie weighs too much for his height.
b. Billie weighs too little for his height.
c. Billie is in the 90th percentile.
d. Billie is in the 50th percentile, or about average.

Bibliography

American Institute for Cancer Research: Taking a Closer Look at Phytochemicals E57 TLP/E68. American Institute for Cancer Research, Washington, DC, 1995.

Garn, SM and Leonard, WR: What did our ancestors eat? Nutr Rev 47:11, 1989.

Ocean Spray Foodservice: Neutraceuticals: Eating for health means more than vitamins and minerals. Healthline 4:2, Fall 1995.

Subcommittee on the Tenth Edition of the RDAs. Food and Nutrition Board. Commission on Life Sciences. National Research Council: Recommended Dietary Allowances. National Academy Press, Washington, DC, 1989.

CHAPTER 2

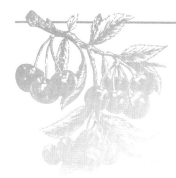

Individualizing Client Care

LEARNING OBJECTIVES

After completing this chapter, the student should be able to:
1. Describe methods of nutrition assessment.
2. Demonstrate the use of three common techniques to analyze dietary status.
3. Define the essential features of a dietary exchange system.
4. Identify components of the health belief systems of large cultural groups.
5. Explain the requirements of a Kosher diet.
6. Discuss means of providing culturally competent nutritional care.

What are the tools and techniques you need to learn more about your clients? This chapter reviews the steps of the nursing process. In addition, the terminology and methodology used for measuring and evaluating nutritional status are introduced. Because cultural traditions influence how people regard certain foods and their influence on their health, the last section of this chapter discusses culturally competent care so that students will understand the importance of clients' cultural, religious, educational, and economic backgrounds in defining who they are.

The Nursing Process

The **nursing process** is the modern method of planning, delivering, and evaluating care that is used by nurses throughout the world (Akiwumi, 1994). In the United States, the Joint Commission on the Accreditation of Healthcare Organizations evaluates the use of the nursing process as part of the accreditation procedure. Throughout this book, the fictional case studies integrate the steps of the nursing process: assessment, diagnosis (Table 2–1), desired outcomes, planning, nursing actions, and evaluation (Box 2–1).

TABLE 2–1   Some Nursing Diagnoses Pertinent to Nutritional Needs of Clients

Breast-feeding, effective, ineffective, or interrupted
Constipation, colonic or perceived
Fluid-Volume Deficit
Fluid-Volume Excess
Infant Feeding Pattern, ineffective
Knowledge Deficit
Nutrition, altered, less than body requirements
Nutrition, altered, more than body requirements
Nutrition, altered, risk for more than body requirements
Oral Mucous Membrane, altered
Self-Care Deficit: feeding
Sensory-Perceptual Alterations: visual, gustatory, or olfactory
Swallowing, impaired
Therapeutic Regimen: community, family, or individual, ineffective management

Steps of the Nursing Process

The nursing process provides an orderly, logical problem-solving approach for administering care. It encompasses all significant actions taken by the nurse and forms the foundation of clinical decision making:

Assessment: The nurse collects information (health data).

Diagnosis: The nurse analyzes the assessment data to determine a diagnosis.

Desired outcome: The nurse identifies specific goals for the individual client and then selects appropriate interventions to assist him or her in attaining them.

Planning: The nurse develops a plan of care that includes interventions that help the client to attain the desired outcomes.

Nursing actions/implementation: The nurse implements the interventions identified in the plan of care.

Evaluation: The nurse evaluates the client's progress in attaining the expected outcomes and changes the plan if necessary.

Advantages of the Nursing Process

Among the many advantages of the nursing process approach to client care are the following:

- **Organizing framework:** The nursing process provides a framework for meeting the individual needs of the client, the client's family and significant other(s), and the community.
- **Human response focus:** The nursing process focuses the nurse's attention on the individual human responses of a client or group of clients, and the nurse is thus able to incorporate these responses into a holistic plan of care.
- **Structured decision making:** The nursing process provides an organized, systematic method of solving problems, which may minimize the occurrence of dangerous errors or omissions in caregiving and prevent time-consuming repetition in care and documentation.
- **Client involvement:** The nursing process promotes the active involvement of the client in his or her own health care. Such participation increases the client's sense of control over what is happening to him or her, stimulates problem solving, and promotes personal responsibility, all of which strengthen the client's commitment to achieving identified goals.

BOX 2–1   STEPS IN THE NURSING PROCESS

Assessment is an organized procedure for gathering facts or data necessary to help the client. Usually a history is taken, followed by a physical examination. There are two types of data pertinent to the nursing process, subjective and objective.

The **symptoms** the client recounts are **subjective data** and not verifiable by another. **Objective data** can be observed and verified by someone other than the client. These data are called **signs** obtainable by physical examination or through laboratory tests.

A **nursing diagnosis** is a statement of a client's nursing problem that the nurse is licensed to treat. It stems from the data collected during the nursing assessment. The **North American Nursing Diagnosis Association (NANDA)** studies and approves nursing diagnoses for clinical testing. Table 2–1 lists nursing diagnoses that are often pertinent to nutrition. Many other nursing diagnoses require nutritional interventions as part of the complete care of the client.

After gathering data, the nurse identifies problem areas. The assessment findings are shared with the client, and the problem is defined. For many areas of health maintenance the client's active participation is essential to achieving the desired outcome. If clients do not participate in the nursing diagnostic process and their priorities are not respected, they may not cooperate with the treatment plans. When the treatment plan includes diet changes, the client must choose to follow or ignore the plan several times a day.

The **desired outcome** describes the client who has mastered the nursing problem. Sometimes desired outcomes are called *goals* or *objectives*. They are client-centered, realistic, and measurable, and they contain a deadline.

Directions for nursing care, called **nursing actions/interventions,** should be clear and specific so that a new person assigned to care for a client can proceed without hesitation. A correct nursing action must be likely to produce the desired outcome. A statement justifying the selection of a nursing action to produce a certain outcome is called a **rationale.** The nursing care plans in this text contain statements of rationale to logically link desired outcomes and nursing actions.

Evaluation is the process of comparing the client's status with the established desired outcome. The nurse and client judge whether the problem has been resolved. If not, the nursing process is again set in motion beginning with an assessment.

Terminology

How do health care workers determine whether a client is well nourished or suffering from malnutrition? Before this question can be answered, two terms need to be defined. **Nutritional status** refers to the condition of the body as it relates to the intake and use of nutrients. All members of the health care team have a role to play in the effective evaluation of a client's nutritional status. **Dietary status** tells what a client is eating. While a client's dietary status may be adequate, his or her nutritional status may nevertheless be poor. An evaluation of a client's dietary status can help determine the reason for this poor nutritional status, or it may rule out poor diet as the source of the client's problem.

Two levels of methodology are commonly used to identify clients at nutritional risk. Table 2–2, a screening form, is an example of the first level of nutritional care. A nutritional screening should be sufficiently concise so that the information can be

---

Nutritional status—The condition of the body as it relates to the intake and use of nutrients.

Dietary status—Description of what a person has been eating.

TABLE 2–2 Nutritional Screening Form

Name _____ Date _____ Adm. Date _____	
Sex _____ Birthdate _____ Physician's Name _____	
Adm Dx. _____	

Diet. *Information*	Diet order _____ Date Prescribed _____ Aceepts all major groups _____ Feeds self _____ Type of assistance needed _____
Physical	Height _____ Weight _____ Healthy body weight % _____ Weight change in last 3 months _____ Chewing ability _____ Weight history _____ Swallowing ability _____ Hearing _____ Vision _____ Bowel function _____ Bladder function _____ Edema _____ Nausea _____ Pressure ulcer _____ Stage _____ Allergies _____
Laboratory	Blood glucose _____ Albumin _____ Potassium _____ Lymphocytes _____ Hemoglobin _____ Hematocrit _____ Cholesterol _____
Medications	Insulin _____ Diuretics _____ Laxatives _____ Vit/min supp _____ Antibiotics _____ Thyroid _____ Anticoagulants _____ Antidepressants (MAO) _____ Antabuse _____ Flagyl _____ Lithium _____

If the above identifies a problem, continue with in-depth assessment.

_____ *(Signature)* _____ *(Date)*

gathered in 5 to 10 minutes. The second level of care is a **nutritional assessment,** which includes a physical examination, anthropometric measurements, laboratory data, and food intake information. It is more comprehensive than a nutritional screen, and it is done to determine a client's nutrient stores. Usually all members of the health care team are involved in a nutritional assessment, including the physician, dietitian, nurse, and social worker. A common source of confusion among nurses is caused by the term *assessment.* The phrase *nutritional assessment* is used differently by physicians and dietitians than by nurses. A "nutritional assessment" is the evaluation of a client's nutritional status (nutrient stores) based on a physical examination, anthropometric measurements, laboratory data, and food intake information. Because a comprehensive nutritional assessment requires a large investment of health care resources, it is usually completed only on clients at a high nutritional risk. For example, surgeons may order a comprehensive nutritional assessment prior to surgery to determine if a client can tolerate a procedure better after nutritional rehabilitation.

Subjective Data

In a nutritional assessment, subjective data include knowledge of nutrition, recounted intake of food, and reported height and weight. The subjective data listed in Table 2–3 are appropriate for assessment purposes. When more detailed food intake information is required, the five techniques listed in Table 2–4 may be used. Some of the advantages and disadvantages of each are given.

Objective Data

A physical examination can include general appearance, anthropomorphic measurements, and laboratory or other diagnostic tests. Table 2–3 lists objective data relevant to a nutritional assessment.

General Appearance

Well-nourished people look healthy and usually have an optimistic perspective. A list comparing the

TABLE 2–3 Sample Subjective and Objective Nutritional Data

Subjective	Objective
Usual diet and fluid intake	Accurate actual height and weight
Number of meals per day	Body build or frame
Last meal: time, foods, and amounts	Skin turgor and/or dryness
Food and nutrient supplements	Condition of teeth and gums
Appetite	Hair quantity and quality
Problems with digestion and/or elimination	Body fat measurements
Allergies or food intolerances	Complete blood count
Chewing and/or swallowing problems	Serum albumin
Use of dentures	Serum electrolytes
Usual weight and recent changes	
Likes and dislikes	

appearance of a well-nourished individual with one less well nourished is shown in Table 2–5. A person need not display all the abnormal signs to be regarded as malnourished.

Anthropometric Data

For clinical purposes, body size, weight, and proportions are determined by **anthropometry,** the science of measuring the body. Such measurements are used to determine growth, body composition, and nutritional status. The body's kilocalorie and protein stores can be determined by these measurements. Collection of anthropometric data on height and weight, triceps skinfold, midarm circumference, abdominal circumference, and waist and hip measurements are described briefly. Other measurements can be selected.

Height and Weight

Height may be measured in inches or centimeters. Adults and older children are measured standing

TABLE 2–4 Commonly Used Techniques to Obtain Food Intake Information

Technique	Comments
Comparison with the Food Pyramid Model Health care provider asks client what he or she eats and compares this reported food intake with the Food Pyramid model.	Can be used to screen many clients quickly. Does not require a trained interviewer. Is not comprehensive. May overlook some clients who would benefit from nutritional care.
Food Frequency Health care provider requests client to fill out a questionnaire asking about usual food intake during specified times such as "What do you usually eat for breakfast?"	Questionnaire can be tailored to particular nutrients of interest (e.g., lactose, gluten). May assess food usage for any length of time: day, week, month, weekends versus weekdays, summer versus winter, etc. Initial client contact does not require a trained interviewer. May require special resources (e.g., computer database) to evaluate the information collected. Provides limited information on a client's food behaviors such as meal spacing, length of usual mealtime, etc.
Food Records Health care provider asks client to record his or her food intake for a specified length of time (1 or 3 or 7 days).	A motivated client will provide reasonably accurate information. A less highly motivated client will "forget to keep" part or all of the food record. Research shows some clients will change their food habits while keeping a food record; therefore, this technique works poorly to assist in determining a client's dietary and/or nutritional status. This technique works well when a behavior change is desired. May require special resources (e.g., a computer database) to evaluate the information obtained. Client needs to be available for a follow-up visit to review the evaluated food records. Analysis of results is time-consuming.

TABLE 2–4   Commonly Used Techniques to Obtain Food Intake Information (Continued)

Technique	Comments
24-h Dietary Recall Health care provider asks client what he or she has eaten during the previous 24 h.	Is a fairly simple technique. Interviewer should be trained not to ask leading questions. Yields limited information only about the kinds of foods and beverages consumed within the previous 24 h. The previous 24 h may not have been usual for the client. Frequently clients may not remember what they ate and the amounts they ate.
Diet History A diet history is an in-depth interview that yields information about the usual food intake, drug and medication usage, alcohol and tobacco use, financial ability to obtain food, special dietary needs, food allergies and intolerances, weight history, cultural and religious preferences that may influence food selection, ability to chew and swallow foods, previous dietary instructions received, client knowledge about nutrition, and elimination patterns.	Is comprehensive. Requires a trained interviewer who is usually a dietitian. An analysis of the results obtained can usually be provided on the same day the information is collected. Is a good technique for high-risk clients when information is needed to evaluate the need for nutritional support. Is highly dependent on the willingness of the client to reveal information to the interviewer. Client must be a good historian. Is time-consuming.

SOURCE: Adapted from Moore, MC: Pocket Guide, Nutrition and Diet Therapy. Mosby, St. Louis, 1993, p. 10, and from Mason, M, Wenberg, BG, and Welsch, PK: The Dynamics of Clinical Dietetics, p. 10. John Wiley & Sons, New York, 1982.

with head erect; infants and young children, lying on a firm, flat surface.

Weight may be recorded in pounds or kilograms. If required, the scale should be balanced before each measurement. The client should be weighed on the same scale, at the same time of the day, wearing similar clothing each time.

Triceps Skinfold

This measurement of subcutaneous tissue over the triceps muscle in the upper arm provides an estimate of the amount of body fat. The **triceps skinfold** measurement helps to differentiate between a person who is heavy because of muscle mass and one who is heavy because of excess fat.

Practice is needed to take accurate measurements. Often research designs require the same researcher to take all the measurements and record the average of two or three values at each site. Locations other than the triceps can also be used to measure skinfolds. Although nurses usually do not measure skinfolds, they do need to answer clients' questions.

Midarm Circumference

A circle's outside edge is its *circumference*. Since 50 percent of the body's protein stores are located in muscle tissue, the circumference of the midarm provides information about body protein stores.

Body Frame Size

Wrist measurement is one method of categorizing a person's frame. It requires no tools or references. Have the person wrap the thumb and middle finger of one hand around the smallest part of the opposite wrist (Feldman, 1988). The **body frame size** is as designated below. If the thumb and middle finger:

Overlap by 1 cm or more = small frame
Meet = medium frame
Cannot meet by 1 cm or more = large frame

An alternate method is shown in Clinical Calculation 2–1. Elbow width and shoe size also have been used as indices of frame size.

Abdominal Circumference (Girth)

This measurement, in inches or centimeters, is often taken at the umbilicus. **Abdominal circumference (girth)** provides information when an individual is accumulating fluid in the abdominal cavity, a sign called **ascites.** Girth measurements are also taken to monitor growth of a fetus or of abnormal tissue within the abdomen.

Waist and Hip Measurements

At one clinic the most accurate waist measurement was taken at the smallest dimension with the client lying on his back (Jensen, 1992), but in any case a standard procedure should be used. The hips are measured at the largest dimension as the client stands with the feet together.

Body Density Measures

Muscle and fat tissue differ in their rates of metabolism. Therefore, the proportions of each in the body influence whether a person is overweight. These proportions can be determined by several techniques, including underwater weighing and bioelectric impedance.

Underwater Weighing

Underwater weighing compares the person's scale weight with his or her weight underwater. After correcting for lung volume, the proportion of body fat is calculated. Underwater weighing accurately assesses the amount of fat in the body. Because the technique is cumbersome, time-consuming, and requires special equipment, its main use is in research.

Bioelectric Impedance

In this test, the greater electrolyte content and conductivity of the body's fat-free mass is compared to that of fat or bone (Baumgartner, Chumlea, and Roche, 1990). Body composition is predicted from a measure of total body water. The client's fat-free

mass is predicted and his or her percent body fat is determined by comparing his or her body weight with the predicted fat-free mass (Baumgartner, Heymsfield, and Roche, 1995). Results reported are percent body water, percent lean body mass, and percent body fat. Procedures were validated on adults and are not necessarily applicable to children (Wu, et al, 1993) or athletes (Oppliger, 1992). Because **bioelectric impedance** rests upon total body water, any factors disturbing water balance may discredit the results. Examples are diuretic use, excessive sweating, hemodialysis, premenstrual edema, and alcohol consumption within the previous 24 hours.

TABLE 2–5 General Appearance as an Indicator of Nutritional Status

	Normal	*Abnormal*
Demeanor	Alert, responsive	Lethargic
	Positive outlook	Negative attitude
Weight	Reasonable for build	Underweight
		Overweight, obese
Hair	Glossy, full, firmly rooted	Dull, sparse,
		Easily, painlessly plucked
	Uniform color	
Eyes	Bright, clear, shiny	Pale conjunctiva
		Redness, dryness
Lips	Smooth	Chapped, red, swollen
Tongue	Deep red	Bright red, purple
	Slightly rough	Swollen or shrunken
	One longitudinal furrow	Several longitudinal furrows
Teeth	Bright, painless	Cavities, painful, mottled, or missing
Gums	Pink, firm	Spongy, bleeding, receding
Skin	Clear, smooth, firm, slightly moist	Rashes, swelling
		Light or dark spots
		Dry
Nails	Pink, firm	Spoon shaped, ridged spongy bases
Mobility	Erect posture	Muscle wasting
	Good muscle tone	Skeletal deformities
	Walks without pain or difficulty	Loss of balance

CLINICAL CALCULATION 2–1
_____

Determining Body Frame Type

Measure the smallest part of the wrist between the wrist bones and the hand. If the person's height is not known, measure him or her, in feet and inches, without shoes. Taking that information, look at the chart below. Find the person's height on the left and wrist size at the bottom, and compare the shaded area with the boxes at the bottom. As an example, find the frame size of a person who is 5 ft, 4 in and has a wrist circumference of 6 1/4 in. (The person has a medium frame.)

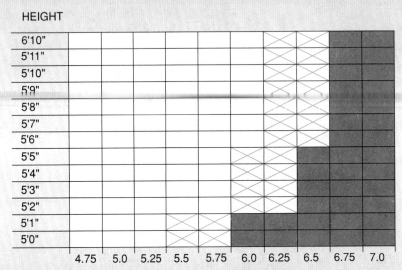

HEIGHT

WRIST MEASUREMENT IN INCHES
(Distance around smallest part of wrist, between wrist bones and hand)

☐ = Small frame

◻ = Medium frame

■ = Large frame

Laboratory Tests

Laboratory data include results from blood, urine, and stool tests. The results of these tests reveal much of what a person has eaten, what his or her body has stored, and how nutrients are being used by the body. Blood can be analyzed for glucose, protein, or fat content. Vitamin and mineral status can be determined by directly examining the blood or indirectly by examining enzymes related to the vitamin or mineral. Many experts doubt that vitamin or mineral body stores can be accurately determined by blood samples. The uncertainty lies in whether the nutrient in the blood reflects body stores, a transport form of the nutrient, or the amount in one specific body compartment.

Laboratory Tests

Good clinical judgment must be used in selecting tests and interpreting results. Some studies have shown a thorough nutritional history and physical examination are as effective in identifying malnutrition as a battery of laboratory tests (Moore, 1993).

Using Nutritional Parameters to Derive a Nursing Diagnosis

The health care provider uses either subjective or objective data, or both, to determine if the client has a problem. The client's data are compared to nutritional parameters. Those in common use include height-weight tables, body mass index, waist-to-hip ratio (WHR), the USOA's Dietary Guidelines, the Food Pyramid, the National Research Council's Recommended Dietary Allowances (RDAs), and the ADA Exchange Lists. No single parameter of comparison is recommended to be used exclusively.

Height-Weight Tables

There are many height-weight tables currently used. Each table is based on a different underlying assumption (see chapter 17, "Weight Control"). This text uses the Metropolitan Life Insurance Table which lists weights for height based on the lowest mortality (Table 2–6). No assurance is given with this table that the specified weights are equated with maximum health. A reliable height-weight table should stipulate shoe heel height and the weight of clothing. The information from height-weight tables is used to calculate a person's percent **healthy body weight (HBW)**. If a range of weights is given, the midpoint of the range is used. Clinical Calculation 2–2 illustrates the process.

Body Mass Index (BMI)

This measure is derived from weight and height (weight in kilograms divided by height in meters

TABLE 2–6   Metropolitan Life Insurance Company Height-Weight Table

| | Height (in Shoes*) | | Men (Indoor Clothing†) | | | | | |
| | | | Small Frame | | Medium Frame | | Large Frame | |
Feet	*Inches*	*Centimeters*	*Pounds*	*Kilograms*	*Pounds*	*Kilograms*	*Pounds*	*Kilograms*
5	2	157.5	128–134	58.2–60.9	131–141	59.5–64.1	138–150	62.7–68.2
5	3	160.0	130–136	59.1 61.8	133–143	60.4–65.0	140–153	63.6–69.5
5	4	162.6	132–138	60.0–62.7	135–145	61.4–65.9	142–156	64.5–70.9
5	5	165.1	134–140	60.9–63.6	137–148	62.3–67.2	144–160	65.5–72.7
5	6	167.6	136–142	61.8–64.5	139–151	63.2–68.6	146–164	66.4–74.5
5	7	170.2	138–145	62.7–65.9	142–154	64.5–70.0	149–168	67.7–76.4
5	8	172.7	140–148	63.6–67.2	145–157	65.9–71.4	152–172	69.1–78.2
5	9	175.3	142–151	64.5–68.6	148–160	67.2–72.7	155–176	70.5–80.0
5	10	177.8	144–154	65.5–70.0	151–163	68.6–74.1	158–180	71.8–81.8
5	11	180.3	146–157	66.4–71.4	154–166	70.0–75.5	161–184	73.2–83.6
6	0	182.9	149–160	67.7–72.7	157–170	71.4–77.3	164–188	74.5–85.5
6	1	185.4	152–164	69.1–74.5	160–174	72.7–79.1	168–192	76.4–87.3
6	2	188.0	155–168	70.5–76.4	164–178	74.5–80.9	172–197	78.2–89.5
6	3	190.5	158–172	71.8–78.2	167–182	75.9–82.7	176–202	80.0–91.8
6	4	193.0	162–176	73.6–80.0	171–187	77.7–85.0	181–207	82.3–94.1

* Shoes with 1-in heels.
† Allow 5 lb.

Table continued on following page

TABLE 2–6   Metropolitan Life Insurance Company Height-Weight Table (Continued)

			Women (Indoor Clothing†)					
Height (in Shoes*)			Small Frame		Medium Frame		Large Frame	
Feet	Inches	Centimeters	Pounds	Kilograms	Pounds	Kilograms	Pounds	Kilograms
4	10	147.3	102–111	46.4–50.0	109–121	49.5–55.0	118–131	53.6–59.5
4	11	149.9	103–113	46.8–51.4	111–123	50.0–55.9	120–134	54.5–60.9
5	0	152.4	104–115	47.3–52.3	113–126	51.4–57.2	122–137	55.5–62.3
5	1	154.9	106–118	48.2–53.6	115–129	52.3–58.6	125–140	56.8–63.6
5	2	157.5	108–121	49.1–55.0	118–132	53.6–60.0	128–143	58.2–65.0
5	3	160.0	111–124	50.5–56.4	121–135	55.0–61.4	131–147	59.5–66.8
5	4	162.6	114–127	51.8–57.7	124–138	56.4–62.7	134–151	60.9–68.6
5	5	165.1	117–130	53.2–59.0	127–141	57.7–64.1	137–155	62.3–70.5
5	6	167.6	120–133	54.5–60.5	130–144	59.0–65.5	140–159	63.6–72.3
5	7	170.2	123–136	55.9–61.8	133–147	60.5–66.8	143–163	65.0–74.1
5	8	172.7	126–139	57.3–63.2	136–150	61.8–68.2	146–167	66.4–75.9
5	9	175.3	129–142	58.6–64.5	139–153	63.2–69.5	149–170	67.7–77.3
5	10	177.8	132–145	60.0–65.9	142–156	64.6–70.9	152–173	69.1–78.6
5	11	180.3	135–148	61.4–67.3	145–159	65.9–72.3	155–176	70.5–80.0
6	0	182.9	138–151	62.7–73.6	148–162	67.3–73.6	158–179	71.8–81.4

* Shoes with 1-in heels.
† Allow 3 lb.
SOURCE OF BASIC DATA: Build Study, 1979, Society of Actuaries and Association of Life Insurance Medical Directors of America, 1980. © 1983 Metropolitan Life Insurance Company.

NOTE: The weights presented are those associated with the lowest mortality. They are not necessarily the weights at which people are healthiest, perform their jobs optimally, or even look their best. From Metropolitan Life, Warwick, RI, with permission.

CLINICAL CALCULATION 2–2

Percent Healthy Body Weight

The formula for calculating percent healthy body weight is:

$$\frac{\text{Client's weight}}{\text{Weight from table}} + 100 = \frac{\text{percent healthy}}{\text{body weight}}$$

For example, according to the height-weight table (Table 2–6), a 5 ft, 5 in woman with a medium frame has a range of 130 to 144 lb, including 3 lb of clothing. Assuming she is 5 ft, 5 in, barefoot, the table is entered at 5 ft, 6 in, to allow for 1-in heels. The midpoint of the range is 137 lb.

If the woman weighed 137 lb, her HBW would be 100 percent. If she weighed 159 lb, her HBW would be 116 percent, calculated as follows:

$$\frac{159 \text{ lb}}{137 \text{ lb}} \times 100 = 116 \text{ percent}$$

A person at 111 to 119 percent HWB is overweight. One at 120 percent or more is obese.

---

squared). **Body mass index** was designed to provide a measure of weight that was independent of height. Although the body mass index has been used as an indicator of obesity, it fails to distinguish adipose from muscle or water weight. Table 2–7 shows weight classifications using body mass indices.

Waist-to-Hip Ratio (WHR)

The waist measurement is divided by the hip measurement. A **Waist-to-Hip Ratio (WHR)** greater than 0.85 in women and greater than 1.0 in men indicates increased risk of problems related to obesity.

TABLE 2–7   Weight Classification Using Body Mass Indices

Weight Classification	Body Mass Index	
	Men	Women
Underweight	<20.7	<19.1
Normal	20.8 to 27.7	19.2 to 27.2
Obese	>27.8	>27.3

Dietary Guidelines

The US Departments of Agriculture and Health and Human Services jointly publish a pamphlet entitled "Nutrition and your Health: Dietary Guidelines for Americans" (Fig. 2–1). The seven guidelines for health promotion and the rationale for each can be found in Clinical Application 2–1. These guidelines are targeted to the healthy general population to assist in the prevention of chronic and degenerative diseases. They do not apply to individuals who need special diets because of disease or conditions that alter normal nutritional requirements.

The Food Pyramid

The **Food Pyramid** illustrates healthful diet choices (Fig. 2–2). Foods are arranged in the following groups: (1) bread, cereal, rice, and pasta; (2) vegetable; (3) fruit; (4) meat, poultry, fish, dry beans, eggs, and nuts; (5) milk, yogurt, and cheese; (6) fats, oils, and sweets. Each group contains foods of similar nutrient content. For example, foods in the milk, yogurt, and cheese group are high in calcium, riboflavin, and protein. Each of the food groups supplies some but not all of the essential nutrients, and some servings from each of the groups should be eaten daily. In terms of quantity, the group at the bottom of the pyramid—bread, cereal, rice, and pasta—should provide the foundation of the diet and supply the most servings eaten. The group at the top of the pyramid—fats, oils, and sweets—should provide the fewest daily servings.

Recommended Dietary Allowances

The **Recommended Dietary Allowances (RDAs)** are the levels of essential nutrients that, on the basis of scientific knowledge, are judged by the Food and Nutrition Board of the National Research Council as adequate to meet the known nutrient needs of practically all healthy persons (Subcommittee on the 10th Edition of the RDAs, 1989). RDAs were designed to be used to plan and evaluate diets for groups of people such as schoolchildren and people living in institutions. Because individual requirements for nutrients are highly variable, consuming less than the RDAs does not necessarily indicate that an individual has a deficiency. The 1989 RDA table appears in Appendix F.

Other governments have published standards appropriate to their populations. The Canadian Council on Nutrition's standards are somewhat different from those of the United States.

Leading experts do not have enough information to list an RDA for two vitamins and five minerals. For these nutrients, only an **Estimated Safe and Adequate Dietary Intake (ESADDI)** has been set by the Food and Nutrition Board. A table listing these amounts appears in Appendix G.

Comparison of an individual's food intake to the RDAs or the ESADDI can be accomplished in two ways. Items can be found in a table of food composition and the separate nutrients hand calculated, or

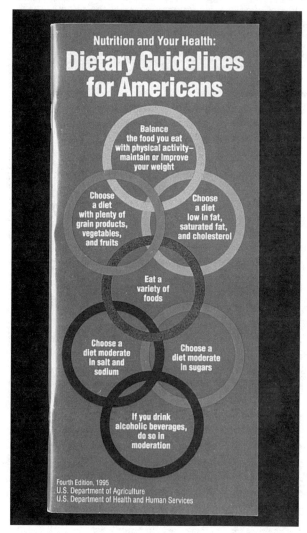

FIGURE 2–1 Nutrition and Your Health: Dietary Guidelines for Americans. This booklet was developed by the US Departments of Agriculture and Health and Human Services. Information on how to put guidelines into practice can be obtained by contacting the Human Nutrition Information Service, USDA, Room 325-A, 6505 Belcrest Road, Hyattsville, MD 20782.

Dietary Guidelines

Guideline	*Rationale*
Eat a variety of foods.	Benefits of eating a wide variety of food include increasing assurance of adequate nutrient intakes, avoiding deficiencies or excesses of any single nutrient, ensuring an appropriate balance of trace minerals, and reducing the likelihood of exposure to contaminants in any single food.
Balance the food you eat with physical activity. Maintain or improve your weight.	The chances of developing health problems are increased when a person is overly fat. Excess body fat is connected with high blood pressure, stroke, heart disease, the most common form of diabetes, certain cancers, and other types of illness.
Choose a diet with plenty of grain products, vegetables, and fruits.	Healthy adults need at least 3 servings of vegetables, 2 servings of fruits, and 6 servings of starches (preferably whole-grain) each day. These foods contain complex carbohydrates, dietary fiber, and other components that are linked to good health.
Choose a diet low in fat, saturated fat, and cholesterol.	Populations like ours with diets relatively high in fat tend to have more obesity and certain types of cancers. A high intake of saturated fat and cholesterol is linked to our increased risk of heart disease.
Choose a diet moderate in sugars.	A significant heatlh problem from eating too much sugar is tooth decay. Contrary to widespread belief, too much sugar in the diet does not cause diabetes or hyperactivity. Sugar provides kilocalories (fuel) but few other nutrients. Thus, diets with large amounts of sugar should be avoided because they often displace other, more healthful foods in the diet.
Choose a diet moderate in salt and sodium.	A high sodium intake may predispose a person to high blood pressure. In populations with low salt intakes, high blood pressure is less common than in populations with diets high in salt. Other factors besides salt intake affect blood pressure. At present there is no way to predict who might develop high blood pressure and who will benefit from reducing dietary salt and sodium. However, most experts consider it wise for most people to eat less salt and sodium than they now eat. Such reduction will benefit those people whose blood pressure rises with salt intake.
If you drink alcoholic beverages, do so in moderation.	People who should **not** drink are children and adolescents, persons who cannot moderate their consumptions, and women who are or want to become pregnant. Alcoholic beverages are high in calories and low in nutrients. Even moderate drinkers who are overweight should decrease their intake of alcohol. Heavy drinkers often develop nutritional deficiencies as well as more serious diseases, such as cirrhosis of the liver and certain forms of cancer. Consumption of alcohol by pregnant women may cause birth defects or other problems during pregnancy; there is no known ''safe'' level of alcohol intake in pregnancy.

to simplify the task, a computer program can be used.

Tables of Food Composition

Food composition tables list foods and the amounts of selected nutrients for a specified volume or weight of the food. The US Department of Agriculture (USDA) publishes a food composition table titled "Nutritive Values of the Edible Part of Foods" (Appendix B). From a practical viewpoint, tables of food composition can be used as a reference to look up the nutritive content of a particular food.

Computerized Diet Analysis

Many computer software programs are available to compare an individual's intake with the RDA. Table 2–8 shows such an analysis. The nutrient database refers to the food composition data, such as is shown in Appendix B, that are stored in the computer program. Not all nutrient databases are equal. For example, some nutrient databases contain blank spaces for one or more of the nutrient values for a given food item. The value may have been deleted in error or was not available to the authors. In either case, the missing data will impact the final value obtained for a given nutrient.

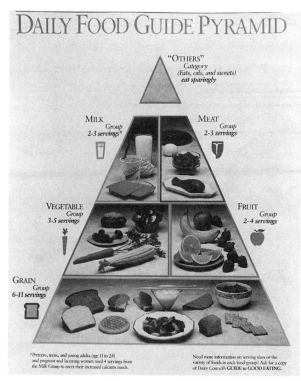

FIGURE 2–2   The Food Pyramid. This guide is commonly used to evaluate the dietary status of individuals and to educate clients about food choices. Courtesy of National Dairy Council®.

TABLE 2–8   Computerized Diet Analysis

RECOMMENDED DIETARY ALLOWANCES			
Name: Jane Smith Age: 7 yrs Sex: Female			
Weight: 51 lb Height: 4 ft, in Moderately Active			
Calories	2000*	Pyridoxine—B6	1.40 mg
Protein	28.0 g	Cobalamin—B12	1.40 mcg
Carbohydrates	290 g†	Folacin	100 mcg
Dietary fiber	20.0‡	Pantothenic	5.00 mg*
Fat-total	66.7 g†	Vit C	45.0 mg
Fat-saturated	22.2 g†	Vit E	7.00 mg
Fat-mono	22.2 g†	Calcium	800 mg
Fat-poly	22.2 g†	Copper	1.50 mg*
Cholesterol	mg†	Iron	10.0 mg
Vit A—Carotene	RE	Magnesium	170 mg
Vit A—preformed	RE	Phosphorus	800 mg
Vit A—total	700 RE	Potassium	1600 mg*
Thiamin—B1	1.00 mg	Selenium	30.0 mcg
Riboflavin—B2	1.20 mg	Sodium	2400 mg*
Niacin—B3	13.2 mg	Zinc	10.0 mg

* Suggested values; within recommended ranges.
† Dietary goals.
‡ Fiber = 1 g/100 kcal.
mcg = microgram; 1/1000 mg.

Table continued on following page

TABLE 2–8   Computerized Diet Analysis (Continued)

Jane Smith   (Plus Percent RDA for Jane Smith
Weight: 1880 g (66.3 oz)   Water weight: 1446 g

Calories	1946*	97%	Pyridoxine—B6	1.15 mg	82%
Protein	56.0 g	200%	Cobalamin—B12	3.37 mcg	240%
Carbohydrates	291 g†	100%	Folacin	181 mcg	181%
Dietary fiber	19.2 g‡	96%	Pantothenic	4.00 mg*	80%
Fat-total	67.3 g†	101%	Vit C	86.3 mg	192%
Fat-saturated	20.2 g†	91%	Vit E	14.4 mg	205%
Fat-mono	26.2 g†	118%	Calcium	1067 mg	133%
Fat-poly	16.3 g†	73%	Copper	0.998 mg*	67%
Cholesterol	97.8 mg†		Iron	11.1 mg	111%
Vit A—carotene	154 RE		Magnesium	239 mg	141%
Vit A—preformed	618 RE		Phosphorus	1123 mg	140%
Vit A—total	773 RE	110%	Potassium	2423 mg*	151%
Thiamin—B1	1.05 mg	105%	Selenium	75.6 mcg	252%
Riboflavin—B2	1.57 mg	131%	Sodium	1934 mg*	81%
Niacin—B3	11.7 mg	89%	Zinc	7.80 mg	78%

* Suggested values; within recommended ranges.
† Dietary goals.
‡ Fiber = 1 g/100 kcal.

Calories from protein:	11%	Poly/Sat = 0.8:1	
Calories from carbohydrates:	58%	Sod/Pot = 0.8:1	
Calories from fats:	30%	Ca/Phos = 1.0:1	
		CSI = 25.3	

Jane Smith (Plus Percent RDA for Jane Smith)

	Items Analyzed:	Code		Items Analyzed:	Code
2 cup	Skim milk/nonfat milk	73	1 tbs	Tomatoes, fresh, chpd.	640
0.5 ea.	Orange, avg, 2 5/8-in diam.	263	0.25 cup	Broccoli, frzn., ckd., chpd.	420
0.5 ea.	Bagel, plain, 3.5-in diam.	975	1 oz	Beef rib, oven rst., lean	786
1 tbs	Cream cheese	20	0.25 cup	White rice, instant, prepd.	1271
0.4 cup	Cream of Wheat cereal, ckd.	1232	1 ea.	Dinner rolls, commercial	1131
0.5 ea.	Banana, peeled weight	190	1 tsp	Olive oil	1482
1 ea.	Celery, raw, 1 g outer stalk	448	3 tsp	Margarine, reg/soft, 80% fat	1472
1.75 tbs	Peanut butter, smooth	1561	1.5 cup	Cola beverage, regular	1406
0.5 oz	Swiss cheese	147	2 ea.	Jelly, 1 packet	1637
2 tsp	Salad dressing, mayo type	1497	1 cup	Popcorn, plain, air-popped	1289
1 pce	Italian bread, slice	989	1 ea.	White sugar, 1 packet	1647
0.5 cup	Ice cream, regular, vanilla	130	2 ea.	Apple w/peel, 2.75-in diam.	154
0.25 cup	Butterhead lettuce, chpd.	488	1.25 oz.	Hard candy, all flavors	1612
1 tbs	Ranch salad dressing	1499	1.5 tsp	Peanuts, dried, unsalted	1557
			0.25 tsp	Salt	1710

TABLE 2–8   Computerized Diet Analysis (Continued)

Name of analysis: Jane Smith
Recommendations for: Jane Smith

	Percentage of Recommended Amounts	
	0 20 40 60 80 100 120 140	
Calories		(97)
Protein		>>200>
Carbohydrates		(100)
Dietary fiber		(96)
Fat—total		(101)
Fat—saturated		(91)
Fat—mono		(118)
Fat—poly		(73)
Vit A—total		(110)
Thiamin—B1		(105)
Riboflavin—B2		(131)
Niacin—B3		(89)
Pyridoxine—B6		(82)
Cobalamin—B12		>>240>
Folacin		>>181>
Pantothenic		(80)
Vit C		>>192>
Vit E		>>205>
Calcium		(133)
Copper		(67)
Iron		(111)
Magnesium		(141)
Phosphorus		(140)
Potassium		>>151>
Selenium		>>252>
Sodium		(81)
Zinc		(78)

Computerized diet analysis programs can save time, but even with excellent databases, the information gained from such a program needs interpretation. The only scientifically correct statement is that the intake for a given period does or does not meet the RDA. It is inappropriate to base a judgment of nutritional or dietary status solely on a comparison to the RDA.

American Dietetic and Diabetes Associations Exchange Lists

The American Dietetic Association and the American Diabetes Association jointly publish a food guide commonly called the *ADA Exchange Lists.* These lists can be used in clinical practice to aid in meal planning. The **Exchange lists** are sometimes used to assist clients in weight control. Recent changes in dietary prescriptions for patients with diabetes are discussed in Chapter 18. The ADA Exchange Lists are revised and updated about every 10 years. The last revision was in 1995. It is possible to approximate a client's carbohydrate, fat, protein, and kilocalorie intake with exchange lists. Exchange lists are used not only for calculating a client's food intake but also for education, meal planning, and counseling.

There are six basic exchange lists: (1) starch; (2) fruit; (3) milk in three groups, skim, low fat, and whole; (4) vegetable; (5) meat in four groups, very lean, lean, medium fat, and high fat; and (6) fat in three groups, monounsaturated, polyunsaturated, and saturated. Table 2–9 identifies typical foods in each exchange list. In addition, some foods are considered "free." Free foods are on a separate list. The complete exchange lists appear in Appendix A.

Foods are placed on each list based on their energy nutrient composition because foods within each list contain similar nutrient composition. For example, corn is on the starch list because it is closer in composition to a slice of bread than to green beans. Table 2–10 shows the amount of carbohydrate, protein, fat, and kilocalories in one exchange on each list. As you can see from the table, one exchange on the fruit list is not equal to one exchange on the starch list. To correctly use this method of meal planning, it is necessary for clients to choose the correct number of items from each appropriate list.

Understanding the meaning of the term **exchange** is important. In this context, the term exchange means only and precisely a defined quantity of food within an exchange list. For example, one exchange of bread is one slice (a defined quantity). Individual food items within an exchange list are essentially equal to each other in nutrient composition and can thus be exchanged or "swapped" for each other. This is possible because portion sizes for various items were adjusted at the time the lists were created. Lists were created to make each exchange approximately equal. For example, Table 2–11 shows items equal to one starch exchange.

Exchange lists can be adapted for any prescribed kilocalorie, protein, fat, or carbohydrate level. Exchange lists should always include a specific meal plan for the client to follow. A *meal plan* is a food guide that shows the number of choices or exchanges the client should eat at each meal or snack.

TABLE 2–9   Typical Foods in Each Exchange List

Exchange List	Food Items
Starch	Cereals, grains, pasta, dried beans, peas, lentils, starchy vegetables, bread, crackers
Meat	Beef, pork, veal, poultry, fish, wild game, cheese, eggs, tofu, peanut butter
Fruit	Fresh, frozen, or unsweetened canned fruit; dried fruit; fruit juice
Vegetable	Raw or cooked nonstarchy vegetables, vegetable juices
Milk	Milk, yogurt, evaporated milk, powdered milk
Fat	Avocado, margarine, mayonnaise, nuts, seeds, oil, salad dressing, bacon, coconut, powdered coffee whitener, cream, sour cream, whipped cream, cream cheese, salt pork

TABLE 2–10   Energy Composition of the Six Exchange Lists

Exchange List	CHO (g)	Protein (g)	Fat (g)	Calories
Starch	15	3	0–1	80
Meat				
Very lean	0	7	0–1	35
Lean	0	7	3	55
Medium fat	0	7	5	75
High fat	0	7	8	100
Vegetables	5	2	0	25
Fruit	15	0	0	60
Milk				
Skim	12	8	0–3	90
2 percent	12	8	5	120
Whole	12	8	8	150
Fat (all)	0	0	5	45

SOURCE: The exchange lists are the basis of a meal planning system designed primarily for people with diabetes and others who must follow special diets. The exchange lists are based on principles of good nutrition that apply to everyone. © With permission 1995 American Diabetes Association and American Dietetic Association.

Table 2–12 illustrates two different meal plans for two different kilocalorie levels. One example is provided for distributing the various exchanges among the meals. It is also possible to calculate two different meal plans for the same kilocalorie level. Table 2–13 illustrates two 1200-kilocalorie meal plans.

Using exchange lists and following a meal plan allows the patient a variety of food choices. This method can also be used to control the distribution of nutrients throughout the day. For clinical reasons, many clients need to modify meal frequency.

Desired Outcomes

Several examples of **desired outcome** or goal or objective statements are given in Table 2–14. Correctly and incorrectly formulated outcomes are shown with a critique of the faulty ones.

Nursing Actions

After the nursing diagnosis has been made, the nurse decides how best to treat the client. The nurse can help clients receive optimal nutritional care by referring clients to nutritional services or providing care directly. Some of the reasons for not being able to address a particular client's needs include lack of

TABLE 2–11 Examples of One Starch Exchange

Puffed cereal	1 1/2 cups
Bread	1 slice
Corn, whole kernel	1/2 cup
Rice, cooked	1/3 cup

TABLE 2–12 1500- and 1800-kcal Meal Plan Using Exchanges for 1 Day

	1500 kcal	1800 kcal
Starch	7	7
Meat, lean	1	3
Meat, medium	3	3
Vegetable	4	5
Fruit	3	5
Milk, skim	2	2
Fat	6	7

DISTRIBUTION OF EXCHANGE THROUGHOUT THE DAY

	1500-kcal Meal Plan			
	Breakfast	Lunch	Dinner	Snack
Starch	2	2	2	1
Meat, lean	0	1	0	0
Meat, medium	0	0	3	0
Vegetable	0	2	2	0
Fruit	1	1	1	0
Milk, skim	1	0	0	1
Fat	2	2	2	0

TABLE 2–13 Two 1200-kcal Meal Plans Using Exchanges for 1 Day

Exchanges	Meal Plan 1	Meal Plan 2
Starch	5	6
Meat, lean	4	1
Meat, medium	1	3
Vegetable	2	4
Fruit	3	2
Milk, skim	2	1
Fat	4	4

resources (including time), lack of knowledge, and the wasteful practice of duplicating existing services and information.

The referral system has two functions. First, it ensures that the client gets comprehensive care. Second, it informs clients about the service of a nutrition program by making them aware of their need for and the benefits of that service. In the event that the nurse decides to treat the client directly, an efficient approach is to utilize the same nutritional parameter to educate the client as used during the assessment. Some of the roles the nurse assumes to resolve the client's nursing problems are discussed in Box 2–2.

Evaluation of Nutritional Care

When the deadline stated in the desired outcome arrives, the nurse and the client decide if the objective has been met. If not, they explore the reasons: unrealistic expectations, not enough time elapsed, of nursing actions not appropriate or not implemented.

A diet can be quickly measured against three criteria: balance, moderation, and variety. A **balanced diet** includes foods from each of the five food groups daily. The five major food groups are those in the Food Pyramid with the exception of fats, oils, and sweets. *Moderation* means avoiding too much or too little of any one food or food group. *Variety* means eating many different foods within each food group.

TABLE 2–14 Correctly and Incorrectly Stated Desired Outcomes

Correct	Incorrect	Critique of Incorrect
Client will lose 2 lb per week for the next 4 weeks.	Client will lose 20 lb in 2 weeks.	Not realistic
	Client will lose 20 lb.	No deadline
Client will consume a vegetable rich in vitamin A every other day for the next 6 weeks.	Client will increase intake of vitamin A.	Not measurable
	Teach client to consume vegetables rich in vitamin A.	Not client centered

BOX 2–2   NURSING ROLES PERTINENT TO NUTRITION

Nurses classify their functions into roles. Although often divided for discussion, the roles may be mingled in a single client interaction.

Nurses are *care providers*. They monitor clients' food intake and report and record deficits. Nurses coordinate clients' diagnostic tests and promote compensatory food and fluid intake when tests are completed. Nurses also prepare clients and their surroundings for meals, prepare food served for self-feeding, or feed clients who are unable to feed themselves.

Nurses are *teachers*. They provide information and coach clients in required skills to maximize nutritional care. To accomplish this, the nurse may have to assess feelings and motor skills. A variety of materials using visual, auditory, and psychomotor approaches will permit working with the client's preferred learning style.

This may be done one to one or in groups and possibly using supplementary materials and techniques. If printed materials are used, the reading level should be appropriate, often two to four grades lower than the person's achieved educational level (Wells, 1994). A general rule for health education materials is that they should be written at a maximum of the eighth-grade reading level (Estey, 1991). Pilot Testing the material on its intended audience will reveal weaknesses. Self-paced learning programs have been effective in guiding clients, even children, to acquire necessary information (Shannon, et al, 1995). Since the learning takes place over an extended time, the program provides its own reinforcement.

Often the desired outcome of teaching is behavior change, not increased knowledge. In one situation, blood cholesterol levels were used to evaluate instruction. Multiple sessions produced a better result than a single lesson (Byers, et al, 1995).

As a *counselor* the nurse assists the client to make decisions affecting his or her health. A counselor focuses on attitudes, feelings, and behaviors to encourage the client in achieving self-control. Especially when the client displays self-destructive behaviors, the nurse may need special training to confront specific behaviors, to remain nonjudgmental, and to avoid speculating on reasons for the client's behavior (Sutherland, 1995). The nurse needs to ensure that the client receives a diet that he or she is willing to follow and that is adapted to his or her home situation. Studies have shown that facilitation skills of customizing, adapting, and including the client in decision making exert the strongest force on client satisfaction and intention to comply with diet counseling (Trudeau and Dube, 1995). An imperfect diet that is followed is preferable to a perfectly designed one that is ignored. The nursing role of counselor contrasts with that of the teacher who helps the client to acquire new knowledge and skill.

A nurse acts as a *client advocate* when protecting and supporting the client's rights. Basic to these rights is the client's right to choose after having been informed of treatment options, risks, and expected outcomes.

Modern health care requires the cooperation of many individuals of varied professions. Nurses function as *health team members*. Nutrition instruction can be provided effectively by physicians, nurses, or dietitians (Peiss, Kurleto, and Rubenfire, 1995). The client or his or her surrogate functions as a member of the health care team, also. Clients are more knowledgeable, assertive, and independent than in the past. These attributes can be used to maximize their health.

Impact of Culture

Culture is the learned, shared, and transmitted values, beliefs, and norms of a particular group that guide their thinking, decisions, and actions in patterned ways (Leininger, 1991). Although national, ethnic, and religious groups are prime examples of cultures, other alliances such as colleges, corporations, professions, political parties, and service clubs also imbue their members with values and norms. Health practices unite persons with others of similar habits, such as athletes or vegetarians. From this perspective some aspects of culture are imposed at birth, but other aspects are voluntarily selected. An individual's food choices may be influenced by ethnicity and religion.

Even when individuals share a similar heritage, differences exist. Diseases and dietary preferences vary among people of Cuban, Puerto Rican, and Mexican descent (Loria, et al, 1995). To assume that because an individual is a member of a group, that the individual has adopted the group's lifestyle is to stereotype the person.

Ethnocentrism

The belief that one's own view of the world is superior to that of anyone else's is **ethnocentrism.** The dominant cultural groups in the United States have been white descendants of northern Europeans, middle class, and Protestant. Education, work, punctuality, independence, and a future orientation are important values of the dominant culture and undergird the health care system. Providers have tried, often unsuccessfully, to deliver this version of health care to clients without regard to the clients' cultures. If the clients fail to achieve goals that have been imposed on them, they have been labeled as "noncompliant" (Wuest, 1995). Another example of ethnocentrism from the past is calling an inability to communicate in the dominant culture's language "altered communication" (Eliason, 1993; Levine, Ortmann, and Lunney, 1994).

Postulating a single standard of health regardless of ethnicity is questionable because health care research has systematically excluded large subgroups of the population. For example, Caucasians tend to excrete caffeine faster than Asians (Kudzma, 1992). Because waist-to-hip ratio norms used to identify high risk for cardiovascular disease are based on white populations, they may not be appropriate for other racial groups (Croft, et al, 1995).

Acculturation

The process of adopting the values, attitudes, and behavior of another culture, **acculturation,** often is a disadvantage, for example, Latino women most acculturated into norms of the United States were least likely to initiate and to continue breast-feeding (Rassin, et al, 1994).

The major disease affecting widely scattered indigenous populations undergoing acculturation is non-insulin-dependent diabetes mellitus (NIDDM). The Pima Indians in Arizona have the highest reported prevalence of the disease (McCance, et al, 1994). Native residents of Canada and Australia have a higher incidence of NIDDM than their general populations (Daniel and Gamble, 1995; D'Alessio, 1995). The death rate from diabetes for native Hawaiians is more than three times that of the general US population. Mortality from heart disease, which is related to diabetes, is 44 percent higher than that of the US population (Mokuau, Hughes, and Tsark, 1995).

Culturally Competent Care

Knowledge and acceptance of, and respect for, another's culture are necessary to provide culturally competent care. The goal is a treatment plan that blends the client's cultural beliefs and practices with those of modern medicine. Clinical Application 2–2 illustrates the adaptation of diabetic teaching to Native American mythology.

Food selection and preparation are heavily influenced by culture. Items considered appropriate for human consumption vary by culture, including economic and geographic constraints. The Seminole language, for instance, has no word for "vegetables," and it is translated as "weeds" (Nelson, et al, 1983). Rituals of preparation may be culturally determined. Foods may be culturally endorsed treatments for disease. A certain food traditionally given to a sick person as a child may later evoke comfort to an adult. The following brief summaries describe traditional food beliefs of five cultural groups and suggest possible applications for adapting nutritional needs to their beliefs.

African Americans

Some African Americans prepare stews from pork and greens such as dandelion, turnip, and collard.

CLINICAL APPLICATION 2–2

Using Ojibway Mythology in Diabetic Teaching

The Native American adage to walk in another's moccasins offers insight into culturally competent care. A program in Toronto capitalized upon Ojibway mythology to provide instruction on the self-care of diabetes. The program was organized at the request of Native Canadians and included daylong educational workshops. These sessions were conducted by an elder, and all participants sat in a circle. The circle confers equal status on every individual and represents harmony with nature. The beginning focus was on Nanabush, a legendary teacher of the Ojibway who symbolizes moderation and balance. Traditional narratives show him conversing with Diabetes. The moral of the story is to learn about "Diabetes," to live with him, and to control one's life through spiritual strength. Workshop activities included exercise breaks and a buffet lunch that allowed participants to choose their meals. Practitioners learned that avoiding a rigid diet prescription would enhance the individual's freedom, which was highly valued among the Ojibway (Hagey, 1984).

The meat and greens are cooked together as one-pot dinners to tenderize the meat and flavor the vegetables. Other foods often served are dried beans, sweet potatoes, rice, grits, cornbread, and specialty gravies (red-eye, sausage, or cream). The Food Pyramid supports the use of beans, rice, and sweet potatoes cooked without a lot of fat, such as by steaming. Other methods of preparing traditional foods to decrease fat consumption are to bake, braise, broil, or grill them instead of frying them. Fat-free broths can be substituted for rich gravies.

Mexican Americans

Corn is the staple crop of Mexico. When corn is served with beans, the combination provides adequate protein. Vegetables and meat usually are incorporated into a main dish and served with salsa. Foods are often stewed or fried in oil or lard. Fruits are popular. Sweet foods, such as yeast pastries, are common in the traditional Mexican diet, and sugar is often added to foods.

A health belief that may influence a Mexican American's food choices is the "hot-cold" system. Illness and physiological conditions are categorized as "hot" or "cold." Foods of the opposite category are eaten in an attempt to return balance to the body. The categories vary widely by region so the practical procedure is to ask clients what foods they would like to eat.

To implement the Food Pyramid, traditional Mexican foods can be used with some changes in preparation—for example, boiled instead of refried beans, grilled instead of fried beef, or diet drinks instead of lemonade or soda. Continued use of starches and fruits should fulfill the Food Pyramid requirements while keeping tradition viable.

Native Hawaiians

Before the arrival of Westerners, native Hawaiians consumed a diet of taro (a starch root similar to potato), sweet potatoes, breadfruit, fruit, greens, and seaweed. Fat content was about 10 percent of kilocalories. Foods were eaten raw or steamed.

An experiment offering as much as desired of their traditional foods and limited amounts of fish and chicken produced astounding results in 3 weeks. Average energy intake decreased 41 percent. Average weight loss was 17.1 pounds (7.8 kilograms). Serum cholesterol decreased 14 percent (Shintani, et al, 1991). Reverting to a pre-Western diet dramatically altered risk factors for diabetes mellitus and heart disease.

Chinese Americans

Two major regions distinguish Chinese cooking. Because northern China produces wheat noodles and dumplings are usually served, whereas southern China produces rice. Meats are cut into bite-sized pieces in the kitchen. Poor sanitation led to avoidance of cold water and raw fruits and vegetables. Fruits and vegetables are quickly cooked, and thus they retain a crisp texture. Dairy products are rarely used.

Chinese medicine views sickness as an imbalance between yin and yang forces, compared by some to the parasympathetic and sympathetic nervous systems. Certain illnesses, foods, and medicines are categorized as *yin* or *yang*. Yin, or "cold," foods include pork, most vegetables, boiled foods, cold foods, and white foods. *Yang*, or "hot," foods include beef, chicken, eggs, fried foods, hot foods, and red foods. Noodles and soft rice are neutral, neither yin nor yang.

To maintain fluid intake, Chinese Americans would prefer hot tea to ice water. To increase calcium intake, green leafy vegetables or tofu would be accepted more readily than milk. Family members may cook food at home to provide the hospitalized client with hot or cold foods (Chan, 1995). Since yin and yang cover various categories of foods, cooking methods, and colors, the perceptive nurse or dietitian can tactfully suggest items or procedures that also fit the diet prescribed by Western medicine. Clinical Application 2–3 relates such a case.

Jewish Americans

Some Jewish foods have been adopted by the general American public: bagels with cream cheese, pastrami on rye, and kosher dill pickles. Orthodox Jews interpret dietary laws most stringently. There are three key characteristics of kosher food preparation: (1) Only designated animals can be eaten; (2) Some of those animals must be ritually slaughtered and dressed; (3) Dairy products and meats are not eaten at the same meal. Separate cooking and serving utensils are used for dairy meals and meat meals. Dairy foods may be eaten before the meat but not until 1 to 6 hours afterward. Fruits, vegetables, and starches need no special preparation and can be served with either meat or dairy meals.

When a preplanned kosher meal is unavailable, a cottage cheese fruit plate is a good choice. The cottage cheese should be transferred to a paper plate with plastic utensils so that neither the plate nor the utensils have touched meat. If bread or crackers are served, labels must indicate they contain no meat products.

Table 2–15 lists the characteristic eating patterns of selected cultural groups with suggested means of decreasing fat intake. Table 2–16 lists selected religious customs that affect food intake.

Summary

The assessment of nutritional status includes subjective data (knowledge of nutrition, usual intake) and objective data (general appearance, anthropometric data, body density measures, and diagnostic tests). Nursing diagnoses are derived by comparing the client's data with nutritional parameters (height–weight tables, body mass index, US Dietary Guidelines, the Food Pyramid, and Recommended Dietary Allowances). Diet prescriptions and instructions may use the American Dietetic Association and American Diabetes Association Exchange Lists.

To avoid stereotyping individuals because of their ethnic or religious affiliations, the best practice is to ask clients to describe their dietary preferences. Nurses can then design nursing action that will be meaningful to the client.

> ### CLINICAL APPLICATION 2–3
> #### Bridging Yin and Yang Beliefs and the Germ Theory of Disease
>
> A Chinese infant was experiencing repeated bouts of diarrhea. Several tests were performed, and changes were made in the child's formula to no avail. Finally a nurse made a home visit. She discovered several bottles of home-prepared formula on the windowsill, while others were in the refrigerator. The family lived in an apartment in New York without air-conditioning, and it was midsummer. When she was asked about the procedure used to store the formula, the mother stated that because childbirth is regarded as a cold condition and she should therefore avoid cold, her husband was taking the day's bottles from the refrigerator before he left for work in the morning so they would be "warm." The nurse explained that storage at room temperature permitted bacteria to grow in the formula, which was the cause of the baby's diarrhea. Together, the mother and nurse searched for another procedure to bridge the cultural belief and the germ theory of disease. The mother decided to don a coat, hat, and gloves before opening the refrigerator to retrieve each bottle. The nurse wisely guided the mother to a solution that left her belief system intact. The infant suffered no further episodes of diarrhea (Jackson, 1993).

TABLE 2–15   Characteristic Eating Patterns of Selected Cultural Groups

Group	Grains and Starches	Fruits	Vegetables	Meat and Meat Substitutes	Milk and Milk Substitutes	To Decrease Fat
Latinos						
Mexicans	Tortillas, corn products, potatoes, corn		Chili peppers, tomatoes, onions, beets, cabbage, pumpkins, string beans	Meat, poultry, eggs; pinto, calico, garbanzo beans	Cheese (milk seldom consumed)	Encourage: • Salsa as dip or topping • Baked corn tortillas, especially stuffed with chicken to make tamales, tostados, or enchiladas • Rice with chicken or beans • Reduced-fat cheeses Discourage: • Fried tortillas • Sour cream and regular cheese as toppings • Refried beans that are cooked in lard • Deep-fried foods such as chimichangas
Puerto Ricans	Platanos (starchy vegetable that looks like a large banana), Puerto Rican bread (resembles Italian bread), rice, viands (starchy vegetable whose roots and tubers are peeled, boiled, and eaten as a side dish)	Guava, canned peaches, pears, fruit cocktail	Beets, eggplant, carrots, green beans, onions	Legumes (especially red kidney beans), eggs, pork, chicken, cod, fish, pigeon, peas, garbanzo beans	Milk seldom consumed, flan (custard)	
Cubans	Rice		Green peppers, onions, tomatoes	Black beans, pork, chicken, chorizo, (a highly seasoned sausage)	Milk seldom used	
Italians	Pasta, yeast breads, starchy root vegetables		Green peppers, onions, tomatoes	Spiced sausages, fish, tomato-based meat sauces	Cheese (milk seldom consumed— high incidence of lactose intolerance in Italians)	Encourage: • Salad with no-fat dressing • Minestrone soup • Pasta with tomato or clam sauce • Grilled meat or seafood Discourage: • White sauces made with cream, butter, cheese • Breaded and fried meats and vegetables • Sausages and other fatty meats such as prosciutto (spiced ham)
Southern Black Americans	Cornbread, biscuits, white bread, butter beans, corn, sweet potatoes, grits, rice, white potatoes, corn, yams	Melons, bananas, peaches	Kale, collards, and mustard greens, okra, tomatoes, cabbage, summer squash	Catfish, pork, chicken, black-eyes peas, other dried beans and peas	Buttermilk, evaporated milk, ice cream (high incidence of lactose intolerance in blacks)	Encourage: • Baked fish and chicken • Steamed vegetables • Fresh melon • Grilled foods
Asians						
Southern Chinese	Rice	All	Mushrooms, bean sprouts, Chinese greens, bok choy	Beef, pork, poultry, seafood	Limited except for ice cream	Encourage: • Hot and sour soup; wonton soup • Steamed (not fried) dumplings • Lightly stir-fried chicken or seafood • Steamed whole fish • Steamed vegetables; steamed rice
Northern Chinese	Wheat, millet seed used in noodles, bread, dumplings		Chinese greens, bamboo, alfalfa sprouts, bok choy	Beef, poultry, seafood, eggs, tofu, soybeans	None (high incidence of lactose intolerance among all Chinese)	

TABLE 2–15   Characteristic Eating Patterns of Selected Cultural Groups (Continued)

Group	Grains and Starches	Fruits	Vegetables	Meat and Meat Substitutes	Milk and Milk Substitutes	To Decrease Fat
Japanese	Rice, most other complex carbohydrates		All	Fish, beef, pork, eggs, poultry, shellfish, soybean products	None (high incidence of lactose intolerance among all Japanese)	Discourage: • Egg rolls • Crispy fried noodles • Fried rice • Deep-fried entrees • Spareribs • Tempura
Middle Eastern	*Europeans* Pita bread Bulgar, dark breads, wheat breads, potatoes	All	Grape leaves All, especially, onions, carrots, beans	Lamb, chicken, goat, legumes Beef, pork, poultry, fish, shellfish, eggs, sausages	Yogurt All cheese and milk products	Encourage: • Lean beef, pork, poultry • Broiled, poached, or steamed meats • Wine- and tomato-based sauces • Consomme Discourage: • Creamed soups and sauces • Sausages • Whole milk and whole-milk products • Fried potatoes • Sour cream

TABLE 2–16   Selected Religious Customs that Affect Food Intake

Religion	Restricted Food and Beverages
Buddhism	1. All meat.
Catholicism	1. Meat prohibited by some denominations on holy days such as Good Friday and Ash Wednesday. 2. Alcoholic beverages by some denominations.
Hinduism	1. Beef, pork, and some fowl.
Islam	1. All pork and pork products. 2. All meat must be slaughtered according to ritual letting of blood. 3. Coffee and tea. 4. All alcoholic beverages.
Orthodox Judaism	1. All pork and pork products. 2. All fish without scales and fins. 3. Dairy products should not be eaten at the same meal that contains meat and meat products. 4. All meat must be slaughtered and prepared according to Biblical ordinances. Since blood is forbidden as food, meat must be drained thoroughly. 5. Bakery products and prepared food mixtures must be prepared under acceptable kosher standards. 6. Leavened bread and cake are forbidden during Passover.
Seventh-Day Adventist	1. All pork and pork products. 2. Shellfish. 3. All flesh foods (some members). 4. All dairy products and eggs (some members) 5. Blood. 6. Highly spiced foods. 7. Meat broths. 8. All alcoholic beverages. 9. Coffee and tea.

Case Study 2–1   A student in a beginning nutrition course is showing a friend the textbook. "You could help me improve my diet," the friend says. "I know I am not eating right." At the time the friend was eating a chocolate bar.

The student asks the friend to list what he has eaten during the past 24 hours. From the friend's list, the student gathers the following data:

Breakfast: Orange juice, black coffee
Lunch: Yogurt and graham crackers
Midafternoon snack: Chocolate bar
Dinner: Pork chop, green salad, French dressing, diet cola

Comparing the friend's intake to the Food Pyramid, the student finds the following:

	Number of Servings	
	Friend's Intake	*Food Pyramid*
Fats, oils, sweets	2	Use sparingly
Milk, yogurt, cheese	1	2–3
Meat, poultry, fish, dried beans, eggs, nuts	1	2–3
Vegetables	1	3–5
Fruits	1	2–4
Bread, cereal, rice, pasta	1	6–11

In this situation the student may not formalize a nursing care plan for the friend. The following plan illustrates the thought process involved in developing a nursing care plan for this case

NURSING CARE PLAN

Assessment

Subjective Data   Client expresses need for instruction in healthy diet. A 24-hour recall shows fewer than the recommended Food Pyramid servings in all categories except fats, oils, and sweets.

Objective Data   Client is observed eating a chocolate bar at 3 P.M.

Nursing Diagnosis   Knowledge deficit related to Food Pyramid is evidenced by verbalization to nutrition student.

Desired Outcomes/ Evaluation Criteria	Nursing Actions	Rationale
Friend will keep a food record for 3 days.	Instruct friend to list everything he eats or drinks for 3 days.	Food record will accumulate facts about the friend's food intake to use as an instructional tool.
Friend will read the section discussing the Food Pyramid in student's textbook by this evening.	Lend friend textbook to read.	Providing literature utilizes expert opinion to reinforce the student's teaching. Reading and seeing illustration elicits active participation by the friend and employs senses other than hearing.
Friend will meet with student in 4 days to compare food record to Food Pyramid and design a plan of action.	Meet with friend in 4 days to sort and analyze food record data. Provide apples at meeting to model healthy snack food.	Setting follow-up visit just after food record is completed will maintain the friend's interest. Modeling desirable behavior is a way to encourage change.

Study Aids

Chapter Review

1. Which one of the following statements about a nutrient analysis calculated by a computer is correct:
   a. The results obtained will not vary from one nutrient database to another.
   b. Nutrient databases using the RDA to compare and analyze results may not be appropriate for a certain client.
   c. The results obtained are self-explanatory and need not be explained to the client.
   d. The results are always more accurate than that obtained from manual calculations using a table of food composition.

2. Which of the following is not a part of the US Dietary Guidelines?
   a. Choose a diet low in fat, saturated fat, and cholesterol.
   b. Eliminate salt and sugar from the diet.
   c. Maintain a healthy weight.
   d. Vary the foods you consume.

3. Which statement about the use of the ADA Exchange Lists is true?
   a. Two starch exchanges can be substituted for two meat exchanges.
   b. Exchange lists are used to calculate an individual's RDA.
   c. An exchange is a defined quantity of food on a particular exchange list.
   d. All 1200-kilocalorie meal plans contain six starch exchanges and only lean meat exchanges.

4. Which of the following is true of the traditional Chinese yin and yang health belief system?
   a. A cold, or yin, condition is balanced by consuming hot, or yang, foods.
   b. A hot condition is flushed with large quantities of cold water.
   c. Rice is considered magical and is consumed at every meal.
   d. Yang, or hot, foods include only foods served hot.

5. Adherents to strict kosher regulations
   a. Avoid cheese and cheese products.
   b. Eat certain cuts of pork.
   c. Keep separate utensils and dishes for meat and dairy meals.
   d. Serve lobster, clams, and shrimp only on festive occasions.

Clinical Analysis

1. Ms. G has just been diagnosed with NIDDM. She is a Native American who has left her reservation for employment in town. Which of the following actions by the nurse shows respect for Ms. G's culture?
   a. Instructing her to increase her intake of vegetables.
   b. Telling her to lose weight and avoid alcohol and fast-food restaurants.
   c. Giving Ms. G an instruction sheet based on the ADA exchange system.
   d. Asking Ms. G how she sees diabetes in her life.

2. Mr. P is a 65-year-old widower whose physician is recommending weight loss. Mr. P has had little experience with grocery shopping or cooking. Which of the following systems for instructing Mr. P would the nurse select to offer the best chance of success?
   a. A computerized diet analysis program
   b. The Food Pyramid
   c. The ADA Exchange Lists
   d. The current RDA table

3. Ms. E attended a community health fair where she entered her recalled intake for the previous 24 hours into a computer for analysis. Based on the printout she was given, she now thinks she should begin taking vitamin and mineral supplements. A friend who is a nurse correctly gives her this advice:
   a. A 1-day diet recall is an inadequate base to begin the supplements.
   b. Ms. E should recalculate the recalled intake by hand to verify the accuracy of the computer printout.
   c. The RDAs on which computer programs are based are intended for only the 50 percent of the population who are obsessed with health.
   d. Undoubtedly, the operators of the computer at the fair had a product to sell: "Let the buyer beware."

Bibliography

Akiwumi, A: In search of the 21st century nurse for Ghana. International Nursing Review 41:118, 1994.

American Dietetic Association and American Diabetes Association: Exchange Lists for Meal Planning. American Dietetic Association and American Diabetes Association, Chicago and Alexandria, VA, 1995.

Baumgartner, RN, Chumlea, WC, and Roche, AF: Bioelectric impedance for body composition. Exercise and Sport Sciences Reviews 18:193, 1990.

Baumgartner, RN, Heymsfield, SB, and Roche, AF: Human body composition and the epidemiology of chronic disease. Obesity Research 3:73, 1995.

Broderick, E, et al: Baby bottle tooth decay in Native American children in Head Start Centers. Public Health Reports 104:50, 1989.

Byers, T, et al: The costs and effects of an nutritional education program following work-site cholesterol screening. Am J Public Health 85:650, 1995.

Chan, JYK: Dietary beliefs of Chinese patients. Nurs Stand 9:30, 1995.

Croft, JB, et al: Waist-to-hip ratio on a biracial population: Measurement, implications, and cautions for using guidelines to define high risk for cardiovascular disease. J Am Diet Assoc 95:60, 1995.

D'Alessio, V: Running a band-aid service. Nurs Stand 9:22, 1995.

Diabetes Care and Education Dietetic Practice Group of the American Dietetic Association: Chinese American Food Practices, Customs, and Holidays. The American Dietetic Association and American Diabetes Association, Chicago and Alexandria, VA, 1990.

Diabetes Care and Education Dietetic Practice Group of the American Dietetic Association: Jewish Food Practices, Customs, and Holidays. The American Dietetic Association and American Diabetes Association, Chicago and Alexandria, VA, 1989.

Diabetes Care and Education Dietetic Practice Group of the American Dietetic Association: Mexican American Food Practices, Customs, and Holidays. The American Dietetic Association and American Diabetes Association, Chicago and Alexandria, VA, 1989.

Diabetes Care and Education Dietetic Practice Group of the American Dietetic Association: Soul and Traditional Southern Food Practices, Customs, and Holidays. The American Dietetic Association and American Diabetes Association, Chicago and Alexandria, VA, 1995.

Daniel, M, and Gamble, D: Diabetes and Canada's aboriginal peoples; the need for primary prevention. International Journal of Nursing Studies 32:243, 1995.

Eliason, MJ: Ethics and transcultural nursing care. Nursing Outlook 41:225, 1993.

ESHA Research: Food Processor Plus. Salem, OR, 1994.

Estey, A, Musseau, A, and Keehn, L: Comprehension levels of patients reading health information. Patient Education and Counseling 18:165, 1991.

Feldman, EB: Essentials of Clinical Nutrition. FA Davis, Philadelphia, 1988.

Grootenhuis, PA, et al: A semiquantitative food frequency questionnaire for use in epidemiologic research among the elderly: Validation by comparison with dietary history. J Clin Epidemiol 48:859, 1995.

Hagey, R: The phenomenon, the explanations and the responses: Metaphors surrounding diabetes in urban Canadian Indians. Soc Sci Med 18:265, 1984.

Hahn, NI: Variety is still the spice of a healthful diet. J Am Diet Assoc 95:1096, 1995.

Jackson, LE: Understanding, eliciting and negotiating clients' multicultural health beliefs. Nurse Practitioner 18:30, 1993.

Jensen, M: Research techniques for body composition assessment. J Am Diet Assoc 92:454, 1992.

Kudzma, EC: Drug response: All bodies are not created equal. Am J Nurs 92(12):48, 1992.

Kushner, RF: Bioelectrical impedance analysis: A review of principles and applications. J Am Coll Nutr 11(2):199, 1992.

Larson, E: Exclusion of certain groups from clinical research. Image 26:185, 1994.

Leininger, M: The theory of culture care diversity and universality. In Leininger, M (ed): Culture Care Diversity and Universality: A Theory of Nursing. National League for Nursing Press, New York, 1991.

Levine, MA, Ortmann, D, and Lunney, M: Nursing diagnosis in crosscultural settings. Nursing Diagnosis 5:158, 172, 1994.

Loria, CM, et al: Macronutrient intakes among adult Hispanics: A comparison of Mexican Americans, Cuban Americans, and mainland Puerto Ricans. Am J Public Health 85:684, 1995.

McCance, DR, et al: Birthweight and non-insulin dependent diabetes: Thrifty genotype, thrifty phenotype, or surviving small baby genotype? Br Med J 308:942, 1994.

Moggatt, MEK: Current status of nutritional deficiencies in Canadian aboriginal people. Can J Physiol Pharmacol 73:754, 1995.

Mokuau, N, Hughes, CK, and Tsark, JAU: Heart disease and associated risk factors among Hawaiians: Culturally responsive strategies. Health and Social Work 20:46, 1995.

Moore, MC: Pocket Guide, Nutrition and Diet Therapy. Mosby, St Louis, 1993.

National Research Council: Diet and Health: Implications for Reducing Chronic Disease Risk. Report of the Committee on Diet and Health, Food and Nutrition Board, Commission on Life Sciences. National Academy Press, Washington, DC, 1989.

Nelson, M, et al: Problem of changing food habits: Reaching disadvantaged families through their own food cultures. In Karp, RJ (ed): Malnourished Children in the United States. Springer, New York, 1993.

Opplinger, RA, Nielsen, DH, Shetler, AC, et al: Body composition of collegiate football players: Bioelectrical impedance and skinfolds compared to hydrostatic weighing. Journal of Orthopedic and Sports Physical Therapy 15:187, 1992.

Pacy, PJ, et al: Body composition measurement in elite heavyweight oarswomen: A comparison of five methods. Journal of Sports Medicine and Physical Fitness 35:67, 1995.

Peiss, B, Kurleto, B, and Rubenfire, M: Physicians and nurses can be effective educators in coronary risk reduction. J Gen Intern Med 10:77, 1995.

Pichert, JW, and Elam, P: Readability formulas may mislead you. Patient Education and Counseling 7:181, 1985.

Rassin, DK, et al: Acculturation and the initiation of breastfeeding. J Clin Epidemiol 47:739, 1994.

Rooubenoff, R, Dallal, GE, and Wilson, PWF: Predicting body fatness: The body mass index vs estimation by bioelectrical impedance. Am J Public Health 85:726, 1995.

Shannon, BM, et al: Reduction of elevated LDL-cholesterol levels of 4- to 10-year old children through home-based dietary education. Pediatrics 94:923, 1994.

Shintani, TT, et al: Obesity and cardiovascular risk intervention through the ad libitum feeding of traditional Hawaiian diet. Am J Clin Nutr 53:1647S, 1991.

Stephens, ST: Patient education materials: Are they readable? Oncology Nursing Forum 19:83, 1992.

Subcommittee on the Tenth Edition of the RDAs. Food and Nutrition Board. Commission on Life Sciences. National Research Council: Recommended Dietary Allowances. National Academy Press, Washington, DC, 1989.

Sutherland, JA: The Johari window: A strategy for teaching therapeutic confrontation. Nurse Educ 20:22, 1995.

Trudeau, E, and Dube, L: Moderators and determinants of satisfaction with diet counseling for patients consuming a therapeutic diet. J Am Diet Assoc 95:34, 1995.

Vahabi, M, and Ferris, L: Improving written patient education materials: A review of the evidence. Health Education Journal 54:99, 1995.

Wells, JA: Readability of HIV/AIDS educational materials: The role of the medium of communication, target audience, and producer characteristics. Patient Educ Couns 24:249, 1994.

Wu, Y: Cross-validation of bioelectrical impedance analysis of body composition in children and adolescents. Phys Ther 73:320, 1993.

Wuest, J: Removing the shackles: A feminist critique of noncompliance. Nurs Outlook 41:217, 1993.

CHAPTER 3

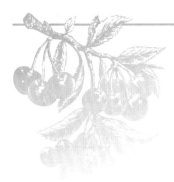

Carbohydrates

LEARNING OBJECTIVES

After completing this chapter, the student should be able to:

1 Describe the types of carbohydrates and identify food sources and individual needs.
2 List the major functions and storage methods in the human body for carbohydrates.
3 Discuss dietary fiber and list its functions and food sources.
4 Describe the relationship between carbohydrates and dental health.
5 List the carbohydrate content (in grams) of each appropriate exchange list.
6 List two dietary recommendations relating to carbohydrates.

Nature of Carbohydrates

Carbohydrates, along with fats and proteins, provide the body's basic fuel or energy needs. Carbohydrates, however, are the recommended major source of energy; they break down rapidly and are therefore readily available for use by the body. In this chapter we discuss the role of carbohydrates in the body and their relationship with the other energy nutrients. We also consider carbohydrates in the diet and health issues related to carbohydrate intake.

Carbohydrates are manufactured by green plants during a complex process known as **photosynthesis.** In this process, sugars and starches are formed in the plant by the combination of carbon dioxide from the air and water from the soil. Sunlight and the green plant pigment called **chlorophyll** are necessary for this conversion to occur. Through photosynthesis the sun's energy is transformed into food energy in the form of carbohydrates.

Carbohydrates may be divided into two major groups: sugars and starches. The chemical structure of each carbohydrate determines whether it is classified as a sugar or starch. Sugars have the simplest chemical structure, while starches are more *complex.* Thus sugars are frequently referred to as **simple carbohydrates** and starches as **complex carbohydrates.** The terms sugar, starch, simple, and complex all refer to the intricacy of the chemical structure of the carbohydrate.

Composition of Carbohydrates

To understand the composition of carbohydrates, three terms need to be defined: molecule, element, and atom. A **molecule** is the smallest quantity into which a substance may be divided without loss of its characteristics. For example, water's formula is H_2O. If the hydrogen atoms are pulled apart from the oxygen atom, the resulting products are the two gases hydrogen and oxygen, which bear no resemblance to water. Molecules are made of elements. In the case of water, H_2O, the elements are hydrogen and oxygen. An **element** is a substance that cannot be separated into simpler parts by ordinary means. An **atom** is the smallest particle of an element, which retains its physical characteristics.

Classification of Carbohydrates

Carbohydrates are composed of the elements carbon, hydrogen, and oxygen. The ratio of hydrogen to oxygen is the same as that for water, two parts of hydrogen to one part of oxygen. The simplest carbohydrates have the formula $C_6H_{12}O_6$, or six molecules each of carbon and oxygen and twelve molecules of hydrogen. Carbohydrate is frequently abbreviated CHO.

Carbohydrates are classified as either simple or complex. Simple carbohydrates include monosaccharides and disaccharides. Complex carbohydrates are called polysaccharides.

Simple Carbohydrates

Simple sugars can be either monosaccharides or disaccharides. Mono- means one, di- means two, and saccharide means sweet. A **monosaccharide** contains one molecule of $C_6H_{12}O_6$. A **disaccharide** is composed of two molecules of $C_6H_{12}O_6$ joined together (minus one unit of H_2O). When the body joins two molecules of monosaccharides together, a molecule of water is released at the same time.

Monosaccharides

The monosaccharides are the building blocks of all other carbohydrates. The three monosaccharides of importance in human nutrition are *glucose, fructose,* and *galactose.* Note the *-ose* ending for each of these

---

Photosynthesis—Process by which plants containing chlorophyll are able to manufacture carbohydrates from carbon dioxide and water using the sun's energy.

Molecule—The smallest quantity into which a substance may be divided without loss of its characteristics.

Element—A substance that cannot be separated into simpler parts by ordinary means.

Atom—Smallest particle of an element that has all the properties of the element. An atom consists of the nucleus, which contains protons (positively charged particles), neutrons (no-charge particles), and surrounding electrons (negatively charged particles).

Monosaccharide—A simple sugar composed of one unit of $C_6H_{12}O_6$; examples include glucose, fructose, and galactose.

Disaccharide—A simple sugar composed of two units of $C_6H_{12}O_6$ joined together; examples include sucrose, lactose, and maltose.

sugars. All monosaccharides and disaccharides end with the letters "o-s-e."

GLUCOSE   The monosaccharide **glucose** is commonly called the *blood sugar* because it is the major form of sugar in the blood. Normal **fasting blood sugar** (FBS) is 70 to 100 milligrams per 100 milliliters of serum or plasma. No matter what form of sugar is consumed, the body readily converts it to glucose, which it obtains mostly from the breakdown of more complex carbohydrates. Glucose is present in only small amounts in some fruits and vegetables and is moderately sweet.

Another name for glucose is **dextrose.** A common practice in almost all health care facilities is to place clients on intravenous feedings. **Intravenous** simply means within or into a vein. The most common intravenous feeding is D₅W, used primarily to deliver fluids to the client. The abbreviation D₅W means that the solution contains 5 percent dextrose (glucose) and water.

FRUCTOSE   Found in fruits and honey, **fructose** is commonly referred to as the honey sugar. It is the sweetest of all the monosaccharides. Relatively new on the list of sweeteners is **high-fructose corn syrup.** Fructose is used extensively in soft drinks, canned foods, and a number of other processed foods. The human body readily converts fructose to glucose after ingestion.

Dietary treatment for some diseases includes restricting many forms of concentrated sugars from the diet. Because fructose is now so prevalent in our food supply, nurses need to teach clients that fructose is a form of concentrated sugar.

GALACTOSE   The monosaccharide **galactose** comes mainly from the breakdown of the milk sugar lactose. Yogurt and unaged cheese may contain free galactose. It is the least sweet of all the monosaccharides. The body converts galactose into glucose after ingestion.

Disaccharides

When two monosaccharides are linked together, a disaccharide is formed. The three disaccharides of importance are *sucrose, lactose,* and *maltose.*

SUCROSE   The most prevalent disaccharide, **sucrose,** is ordinary white table sugar made commercially from sugar beets and sugar cane. Brown, granulated, and powdered sugars are all forms of

sucrose. Sucrose is also found in molasses, maple syrup, and fruits. The two monosaccharides joined together to form sucrose are glucose and fructose. The total average daily intake of both sucrose and fructose is considered excessive and has been approximated to be 80 grams a day or 18 percent of energy intake. (National Research Council, 1989). See Clinical Calculation 3-1 for an explanation of converting grams of simple sugars to teaspoons of sugar. This calculation is designed to help you learn to read and interpret food labels.

LACTOSE   Because it occurs naturally only in milk, **lactose** is commonly referred to as the milk sugar. Lactose is the least sweet of the disaccharides. The two monosaccharides that make up lactose are glucose and galactose.

MALTOSE   The disaccharide **maltose** is produced when starches are broken down by the body into simpler units. This disaccharide is present in malt, malt products, beer, some infant formulas, and sprouting seeds. Maltose consists of two units of glucose joined together.

Complex Carbohydrates

Complex carbohydrates are called **polysaccharides.** Poly- means *many,* and polysaccharides are many molecules of $C_6H_{12}O_6$ joined together, with many molecules of water released. Polysaccharides can be composed of various numbers of monosaccharides and disaccharides. The three types of complex carbohydrates of nutritional importance are starch, glycogen, and fiber. See Table 3–2 for a summary of the composition of carbohydrates.

Starch

Starch is the major source of carbohydrate in the diet. Starch is found primarily in grains, cereals, breads, pasta, starchy vegetables, and legumes. Legumes include dried peas and beans such as black beans, pinto beans, kidney beans, navy beans, soybeans, black-eyed peas, split green or yellow peas, chick peas (garbanzo beans), and lentils. Many consumers erroneously believe that complex carbohydrate foods are fattening. In fact, gram for gram, fat has more than twice the kilocalories as carbohydrates. Strictly speaking, all **starches** yield simple sugars on digestion; starchy foods are mostly low in fat and high in carbohydrates and some starchy foods contain much fiber (discussion follows).

Converting Grams of Sugar into Teaspoons of Sugar

The average American's intake of sugar is considered excessive and has been approximated to be 80 g of sugar per day and 18 percent of kcal (National Research Council, 1989).

The expression "eighty grams of sugar" does not mean much to the average American consumer, since most Americans are unfamiliar with the metric system. Many food labels use the metric system to list the nutritional content of a product. To convert grams of sugar to its equivalent in teaspoons, remember one teaspoon of sugar contains 4 g of carbohydrate.

$$\frac{80 \text{ g of sugar}}{4 \text{ g of sugar per tsp}} = 20 \text{ tsp of sugar}$$

Eighty grams of sugar is equal to 20 tsps. Table 3–1 lists sweeteners that also contain 4 g of carbohydrate per tsp. Figure 3–1 provides another opportunity to convert grams of sugar to teaspoons of sugar.

TABLE 3–1   Sweeteners that Contain 4 Grams of Carbohydrates per Teaspoon

Molasses
Granulated sugar
Powdered sugar
Syrup
Brown sugar
Jam
Marmalade
Honey
Jelly

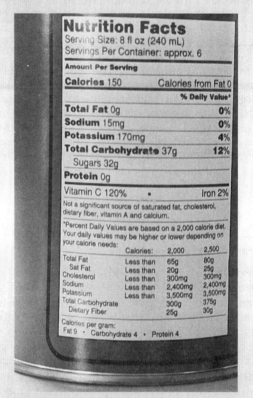

FIGURE 3–1   Nutrition facts on a label. Use this photograph as you read Clinical Calculation 3–1.

TABLE 3–2   Composition of Carbohydrates

Elements	C (carbon)
	H (hydrogen)
	O (oxygen)
Molecule	$C_6H_{12}O_6$
Monosaccharide (simple)	One unit of $C_6H_{12}O_6$
Disaccharide (simple)	Two units of $C_6H_{12}O_6$ minus one unit of H_2O
Polysaccharide (complex)	Many units of $C_6H_{12}O_6$ minus many units of H_2O

Dextrose—Another name for the simple sugar glucose.

High-fructose corn syrup (HFCS)—A common food additive used as a sweetener; made from fructose.

Polysaccharide—Complex carbohydrates composed of many units of $C_6H_{12}O_6$ joined together; examples important in nutrition include starch, glycogen, and fiber.

Glycogen

The polysaccharide **glycogen** is commonly called *the animal starch*. It is a starchlike substance in the liver and muscle tissues that is changed to glucose as needed for muscular work and for liberating heat. Glycogen represents the body's carbohydrate stores. Liver glycogen helps sustain blood glucose levels during sleep.

The typical human body has an available store of glucose in the form of glycogen for about one day's energy needs. The body's ability to store carbohydrates in the form of glycogen is limited, so adequate intake of dietary carbohydrates is essential. When a person stores glycogen, water is also stored. Each glycogen molecule attracts many molecules of water because of the way the elements are arranged. With glycogen stores completely filled, the average person will store about 4 pounds of water after eating.

Dietary Fiber

Dietary fiber refers to foods, mostly from plants, that the human body cannot break down or digest. It is eliminated from the body in the form of fecal material. Sometimes called roughage or bulk, fiber adds almost no fuel or energy value to the diet, but it does add volume.

Experts recommend that a healthy adult eat 20 to 35 grams of dietary fiber a day. In the United States, usual intakes of dietary fiber average about 11 grams per day, so few people ingest the recommended levels (Slavin, 1995).

Eating too much fiber can cause problems. Much evidence suggests that eating more than 50 grams of fiber a day can interfere with mineral absorption, which can lead to problems like anemia and osteoporosis. The current recommendation is that a desirable fiber intake be achieved *not* by adding fiber concentrates to the diet, but by the consumption of fruits, vegetables, legumes, and whole-grain cereals, because they are excellent sources of fiber that also provide minerals and vitamins.

Fiber is classified as either **soluble** or **insoluble. Solubility** is defined as the ability of one substance to dissolve into another. For example, oil does not dissolve in water, so oil is insoluble in water. Insoluble fiber does not dissolve in water, whereas soluble fiber does. Both types of fiber react differently in the body and are needed for different reasons.

SOLUBLE FIBER   Examples of sources of soluble fibers include beans, oatmeal, barley, broccoli, and citrus fruits. Oat bran is a good source of soluble

TABLE 3–3   Food Sources and Reported Benefits of Fiber

	Insoluble Fiber	Soluble Fiber
Solubility	Does not dissolve in water	Dissolves in water
Food Sources	Wheat bran	Oatmeal
	Corn bran	Oat bran, barley
	Vegetables	Some fruits such as
	Nuts	apples, oranges
	Fruit skins	Broccoli
	Some dry beans*	Some dry beans*
Reported Benefit	Promotes regularity	May help reduce cholesterol levels
	May help reduce risk of some forms of cancer	May assist in regulating blood sugar levels
	May reduce risk of diverticular disease	May promote weight loss by increasing satiety†

* Current laboratory methods to assay soluble fiber content of individual foods are imprecise. This is the subject of much research.
† Satiety is defined as the sensation of fullness after eating.

fiber. Soluble fibers dissolve in water and thicken to form gels. The reported health benefits of soluble fibers include reduced cholesterol levels, regulated blood sugar levels, and weight loss (by helping dieters control their appetites).

INSOLUBLE FIBER   Examples of sources of insoluble fibers include the woody or structural parts of plants, such as fruit and vegetable skins, and the outer coating (bran) of wheat kernels. Insoluble fibers have been reported to promote regularity of bowel movements and reduce the risk of diverticular disease and some forms of cancer. Table 3–3 relates the solubility of each type of fiber to food sources and lists the reported health benefits attributed to each.

Functions of Carbohydrates

Carbohydrates play the following roles in the body: they provide fuel, spare body protein, help prevent ketosis, and enhance learning and memory processes.

Provide Fuel

Carbohydrates, fats, and proteins provide the body's basic fuel or energy needs. *Energy* is defined as the capacity to do work. To understand the concept of energy, it may be helpful to think of the human body as a machine. Just as gasoline is a car's fuel, so carbohydrates, proteins, and fats are the human machine's fuel. Without fuel, a car will not operate; without a fuel source over an extended period of time, death by starvation is the result for the human machine. Just as you cannot easily substitute something other than gasoline for your car (if you have a gasoline engine), you cannot efficiently substitute something other than carbohydrate, protein, and fat for fuel in your body.

The brain, other nervous tissue, and the lungs use carbohydrate as a primary source of fuel. In addition, the brain cannot store carbohydrate. This means that the brain must have an uninterrupted source of carbohydrate on an ongoing basis. This has many clinical implications, which will be discussed throughout this book.

Spare Body Protein

When we eat an inadequate amount of carbohydrates, our bodies suffer. We must have a continuous supply of glucose for all cells to function, particularly those of the central nervous system. Remember, our glycogen stores are limited. But the body can convert protein to glucose. An adequate supply of dietary carbohydrates spares body protein stores from being partially converted into glucose and allows protein to be used for growth and repair of body tissue. This principle has important ramifications for human nutrition, which will be discussed throughout the text.

Help Prevent Ketosis

A balanced intake of energy nutrients is vital. If a person's carbohydrate intake is too low, the body will break down stored fat to meet its fuel needs. The human machine cannot handle the excessive breakdown of stored body fat because the body lacks the necessary equipment. As a result, partially broken-down fats accumulate in the blood in the form of ketones and the person is said to be in a state of **ketosis.** Fatigue, nausea, and a lack of appetite are some of the undesirable consequences of ketosis. Coma and death have occurred in severe cases. The presence of ketosis is easily determined by testing for the presence of **acetone** or **diacetic acid** in the urine. Acetone and diacetic acid are **ketone bodies.** A minimum of 50 to 100 grams of carbohydrate each day is usually enough to prevent ketosis.

Learning and Memory Enhancement

Considerable evidence exists that blood glucose concentrations regulate several brain functions. Glucose enhances learning and memory in healthy, aged humans. The process by which memory formation is regulated involves glucose and is a major focus of current research.

Consumption Patterns

Most of the world's population subsist primarily on carbohydrates. Foods rich in carbohydrates are easily grown in most climates, are low in cost, and are easily stored. They do not require refrigeration or electricity, and their shelf life may stretch to years. In Asia, where rice is a dietary staple, carbohydrates provide as much as 80 percent of the fuel in the diet.

Several trends reveal important information about the consumption of carbohydrates. For example, the percentage of fuel available from carbohydrates has decreased from 57 percent from the period covering 1909 to 1913 to 46 percent in 1985. Americans are eating less carbohydrate and more fat and protein as a percentage of total kilocaloric intake. In addition, in 1909 Americans obtained about 66 percent of their total carbohydrate intake from starches such as corn, potatoes, wheat, and beans, and about 33 percent of their carbohydrates from sugars such as table sugar, maple sugar, molasses, jelly, and jam. By 1980, sugars furnished more than 50 percent of the carbohydrates in the food supply.

Glycogen—A polysaccharide commonly called the animal starch; the form in which carbohydrate is stored in liver and muscle tissue formed in the body from glucose.

Dietary fiber—Material in foods, mostly from plants that the human body cannot break down or digest.

Soluble—Able to be dissolved in another substance.

Insoluble—Incapable of being dissolved.

Ketosis—The physical state of the human body with ketones elevated in the blood and present in the urine, as may occur with consumption of an extremely low carbohydrate diet.

Ketone bodies—Compounds such as acetone and diacetic acid that are formed when fat is metabolized incompletely.

Relationship to Dental Health

Several studies have shown a relationship between carbohydrate consumption and dental caries. **Dental caries** is defined as the gradual decay of the teeth. A dental cavity is a hole in a tooth caused by dental caries. Dental caries results from four interactions: a genetically susceptible tooth, bacteria, carbohydrate, and time. All four of these factors must occur simultaneously for a cavity to form, as Figure 3–2 illustrates.

Genetic Susceptibility

Diet is not the sole contributor to health. Considerable genetic variability exists in the population. Even dental caries or a cavity is subject to genetic influences. Thus, one individual's teeth may be more genetically susceptible or prone than another's to caries. **Genetic susceptibility** is the likelihood of an individual developing a given trait as determined by heredity. This is one reason why each client must be evaluated as a unique individual.

Other Factors Related to Cavity Formation

Bacteria, carbohydrate-containing foods, and the length of time that teeth are exposed to sugars influence cavity formation. Bacteria normally present in the mouth interact with dietary carbohydrates and produce acids. The acids, not the sugar, cause decay (see Fig. 3–3). All types of sugars can promote cavity formation, including fructose, glucose, maltose, lactose, and sucrose. A strong relationship exists between the length of time sugars are actually present in the mouth and the development of caries. For example, sticky foods like caramels and raisins, which adhere to the tooth surface for longer periods, can lead to tooth decay in susceptible people. Sipping sweetened beverages continually throughout the day can also lead to tooth decay. Clinical Application 3–1 discusses a common health care problem known as nursing-bottle syndrome.

Certain foods may help counteract the effects of the acids produced by oral bacteria. Aged cheese (cheddar, swiss, blue, monterey jack, brie, gouda), as well as processed American cheese, may inhibit tooth decay. Cheese stimulates the production of saliva. Chewing fibrous foods such as apples or celery stimulates the production of generous amounts of saliva. Saliva helps clear the mouth of food and counteracts acid production. Because saliva production is increased during a meal, sugars eaten with a meal are less likely to cause decay than those eaten between meals.

Food Sources

As indicated earlier, carbohydrates consist of two groups: sugars and starches. All starches contain fiber; however, all starches do not provide equal amounts of fiber.

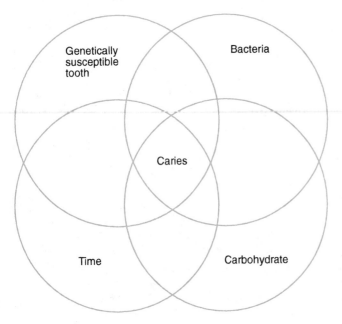

FIGURE 3–2 Interactions necessary for dental caries formation. Each of these four variables is necessary for a cavity to form. We cannot control our genetic susceptibility for cavities, and bacteria are always present in our mouths and difficult to eliminate. However, we can control the length of time carbohydrate-containing foods are in our mouths and the kinds and amounts of carbohydrates we eat.

DENTAL CARIES

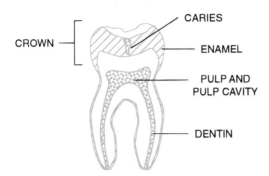

ACID BREAKS DOWN THE ENAMEL
THAT COVERS THE CROWN
OF THE TOOTH

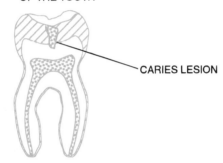

DECAY PENETRATES THE DENTIN,
THE LAYER UNDER THE ENAMEL,
CAUSING THE CAVITY

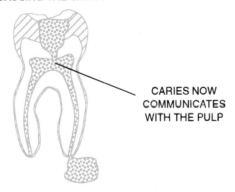

THE CAVITY, IF NOT REPAIRED,
SPREADS INTO THE PULP OF THE
TOOTH. THIS MAY CAUSE INFLAMMATION
AND AN ABSCESS. THEN THE TOOTH
MAY HAVE TO BE EXTRACTED.

FIGURE 3–3 The process of cavity formation. (From Thomas, CL [ed]: Taber's Cyclopedic Medical Dictionary, ed 18. FA Davis, Philadelphia, 1997, p 321, by Beth Anne Willert, MS, Dictionary Illustrator with permission.)

CLINICAL APPLICATION 3–1

Nursing-Bottle Syndrome

Nursing-bottle syndrome is a dental condition caused by the frequent and prolonged exposure of an infant or young child to liquids containing sugars. Milk, formula, fruit juice, or other sweetened drinks can all cause rampant dental caries.

Typically, nursing-bottle syndrome occurs when a caretaker habitually puts a baby to bed with a bottle of milk, juice, or other sweetened liquid. During sleep the flow of saliva decreases, which allows the liquids from the nursing bottle to pool around the teeth, undiluted, for extended periods. Mothers need to be cautioned against this practice.

Sugars

Sugar, as mentioned in Clinical Calculation 3–1, contains 4 grams of carbohydrates per teaspoon. When determining a person's sugar consumption, we consider not only the simple sugars such as honey, jam, and jelly but also the sugars present in carbonated beverages, ice cream, sherbet, cakes, pies, cookies, and donuts. Tables of Food Composition may be used to approximate the actual intake a person may have from combination foods (see Appendix A). Simple sugar intake can be estimated using the value of 4 grams of carbohydrates per teaspoon (see Table 3–1).

Starches

Starches provide complex carbohydrates and are important sources of fiber and other nutrients. Figure 3–4 illustrates a typical cereal grain. Its main parts, the germ, bran, and endosperm, are labeled. Most of the nutrients in cereal are in the bran and germ.

Emphasis on Whole Grain

During the **milling** of grain, the germ and bran from the grain kernel are removed. Products made

---

Genetic susceptibility—The likelihood of an individual developing a given trait as determined by heredity.

Bacteria—Single-celled microorganisms that lack a true nucleus; may be either harmless to humans or disease producing.

Milling—The process of grinding grain into flour.

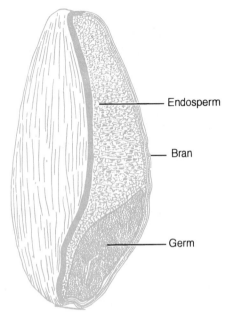

FIGURE 3–4   A grain of wheat. The most nutritious parts of a grain of wheat are the bran and the germ, which are removed during the milling of grain. For this reason, the use of whole-grain products should be encouraged.

from the milling process are said to be refined. White flour results from the milling of wheat, white rice from the milling of rice. Oat products are not normally milled. Refined cereals and bread products are not as nutritious as their whole-grain counterparts since the bran and germ contain appreciable vitamins, minerals, and fiber. The nutritive value of cereal depends on the amount of bran and germ retained during the milling process. For this reason, the use of whole grains should be encouraged whenever possible.

Enrichment

The addition of nutrients previously present in a food but removed during food processing or lost during storage is called **enrichment.** Enrichment of bread and white flour is mandatory in about two-thirds of the United States, but in fact nearly all white bread in the United States is enriched with certain B vitamins and iron (National Research Council, 1989). Other enriched products include macaroni, noodles, spaghetti, and ready-to-eat cereals. Enriched products are not nutritionally equal to their whole-grain counterparts because not all of the nutrients lost during the milling process are replaced. The fiber lost during the milling of whole-

grain products, for example, is not replaced by enrichment. If a person will not eat whole grains, encourage him or her to select enriched grain products.

Exchange List Values

The concept of exchange lists was introduced in Chapter 2. In this section we will focus on those exchange lists that contain carbohydrates. A complete copy of the exchange lists is located in Appendix A. Exchanges that include carbohydrates are the starch and/or bread, vegetable, fruit, and milk lists.

Starch/Bread Exchange List

One American Dietetic Association/American Diabetes Association (ADA) exchange of starch contains approximately 15 grams of carbohydrates. For example, each of the food items in Figure 3–5 is equal to one starch exchange. Whole-grain products average about 2 grams of fiber per serving. Some foods are higher in fiber (Table 3–4). As a general rule, 1/2 cup of cooked cereal, grain, or pasta or 1 ounce of a bread product is one starch exchange.

Vegetable Exchange List

Either raw or cooked vegetables are also good sources of carbohydrates. Vegetables contain between 2 and 3 grams of fiber per serving. One vegetable exchange contains approximately 5 grams of carbohydrates. Table 3–5 defines one vegetable exchange. Vegetables also contribute vitamins and minerals to the diet.

Fruit Exchange List

Fruits are another source of carbohydrates. One ADA exchange of fruit contains approximately 15 grams of carbohydrates. Many fruits are excellent sources of fiber (Table 3–6) and contain vitamins and minerals.

Milk Exchange List

Milk, with its lactose content is an important source of carbohydrates. One cup of milk contains 12 grams of carbohydrates. Skim, whole, and 2 percent milk all contain approximately equal amounts of carbohydrates. Eight ounces of plain low-fat yogurt (with added nonfat milk solids), 1/3 cup dry nonfat milk, 1/2 cup evaporated milk, and 1 cup of buttermilk are all equal to 1 cup of milk.

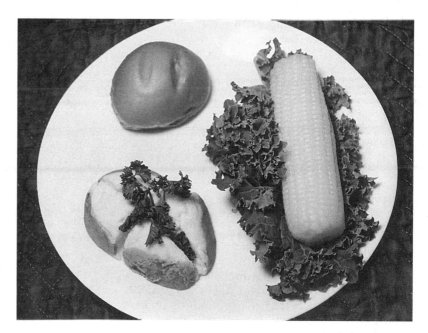

FIGURE 3–5 Each of these foods is equal to one starch exchange. An exchange is a defined quantity of a food item. One dinner roll, one small potato, and one medium ear of corn are all defined quantities (amounts) of food.

TABLE 3–4   Selected Starch Exchanges

Bran cereals*	1/2 cup
Cooked cereal	1/2 cup
Ready-to-eat, unsweetened cereals	3/4 cup
Sugar-frosted cereal	1/2 cup
Beans and peas (cooked)*	1/3 cup
Corn, whole kernel*	1/2 cup
Potato, baked	1 small (3 ounces)
Whole wheat bread	1 slice (1 ounce)

General rule: ½ cup of cereal, grain, or pasta or 1 oz of a bread product is equal to one starch exchange.
* Higher in fiber.

TABLE 3–6   Selected Fruit Exchanges

Apple (raw, 2 in across)	1 apple
Banana (small)	1 banana
Blueberries*	3/4 cup
Grapefruit (medium)	1/2 grapefruit
Nectarine (1 1/2 in across)*	1 1/2 nectarine
Strawberries (raw, whole)*	1 1/4 cup
Prunes (dried)*	3 medium
Orange (2 1/2 in across)	1 orange
Orange juice	1/2 cup

* Contain 3 or more g of fiber.

TABLE 3–5   Vegetable Exchanges

1/2 cup of cooked vegetables
1/2 cup of vegetable juice
1 cup of raw vegetables

Enrichment—The addition of nutrients previously present in a food but removed during food processing or lost during storage.

TABLE 3–7   Carbohydrate and Fiber Content of ADA Exchanges

	Carbohydrate (g)	Fiber (g)
Milk	12	0
Fruit	15	2*
Starch	15	2*
Vegetable	5	2–3

* Unless identified as a food with 3 or more g of fiber per serving.

Estimating the Fiber Content of Foods

Table 3–7 lists the carbohydrate and approximate fiber content in one serving from each of the carbohydrate-containing exchange lists. Because the fiber content of starches, fruits, and vegetables is highly variable, using the exchange list to approximate a client's fiber intake provides only an estimate. For example, 1/3 cup of All Bran cereal contains 10 grams of fiber. This is several more grams than would have been approximated if the exchange list value of 2 grams had been used.

The fiber values given in Table 3–7 may be useful to screen large numbers of clients to identify individuals with a potential fiber deficiency. If a more accurate intake of a client's fiber intake is necessary, other techniques include using a computerized nutritional analysis or looking up individual food items in a Table of Food Composition (Appendix B).

Dietary Recommendations

There is no recommended dietary allowance for carbohydrates. According to the 1989 edition of *Diet and Health*, the following minimal recommendations relating to carbohydrate-containing food groups were published:

1. Every day, eat five or more servings of a combination of vegetables and fruits, especially green and yellow vegetables and citrus fruits. (One serving equals 1/2 cup cooked or 1 cup raw.)
2. Increase intake of starches and other complex carbohydrates by eating six or more daily servings of a combination of breads, cereals, and legumes. (One serving equals one slice of bread or 1/2 cup cooked cereal, grain, or pasta.)

If individuals consume the recommended number of servings of fruits, vegetables, and starches, they will most likely be taking in the recommended amount of dietary fiber. Additionally, if individuals follow the Food Pyramid guide, the total carbohydrate intake should approximate 50 percent of kilocalories with no more than 10 percent of kilocalories from sugar.

Summary

Carbohydrates are divided into groups: sugars and starches. All carbohydrates are composed of one or more units of $C_6H_{12}O_6$ singly or joined together. The average American's intake of sugars is considered excessive, while the intake of starches is considered low. Many Americans would also benefit by increasing their fiber intake with the consumption of more starches, fruits, and vegetables. The use of whole-grain starches should be encouraged. Dietary carbohydrates promote tooth decay in susceptible individuals. The ADA Exchange Lists that contain carbohydrates are the starch, vegetable, fruit, and milk lists.

Adverse consequences follow inadequate carbohydrate consumption. The human body must have a continuous source of glucose for proper central nervous system function, but its glycogen stores are limited. Therefore, when there is no carbohydrate in the diet and the body uses protein or fat for a fuel source, the body in effect cannibalizes itself for glucose. Muscle and organ mass are lost in the process. A minimum of 50 to 100 grams of carbohydrate a day is usually adequate to prevent these consequences.

Case Study 3–1   The nurse was in Ms. D's room when her tray and menu for the following day arrived. Ms. D, a 22-year-old, 5-ft 6-in, 142-lb client, was having some trouble manipulating her pencil because she had a cast on her right arm. Ms. D was on a general diet, and the nurse offered to assist her in marking her menu. As the nurse read the menu, Ms. D indicated her selections. The client selected eggs and bacon for breakfast, a double order of chicken for lunch, and a double order of roast beef for dinner. Ms. D refused all milk, fruit, vegetables, and starches. When the nurse questioned Ms. D as to why she refused these items, she stated, "I am following a high-protein diet to lose weight." Upon

further questioning, the nurse learned that the client has been following this diet for about 2 weeks. In addition, laboratory analysis of her urine was positive for ketones.

Applying the principles learned in the nursing process, a nurse might construct a nursing care plan similar to the one illustrated below. Remember, however, that real clients may have more complex needs and problems and that other nurses may devise other equally valid and effective interventions.

NURSING CARE PLAN FOR MS. D

Assessment

Subjective Data	Refuses foods containing CHO
Objective Data	Ketone bodies in urine
	Height 5 ft, 6 in
	Weight 142 lb

Nursing Diagnosis Nutrition, altered: Less than body requirements for CHO, related to knowledge deficit as evidenced by refusal to select CHO-containing foods on menu and urine positive for ketones.

Desired Outcome/ Evaluation Criteria	Nursing Actions	Rationale
Client will state at least one reason why she needs CHO by midnight tonight (date).	Encourage client to consume milk, vegetables, fruits, and starches. Refer to dietitian for instruction on normal nutrition and possible appropriate weight reduction strategies.	Explaining the reason carbohydrates are necessary in the diet may motivate the client to eat carbohydrates. Milk, vegetables, fruits, and starches are all good sources of carbohydrates. The nurse may need to educate the client about dietary sources of carbohydrates.
Client will select at least 100 g of CHO on menu each day beginning tomorrow (date).	Assist with daily menu selections.	The minimum daily recommended intake to prevent ketosis is 50 to 100 g of carbohydrates. Helping the client fill out his or her menu is a good method to determine if the client understands the dietary sources of carbohydrates.
Client will consume at least 100 g of CHO each day beginning the day after tomorrow (date).	Document food intake (may be called a calorie count).	Directly observing a client's food intake and documenting the observations made are necessary to evaluate if the approach taken by nursing was successful.

Study Aids

Chapter Review

1. The following are all monosaccharides except:
   a. Glucose
   b. Lactose
   c. Fructose
   d. Galactose

2. _____ is (are) the body's carbohydrate stores.
   a. Polymers
   b. Glycogen
   c. Soluble fiber
   d. Ketones

3. Eight grams of simple carbohydrate is equal to _____ teaspoon(s) of sugar.
   a. 1
   b. 2
   c. 3
   d. 8

4. One cup of milk contains approximately _____ grams of carbohydrates:
   a. 5
   b. 8
   c. 10
   d. 12

5. The following practice is the most likely to promote cavity formation:
   a. Eating apples between meals
   b. Skipping meals
   c. Slowly sipping a soft drink continually throughout the day
   d. Eating a piece of cake as part of a meal

Clinical Analysis

1. Mrs. D is trying to lose weight and complains of hunger. She asks the nurse to recommend fruit exchanges that "have a large volume." Which of the following would you recommend?
   a. Orange juice
   b. Prunes
   c. Strawberries
   d. Raisins

2. Ms. B takes Dolores, who is 18 months old, to the clinic for a routine checkup. The nurse notices that Dolores has rampant dental caries. This can usually be attributed to:
   a. Feeding the child only liquids and not enough solids
   b. Feeding the child all solids and not enough liquids
   c. The occasional ingestion of candy
   d. Dolores's caretaker putting her to bed for a nap or a night's sleep with a bottle of milk or juice

3. Mr. P has a high-fiber diet order. The nurse should encourage the intake of:
   a. Milk, yogurt, and ice cream
   b. Eggs, cheese, and chicken
   c. Fruits, vegetables, and starches
   d. Margarine, salad dressings, and oils

Bibliography

American Dietetic and Diabetic Associations: Exchange Lists for Meal Planning. The American Dietetic Association, Chicago, 1995.

Gold, PE: Role of glucose in regulating the brain and cognition. Am J Clin Nutr 61(Suppl): 9875–9955, 1995.

National Research Council: Diet and Health. National Academy Press, Washington, DC, 1989.

Pennington, JA and Church, HW: Food Values of Portions Commonly Used, ed 14. Harper & Row, New York, 1985.

Slavin, JL: Health benefits of soy fiber, The soy connection 2:1. United Soybean Board, Chesterfield, MD, 1995.

Subcommittee on the Tenth Edition of the Recommended Dietary Allowances: National Research Council: Recommended Dietary Allowances, ed 10. National Academy Press, Washington, DC, 1989.

Thomas, CL (ed): Tabers Cyclopedic Medical Dictionary, ed 18. FA Davis, Philadelphia, 1997.

United Dairy Industry of Michigan: Tooth decay: Protective effect of certain cheeses. Nutrition Reports 1:3, 1995.

CHAPTER 4

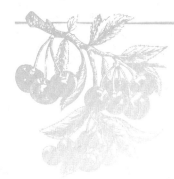

Fats

LEARNING OBJECTIVES

After completing this chapter, the student should be able to:

1 Describe the different types of fats and identify food sources for each.
2 Identify how fats are classified and discuss their physical properties.
3 List the major functions of fats both in the diet and in the body.
4 Discuss the relationship of cholesterol, saturated fat, polyunsaturated fat, and monounsaturated fat to health.
5 List three current recommendations of the Food and Nutrition Board of the National Research Council that pertain to fats.
6 Correctly interpret a food label for a margarine or salad dressing.

The descriptive name for fats of all kinds is **lipids.** You will see the term lipid used in client's medical records. The group of lipids includes true fats and oils, and related fat-like compounds such as **lipoids** and **sterols.** Fats and oils are present in the body and also found in foods. Fats are typically thought of as solids, while oils are regarded as liquids. For example, your body produces oil adjacent to your hair. Not as readily apparent to some people is the layer of fat beneath the skin, which is solid. At room temperature, dietary fats such as lard and butter are solid, whereas corn and olive oils are liquid.

Lipids exhibit the physical property of insolubility in water, and are greasy to the touch. When two insoluble substances are mixed together, they separate readily, the classic example being that of vinegar and oil. You can shake the vinegar and oil combination repeatedly, and it will still separate after the agitation stops.

Composition

Lipids are composed of the elements carbon, hydrogen, and oxygen. These are the same three elements that make up carbohydrates, but the proportion of oxygen to carbon and hydrogen is lower in fats. The implications of this will be discussed later in the chapter. The basic structural unit of a true fat is one molecule of **glycerol** joined to one, two, or three fatty acid molecules. Glycerol is thus the backbone of a fat molecule.

A **fatty acid** is composed of a chain of carbon atoms with hydrogen and a few oxygen atoms attached. The fatty acid chains joined to the glycerol molecule vary in length (depending on the number of carbon atoms present) and composition. The different taste, smell, and physical appearance of each fat results from the variety of fatty acids and their physical arrangement in the fat molecules. Beef tastes, smells, and looks different from chicken because of the difference in fatty acid composition. All fats contain fatty acids.

Number of Fatty Acids

A fat can have from one to three fatty aids. As you will see, the number of fatty acids a fat contains has important implications for both diet and health.

Monoglycerides and Diglycerides

When a single fatty acid is joined to a glycerol molecule, the resulting fat is called a **monoglyc-** eride. When two fatty acids are joined to a glycerol molecule, the fat is called a **diglyceride.** The terms monoglyceride and diglyceride are commonly seen on food labels.

Triglycerides

When three fatty acids are joined to a glycerol molecule, a **triglyceride** is formed. Most of the fat found in our diets and in the body is in the form of triglycerides. Excess triglycerides are stored in the specialized adipose cells that make up **adipose tissue.** The human body has a virtually unlimited capacity to store fat. Figure 4–1 illustrates the structure of monoglycerides, diglycerides, and triglycerides.

Length of Fatty Acid Chain

Fatty acids vary in the length of their fatty acid chains. The length of each fatty acid chain is determined by the number of carbon atoms present and can vary from 2 to 24 carbons. The length of the fatty acid chain determines how the body transports the fat in the body, since fatty acid chains of short length (<6 carbon atoms) and medium length (8 to 12 carbon atoms) are processed differently than fats with longer chains. This has implications for diet in many diseases.

Degree of Saturation

The terms saturated, unsaturated, monounsaturated, and polyunsaturated have become household words. Consumers and clients ask sophisticated questions about fats and turn to all health care professionals to define and explain the terminology. Technically, all of these terms refer to the chemical structure of fatty acids, based on the degree of hydrogen atom saturation.

The degree of saturation of a fatty acid depends on the extent to which hydrogen is joined to the carbon atoms that are present. A saturated fatty acid is filled with as many hydrogen atoms as the carbon atoms can bond with, and has no double bonds between carbons. In this case, a **double bond** describes the type of chemical connection between two neighboring carbon atoms, each lacking one hydrogen atom. In an unsaturated fatty acid, the carbon atoms are joined together by one or more of such double bonds.

Wherever a double bond occurs, another hydrogen atom could potentially "join" the chain. In other words, the fatty acid chain is lacking hydrogen

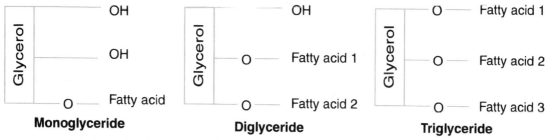

FIGURE 4–1 Monoglycerides, diglycerides, and triglycerides. A monoglyceride has one fatty acid attached to the glycerol molecule, a diglyceride has two fatty acids attached to the glycerol molecule, and a triglyceride has three fatty acids attached to the glycerol molecule.

atoms and is thus less saturated than a chain that is completely filled. A fatty acid with only one carbon-to-carbon double bond is monounsaturated. A fatty acid with more than one carbon-to-carbon bond is polyunsaturated. See Figure 4–2 for a structural comparison of saturated, monounsaturated, and polyunsaturated fatty acids.

In addition to the fats in the body, the fats found in foods are combinations of saturated and unsaturated fatty acids. They are designated as follows:

Saturated fat: Composed mostly of saturated fatty acids

Unsaturated fat: Composed mostly of unsaturated fatty acids

Monounsaturated fat: Composed mostly of monounsaturated fatty acids

Polyunsaturated fat: Composed mostly of polyunsaturated fatty acids

Physical Properties and Food Sources

Saturated Fats

Saturated fats are likely to be solid at room temperature and usually occur in products of animal origin such as meat, poultry, and whole milk. The exceptions are the tropical coconut and palm-kernel oils, and cocoa butter, which are of vegetable origin. See Tables 4–1 and 4–2 for a more complete list of foods containing saturated fat. Saturated fats become rancid very slowly because the chemical bond between carbon and hydrogen is very stable. A **rancid** fat has an offensive odor and taste caused by the partial chemical breakdown of the fat's molecular structure. Products made with saturated fats have a long **shelf life** because the fat in the product is stable. Saturated fats have been targeted for reduction in the av-

erage American's diet by the Committee on Diet and Health of the National Research Council.

Unsaturated Fats

Unsaturated fats are likely to be liquid at room temperature, to be of plant origin, and to become rancid more quickly than saturated fats. The double carbon bonds in unsaturated fatty acids are very unstable and therefore easily broken. For this reason, many convenience products have been made with saturated fats to lengthen their shelf life. The food industry is slowly changing this practice; increasingly, more convenience products are being made with unsaturated fats. Examples of unsaturated fats are corn, cottonseed, safflower, soybean, and sunflower oils. See Table 4–3 for a more complete list of unsaturated fats.

Hydrogenation

Commercial food processing frequently involves taking a fat of vegetable origin (unsaturated) and

---

Lipid—Any one of a group of fats or fat-like substances that are insoluble in water; includes true fats (fatty acids and glycerol), lipoids, and sterols.

Glycerol—The backbone of a fat molecule.

Fatty acid—Part of the structure of a true fat.

Triglyceride—Three fatty acids joined to a glycerol molecule.

Adipose tissue—Aggregation of fat cells; technical name for fat tissue.

Double bond—A type of chemical connection in which a fatty acid has only two neighboring carbon atoms, each lacking one hydrogen atom.

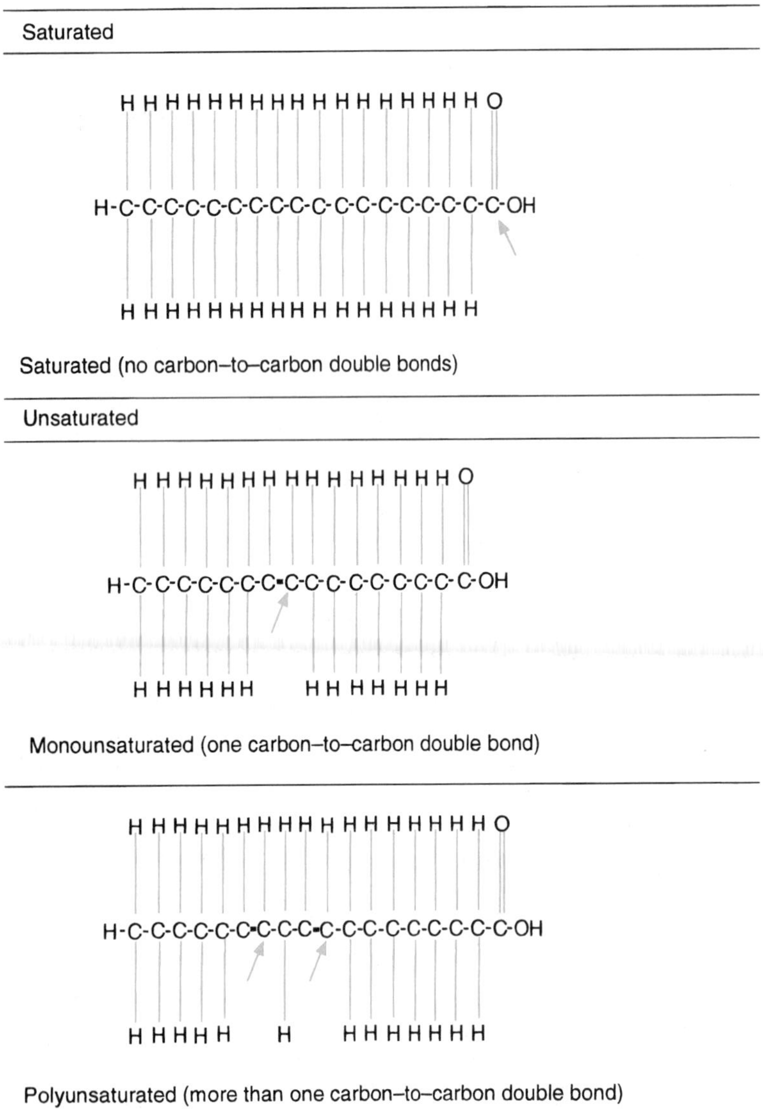

Saturated

H H H H H H H H H H H H H H H H H O
| | | | | | | | | | | | | | | | | ‖
H·C·C·C·C·C·C·C·C·C·C·C·C·C·C·C·C·C·OH
| | | | | | | | | | | | | | | | |
H H H H H H H H H H H H H H H H H

Saturated (no carbon–to–carbon double bonds)

Unsaturated

H H H H H H H H H H H H H H H O
| | | | | | | | | | | | | | | ‖
H·C·C·C·C·C·C·C·C•C·C·C·C·C·C·C·C·OH
| | | | | | | | | | | | | | | |
H H H H H H   H H H H H H

Monounsaturated (one carbon–to–carbon double bond)

H H H H H H H H H H H H H H H H H O
| | | | | | | | | | | | | | | | | ‖
H·C·C·C·C·C·C•C·C·C•C·C·C·C·C·C·C·C·OH
| | | | | | | | | | | |
H H H H H   H   H H H H H H

Polyunsaturated (more than one carbon–to–carbon double bond)

FIGURE 4–2 Saturated, monounsaturated, and polyunsaturated fatty acids. A saturated fatty acid has no carbon-to-carbon double bonds. A monounsaturated fatty acid has one carbon-to-carbon double bond. A polyunsaturated fatty acid has more than one carbon-to-carbon double bond.

TABLE 4–1   Food Sources of Saturated Fats

Meat products	Visible fat and marbling in beef, pork, and lamb, especially in prime-grade and ground meats, lard, suet, salt pork
Processed meats	Frankfurters
	Luncheon meats such as bologna, corned beef, liverwurst, pastrami, and salami
	Bacon and sausage
Poultry and fowl	Chicken and turkey (mostly beneath the skin), cornish hens, duck, and goose
Whole milk and whole-milk products	Cheeses made with whole milk or cream, condensed milk, ice cream, whole-milk yogurt, all creams (sour, half-and-half, whipped)
Plant products	Coconut oil, palm-kernel oil, cocoa butter
Miscellaneous	Fully hydrogenated shortening and margarine, many cakes, pies, cookies, and mixes

TABLE 4–2   Selected Foods High in Cholesterol and/or Saturated Fat

Foods	Amount	Cholesterol (mg)	Saturated Fat (mg)
Liver	3 oz	410	2.4
Cream puff	1	228	10.0
Baked custard	1 cup	213	7.0
Egg, hard cooked	1	215	5.0
Waffles, homemade	2	204	8.0
Coconut custard pie	1 pce	183	8.0
Cheesecake	3.25 oz	170	10.0
Shrimp, boiled	6 lg	167	0.2
Eggnog, commercial	1 cup	149	11.0
Bread pudding/raisins	1 cup	142	4.5
Whole milk	1 cup	124	5.0
Ground beef, 21 percent fat	3 oz, cooked	76	7.0

TABLE 4–3   Food Sources of Unsaturated Fats

Foods High in Monounsaturated Fatty Acids	Foods High in Polyunsaturated Fatty Acids
Canola, olive, peanut oils	Corn, cottonseed, mustard seed, safflower, sesame, soybean, and sunflower seed oils
Almonds, avocados, cashews, filberts, olives, and peanuts	Halibut, herring, mackerel, salmon, sardines, fresh tuna, trout, whitefish

adding hydrogen to either extend the fat's shelf life or make the fat harder. This process of adding hydrogen to a fat is called **hydrogenation.** If only some of the fat's double bonds have been broken by hydrogenation, the product becomes "partially hydrogenated." If all of the double bonds are broken, the product becomes "completely hydrogenated." Completely hydrogenated fats are highly saturated fats. That is, they have no carbon-to-carbon double bonds. For example, a completely hydrogenated corn oil is closer to lard in saturation than a partially hydrogenated corn oil. All vegetable spreads, such as corn oil margarine, have been hydrogenated to some extent. If these spreads had not been hydrogenated, they would be liquids (except for the saturated tropical oils). Clients are usually advised to avoid products that contain completely hydrogenated fats when the therapeutic goal is to decrease saturated fat intake.

Classification

Lipids can be classified according to three criteria: whether the fat is emulsified or nonemulsified, whether the fat is visible or invisible, and/or whether the fat is simple or compound.

Emulsified or Nonemulsified Fats

Fats can be classified as emulsified or nonemulsified. The term **emulsion** is applied to a liquid dispersed in another liquid with which it does not usually mix. The body emulsifies dietary fat so that it can be transported throughout the body by the blood, which is water-based. Emulsification takes place in the small intestine through the action of bile salts during the digestive process.

Visible or Invisible Fats

Dietary fat can be classified as either **visible fat** or **invisible fat** according to whether it can or cannot

---

Shelf life—The time a product can remain in storage without deterioration.

Hydrogenation—The process of adding hydrogen to a fat to make it more highly saturated.

Visible fat—Dietary fat that can be easily seen, such as the fat on meat or in oil.

Invisible fat—Dietary fats that cannot be seen easily; hidden fats in foods such as baked goods, peanut butter, emulsified milk, and so forth.

be seen. About 40 percent of dietary fat is ingested as visible fat. This 40 percent includes vegetable oils, butter, margarine, lard, mayonnaise, salad dressings, visible fat on meats, and shortening. If a person is trying to decrease the fat content of his or her diet, it is prudent to eliminate visible fats first. Invisible fats cannot be identified as readily. These fats are present in grains, egg yolks, poultry, emulsified milk and milk products, the marbling in meat, and many baked goods and snacks. Invisible fat accounts for the remaining 60 percent of fat in the American diet. Even if clients eliminate all visible forms of fat from their diet, large amounts of invisible fat may be present. Clients should be taught to identify the invisible forms of fat.

Simple or Compound Fats

Fats are also classified as simple or compound. **Simple fats** are lipids that have only fatty acids or a hydroxyl molecule joined to glycerol. Think of the hydroxyl molecule as being just a simple chemical "filler." Monoglycerides, diglycerides, and triglycerides are all simple fats.

When one of the fatty acid chains joined to the glycerol molecule is replaced by a protein, the result is a **compound fat.** This structure is then called a **lipoprotein.** Lipoproteins are composed of fat, protein, and fat-related components. They transport fat in the blood stream. The human body makes four types of lipoproteins: chylomicrons, very low-density lipoproteins (VLDL); low-density lipoproteins (LDL), and high-density lipoproteins (HDL). As is evident by their names, the lipoproteins vary in density. The higher the protein content of the lipoprotein, the greater the density. Lipoproteins also vary in the proportional amounts of fat and protein each contains. The type and amount of lipoproteins in a person's blood can protect them from, or predispose them to, heart disease. This is discussed further in the chapter on cardiovascular disease.

Functions of Fats

Lipids are important in the diet and serve many functions in the human body. Fats in food serve as a fuel source, carry the essential fatty acids, act as a vehicle for fat-soluble vitamins, and help add satiety to the diet. Fats in the body supply fuel to most tissues, function as an energy reserve, insulate the body, support and protect vital organs, lubricate body tissues, insulate nerve fibers, and form an integral part of cell membranes.

Fats in Food

Fuel Source

Fats are the major dietary source of fuel. Because fats have proportionately more carbon and hydrogen and less oxygen than carbohydrates, they have a greater potential for the release of energy. In practical terms, this means that fats are a concentrated source of fuel or kilocalories. Fats furnish more than twice the kilocalories, gram for gram, as carbohydrates. Each gram of fat yields 9 kilocalories, so 1 teaspoon of fat, which is equivalent to 5 grams of fat, will yield 45 kilocalories. Compare this with carbohydrates, each gram of which yields only 4 kilocalories. A teaspoon of sugar contains 4 grams of carbohydrate and will therefore yield only 16 kilocalories.

Vehicle for Fat-Soluble Vitamins

In foods, fats act as a vehicle for vitamins A, D, E, and K. In the body, fats assist in the absorption of these fat-soluble vitamins.

Satiety Value

Fats also contribute flavor, **satiety,** and palatability to the diet. They supply texture to food, trap and intensify its flavor, and enhance its odor. Consider for a moment the different sensations felt when eating 2 cups of ice cream versus eating six apples.

Sources of Essential Fatty Acids

An essential nutrient must be supplied by the diet because the body cannot manufacture it. Fat contains the essential fatty acid **linoleic acid.** Linoleic acid strengthens cell membranes and has a major role in the transport and metabolism of cholesterol. Two necessary fatty acids, gamma-linolenic (γ-linolenic) acid and arachidonic acid, can be synthesized by the body from linoleic acid. These fatty acids taken together prolong blood clotting time, hasten fibrolytic activity, and are involved in the development of the brain. **Prostaglandins,** compounds with extensive hormone-like actions, require arachidonic acid for synthesis. A group of fatty acids such as alpha-linolenic (α-linolenic) is now considered essential.

A deficiency of linoleic acid can occur in infants and hospitalized clients under certain conditions.

Linoleic acid deficiency was first observed in infants fed formulas deficient in linoleic acid. Drying and flaking of the skin has been observed (Wiese, Hansen, and Adam, 1958). This deficiency was again observed in the early 1970s in hospitalized clients fed exclusively with intravenous fluids containing no fat. The symptoms included scaly skin, hair loss, and impaired wound healing. Linoleic acid deficiency is still seen occasionally with artificial feeding.

Fats in the Body

Fuel Supply

Fat serves as fuel to supply needed energy for all tissues except in the central nervous system. Glucose is the preferred energy form of the brain.

Fuel Reserve

Fat also functions as the body's main fuel or energy reserve. Excess kilocalories consumed are stored in specialized cells called **adipose cells.** When an individual does not eat enough food to meet the energy demands of the body, the adipose cells release fat for fuel.

Organ Protection

Fatty tissue cushions and protects vital organs by providing a supportive fat pad that absorbs mechanical shocks. Examples of organs supported by fat are the eyes and kidneys.

Lubrication

Fats also lubricate body tissue. The human body manufactures oil in structures called **sebaceous glands.** Secretions from the sebaceous glands lubricate the skin to retard loss of body water to the outside environment.

Insulation

The subcutaneous layer of fat beneath the skin helps to insulate the body by protecting it from excessive heat or cold. A sheath of fatty tissue surrounding nerve fibers provides insulation to help transmit nerve impulses.

Cell Membrane Structure

Fat serves as an integral part of cell membranes, helps transport nutrient materials and metabolites, and provides a barrier against water-soluble substances.

Cholesterol

Cholesterol is not a true fat, but belongs to a group called **sterols.** Cholesterol is a component of many of the foods in our diet. In addition, the human body manufactures about 1000 milligrams of cholesterol a day, mainly in the liver. The liver also filters out excess cholesterol and helps to eliminate it from the body.

Functions

Cholesterol has several important functions: It is a component of bile salts that aid digestion; it is an essential component of all cell membranes; it is found in brain and nerve tissue and in the blood. Cholesterol is necessary for the production of several hormones, including cortisone, adrenalin, estrogen, and testosterone. A **hormone** is a substance produced by the endocrine glands and secreted directly into the bloodstream. Hormones stimulate functional activity or the secretion of another hormone in various organs and cells.

Blood Cholesterol Levels

An elevated level of cholesterol in the blood is a major risk factor for coronary artery disease. Lowering blood cholesterol levels reduces the risk of heart attacks due to coronary disease. Individuals with cholesterol levels between 200 and 239 milligrams per deciliter have a borderline to high risk. A cholesterol level in excess of 240 milligrams per deciliter places the individual in the high-risk category. The consumption of cholesterol is considered to be less

---

Lipoprotein—A fat and protein complex in which one of the fatty acids joined to the glycerol molecule is replaced by a protein; may combine with cholesterol, phospholipids, and triglycerides.

Satiety—The feeling of satisfaction after eating.

Linoleic acid—An essential fatty acid.

Prostaglandins—Long-chain, unsaturated fatty acids mostly synthesized in the body from arachidonic acid; have hormone-like effects.

Cholesterol—A fat-like substance made in the human body and found in foods of animal origin

of a risk factor for coronary heart disease than the consumption of saturated fats (National Research Council, 1989a).

Food Sources

Cholesterol is present in the foods we eat. In fact, many of the products sold in supermarkets are targeted to shoppers interested in controlling their blood cholesterol level through diet. Cholesterol occurs naturally in all animal foods and is produced only in liver tissue. When we ingest animal products, we also ingest the cholesterol the animal made. For this reason, The American Heart Association recommends that a healthy woman eat no more than 6 ounces of lean meat per day and a healthy man no more than 7 ounces of lean meat per day.

Table 4–2 lists selected foods high in cholesterol. Note that one egg supplies about 215 milligrams of cholesterol. Eggs are the major contributor of cholesterol in the average American's diet. The American Heart Association recommends that consumers limit their intake of egg yolks to no more than four per week.

Fats in the American Diet

Fat available in the food supply increased from an average of 124 grams per day per person in 1909 to 172 grams per day per person in 1985. There are approximately 5 grams of fat in a teaspoon; therefore, 124 grams converts to 25 teaspoons of fat and 172 grams to 34 1/2 teaspoons. Thus, as of 1985, Americans were eating about 9 1/2 more teaspoons of fat per day than they did in 1909. The relative proportion of fat from saturated versus polyunsaturated sources has also changed. The intake of animal fat from red meat has declined while that of vegetable fat has risen. Americans are also consuming less whole milk and more low-fat milk. Notwithstanding, fat intake in the American diet is still considered excessive. Recent estimates indicate that Americans derive approximately 37 percent of their total caloric intake from fat, whereas most experts agree that less than 30 percent of total caloric intake should be derived from fat.

Calculating the amount of fat as a percentage of total kilocalories is a convenient way of evaluating the level of fat in a food item. Clinical Calculation 4–1 demonstrates how to calculate the percent of kilocalories from fat in a food item. If a food item contains more than 30 percent fat, it should be balanced with other items that contain less fat, such as

---

CLINICAL CALCULATION 4–1

Percent of Kilocalories from Fat

The following formula can be used to determine the percentage of kilocalories from fat in many packaged foods:

$$\frac{\text{Kilocalories from fat per serving}}{\text{*Kilocalories per serving}} \times 100 = \text{percent kilocalories from fat}$$

Example: kilocalories from fat = 30
kilocalories per serving = 90

$$\frac{30}{90} = 0.33 \times 100 = 33 \text{ percent kilocalories from fat}$$

*Food labeling regulations require manufacturers to list both the number of kilocalories in a serving and the number of kilocalories from fat.

---

fruits and vegetables. What is important is "balance." The main objective is to reduce overall fat intake.

Dietary Recommendations Concerning Fat

There is no RDA for fat. The Food and Nutrition Board's Committee on Diet and Health recommends that the fat content of the US diet not exceed 30 percent of kilocaloric intake. They also recommend that less than 10 percent of kilocalories should be provided from saturated fatty acids and that dietary cholesterol should be less than 300 milligrams per day. Some fat is needed to provide linoleic acid, an essential fatty acid. The Food and Nutrition Board of the National Research Council recommends a minimum adequate intake of linoleic acid as opposed to a set amount. The minimum adequate amount of linoleic acid is 1 to 2 percent of total dietary kilocalories. The healthy adult can obtain this amount from about 1 teaspoon of oil per day. For infants consuming 100 kilocalories per kilogram, this would correspond to a daily intake of 0.2 grams per kilogram of body weight.

Fat Intake and Health

Dietary Fat

Excess dietary fat has been associated with an increased risk of cardiovascular disease, the develop-

TABLE 4–4 Recommended Maximum Fat Intake at Selected Kilocalorie Levels

Kilocalorie Level	Total Fat (g)
1200	40
1500	50
1600	53
1800	60
2000	67
2200	73
2400	80
2500	83

ment of obesity, and an increased risk of certain cancers, especially cancers of the colon and prostate. Although it is difficult to predict exactly which conditions will lead to a disease in a particular individual, scientists have been able to develop a list of factors closely associated with particular diseases in large population groups. These factors are called risks. Saturated fat increases the risk of coronary heart disease independent of other factors. High dietary cholesterol also contributes to the development of atherosclerosis and increased coronary heart disease risk in the population, but to a lesser extent. Table 4–4 shows the maximum recommended grams of fat an individual should consume at selected kilocaloric levels.

Monounsaturated Fats

Recently, the health benefits of monounsaturated fatty acids have been newsworthy. The Committee on Diet and Health of the National Research Council recommends that the average American increase his or her intake of monounsaturated fats. There is some evidence that individuals with a high intake of monounsaturated fats, a low intake of saturated fats, and a low total fat intake may have a decreased risk of colorectal cancer (National Research Council, 1989b).

Polyunsaturated Fats

The Committee on Diet and Health of the National Research Council does not recommend that the average American increase his or her intake of polyunsaturated fat. At very high levels of polyunsaturated fat intake, animal studies consistently show an increase in colon and mammary cancers. Observations in humans have shown that a polyunsaturated fat intake of less than 10 percent of kilocalories does not increase the population's risk of cancer. Box 4–1 discusses the renewed interest in one type of polyunsaturated fatty acid.

Body Fat

Both the amount of body fat and its location are related to health risk. Many experts feel that the ratio of body fat to total weight is more important than total weight. Healthy ranges for body fat are between 15 and 19 percent for men and between 18 and 22 percent for women. A high percentage of body fat has been associated with increased risk of disease, even when total body weight is normal. The location of excess body fat is also important. Excessive fat on the lower body, specifically on the hips and thighs, appears to be less dangerous than excessive fat on the abdomen and upper body, which is associated

---

BOX 4–1 *CIS* VERSUS *TRANS* DOUBLE BOND CONFIGURATION

There is controversy regarding *cis* configuration double bonds and the *trans* configuration double bonds in fatty acids. As illustrated in Figure 4–3, a *cis* configuration double bond between carbon atoms in a fatty acid has a kink or bend. As illustrated in Figure 4–3, a *trans* configuration double bond between carbon atoms in a fatty acid is straighter. There is some evidence that the *trans* configuration is detrimental in that it contributes to an increased risk of cardiovascular disease. If the goal is to decrease consumption of fatty acids with relatively large amounts of *trans* configuration, it is desirable to decrease consumption of hydrogenated foods. Examples of hydrogenated foods include margarine and many commercially processed foods such as some cake mixes and frozen items. Another way to decrease intake of the *trans* configuration of fatty acids is to substitute monounsaturated fat for hydrogenated margarine. Figure 4–4 shows how olive oil can be substituted for margarine and served with bread.

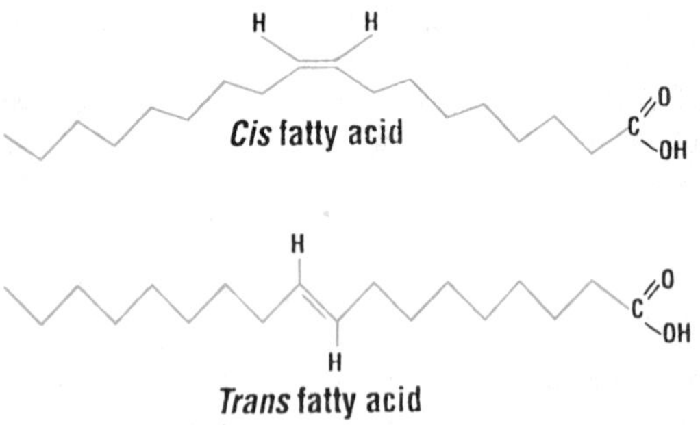

Cis fatty acid

Trans fatty acid

FIGURE 4–3   A *cis* fatty acid and a *trans* fatty acid. Whenever there is a change from *cis* to *trans* configuration in a fatty acid, the three-dimensional shape of the molecule is altered.

with a much higher risk of diseases such as cancer, heart disease, and diabetes. The exchange lists in the next section can be used to assist in planning meals low in fat.

Exchange Lists

Exchange categories that include fat are the milk, meat, and fat lists. The amount of fat in one exchange of meat or milk varies within the list. Some foods not listed on the exchange lists are also high in fat. Many of these foods may be found in the Nutritive Values of Edible Parts of Food tables (see Appendix B).

Milk Exchange List

The fat content of milk varies according to the type of milk consumed. Table 4–5 shows the grams of fat and percent of kilocalories from fat in one milk exchange for each kind of milk. Whole milk and 2 percent milk contain saturated fat and cholesterol. The protein, carbohydrate, vitamin, and mineral content of whole, 2 percent, and skim milk are comparable. Skim milk is thus a nutritional bargain.

Meat Exchange List

The meat exchange list is divided into four subgroups: one very lean meat exchange contains less than 1 gram of fat; one lean meat exchange contains 3 grams of fat; one medium-fat meat exchange contains 5 grams of fat; and one high-fat meat exchange contains 8 grams of fat. Table 4–6 lists selected food examples from each of these meat exchanges.

Many patients have misconceptions about meat. Some patients avoid all red meat because they believe that all red meat contains excessive fat. Many beef and pork products are not excessively high in fat. Figure 4–5 compares prized 1940s hogs with 1990s hogs, and Figure 4–6 compares 1940s steers with 1990s steers. In both figures, note how much leaner the 1990s animals appear than the 1940s animals. Many consumers are not aware of the lean cuts of beef or pork. Conversely, not all fish and poultry items are lean meat exchanges.

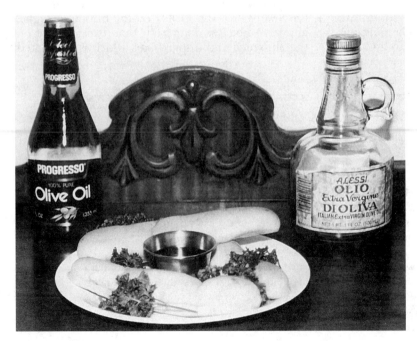

FIGURE 4–4   Many restaurants serve olive oil instead of butter and margarine with bread. Olive oil is a monounsaturated fat and contains insignificant trans fatty acids.

TABLE 4–5 Grams of Fat in One Milk Exchange

Type	Fat (g)	Percent Kilocalories From Fat
Whole milk	8	48
2 percent (low fat)	5	38
Skim milk	Trace	<1

Different methods of food preparation can greatly influence the fat content of these foods. Some clients have the misconception that if they eat only lean meats, they can eat as much as they like. This is not true because all meat contains fat. The total amount of meat any healthy individual should eat each day is between 6 and 7 ounces.

Meat exchanges are usually one ounce, but an average portion is three ounces. Table 4–7 totals the fat content of three meat exchanges. Typically, meats such as prime rib are eaten in large amounts (from 6-ounce to 16-ounce servings). Teaching a client meat portion sizes is usually indicated when the goal is to decrease a client's fat intake.

Whether the meat is classified as a very lean, lean, medium-fat, or high-fat meat exchange, the grams of fat in each exchange are calculated based on the following assumptions:

- Visible fat on meat is not consumed.
- Meat is weighed after cooking.
- Meat is baked, boiled, broiled, grilled, or roasted (unless indicated otherwise).

Since 1994 food labeling regulations have become more comprehensive. Regarding the fat content of meat, poultry, seafood, and game meats, two terms now have legal definitions: "lean" and "extra lean." The term "lean" can be used on meat, poultry, seafood, or game meat product only if the product contains less than 10 grams of fat, less than 4 grams of saturated fat, and less than 95 milligrams of cholesterol per 100-gram serving (3 1/2 ounces). The legal term "lean" will thus equal the ADA exchange list definition for a lean meat exchange. The term *extra lean* can be used only if the product contains less than 5 grams of fat, less than 2 grams of saturated fat, and less than 95 milligrams of cholesterol per serving and per 100 grams (3 1/2 ounces) (US Food and Drug Administration, 1992).

Fat Exchange List

Each fat exchange provides 5 grams of fat. Figure 4–7 illustrates three fat exchanges. The fat list is sub-

TABLE 4–6 Examples of Very Lean, Lean, Medium-Fat, and High-Fat Meat Exchanges

Each of the Following is 1 Very Lean Meat Exchange and Contains Less Than 1 g of Fat:		
Poultry:	Chicken or turkey (white meat, no skin)	1 oz
Fish:	Fresh or frozen cod, flounder, haddock	1 oz
Game:	Venison	1 oz
Cheese:	Nonfat cottage cheese	1/4 cup
	Fat-free cheese	1 oz
Other:	Egg whites	2
	Hot dogs with less than 1 g of fat	1 oz
	Egg substitute	1/4 cup

Each of the Following is 1 Lean Meat Exchange and Contains 3 g of Fat:		
Beef:	Round, sirloin, or flank steak	1 oz
Fish:	Salmon (fresh or frozen)	1 oz
Pork:	Tenderloin	1 oz
Veal:	Lean chop or roast	1 oz
Poultry:	Chicken, dark meat, no skin	1 oz
Game:	Goose, no skin	1 oz
Cheese:	4.5 percent fat cottage cheese	1/4 cup
	Cheeses with less than 3 g of fat per oz	1 oz
Other:	Hot dogs with less than 3 g of fat per oz	1 oz
	Processed lunch meat with less than 3 g of fat per oz	1 oz

Each of the Following is 1 Medium-Fat Meat Exchange and Contains 5 g of Fat:		
Beef:	Ground beef, corned beef	1 oz
Pork:	Chops	1 oz
Poultry:	Chicken, dark meat, with skin	1 oz
Fish:	Any fried fish product	1 oz
Cheese:	Mozzarella	1 oz
Other:	Egg (high in cholesterol)	1
	Tofu	1/2 cup

Each of the Following is 1 High-Fat Meat Exchange and Contains 8 g of Fat:		
Pork:	Spareribs, pork sausage	1 oz
Cheese:	All regular cheeses such as cheddar, Swiss, and American	1 oz
Other:	Bologna	1 oz
	Knockwurst, bratwurst	1 oz
	Bacon	3 slices

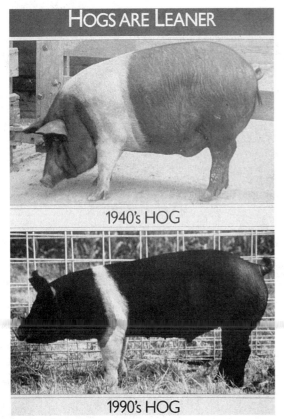

HOGS ARE LEANER

1940's HOG

1990's HOG

FIGURE 4–5 The fat content of hogs has decreased during the last 50 years. Consumers are increasingly demanding leaner red-meat products, and farmers are responding. (From the National Live Stock and Meat Board, 444 North Michigan Ave., Chicago, IL 60611, with permission.)

need not avoid eating out, but they do need to make wise food choices.

Food labeling regulations spell out what terms may be used to describe the level of fat in a food and how they can be used. "Fat-free" on a food label means that the food contains no more than 0.5 grams of fat per serving. Synonyms for "free" include "without," "no," and "zero." These terms can legally be used on a food label only if the product contains no amount of—or only trivial or "physiologically inconsequential" amounts of—fat, saturated fat, and cholesterol.

Low-fat is legally defined as a food that contains no more than 3 grams of fat in a serving. *Low saturated fat* is legally defined as a food that contains no more than 1 gram of saturated fat per serving. *Low cholesterol* is defined as a food that contains less than 20

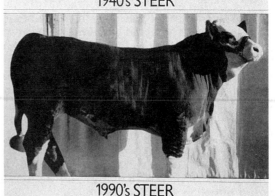

CATTLE ARE LEANER

1940's STEER

1990's STEER

FIGURE 4–6 For beef, the ideal 1940s market animal was short-legged, short and deep in body, and exhibited good evidence of body fat. By the 1980s and 1990s, improved breeding techniques and animal nutrition resulted in a dramatic change in the characteristics of the typical beef animal. Muscle now replaces much of the fat in today's beef animal. (From the National Live Stock and Meat Board, 444 North Michigan Ave., Chicago, IL 60611, with permission.)

divided into two groups: unsaturated fats and saturated fats. Table 4–8 lists selected exchanges from each group.

Additional Food Sources of Fat

Snack foods including crackers, cakes, pies, donuts, and cookies may be high in fat. Often potato chips, gravies, cream sauces, soups, pizza, tacos, and spaghetti are high in fat. Microwave popcorn is higher in fat than air-popped popcorn (without added fat).

A low-fat meal is possible at a fast-food restaurant. However, many of the specialty fast-food hamburgers are high in fat. A small hamburger is the best "burger" choice. A small side salad with low-fat dressing is a better low-fat choice than french fries. Skim milk is lower in fat than either a milk shake or whole milk. Consumers who desire low-fat foods

TABLE 4–7   Total Fat in Three Meat Exchanges

Meat	Subgroup	Grams of Fat/Exchange	Grams of Fat Per Serving
Cod	Very lean	1	3
Sirloin steak	Lean	3	9
Hamburger patty, broiled*	Medium fat	5	15
Spareribs**	High fat	8	24

* About 4 oz raw
** Boneless

milligrams per serving. Synonyms for low include "little," "few," and "low source of." Additionally, serving sizes listed on food labels are standardized to make nutritional comparisons of similar products easier.

Summary

The group name for all fats is lipids. Lipids include true fats and oils and related fat-like compounds such as lipoids and sterols. Lipids are insoluble in water and greasy to the touch.

Hydrogen, oxygen, and carbon are the primary elements in fats. Gram for gram, fats contain more than twice the kilocalories as carbohydrates. All fats contain fatty acids. The number of fatty acids in a fat determines whether it is a monoglyceride, a diglyc-

eride, or a triglyceride. Most fats in foods and in body stores are triglycerides. The length of a fatty acid chain determines how the body transports fat. The degree of hydrogen atom saturation or the presence or absence of carbon-to-carbon double bonds determine whether a fatty acid is saturated or unsaturated.

Fats are labeled according to the amount and type of fatty acids they contain as saturated, unsaturated, monounsaturated, or polyunsaturated. Fats can also be classified as emulsified or nonemulsified, visible or invisible, and simple or compound. Fats serve many important functions in our diets and our bodies.

Americans currently derive about 37 percent of their kilocalories from fat. Many experts feel this is excessive. Excess fats in our diets relate to cardiovascular disease, obesity, and some types of cancer.

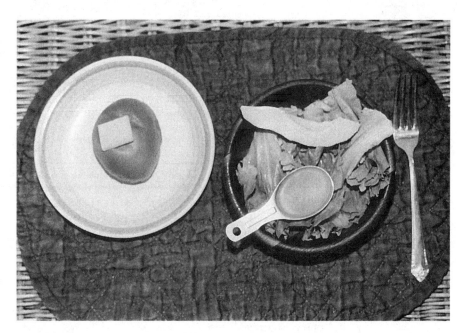

FIGURE 4–7 One tsp of margarine, 1 tsp of regular French dressing, and 1/8 of an avocado are each equal to one fat exchange.

TABLE 4–8   Examples of Monounsaturated, Polyunsaturated, and Saturated Fat Exchanges

Each of the Following is 1 Fat Exchange High in Monounsaturated Fatty Acids and Contains 5 g of Total Fat:	
Olives, stuffed	10 large
Canola oil	1 tsp
Peanut butter	2 tsp
Pecans	4 halves

Each of the Following is 1 Fat Exchange High in Saturated Fatty Acids and Contains 5 g of Total Fat:	
Bacon	1 slice (20 slices/lb)
Butter, stick	1 tsp
Cream cheese, regular	1 tbsp (1/2 oz)
Cream cheese, reduced-fat	2 tbsp (1 oz)
Sour cream, regular	2 tbsp
Sour cream, reduced-fat	3 tbsp

Each of the Following is 1 Fat Exchange High in Polyunsaturated Fatty Acids and Contains 5 g of Total Fat:	
Margarine: stick or tub	1 tsp
Mayo, regular	1 tsp
Corn oil	1 tsp
Pumpkin seeds	1 tbsp
English walnuts	4 halves

Cholesterol is a fat-like substance that is present in food and produced by the human body. Many Americans would benefit from decreasing their cholesterol and saturated fat intake. The ADA exchanges that contain fat are the milk, meat, and fat lists. The current recommendations are that the fat content of the diet should not exceed 30 percent of kilocaloric intake, less than 10 percent of kilocalories should be provided from saturated fats, and dietary cholesterol should be less than 300 milligrams per day.

Case Study 4–1

Mr. D had his cholesterol level analyzed during a routine physical examination. The nurse employed in the office of Mr. D's doctor is responsible for the following:

1. Scheduling the patient for follow-up with the physician
2. Developing a nursing care plan that addresses the patient's nursing problem to complement the medical diagnosis

Mike Rod, the nurse, scheduled the appointment. Mr. D was instructed by the nurse to write down all food he consumed for 1 day prior to the appointment. The client was advised to choose a typical day to record his food intake to provide a more accurate analysis of his usual diet. Mr. D arrived on the appropriate day and handed his food record to the nurse for review. Mike calculated the grams of fat in Mr. D's food record based on a combination of ADA exchanges and a table of food composition similar to the table in the Appendix. Mr. D's food record and Mike's calculations are as follows:

Food	Grams of Fat
11:00 AM Restaurant	
Salad bar:	
Assorted vegetables and lettuce	0
2 tbsp blue cheese dressing	10 (2 fats)
1 oz shredded cheese	8 (1 high-fat meat)
1 oz diced ham	3 (1 lean meat)
1/2 cup potato salad	10*
Dinner roll	0
1 tsp butter	5 (1 fat)
1 cup clam chowder	7*

7:00 PM Restaurant	
4 oz hamburger, ckd. weight	20 (4 medium-fat meats)
1 oz cheese	8 (1 high-fat meat)
1 tbsp mayo	15 (3 fats)
Bun	0
6 onion rings	15*
Tossed salad	0
2 tbsp blue cheese dressing	10 (2 fats)
11:00 PM Home	
1 cup 2 percent milk	5 (1 two-percent milk)
1 orange	0
	116 g of fat

*Values obtained from a table of food composition.

The physician has just seen the client, reviewed Mr. D's food record and Mike's calculations, and determined that the client's elevated cholesterol level is secondary to his dietary habits. Mr. D.'s cholesterol level was 225 mg/dL, he weighed 135 lb, and is 5 ft, 6 in tall. Mr. D stated, "I cannot understand why my cholesterol is elevated. My weight is stable. I always select the salad bar for lunch, avoid sweets, and drink low-fat milk."

NURSING CARE PLAN FOR MR. D

Assessment

Subjective Data	Admitted knowledge deficit
	Food record for 1 day contained 116 grams of fat
Objective Data	Cholesterol level: 225 mg/dL
	Height: 5 ft, 6 in
	Weight: 135 lb

Nursing Diagnosis Nutrition, altered: more than body requirements related to knowledge deficit as evidenced by admitted lack of understanding and a cholesterol level of 225 mg/dL.

Desired Outcome/ Evaluation Criteria	Nursing Actions	Rationale
Cholesterol level of <200 mg/dL in 3 months.	Remind the client to have his serum cholesterol level checked in 6 weeks per standing physician's order.	Individuals with a cholesterol level <200 mg/dL are at a lower risk of cardiovascular disease.

Table continued on following page

Desired Outcome/ Evaluation Criteria	Nursing Actions	Rationale
Client will keep a diary over the next 3 months.	Instruct the client on efficient means of recording. Review food records with him at 6-week intervals.	Keeping food records will remind the client of the importance of decreasing his or her fat intake. Reviewing them with the nurse permits positive reinforcement and correction of misperceptions.
Client will decrease his visible fat intake.	Review visible dietary sources of fat with the client; concentrate on blue cheese dressing, butter, and mayonnaise. Suggest alternatives to using visible fats. Review the diet selected by the physician with the client.	It is prudent to eliminate visible fats first from an individual's diet as they are easily identifiable.
	Tell client to call the nurse if he is having trouble interpreting dietary instructions at home.	Offers the client support between visits.

Study Aids

Chapter Review

1. The body is able to store _____ in unlimited amounts.
   a. Dextrose
   b. Glycogen
   c. Fat
   d. Protein

2. The most common form of fat found in both the body and food is:
   a. Monoglycerides
   b. Diglycerides
   c. Triglycerides
   d. Cholesterol

3. Polyunsaturated fats are:
   a. Solid at room temperature
   b. Unlikely to become rancid
   c. Primarily of animal origin
   d. Composed of many double carbon bonds

4. According to the Committee on Diet and Health, the average American would benefit by increasing his or her intake of which of the following fats?
   a. Corn oil
   b. Olive oil
   c. Safflower oil
   d. Lard

5. One ounce of cheddar cheese contains 9 grams of fat and 115 kilocalories. What percent of kilocalories come from fat?
   a. 9
   b. 18
   c. 40
   d. 70

Clinical Analysis

1. Mrs. S, 50 years old, has a cholesterol level of 233 milligrams per deciliter. She weighs 125 pounds and is 5 feet, 5 inches tall. The dietitian has approximated her body fat content to be 35 percent. When taking a nursing history, the nurse asks Mrs. S if she eats any foods that may be related to her elevated cholesterol level. Which of

the following groups of foods are most related to an elevated cholesterol level?
a. Vegetable oils such as corn, cottonseed, and soybean
b. Fruits and vegetables
c. Starches such as bread, potatoes, rice, and pasta
d. Animal fats such as butter, meats, lard, and bacon

2. Mr. B is a new client whose cholesterol level is 215 milligrams per deciliter. Mr. B's cholesterol level:
a. Places him in the low-risk category
b. Places him in the borderline to high-risk category
c. Places him in the high-risk category
d. Is sufficiently elevated enough for him to be a good candidate for drug therapy

3. When Mrs. L describes her regular intake of foods, you observe that her diet is especially low in monounsaturated fats. Which of the following oils would you recommend be used in place of corn oil?
a. Sunflower seed
b. Soybean
c. Canola
d. Cottonseed

Bibliography

American Dietetic and Diabetic Associations: Exchange Lists for Meal Planning. American Dietetic Association, Chicago, 1995.

American Institute for Cancer Research: Dietary Guidelines to Lower Cancer Risk. American Cancer Society, Washington, DC, 1990.

Consensus Conference: Lowering blood cholesterol to prevent disease. JAMA 253:2080, 1985.

Etherton-Kris, PM and Nicolosi, RJ: Trans Fatty Acids and Coronary Heart Disease Risk. International Life Sciences Institute, Washington, DC, 1995.

Lichtenstein, AH: Trans fatty acids and hydrogenated fat—What do we know? Nutrition Today 30:102, 1995.

National Research Council: Diet and Health. National Academy Press, Washington, DC, 1989.

National Research Council: Recommended Dietary Allowances. National Academy Press, Washington, DC, 1989.

Neuringer, M and Connor, WE: n-3 Fatty acids in the brain and retina: Evidence for their essentiality. Nutr Rev 44:285, 1986.

Report of the Expert Panel on Detection, Evaluation, and Treatment of High Blood Cholesterol in Adults: Cholesterol Education Program. National Heart, Lung, and Blood Institute, National Institutes of Health, Bethesda, 1987.

US Department of Health and Human Services: The Surgeon General's Report on Nutrition and Health. DHHS Publication No. (PHS) 88-55 210, Washington, DC, 1988.

US Food and Drug Administration: Backgrounder. BG 92-4. December 10, 1992.

Wiese, HF, Hansen, AE, and Adam, DJD: Essential fatty acids in infant nutrition. J Nutr 58:345, 1958.

CHAPTER 5

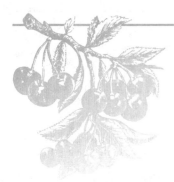

Protein

LEARNING OBJECTIVES

After completing this chapter the student should be able to:

1 Discuss the functions of protein in a healthy and in an ill human body.
2 Explain the difference between complete and incomplete proteins and give examples of food sources of each.
3 Define anabolism and catabolism, and list possible anabolic and catabolic conditions.
4 List the grams of protein in each exchange list containing significant amounts of protein.
5 Calculate the protein allowance for a healthy adult when given the person's healthy body weight.
6 Design a daily meal plan containing adequate protein intake for a healthy adult.

The importance of protein in nutrition and health was first emphasized by an ancient Greek who called this nutrient "proteos," meaning primary, or taking first place. Protein is essential for body growth and maintenance. If kilocaloric need is inadequate to support fuel requirements, dietary protein may be used for energy rather than for tissue growth and maintenance. If protein is eaten in excess it can contribute to body fat stores.

Proteins are the building blocks of blood and bone and all other tissues. Protein is a structural part of every cell. In fact, almost half the dry weight of the cells is protein. It is second only to water in amounts present in the body. A description of some of the tissues composed of protein appears in Clinical Application 5–1.

Composition of Proteins

Proteins are composed of carbon, hydrogen, oxygen, and nitrogen and make up the greater part of plant and animal tissue. Phosphorus, sulfur, iron, and iodine often form part of the protein molecule, but nitrogen is the element that distinguishes proteins from carbohydrates and fats. Proteins are made up of smaller building blocks called amino acids.

Amino Acids

The chemical elements carbon, hydrogen, oxygen, and nitrogen combine in a specific arrangement to form **amino acids.** The amino acids, in turn, are linked in an exact order to make a particular protein. Amino acids are linked together by **peptide bonds.** A chain of two or more amino acids joined together by peptide bonds is called a **polypeptide.** A single protein may consist of a polypeptide of fifty to thousands of amino acids. Scientists have estimated that the body contains up to 50,000 different proteins of which only about 1000 have been identified. Thus, an enormous variety of combinations are possible.

To visualize these combinations, examine Figure 5–1, a schematic representation of the beef insulin molecule. It might also help to think of the elements as the letters of the alphabet and amino acids as words. There are countless ways to make words, or amino acids, from the 26 letters (the elements). Words put into a certain order make up sentences that have a specific and unique meaning. In this comparison, a sentence is a protein. Each protein has a specific and unique sequence of amino acids. To complete the analogy of language to anatomy, see Table 5–1.

Primitive people sometimes drank the blood of an admired animal or brave enemy in the hope of gaining the qualities of that particular creature. In a way we do become what we eat. This is not literally true, of course: We do not turn into a steer or a hog after eating beef or pork. Instead, the animal proteins are disassembled in the digestive process into the component amino acids and then reassembled to form human proteins (see Chapter 10, "Digestion, Absorbtion, Metabolism, and Excretion").

CLINICAL APPLICATION 5–1

Examples of Protein in the Human Body

Most of the cells of the body require periodic maintenance or replacement. Even bone tissue undergoes change in the healthy adult. However, the body cannot repair tooth decay; hence the need for dental fillings.

Scar tissue: The healing of the simplest wound requires proteins. Many blood clotting factors, such as the protein prothrombin, form a blood clot. The fibrin threads that form the mesh to hold the scar tissue in place are composed of protein. The white blood cells which dispose of the waste products of the injury and the healing process are also proteins.

Hair growth: Hair cells are dead. Hence, haircuts do not hurt. The new growth of hair does require protein building blocks, however. One sign of malnutrition is hair that can be easily and painlessly plucked.

Blood albumin: Albumin is a transport protein that carries nutrients or elements to where they are needed. Albumin plays a significant role in medication absorption and metabolism (see Chapter 16). In addition to transporting substances to all the cells of the body, albumin also has functions relating to water balance.

Hemoglobin: Another transport protein, hemoglobin, is the oxygen-carrying part of the red blood cell. The **globin** part of this molecule is a simple protein.

Amino acid—Organic compounds that are the building blocks of protein and products of protein digestion.

Peptide bond—Chemical bond that links two amino acids in a protein molecule.

Polypeptide—Chain of amino acids linked by peptide bonds that form proteins.

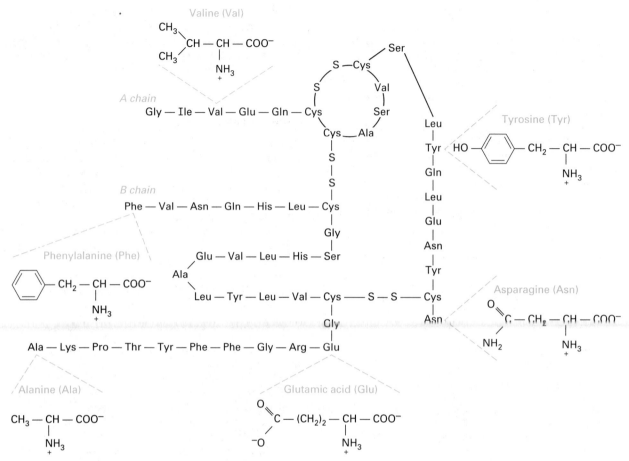

FIGURE 5–1 Beef insulin molecule. The central core represents the amino acids in correct sequence. The six exploded views depict the composition of the individual amino acids. (Adapted from Solomons, TWG: Fundamentals of Organic Chemistry, ed 4. John Wiley & Sons, New York, 1994, and Schumm, DE: Essentials of Biochemistry. FA Davis, Philadelphia, 1988.)

TABLE 5–1   Comparison of Language and Anatomy

Component of Language	Component of Anatomy
Letters	Elements such as carbon, hydrogen, oxygen, nitrogen, sometimes sulfur
Word	Amino acid
Sentence	Protein
Paragraph	Cell
Chapter	Tissue
Book	Organ
Books on a given subject	System
Library	Human body

Precision is necessary to manufacture proteins. A slight error in the construction of a protein, such as occurs in sickle-cell disease, can have severe consequences. Sickle-cell disease is detailed in Clinical Application 5–2.

Twenty-four amino acids have been identified as being important in the body's metabolism. These amino acids are classified as either essential or nonessential.

Essential Amino Acids

As with other nutrients, the body's inability to construct an amino acid is the basis for classifying an amino acid as essential. Histidine has more recently been added to the list of **essential amino acids** for both children and adults.

Sickle-Cell Disease

Normal hemoglobin is an important blood protein consisting of 146 amino acids combined in a specific order. In the hemoglobin of a person with sickle-cell disease, one amino acid, glutamine, has been replaced by valine at one specific location on the protein chain.

Sickle-cell disease is a hereditary condition in which the red blood cells become rigid and crescent-shaped. These abnormal cells tend to clump together and block small blood vessels in many different organs. In sickle-cell disease the body is 99.3 percent correct in manufacturing the red blood cell. However, death results from the 0.7 percent error. No cure is known, and most clients die by the age of 50.

Other amino acids are conditionally essential or can become acquired essential depending on the biochemical needs of the body. Table 5–2 lists the amino acids that have been classified as essential, conditionally and/or acquired essential, and nonessential. Acquired essential amino acids become essential in premature infants, in states of genetic and acquired disorders, and/or during severe stress. A very high intake of particular amino acids can cause other amino acids to become essential.

TABLE 5–2 Essential, Conditionally and/or Acquired Essential, and Nonessential Amino Acids

Essential	Conditionally Essential and/or Acquired Essential	Nonessential
Lysine	Cysteine*	Alanine
Threonine	Tyrosine	Glutamic acid
Histidine	Arginine	Aspartic acid
Isoleucine	Citrulline†	Glycine
Leucine	Taurine‡	Serine
Methionine	Carnitine§	Proline
Phenylalanine		Glutamine
Tryptophan		Asparagine
Valine		

* Also called cystine.
† Not used in protein synthesis but critical in the urea cycle.
‡ Not used in protein synthesis but essential in retinal functioning, particularly in young children.
§ In newborns, can enhance the use of fat as an energy source; can be made from lysine and methionine in adults.

All essential amino acids must be available in the body simultaneously and in sufficient quantity for synthesis of body proteins. These amino acids may come from food or from the body's own cells as they age and are broken down and replaced.

Conditionally and/or Acquired Essential Aminoacids

Under certain conditions some amino acids, not normally essential, become essential. For example, cysteine and tyrosine become indispensable in immaturity, in metabolic disorders, and/or during severe stress. A high intake of cysteine and tyrosine can reduce the requirements for the essential amino acids methionine and phenylalanine.

Nonessential Amino Acids

Nonessential amino acids are those that the body can build in suitable quantities to meet its needs. Often they are derived from other amino acids. Nonessential amino acids are necessary for good health but under normal conditions, adults do not have to obtain them from food. One nonessential amino acid, aspartic acid, is combined with phenylalanine to make aspartame, a sugar substitute.

Functions in the Body

There are five major functions of protein in the body. Protein is required for maintenance and growth, for the regulation of body processes, for the development of immunity, for energy in some circumstances, and for proper water balance. Table 5–3 lists these functions and one example of each.

Maintenance and Growth

Because protein is a part of every cell (half the dry weight), adults as well as growing children require adequate protein intake. As cells of the body wear out, they must be replaced.

Essential amino acid—Amino acid that cannot be manufactured by the human body; must be obtained from food or artificial feeding.

Nonessential amino acid—Amino acid that can be synthesized by the body in sufficient quantities for health.

TABLE 5–3   Functions of Protein in the Body, with Examples

Function	Example
Maintenance and growth	Hair growth
Regulation of body processes	Glucagon (actions opposite those of insulin)
Immunity	Antibodies against measles
Energy source	If adequate carbohydrate and fat are lacking
Contribution to fluid balance	Albumin draws fluid back into capillaries from between the cells

---

CLINICAL CALCULATION 5–1

Nitrogen Balance Studies

To calculate an individual's nitrogen balance, the amount of nitrogen in the foods he or she consumes is compared with the amount of nitrogen excreted in the urine. (Other potential losses are estimated.) Protein is approximately 16 percent nitrogen, so to calculate the nitrogen content in the foods, the amount of protein consumed (in grams) is multiplied by 0.16. Thus, a person who ingests 50 g of protein has a nitrogen intake of 8 g. To be in nitrogen equilibrium, he or she would therefore be expected to excrete or lose 8 g of nitrogen.

Anabolism versus Catabolism

Two terms that refer to the building up or the breaking down of body tissues are anabolism and catabolism. **Anabolism** is the building up of tissues as in growth or healing. **Catabolism** is the breaking down of tissues into simpler substances that the body can use or eliminate. Both of these processes are going on simultaneously in the body. For example, tissue proteins are constantly being broken down into amino acids, which are then reused for building new tissue and repairing old tissue. However, anabolism and catabolism are not always in balance. At times, one process may dominate the other.

Nitrogen Balance

Foods containing protein are the body's only external source of nitrogen. Nitrogen is excreted in the urine, feces, and sweat, and is sometimes lost through bleeding or vomiting. A person is in *nitrogen equilibrium* when the amount of nitrogen eaten is equal to the amount excreted. (See Clinical Calculation 5–1.) A healthy adult at a stable body weight is usually in nitrogen equilibrium. Under certain circumstances, however, **nitrogen balance** may be either positive or negative.

POSITIVE NITROGEN BALANCE   Positive nitrogen balance exists when a person consumes more nitrogen than is excreted. In other words, the body is building more tissue than it is breaking down. This finding is desirable during periods of growth such as infancy, childhood, adolescence, and pregnancy.

NEGATIVE NITROGEN BALANCE   Negative nitrogen balance exists when a person consumes less nitrogen than is excreted. Here, the person is receiving insufficient protein, and the body is breaking down more

tissue than it is building. Situations marked by negative nitrogen balance include undernutrition, illness, and trauma.

Although skipping food for one day may create negative nitrogen balance, noticeable physical signs are not likely to occur. However, prolonged negative nitrogen balance can adversely affect the growth rate in children (Fig. 5–2).

Disruption of body integrity, whether by surgery, burns, or fractures, causes an acute protein loss. Bed rest alone is estimated to cause a loss of an estimated 8 grams of protein per day. People who are well nourished before the disruption are better prepared to weather the resulting catabolism. Poorly nourished people are at an increased risk of weight loss, anemia, or infection.

Severe undernutrition results in specific clinical pictures. Protein-calorie malnutrition is discussed in Clinical Application 5–3.

Regulation of Body Processes

Protein contributes to the regulation of body processes. It is necessary for the manufacture of hormones, enzymes, and the nucleus of every cell. Table 5–4 lists the three kinds of regulators and gives examples of each.

Hormones

Hormones are chemicals secreted by various organs to regulate body processes. Hormones are secreted directly into the bloodstream rather than within an organ. **Insulin** and **glucagon** are two important protein hormones that help to control glucose metabolism.

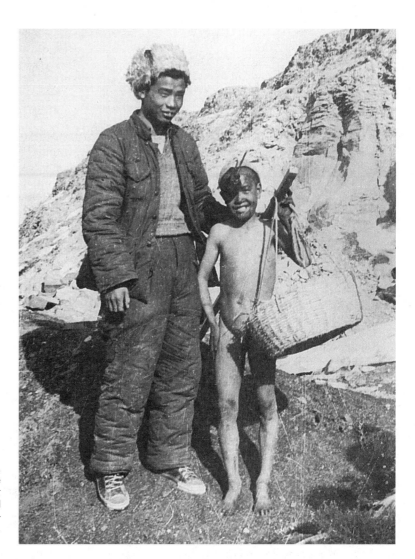

FIGURE 5–2 Two Asian boys of the same age. The boy on the right worked in a mine and ate protein-poor food. The boy on the left lived for 4 years at a boarding school, where he received better food. (Courtesy of the Food and Agriculture Organization of the United Nations, Rome, Italy.)

Enzymes

The body also makes specialized proteins called **enzymes.** Enzymes are crucial to many body processes, such as digestion. The breakdown of foods in the stomach and small intestine involves enzymes, which act as **catalysts.** Catalysts influence the speed at which a chemical reaction takes place, but do not actually enter into the reaction. Without the aid of en-

Catabolism—The breaking down of body compounds or tissues into simpler substances; the destructive phase of metabolism.

Nitrogen balance—The difference between the amount of nitrogen ingested and that excreted each day; the intake of more protein than is used produces positive nitrogen balance, and the intake of less protein produces negative nitrogen balance.

Enzyme—Complex protein produced by living cells that acts as a catalyst.

Catalyst—Substance that speeds a chemical reaction without entering into, or being changed by, the reaction.

Anabolism—The building up of body compounds or tissues by the synthesis of more complex substances from simpler ones; the constructive phase of metabolism.

zymes, many of the processes in the body would proceed too slowly to be effective.

Think of an enzyme as a dating service. Just as a dating service provides an opportunity for two people to meet and react in some fashion with each other, an enzyme provides a place (its surface) for two substances to meet and react with each other. If it were not for enzymes, these two substances would be less likely to encounter one another, and basic body functioning would be impossible.

Enzymes are necessary for health. Lack of a spe-

TABLE 5–4   Examples of Regulators of Body Processes

Regulator	Examples
Hormones	Insulin, thyroid hormone
Enzymes	Lactase, Sucrase
Nucleoproteins	DNA, RNA

cific enzyme can have devastating effects on health, even on life itself. As an example, a disease called **phenylketonuria** is discussed in Clinical Application 5–4.

Nucleoproteins

Nucleoproteins are the third example of regulatory proteins. The center or nucleus of every cell contains nucleoproteins. Their function is to direct the maintenance and reproduction of the cell. Two well-known nucleoproteins are DNA and RNA.

DNA **Deoxyribonucleic acid** (DNA) is present in all body cells of every species. It is the basic component of **genes,** which serve as patterns to guide reproduction.

RNA **Ribonucleic acid** (RNA) is another nucleoprotein present in all living cells. It controls the manufacturing of cellular protein. Each of the common amino acids has its own RNA to transport it to the correct location in the protein chain.

Immunity

A specific protein called an **antibody** is produced in the body in response to the presence of a foreign substance or a substance that the body senses to be foreign. Antibodies provide **immunity** to certain diseases and other toxic conditions. A specific antibody is created for each foreign substance. Thus, if a person is exposed to a certain kind of disease-producing bacteria, the body creates an antibody that will only neutralize the harmful effects of that particular species or strain of bacteria. For some diseases, once the body has produced antibodies, it can respond quickly to another attack, making the individual immune. All antibodies belong to a group of blood proteins called **immunoglobulins.**

Energy Source

Protein is a backup energy source. When the body has insufficient carbohydrate for energy, it will obtain energy from its own tissues. That is, the body converts its own muscle protein into energy. To spare protein for tissue building, adequate carbohydrate intake is necessary. The amount of energy obtained from a gram of protein is the same as the amount obtained from a gram of carbohydrate, 4 kilocalories.

Classification of Food Protein

Few foods contain solely protein. Most foods embody various combinations of protein, fat, and carbohydrates. Nevertheless, some foods are better sources of protein than others.

Protein foods are classified according to the number and kinds of amino acids they contain. **Complete proteins** are foods that supply all eight essential amino acids in sufficient quantity to maintain tissue and support growth. **Incomplete proteins** lack one or more of the essential amino acids.

Complete Protein

With few exceptions, single foods containing complete protein come from animal sources such as meat, poultry, fish, eggs, and cheese. Gelatin is an incomplete protein because it lacks the essential amino acid tryptophan.

Sources Containing Complete Protein

Both meat and milk products are good sources of complete protein. An adult following the Food Pyra-

mid would consume daily two or three servings from the meat group and two or three servings from the milk group.

The Food Pyramid categorizes cheese with milk, whereas the Exchange Group system places it with meat.

Exchange Groups Containing Complete Protein

Each exchange of meat contains 7 grams of protein regardless of the amount of fat. All beef is not high in fat and all fish or poultry is not low in fat. Figure 5–3 shows a 3-ounce portion of beef tenderloin equal to 3 lean meat exchanges.

Each milk exchange furnishes 8 grams of protein. Examples of one milk exchange are 1 cup of milk, buttermilk, or yogurt, 1/2 cup of canned evaporated milk, or 1/3 cup of dry skim milk. All of these milk products offer equal protein nutrition, but all are not nutritionally equivalent because of their fat content.

Incomplete Protein

Plant foods lack sufficient amounts of one or more of the essential amino acids. Thus, the protein they contain is incomplete.

Sources Containing Incomplete Protein

Grains, vegetables, legumes, nuts, and seeds are valuable sources of incomplete protein. These foods should not be avoided because of the term *incom-*

Deoxyribonucleic acid (DNA)—Protein substance in the cell nucleus that directs all cell activities, including reproduction.

Ribonucleic acid (RNA)—A substance which controls protein synthesis in all living cells.

Antibody—A specific protein developed in the body in response to a substance that the body senses to be foreign.

Complete protein—Protein containing all eight (nine for infants) essential amino acids that humans need; usually found in animal sources such as milk, meat, eggs, and fish.

Incomplete protein—Protein lacking one or more of the essential amino acids that humans need; usually found in plant sources such as grains and vegetables

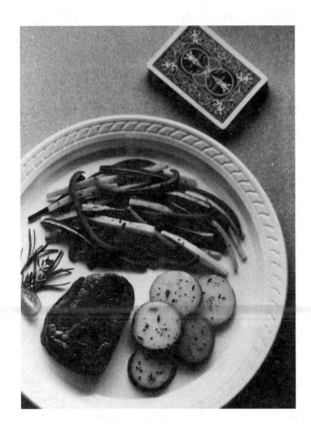

FIGURE 5-3 The 3-oz beef tenderloin pictured equals 3 lean meat exchanges. The standard deck of playing cards is shown for size comparison.

plete. First, they supplement the animal proteins in the diet. Second, a mixture of several different types of plant protein sources can yield all the essential amino acids. In this way, amino acids that are limited in one food will be supplied in one or more of the other foods.

Exchange Groups Containing Incomplete Protein

The vegetable and starch/bread exchanges are sources of incomplete protein. Some vegetables are closer in energy content to a slice of bread than to most vegetables. Vegetables such as corn, peas, and dried beans appear on the Starch/Bread Exchange List. Examples of one vegetable exchange are 1/2 cup of asparagus or 1/2 cup of chopped broccoli. A vegetable exchange contains 2 grams of protein. Examples of one exchange of starch/bread are 1/2 cup of corn, 1 small potato, 1/2 cup of winter squash, 1 slice of bread, 1/2 bagel or 1/2 English muffin, or 3 square graham crackers. A starch/bread exchange contains 3 grams of protein. Table 5–5 lists the protein content of the exchanges that contain protein.

Vegetarian Diets

For vegetarians or other individuals who limit their intake of animal foods, **legumes** are an important protein source. Legumes are plants having roots containing nitrogen-fixing bacteria that "lock" nitrogen into the plant's structure, thus increasing its protein content. Legumes contain two to three times as much protein as most vegetables.

Commonly used legumes are peas, beans, lentils, and nuts. Not all peas and beans are legumes. Figure 5–4 compares the protein content of peas, beans, and nuts. Examples of one exchange of legumes are: 1/2 cup of peas, 1/3 cup of kidney

TABLE 5–5   Grams of Protein per Exchange

Exchange	Grams of Protein
Milk	8
Meat	7
Starch/Bread	3
Vegetable	2

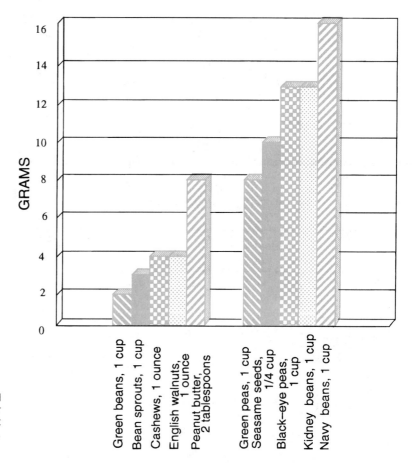

FIGURE 5–4 Protein content of selected food plants. Notice that all foods called peas or beans are not legumes. Green beans offer just 2 g of protein compared with navy beans, which offer 16 g.

beans, or 1/4 cup of baked beans. On the exchange lists, these legumes are classified as starch/bread. Because many legumes are not only low in fat but also high in fiber, they are valued by health-conscious people.

Nuts appear on the fat exchange list. One tablespoon of cashews or 20 small peanuts is one exchange. Peanut butter is on the high-fat meat list; 1 tablespoon equals 1 exchange.

Because grains and legumes lack different amino acids, combining a grain with a legume will substitute for a complete protein. Some favorite combinations such as a peanut butter sandwich or baked beans with brown bread are grain-and-legume combinations. The Mexican burrito, a thin cornmeal bread filled with beans, is another example. Clinical Application 5–5 distinguishes various vegetarian diets.

Textured vegetable protein products from soybeans, peanuts, and cottonseed can enhance the vegetarian diet. The protein is spun into fibers and flavored, colored, and shaped for use as a meat sub-

stitute. Well-processed soybean protein has been demonstrated to have equal quality to animal protein (Young, 1991).

Usually hospital dietitians can provide a balanced vegetarian diet. It is much better, when a nurse encounters a vegetarian client, to inform the dietitian rather than expect the client to select items from a general menu.

Recommended Dietary Allowances

The RDA for adult protein is 0.8 grams of protein per kilogram of body weight. Clinical Calculation 5–2 shows the procedure for calculating this amount based on a person's healthy body weight. Pregnancy and lactation increase the need for protein, as do periods of growth.

During pregnancy and breast-feeding the mother requires additional protein to build new tissue. The "eating for two" advice for pregnant women refers to the quality of foods eaten, not the quantity. Infants

TABLE 5–6　Protein RDA for Healthy Individuals of Various Ages

Age In Years	Grams of Protein per Kilogram of Healthy Body Weight
0–1/2	2.2
1/2–1	1.6
1–3	1.2
4–6	1.1
7–14	1.0
15–18 (Males)	0.9
15–18 (Females)	0.8
19 and older	0.8
Pregnant	Nonpregnant RDA + 10 g
Lactating	
First 6 months	Nonpregnant RDA + 15 g
Remainder	Nonpregnant RDA + 12 g

up to the age of 6 months have the greatest protein requirement in proportion to their body size—2.2 grams per kilogram.

Overeating protein foods can adversely affect a person's health. Excess protein taxes the kidneys, which must excrete the surplus nitrogen. The Committee on Diet and Health recommends that protein intake be no more than twice the RDA. If individuals follow the Food Pyramid, their protein intake should approximate 12 to 20 percent of kilocalories. Table 5–6 displays the protein RDA.

Choosing Protein Foods Wisely

Producing meat is expensive. For every 5 pounds of vegetable or fish protein fed to livestock, only 1 pound of meat protein is produced.

For persons who wish to limit meat intake, Table 5–7 lists equivalent sources of protein. Prices of nationally advertised brands were used, except for cottage cheese, eggs, milk, and steak. Peanut butter provided 10 grams of protein for 11 cents. Water-packed tuna has the most protein per kilocalorie of the foods listed. The most expensive source of 100 grams of protein was bean soup.

Summary

Protein is necessary for tissue maintenance and growth, for the regulation of body processes, for providing immunity, as a backup source of energy, and for water balance. The element that distin-

TABLE 5–7   Comparative Sources of 10 Grams of Protein with Kilocalories and Costs

Food	Portion	Kilocalories	Cost/Amount	Cost/Portion
Peanut butter	2 tbsp	190	$3.09/28 oz	$0.11
Large eggs, poached	1.7	126	$0.89/doz	$0.13
Tuna, canned in water	1 oz	45	$0.85/6.5 oz	$0.13
2 percent milk	1.25 cups	150	$1.99/gal	$0.16
Cottage cheese 2 percent low fat	1/3 cup	68	$1.59/1.5 lb	$0.18
American cheese	1.7 oz	175	$4.97/2 lb	$0.26
Cracked wheat bread	5 slices	325	$1.19/20 oz	$0.27
Boneless sirloin beef steak	1.1 oz	66	$4.39/lb	$0.30
Bologna	2.9 oz	261	$1.99/lb	$0.36
Bean soup, condensed, prepared with water	1.25 cups	213	$0.89/11.5 oz	$0.39

guishes protein from carbohydrates and fats is nitrogen. The body combines carbon, hydrogen, oxygen, and nitrogen in certain ways to form amino acids, which then become the building blocks of various proteins.

Complete protein foods contain all essential amino acids in amounts sufficient to support growth. Complete protein foods usually come from animal sources, especially the meat and milk groups.

Incomplete protein foods are grains, vegetables, legumes, nuts, and seeds. If a person eats a grain product and a legume at the same meal, he or she is likely to receive all essential amino acids.

The normal healthy adult should consume 0.8 grams of protein per kilogram (2.2 pounds) of healthy body weight. A simple method of estimating protein intake uses the Exchange List system. Milk exchanges provide about 8 grams of protein, meat exchanges 7 grams, bread/starch exchanges 3 grams, and vegetable exchanges 2 grams.

Case Study 5–1   Mrs. F is a 72-year-old widow who eats independently in her family homestead. Her usual meals are tea and toast for breakfast, canned fruit and a muffin for lunch, and frozen potpie or canned hash for dinner. She complains that she has been having trouble chewing and has not been eating as much food as she usually does. She does not like milk.

NURSING CARE PLAN FOR MRS. F

Assessment

Subjective Data	Food deficit as evidenced by usual food intake information
	Has trouble chewing
	Does not like milk
Objective Data	Height: 5 ft, 4 in
	Weight: 106 lb
	Wrist circumference: 5.75 in
	Examination of mouth: loose-fitting dentures

Table continued on following page

Nursing Diagnosis	Nutrition altered: less than body requirements for protein and kilocalories, related to difficulty chewing, as evidenced by stated usual intake of 28–32 g of protein per day and body weight 7 percent under minimum for weight and frame.

Desired Outcome/ Evaluation Criteria	Nursing Actions	Rationale
Client will gain 1 lb per week during the next 2 weeks.	Encourage easily chewed sources of complete protein: cheese, eggs, ground meat, fish.	Complete protein foods contain all essential amino acids necessary for tissue building.
Client will increase her total protein intake by 9–13 g per day.	Create a model meal plan with Mrs. F using the Exchange Group system to count grams of protein.	Mrs. F requires 41 g of protein for her healthy body weight. The meal plan she described in her history contains only 28 to 32 g depending on dinner selection.
Client will call for dental appointment within next 2 weeks.	Explore sources of financial assistance for dental care if necessary.	Better fitting dentures would permit Mrs. F a wider variety of foods.

Study Aids

Chapter Review

1. For which of the following functions of protein could other nutrients be substituted?
   a. Energy source
   b. Immunity
   c. Maintenance and growth
   d. Regulation of body processes

2. Which of the following foods is a complete protein?
   a. Baked beans
   b. Broccoli
   c. Beef kabobs
   d. Bread sticks

3. If a person had difficulty purchasing meat to serve every day, which of the following combinations of foods should the nurse suggest as offering the best source of protein?
   a. Applesauce and bran muffins
   b. Bean soup and rye bread
   c. Broccoli and French bread
   d. Carrot-and-raisin salad

4. How much protein should a normal healthy adult consume each day?
   a. 0.8 gram per kilogram of actual body weight
   b. 0.8 gram per kilogram of healthy body weight
   c. 0.8 gram per pound of actual body weight
   d. 0.8 gram per pound of healthy body weight

5. Which of the following persons would the nurse treat as being in a catabolic state?
   a. Adolescent boy who is into body building
   b. Lactating mother
   c. Pregnant woman in the second trimester
   d. Surgical patient, first day after a stomach resection

Clinical Analysis

Mr. P, a 65-year-old widower of 6 months, has been referred to your home health agency for assistance in managing his nutritional intake. He has lost 10 pounds over the past 6 months, although a physical examination within the past month revealed no disease processes requiring treatment.

1. As the nurse assesses Mr. P, which of the following data would she gather first?
   a. List of current medications the client takes.
   b. Blood protein levels analyzed during the recent physical examination.
   c. A description of the procedure Mr. P uses to weigh himself.
   d. Dietary recall of Mr. P's food and fluid intake.

2. Which of the following plans would be most appropriate to increase Mr. P's protein consumption immediately?

a. Refer client to nutrition education program.

b. Have Mr. P apply for meals on wheels.

c. Recommend that Mr. P supplement his meals with one of the milk-based breakfast products.

d. Suggest to Mr. P that he sign up for cooking lessons at the local high school or community college.

3. Which of the following outcomes would indicate achievement of the nutritional objective for Mr. P?

a. A gain in weight of 2 pounds in 2 weeks.

b. An invitation to the nurse to join him for a dinner he has learned to cook.

c. A report by Mr. P that he is eating better.

d. A visual inspection of Mr. P's refrigerator revealing fresh meat and milk products in abundance.

Bibliography

Acosta, PB and Wright, L: Nurses' role in preventing birth defects in offspring of women with phenylketonuria. JOGNN 21:270, 1992.

Bowe, K: Phenylketonuria: An update for pediatric community health nurses. Pediatr Nurs 21:191, 1995.

Brenner, BM, Meyer, TW, and Hostetter, TH: Dietary protein intake and the progressive nature of kidney disease: The role of hemodynamically mediated glomerular injury in the pathogenesis of progressive glomerular sclerosis in aging, renal ablation, and intrinsic renal disease. N Engl J Med 307:652, 1982.

Chandra, RK: Antibody formation in first and second generation offspring of nutritionally deprived rats. Science 190:289, 1975.

Chandra, RK, et al: Nutrition and immunocompetence of the elderly: Effects of short-term nutritional supplementation on cell-mediated immunity and lymphocyte subsets. Nutrition Research 2:223, 1982.

Committee on Diet and Health, Food and Nutrition Board, Commission on Life Sciences, National Research Council: Diet and Health: Implications for Reducing Chronic Disease Risk. National Academy Press, Washington, DC, 1989.

Groff, JL, et al: Advanced Nutrition and Human Metabolism. West Publishing Company, St Paul, 1995.

Hunt, TK: Nutritional requirements of repair. In Ballenger, WF, et al (eds): Manual of Surgical Nutrition. WB Saunders, Philadelphia, 1975.

Janelle, KC and Barr, SI: Nutrient intakes and eating behavior scores of vegetarian and nonvegetarian women. J Am Diet Assoc 95:180, 1995.

Kasprisin, CA and Kasprisin DO: Clinical Human Genetics. Medical Examination, New Hyde Park, NY, 1982.

Lehninger, AL: Biochemistry, ed 2. Worth, New York, 1981.

Schumn, DE: Essentials of Biochemistry. FA Davis, Philadelphia, 1988.

Solomns, TWG: Fundamentals of Organic Chemistry, ed. 4. John Wiley & Sons, New York, 1994.

Subcommittee on the 10th Edition of the RDAs. Food and Nutrition Board. Commission on Life Sciences. National Research Council: Recommended Dietary Allowances, ed 10. National Academy Press, Washington, DC, 1989.

Thomas, PR (ed): Improving Americans Diet & Health. National Academy Press, 1991.

Young, VR: Soy protein in relation to human protein and amino acid nutrition. J Am Diet Assoc 91:828, 1991.

CHAPTER 6

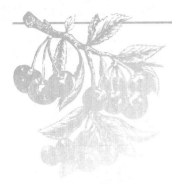

Energy Balance

LEARNING OBJECTIVES

After completing this chapter, the student should be able to:

1 Describe energy homeostasis.
2 List two reasons why the body needs energy.
3 Describe how energy is measured both in foods and in the human body.
4 Discuss the effect of body composition on energy output.
5 Name the energy nutrient that has the highest kilocalorie density and identify two substances usually found in foods with a low kilocalorie density.

For about one-half to three-quarters of the population, the human body automatically regulates energy intake and/or expenditure to maintain energy balance. This feat compensates for varying amounts of energy needed and erratic food intake. The body can also compensate for having less food fuel by conserving energy during food restriction or starvation.

This chapter describes the impact that energy intake and energy expenditure have on energy balance. Topics include energy measurements, factors that can influence the body's need for energy, energy consumption patterns, the kilocaloric and nutrient density of foods, energy allowances, and current recommendations concerning energy consumption.

Homeostasis

The human body seeks balance. **Homeostasis** means equilibrium or balance. Homeostasis, in terms of **energy balance,** results when the number of kilocalories eaten equals the number used to produce energy. An individual is usually in energy balance when a stable body weight is maintained.

Energy Intake

The typical adult eats between 500,000 to 850,000 kilocalories per year. Eating an excess of only 1 percent or 15 extra kilocalories per day would result in a weight gain of 1.5 pounds per year. This equals the kilocalories in 1/3 teaspoonful of butter or one-fourth of a small apple. The individual at a stable healthy weight gives little thought to the amount of food eaten each day, yet the body weight remains constant.

Energy Expenditure

Individuals also expend or use varying amounts of energy daily. **Energy expenditure** is measured by the number of kilocalories that an individual uses to meet the body's demand for fuel. A person uses many more kilocalories to run a marathon than to sleep all day. Physical activity costs energy.

Adaptive Thermogenesis

Energy expenditure frequently adapts to either a large increase or a large decrease in food intake of several days' duration. This adaptive component of energy expenditure is called **adaptive thermogene-** sis. Energy expenditure decreases during food restriction or starvation. Kilocalories are burned more efficiently. An individual trying to lose weight may either lose at a slower rate or stop losing weight. However, overeating for several days will cause an increase in energy expenditure. Energy expenditure has been found to be higher than predicted during the refeeding of previously starved patients (Krahn and Rock, 1993). Adaptive thermogenesis is one example of how the human body evolved to cope with feast-or-famine conditions. When food was scarce, the human body adapted by conserving energy.

Energy Balance

Energy balance exists when energy expenditure equals energy intake. Most individuals are able to maintain a state of energy balance at a healthy body weight. Some people are able to achieve a stable body weight only after the deposition of an excessive amount of body fat. For example, a 120-pound individual (at a healthy body weight) can gain 100 pounds over a period of time and his or her weight will remain at 220 pounds indefinitely. The excessively lean person can also be in a state of energy homeostasis. Researchers do not understand why some people are unable to maintain energy homeostasis at their healthy body weights.

Measurement of Energy

Both the energy (fuel) contained in foods and the amount of energy used by the body can be measured. The methods used to measure energy are fairly universal.

Homeostasis—Tendency toward balance in the internal environment of the body achieved by automatic monitoring and regulating mechanisms.

Energy balance—A situation in which kilocaloric intake equals kilocaloric output.

Energy expenditure—The amount of fuel the body uses for a specified period.

Adaptive thermogenesis—The adjustment in energy expenditure the body makes to either a large increase or a large decrease in kilocalorie intake of several days' duration.

Units of Measurement

The energy content of food is measured in kilocalories, often abbreviated as kcalories or Kcal. A **kilocalorie** is the amount of heat required to raise 1 kilogram of water 1°C. Kilocalories are what lay people and the media call calories. Chemically, a **calorie** is the amount of heat required to raise 1 gram of water 1°C. One kilocalorie contains 1000 times as much energy as one calorie. Kilocalorie is the term used throughout this text.

The joule is another unit increasingly used to measure energy; you may encounter this term as you read scientific journals. One **kilojoule** is the energy required to move a mass of 1 kilogram with an acceleration of 1 meter per second. The kilojoule is equal to 0.239 kilocalories; a kilocalorie equals 4.184 kilojoules.

Energy Nutrient Values

The energy nutrients are carbohydrates, fat, and protein. Alcohol (ethanol) also yields energy. A food's kilocalorie value is determined by its content of protein, fat, carbohydrates, and alcohol. To review:

- 1 gram of carbohydrate = 4 kilocalories (or 17 kilojoules)
- 1 gram of protein = 4 kilocalories (or 17 kilojoules)
- 1 gram of fat = 9 kilocalories (or 37.6 kilojoules)
- 1 gram of alcohol = 7 kilocalories (or 29.3 kilojoules)

Water, fiber, vitamins, and minerals do not provide kilocalories. Clinical Calculation 6–1 demonstrates how to determine the energy content of a food item.

Determination of Energy Values

Foods

The energy content of individual foods is measured by a device called a **bomb calorimeter,** illustrated in Figure 6–1. A bomb calorimeter is an insulated container that has a chamber in which food is burned. The amount of heat (kilocalories) produced by the burning of the food is determined by the change in the temperature of a measured amount of water that surrounds the chamber. All energy in food is in the

---

CLINICAL CALCULATION 6–1

Calculating the Energy Content of a Food Item

If you know the carbohydrate, fat, and protein content of a food item, you can readily calculate the food item's kilocaloric content. Two examples are shown below. One starch exchange contains 3 g of protein and 15 g of carbohydrate. Adding the protein and carbohydrate content in the starch exchange together equals 18.

	Carbohydrate (g)		Protein (g)		Fat (g)		Total (g)
One starch exchange	15	+	3	+	0	=	18

There are 4 kcal in 1 g each of carbohydrate and protein, so all you need to do to obtain the kilocaloric content of the starch exchange is to multiply 4 by 18. Thus there are 72 kcal in one starch exchange. One fat exchange contains 5 g of fat.

	Carbohydrate (g)		Protein (g)		Fat (g)		Total (g)
One fat exchange	0	+	0	+	5	=	5

There are 9 kcal in a gram of fat. To obtain the kilocaloric content of one fat exchange, multiply 5 by 9. Thus one fat exchange contains 45 kcal.

---

form of chemical energy. In a bomb calorimeter, the chemical energy stored in the food sample is transformed into heat energy. The following equation may facilitate understanding of this concept:

$$\text{Protein} + \text{oxygen} = \text{heat energy} + \text{water} + \text{carbon dioxide}$$

(Carbohydrates or fat may be substituted for protein in the above equation.)

Human Body

A process similar to the combustion of food in the bomb calorimeter occurs in the body. The amount of energy the human body uses can be measured directly or indirectly. Direct measurement of energy used by the human body is expensive and used only

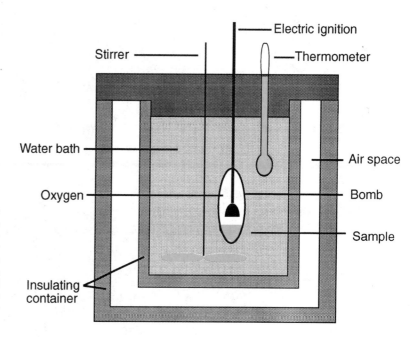

FIGURE 6–1 Cross section of a bomb calorimeter showing essential features. The food sample is completely burned in the inner section; heat produced is absorbed by the known volume of water in the surrounding section. Change in temperature provides the measure of heat produced. (Reproduced by permission from Guthrie, HA: Introductory Nutrition, ed 7. Times Mirror/Mosby College Publishing, St. Louis, 1989.)

in scientific research. Energy is measured directly by placing a person in an insulated heat-sensitive chamber and measuring the heat emitted by the body. Indirect measurement of energy is discussed in Clinical Application 6–1.

Components of Energy Expenditure

The human body requires energy (1) to meet resting energy expenditure needs and (2) to meet physical activity requirements. Resting energy expenditure includes not only the energy (kilocalories) needed to digest, absorb, transport, and utilize nutrients but also the energy required for other involuntary activities. Physical activity includes the energy needed for voluntary activities, those that can be consciously controlled, such as running, walking, and swimming.

Resting Energy Expenditure

Resting energy expenditure (REE) requires more total kilocalories than physical activity in most people. **Resting energy expenditure** represents the energy expended or used by a person at rest. Another

Kilocalorie (kcalorie or Kcal)—a measurement unit of energy; the amount of heat required to raise 1 kilogram of water 1 degree Celsius.

Resting energy expenditure (REE)—The amount of fuel the human body uses at rest for a specified period; often used interchangeably with basal metabolic rate (BMR).

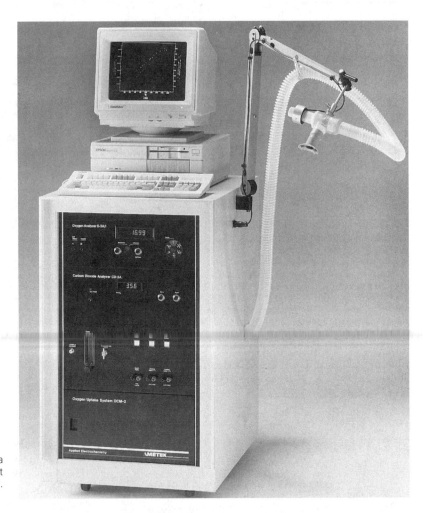

FIGURE 6–2 This device may be called a Respirometer, the Metabolic Measurement System, or a Respiratory Gas Analyzer. (Courtesy of Ametek, Inc., Pittsburgh, PA.)

term still in use in some scientific literature is *basal metabolic rate* (BMR). The major difference between resting energy and basal metabolic rate is that basal metabolic rate is always measured beginning at least 12 hours after the last meal and under certain conditions, such as controlled temperature and humidity. Clinical Application 6–1 discusses the measurement of REE in hospitalized clients. The energy cost to chew, swallow, digest, absorb, and transport nutrients is a component of REE. This component of REE is frequently referred to as the **thermic effect of foods** (TEF). In practice, BMR and REE differ by less than 12 percent and the terms are used interchangeably (Subcommittee on the 10th Edition of the RDAs, 1989).

The kilocalories necessary to support the following contribute to resting energy expenditure:

1. Thermic effect of foods
2. Contraction of the heart
3. Maintenance of body temperature
4. Repair of the internal organs
5. Maintenance of cellular processes
6. Muscular and nervous coordination
7. Respiration (breathing)

REE makes up about 66 percent of total energy requirements in most people.

Body composition influences resting energy expenditure. Individuals of similar age, sex, height, and weight with a higher percentage of lean body mass have a higher REE than those with less lean body mass. It takes more energy, or kilocalories, to support lean body mass (protein) than to support body fat. Muscle tissue requires more kilocalories than does fat tissue, even when muscle tissue is resting. Therefore, the higher a person's body protein content, the more kilocalories he or she can eat and still maintain a stable body weight.

Estimating a person's resting energy expenditure

is commonly done by using the equations found in Table 6–1. These equations take into account age, sex, and weight but ignore differences in body composition, climate, and genetic variability (discussed in the following sections). Although these equations are not completely accurate for individuals, they can serve as a guide for menu planning. The ultimate test of how kilocalories eaten work in the body is to monitor body weight and kilocaloric intake over time.

Age

Resting energy expenditure varies with lean body mass, which varies with age. The highest rates of energy expenditure per pound of body weight occur during infancy and childhood. In adults, REE declines about 2 percent per decade because of a decline in lean body mass. This results in a reduced need for kilocalories. Individuals can retard the decline in lean body mass somewhat by increasing their exercise. An individual who fails either to adjust his or her kilocaloric intake to this reduced need for kilocalories or to increase his or her physical exercise may experience a slow weight gain.

Sex

Differences in body composition between men and women occur as early as the first few months of life.

TABLE 6–1   Equations for Calculating Resting Energy Expenditure

Sex and Age Range (Years)	Equation to Obtain REE in Kilocalories per Day	
Men		
0–3	(60.9 × weight in kilograms)	− 54
3–10	(22.7 × weight in kilograms)	495
10–18	(17.5 × weight in kilograms)	651
18–30	(15.3 × weight in kilograms)	679
30–60	(11.6 × weight in kilograms)	879
> 60	(13.5 × weight in kilograms)	487
Women		
0–3	(61.0 × weight in kilograms)	− 51
3–10	(22.5 × weight in kilograms)	499
10–18	(12.2 × weight in kilograms)	746
18–30	(14.7 × weight in kilograms)	496
30–60	(8.7 × weight in kilograms)	829
> 60	(10.5 × weight in kilograms)	596

SOURCE: Adapted from the Subcommittee on the 10th Edition of the RDAs, 1989, p. 26.

The differences are relatively small until the child reaches age 10. During adolescence, body composition changes radically. Men develop proportionately greater muscle mass than do women, who deposit fat as they mature. Consequently, REE differs by as much as 10 percent between men and women.

Growth

Human growth is most pronounced during the growth spurts that take place during infancy, puberty, and pregnancy. Kilocalories required per kilogram of body weight are highest during these growth spurts. This is because the kilocaloric cost of anabolism is greater than the kilocaloric cost of catabolism.

Body Size

Persons with large bodies require proportionately more energy. A tall individual uses more energy to move his or her body mass over a given distance than a shorter person. This is because a shorter person has less muscular tissue or lean body mass than a taller person.

Genetics

Recent evidence has shown that REE is strongly influenced by the genetic patterns of the individual. Each person is apparently programmed with a need to burn a certain number of kilocalories to meet energy balance. This fact will become apparent to health care workers when counseling two very similar clients. Both clients may be of the same sex, of equal weight, perform similar types of physical activity, and have about the same body fat content. Yet each client may need to eat a different number of kilocalories to maintain a stable body weight. Many individuals have little control over the number of kilocalories required to meet the needs of REE.

Climate

Environmental climate affects REE because kilocalories are needed to maintain body temperature. This pertains to extreme differences in external temper-

---

Thermic effect of foods (TEF)—(diet-induced thermogenesis, specific-dynamic action)—The energy cost to extract and utilize the kilocalories and nutrients in foods; the heat produced after eating a meal.

CLINICAL APPLICATION 6–2

Fever

Heat acts as a catalyst in most chemical reactions. A catalyst is a substance that speeds up a chemical reaction. Fever increases resting energy expenditure by about 7 percent for every 1°F increase in body temperature. Frequently, an individual with a fever is too ill to eat. Fruit juices with added glucose polymers or a nutritional supplement will give the client needed energy.

CLINICAL CALCULATION 6–2

Calculating Resting Energy Expenditure

Sample calculations for a 154-lb, 18- to 30-year-old man's resting energy expenditure:

1. Convert weight in pounds to kilograms.

$$\frac{\text{Weight in pounds}}{\text{Weight in pounds per kilogram}} = \text{weight in kilograms}$$

$$\frac{154}{2.2} = 70 \text{ kg}$$

2. Locate equation from Table 6–1 and perform the calculation

REE = (15.3 × weight in kilograms) + 679
REE = (15.3 × 70 kg) + 679
REE = 1071 + 679
REE = 1750 kcal per day

atures, whether cold or hot. In the United States, most individuals do not need to eat more kilocalories during colder months because the majority of living environments range from 68°F to 77°F. Outside, people usually protect themselves from extreme cold by wearing warm clothes. However, a relatively small increase in REE (2 to 5 percent) is associated with carrying the extra weight of winter clothing and boots. Shivering also causes an increase in REE. Extra kilocalories are also needed by feverish clients. Clinical Application 6–2 discusses the kilocaloric requirements for clients with fevers.

Thermic Effect of Food

The heat produced after eating a meal is called the thermic effect of foods (TEF). An older term for this energy cost is *specific dynamic action* (SDA). Energy is needed to chew, swallow, digest, absorb, and transport nutrients. Metabolism increases after eating. As metabolism increases, more kilocalories are used. Clinical Calculation 6–2 demonstrates the calculation of a typical 18- to 30-year-old, 154-pound man's REE.

According to the Food and Nutrition Board of the National Research Council (National Research Council, 1989), the consumption of protein and carbohydrates results in a much larger thermic effect than the consumption of fat. Fat in food is processed to body fat more efficiently than carbohydrates or protein. If an individual eats an equal number of kilocalories from carbohydrates as from fat, he or she will store fewer of the carbohydrate kilocalories as body fat.

Physical Activity

For most of the US population, the second largest part of total energy expenditure is physical activity. Some very active individuals may need more kilocalories as a result of physical activity than as a result of resting energy expenditure. Figure 6–3 illustrates an athlete who may burn a large amount of kilocalories as a result of training and engaging in competition. Activity factors associated with a range of activity patterns are provided in Table 6–2. The activity factor is multiplied by the REE to calculate kilocaloric requirements. The energy cost of physical activity is frequently referred to as the **thermic effect of exercise (TEE).**

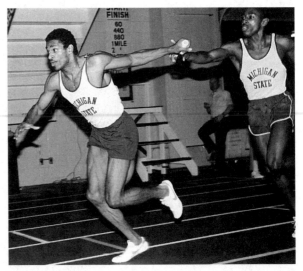

FIGURE 6–3 Trained athletes may burn more kilocalories as a result of physical activity than as a result of their resting energy expenditure. (Courtesy of Sports Information, Michigan State University, East Lansing, MI.)

**TABLE 6–2   Energy Needs
Based on Weight and Activity**

	Energy Needs in Kilocalories per Pound of Body Weight		
	*Sedentary**	*Moderately Active†*	*Active‡*
Overweight	9–11	13	16
Normal weight	13	16	18
Underweight	13	18	18–23

* Patients with severely limited mobility
† Active students, sales clerks, many farm workers
‡ Full-time athletes, unskilled laborers, Army recruits

Energy needs can be calculated based on body weight and adjusted for activity level as shown in Table 6–2. Clinical Calculation 6–3 demonstrates the calculation of daily energy allowance, which includes kilocalories needed for activity. However, calculations of such energy needs are approximations. The most accurate method to determine a client's kilocalorie requirement is to monitor both food intake and body weight over time.

Physical activity can greatly influence energy requirements. For example, a 154-pound man (70 kilograms) will require only 2406 kilocalories on a very sedentary day and up to 3938 kilocalories on a very active day. A 128-pound woman (58 kilograms) will require only 1856 kilocalories on a very sedentary day and up to 3038 kilocalories on a very active day. (Subcommittee of the 10th Edition of the RDAs, 1989.)

CLINICAL CALCULATION 6–3
_____

Calculating Daily Energy Allowance

Sample calculation for a moderately active person at his or her normal weight of 150 lb.

1. Locate the kcal/lb needed from Table 6–2.

    Formula is: Number from table
    × weight in pounds.

2. Perform calculations:

    16 × 150 = 2400 kcal/day

Thus the estimated daily energy need for this person is 2400 kcal.

Thermic Effect of Exercise

Energy expended during exercise is only a portion of the total energy cost of physical activity. Exercise may also affect both REE and the TEF. Some clients' REE increases for up to 48 hours after exercise.

Although the exact reason for this increase in REE is not known, the most plausible explanation is that the glycogen stores need to be refilled. Because exercise depletes glycogen stores, there is an energy cost to refill these stores during the postexercise period.

Adaptive Response to Exercise

An individual with well-developed muscles uses fewer kilocalories to perform a given amount of physical work than an individual with less well-developed muscles. As exercise is repeated, the body learns how to get the job done with the least effort. (This is the body's adaptive response to exercise.) A well-developed muscle performs more efficiently than a less well-developed muscle; thus it uses fewer kilocalories to perform a given physical activity. Also, if an individual loses weight due to increased exercise, he or she will eventually use fewer kilocalories to do a specific activity. Lighter people require fewer kilocalories for a given amount of exercise than heavier people do because it takes fewer kilocalories to move a smaller mass than to move a larger mass.

Exercise and Appetite

Many exercise researchers think that exercise decreases appetite. **Appetite** is defined as a strong desire for food or for a pleasant sensation, based on previous experience, that causes one to seek food for the purpose of tasting and enjoying. After exercise, (the individual) may be satisfied with less food. Some types of exercise release a chemical in the brain called **beta-endorphin.** Beta-endorphin has an effect similar to that of natural morphine. It produces a state of relaxation. In effect, exercise can substitute for overeating in those individuals who eat to decrease stress and tension.

Aerobic Exercise

Aerobic exercise is any activity during which the energy metabolism needed is supported by the oxygen

---

Thermic effect of exercise (TEE)—The number of kilocalories expended above REE as a result of physical activity.

inspired. Aerobic exercises increase physical fitness and involve large muscle groups. Vigorous workouts that last at least 30 minutes, such as fast walking, cycling, swimming, skating, rope jumping, aerobic dancing, hiking, jogging, and rowing require inspired oxygen. Any exercise that raises your pulse to target heart rate is an aerobic activity. To determine your **target heart rate,** see Clinical Application 6–3.

There are many health benefits to aerobic exercise, including:

- Decreased risk of cardiovascular disease
- Better blood sugar control for the people with diabetes
- Decreased risk of obesity
- Reversal or prevention of varicose veins
- Decreased risk of osteoporosis
- Improvement in the quality of sleep
- Better control of hypertension

Anaerobic Exercise

Exercise during which energy needed is provided without the utilization of inspired oxygen is **anaerobic exercise.** Short bursts of vigorous activity, such as resistance or muscle strength training, are forms of anaerobic exercise. The typical example is weight lifting. Anaerobic exercise allows for muscle toning, the building of muscular strength and endurance, and the building of bone mass. This kind of training provides added strength and toughness, which helps to reduce injury during aerobic exercise, prevents lower back problems, and improves overall appearance.

Diet and Activity

A healthy lifestyle is not dependent on diet alone. Physical activity makes a vital contribution to health, function, and performance. The greatest benefit derived from physical activity is gained when moving from sedentary to moderate levels of activity. Only 22 percent of American adults are adequately active. Fully one-fourth are completely sedentary (Blair, 1995). Every American adult should engage in 30 minutes or more of moderate-intensity physical activity on most, preferably all, days of the week (Pale, et al, 1995). Moderate activity means a total of 30 minutes per day of: brisk walking, stair climbing, calisthenics, heavy gardening, or dancing. A person performing these activities for 30 minutes expends 200 kilocalories.

Energy Intake

Historical Trends

Several recent surveys studied the kilocalorie intakes of men and women. Two different surveys found that the average daily energy intakes for men were between 2359 and 2639 kilocalories per day. The average daily reported intakes for women were between 1639 and 1793 kilocalories per day. The average reported intakes for women are of special concern because of the difficulty in incorporating all nutrients at recommended levels in a diet so low in kilocalories. (National Research Council, 1989). The need for the average woman to increase energy output or physical activity is well documented.

Information from the Nationwide Food Consumption Survey has been used to compare energy intakes in 1965 with those in 1977. These data suggest that energy intake declined for both sexes by approximately 10 percent during those 10 to 20 years (National Research Council, 1989). The percentage of overweight men and women has been increasing in spite of the decrease in energy intake. Many experts attribute increased obesity to decreased energy expenditure. We are becoming an increasingly sedentary society. The current recommendation is that the typical person increase physi-

---

CLINICAL APPLICATION 6–3

Determining A Theoretical Target Heart Rate

The theoretical target heart rate is the rate you need to reach to achieve maximal aerobic effect. Determine your theoretical* target heart rate as follows:

1. Subtract your age from the number 220.
2. Multiply this number first by 65 percent and then by 80 percent. The two numbers should represent the range of heart beats per minute that you should try to maintain during aerobic exercise. Example of an 18-year-old woman:

$$220 - 18 = 202$$
$$202 \times 0.65 = 131$$
$$202 \times 0.80 = 161$$

This individual should exercise sufficiently to reach a heart rate of between 131 and 161 beats per minute.

*To monitor your heart rate during exercise, count the number of times your heart beats for 6 seconds and multiply by 10.

cal activity rather than decrease kilocalorie intake below the recommended energy allowance to achieve energy balance.

Kilocaloric Density of Foods

Some foods are more kilocalorically dense than other foods. *Density* is the quantity per unit volume of a substance. **Kilocaloric density** refers to the kilocalories contained in a given volume of a food. Foods with a high water and fiber content have a lower kilocaloric density. Fruits and vegetables such as lettuce, watermelon, and celery are high in water content and low in kilocalories. Grapes have fewer kilocalories than raisins in a given volume because grapes contain more water than raisins.

Fats or foods high in fat have the highest kilocaloric density. Whole-milk products, high-fat meat exchanges, and fat exchanges all contain appreciable fat. Table 6–3 lists several tips for decreasing the kilocaloric density of a diet.

Nutrient Density of Foods

Kilocaloric content alone should not be used to decide whether to include a food in one's diet. The nutrient density of a food is also an important consideration. The **nutrient density** of a food refers to the concentration of nutrients in a food compared with the food's kilocaloric content. If a food is high in kilocalories and low in nutrients, the nutrient density of the food is low. **Empty kilocalories** means that the food contains kilocalories and almost no nutrients. Table sugar is an example of such a food. If a food is low in kilocalories and high in nutrients, the nutrient density of the food is high. Cantaloupe is an example of a food with a high nutrient density—it is low in kilocalories, high in vitamin C, and contains a moderate amount of vitamin A. Skim milk and whole milk are similar in nutrient content. Both types of milk contain about the same amounts of protein, calcium, and riboflavin. Eight ounces of skim milk provides about 90 kilocalories compared with 150 kilocalories in 8 ounces of whole milk. Skim milk thus has a higher nutrient density than whole milk.

Energy Allowances

The recommended dietary allowances for energy are shown in Table 6–4. Differences for age, sex, and body size are factored into the allowances. The kilocalories listed in the table are based on the reference man and woman. For example, the reference 15- to 18-year-old woman weighs 120 pounds and is 64 inches tall. Actual energy requirements may vary widely within any given age group. Genetics may play a role in determining a person's actual energy requirement.

Note in the table that the kilocaloric allowances for both the pregnant and lactating woman are increased. A pregnant woman's energy allowance is 300 kilocalories over and above her nonpregnant allowance; a lactating woman's energy allowance is 500 kilocalories over and above her nonlactating allowance.

TABLE 6–3 Tips for Decreasing the Kilocaloric Density of a Diet

- Use low-fat or nonfat dairy products including skim milk, cheese, and yogurt.
- Brown meats by broiling or cooking in nonstick pans with little or no fat. Avoid fried foods.
- Chill soups, stews, sauces, and broths. Lift off and discard hardened fat.
- Trim all visible fat from meat before cooking.
- Use water-packed, canned foods such as fruits and tuna.
- Use fresh fruits and vegetables often. Try to eat at least 2 1/2 cups of these foods each day.
- Use low-kilocalorie salad dressings.
- When you eat out, do not look at the menu. Instead, have an idea of what you would like to eat before you arrive at the restaurant. Explain to the waitress or waiter what you would like to eat.

Target heart rate—Seventy percent of maximum heart rate (number of heartbeats per minute); the rate at which the pulse should be maintained for at least 20 minutes during aerobic exercise.

Kilocaloric density—The kilocalories contained in a given volume of a food.

Nutrient density—The concentration of nutrients in a given volume of food compared with the food's kilocalorie content.

Empty kilocalories—Food that contains kilocalories and almost no other nutrients.

TABLE 6–4   Recommended Dietary Allowances for Energy

Category	Age or Condition	Weight (kg)	Height (in)	REE† (kcal/day)	Average Energy Allowance (kcal/day)* Per kg ‡	Per day
Infants	0–0.5	6	24	320	108	650
	0.5–1	9	28	500	98	850
Children	1–3	13	35	740	102	1300
	4–6	20	44	950	90	1800
	7–10	28	52	1130	70	2000
Males	11–14	45	62	1440	55	2500
	15–18	66	69	1760	45	3000
	19–24	72	70	1780	40	2900
	25–50	79	70	1800	37	2900
	51+	77	68	1530	30	2300
Females	11–14	46	62	1310	47	2200
	15–18	55	64	1370	40	2200
	19–24	58	65	1350	38	2200
	25–50	63	64	1380	36	2200
	51+	65	63	1280	30	1900
Pregnant 1st trimester						+0
2nd trimester						+300
3rd trimester						+300
Lactating 1st 6 months						+500
2nd 6 months						+500

SOURCE: Adapted from the Subcommittee on the 10th Edition of the RDAs, 1989, p. 33.
* Includes kilocalories needed for physical activity.
† Does not include kilocalories needed for physical activity.
‡ Based on a median age, weight, height, and light-to-moderate activity level.

Dietary Recommendations

All the major national health organizations recommend that individuals maintain a healthy body weight. The American Heart Association recommends maintaining a healthy body weight to decrease the risk of heart and circulatory diseases. The American Cancer Society cites numerous studies suggesting that lower kilocaloric intake may lower the risk of cancer. Most individuals would benefit by monitoring their weight and increasing their energy expenditure and/or decreasing their energy intake as necessary to maintain a healthy body weight.

Summary

Energy balance exists when energy intake equals energy output. A person at his or her stable body weight is usually in energy balance. About one-half to three-quarters of the population have the capability of regulating energy intake and expenditure to accommodate daily variations. When an individual is not in energy balance, he or she is gaining or losing body weight.

The human body needs energy for resting energy expenditure and voluntary physical activity. Energy allowances are calculated by multiplying an individual's resting energy expenditure by a factor for physical activity.

Foods high in water and fiber are low in kilocaloric density. Foods high in fat are high in kilocaloric density. Individuals should try to consume nutritionally dense foods. These foods are low in kilocalories and contain substantial amounts of one or more nutrients.

Americans have been decreasing both their food intake and activity for the past 10 years. The current recommendation is that individuals who gain weight while consuming their energy RDA should increase their activity to maintain energy balance, rather than decrease intake.

Case Study 6–1

The Fairview Nursing Home holds a weekly client care conference. All the facility's residents have their nursing care plans reviewed on a rotating basis, with each client's nursing care plan being reviewed once every 3 months. All members of the health care team are often present at the conference. Team members may include the administrator, the physician, the director of nursing, the staff nurse, the nursing assistant, the activities director, the social worker, the dietitian, and the client or a family member representing the client.

Mr. G has been experiencing a slow weight gain. His weight history follows:

1/89	175 lb
3/89	177 lb
7/89	178 lb
9/89	180 lb
12/89	181 lb

Mr. G is 5 ft, 8 in tall and is 79 years old. He is alert, feeds himself, and has normal bowel and bladder function. Mr. G walks to the dining room three times a day. His favorite activity is watching television. He has good dentition and is on a regular diet. According to the appetite records kept by the nurse's aide, Mr. G's intake is good to excellent. He accepts all the major food groups. Mr G is concerned with his slow weight gain but claims he does not know what to do. To address the slow weight gain problem, the health care team and Mr. G developed the following nursing care plan.

NURSING CARE PLAN

Assessment

Subjective Data Client expressed concern about his slow weight gain.

Objective Data Height is 5 ft, 8 in. Weights and percent healthy body weight:

1/89	175 lb	103 percent healthy body weight
12/89	181 lb	106 percent healthy body weight

Nursing Diagnosis Nutrition, altered: more than body requirements of energy related to knowledge deficit as evidenced by admitted lack of understanding and a gain in healthy body weight of 3 percent over the past year.

Desired Outcome/ Evaluation Criteria	Nursing Actions	Rationale
Client will maintain his present body weight over the next 3 months.	Weigh client once per week.	Monitoring body weight is necessary to determine the success or failure of the care plan.

Table continued on following page

Desired Outcome/ Evaluation Criteria	Nursing Actions	Rationale
Client will select fresh fruits for desserts at 50 percent of all social activities.	Provide encouragement to the client to select fresh fruit at all social activites. Congratulate the client when he is able to refrain from eating rich desserts. Remind the Dietary Department to serve fresh fruit at social functions.	Replacing kilocalorically dense cakes, pies, and cookies with fresh fruit will promote weight maintenance.
Client will keep a food diary and exercise log 1 day per week for the next 3 months.	Review the client's food record with him each week. Note all empty kilocalories consumed. Discuss the client's food selections and exercise log with him. Document results.	Self-monitoring of food intake and exercise will help the client focus on controlling his behaviors. Nurse's review of food records with the client while pointing out kilocalorically dense foods will educate the client about his negative behaviors.
Client will participate in the exercise program provided by the activities director at least seven times per week for the next 3 months.	Encourage the client to attend the exercise program or to walk ten minutes before each meal. Document the activity.	Exercise burns kilocalories and increases body protein content. A high body protein content is associated with increased energy expenditure.

Study Aids

Chapter Review

1. The two components of energy expenditure are _____ and _____ .
   a. Mental activity; physical activity
   b. Thermic effect of exercise; thermic effect of foods
   c. Resting energy expenditure; physical activity
   d. Thermic effect of foods; physical activity

2. Energy homeostasis exists when:
   a. Kilocalories from food intake = kilocalories used for energy expenditure.
   b. Kilocalories used for physical activity = kilocalories used for energy expenditure.
   c. An individual is gaining weight.
   d. Kilocalories from food intake = kilocalories used for resting energy expenditure.

3. A kilocalorie is a measure of:
   a. Weight
   b. Height
   c. Energy
   d. Fatness

4. An individual having well-developed muscle tissue compared with a similar individual who has poorly developed muscles:
   a. Needs to eat less food
   b. Needs to exercise more
   c. May have a higher resting energy expenditure
   d. Will tend to remain in positive energy balance

5. Which of the following foods is the *least* kilocalorically dense?
   a. 1 cup of sugar
   b. 1 cup of margarine
   c. 1 cup of skim milk
   d. 1 cup of celery

Clinical Analysis

1. Mr. I, resident of Sunnybrook Nursing Home, has been experiencing an undesirable slow weight loss. His weight history is as follows:
   Feb   180 pounds

June   175 pounds
Oct   170 pounds

As Mr. I's nurse, you should first:

a. Encourage Mr. I to eat only twice a day.
b. Call the doctor.
c. Wait for the next client care conference to act on this problem.
d. Monitor Mr. I's food intake to determine what he is eating.

2. A teacher has noticed that many students in her fifth grade class are overweight. As a school project, the class kept food records for 3 days. The records were analyzed by a computer software program. Many students were eating less than their recommended dietary allowance for kilocalories. The teacher shared this information with the school nurse and asked her to speak to the class. The school nurse correctly decided that:

a. The teacher is overly concerned since the proportion of overweight students approximates the proportion of overweight adults in the community.
b. The computer program must be in error.
c. All the students need to increase their total intake, including foods from the major food groups.
d. Many students would benefit from an increase in physical activity.

3. A client appears to be totally concerned with the kilocaloric density of foods and not at all concerned with the nutrient density of foods. You need to encourage the consumption of both types of foods. Which of the following behaviors do you need to discourage?

a. The substitution of skim milk for 2 percent milk
b. The avoidance of all red meat
c. Including dark green and yellow fruits and vegetables in the diet
d. Including whole grains in the diet

Bibliography

Bennett, WI: Beyond overeating. N Engl J Med 332:10, 673, 1995.

Blair, SN: Diet and activity: The synergistic merger. Nutrition Today 30:3, 108, 1995.

Cerra, F: Pocket Manual of Surgical Nutrition. CV Mosby, St. Louis, 1984, p. 61.

Hands, ES: Food Finder Food Sources of Vitamins and Minerals. ESHA Research, Salem, 1990.

Krahn DD, et al: Changes in resting energy expenditure and body composition in anorexia nervosa during refeeding. J Am Diet Assoc 93:4, 1993.

National Research Council: Diet and Health: Implications for Reducing Chronic Disease Risk. Report of the Committee on Diet and Health, Food and Nutrition Board, Commission on Life Sciences. National Academy Press, Washington, DC, 1989, p. 110.

Pale, RP: Physical activity and public health. JAMA 273:5, 402, 1995.

Subcommittee on the 10th Edition of the RDAs. Food and Nutrition Board. Commission of Life Sciences. National Research Council: Recommended Dietary Allowances. National Academy Press, Washington, DC, 1989, pp. 24–38.

Thomas, PR (ed): Improving America's Diet and Health: From Recommendations to Actions. Food and Nutrition Board Institute of Medicine. National Academy Press, Washington, DC, 1991.

CHAPTER 7

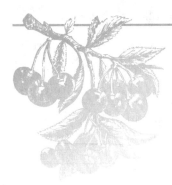

Vitamins

LEARNING OBJECTIVES

After completing this chapter, the student should be able to:

1 Differentiate between fat-soluble and water-soluble vitamins.
2 State the functions of each of the vitamins discussed.
3 Name three food sources for each of the vitamins discussed.
4 List diseases caused by specific vitamin deficiencies and identify associated signs and symptoms.
5 Identify the vitamins considered to be potential public health issues in the United States.
6 Discuss the wise use of vitamin supplements.

Vitamins were first recognized by the effects of their absence. Some deficiency diseases have been known for centuries, but it is only in this century that vitamins have been completely identified and isolated in the laboratory. In this chapter we will consider the importance of vitamins in the body and in the diet, the general functions of vitamins, the classification of vitamins, and the use of vitamin supplements. Each of the vitamins will be discussed from absorption through excretion, including functions, sources, recommended dietary allowances, deficiencies and toxicities, and factors affecting stability.

The Nature of Vitamins

Vitamins are organic substances needed by the body in small amounts for normal metabolism, growth, and maintenance. Organic substances are derived from living matter and contain carbon. Vitamins themselves are not sources of energy nor do they become part of the structure of the body. Vitamins act as regulators of metabolic processes and as **coenzymes** in enzymatic systems.

Specific Functions

Vitamin functions are specific; the bodily processes do not permit substitutes. Thus, vitamins are similar to keys in a lock. All the notches in a key have to fit the lock, or the key will not turn. One vitamin cannot perform the functions of another. If a person does not consume enough vitamin C, for instance, taking vitamin D will not correct the deficiency. Vitamin D is the wrong key for the lock.

Classification

A major distinguishing characteristic among vitamins is their solubility in either fat or water. Vitamins A, E, D, and K are fat soluble. The eight B-complex vitamins and vitamin C are water soluble. See Table 7–1 for a list of the 13 known vitamins.

Recommended Dietary Allowances

The amounts of vitamins recommended by the United States government to meet the needs of almost all healthy individuals are listed by age and physiological status (in Appendix F). Other countries have specified different amounts for their people.

Vitamins A, D, and E were formerly measured in International Units. Clinical Calculation 7–1 sum-

TABLE 7–1 Classification of Vitamins

Fat Soluble	Water Soluble
Vitamin A	B-Complex
Vitamin D	Thiamin
Vitamin E	Riboflavin
Vitamin K	Niacin
	Vitamin B_6
	Folic Acid
	Vitamin B_{12}
	Biotin
	Pantothenic acid
	Vitamin C

marizes the formulae to convert International Units to the newer units of measure.

The vitamins biotin and pantothenic acid are listed in a table of Estimated Safe and Adequate Daily Dietary Intakes (Appendix G). Because less is known about the need for these recently discovered vitamins, the guideline is less rigid.

Fat-Soluble Vitamins

Vitamins A, D, E, and K are more stable than the water-soluble vitamins. They are more resistant to the effects of oxidation, heat, light, and aging. However, the fat-soluble vitamins can be adversely affected by dehydration and sun drying.

Fat-soluble vitamins are absorbed from the intestine in the same way as fats, and, like fats, they can be stored in the body. Because of this storage capacity, excessive intake of fat-soluble vitamins, especially vitamins A and D, can be fatal. Another effect caused by the storage of these vitamins is the slow development of signs of deficiency. Of the fat-soluble vitamins, only vitamin A is considered to be a potential public health issue (US Department of Health and Human Services, 1989).

Vitamin A

Vitamin A comes in two forms: preformed vitamin A, **retinol,** and **provitamin A, carotene.** A

Vitamin—Organic substance needed by the body in very small amounts; yields no energy and does not become part of the body's structure.

Coenzyme—A substance that combines with an enzyme to activate it.

The Elusive International Unit

Formerly, fat-soluble vitamins were measured in International Units (IU), as defined by the International Conference for Unification of Formulae. A unit of vitamin A is not equal to a unit of vitamin D or to a unit of vitamin E. Because the old system is familiar to many people and still appears in laws, on labels, and in research reports, the formulae for conversion of International Units to the newer measures is given below.

Vitamin A

Animal foods—3.3 IU = 1 μg retinol equivalent
Plant foods —10 IU = 1 μg retinol equivalent

Vitamin D

400 IU = 10 μg of cholecalciferol

Vitamin E

1.5 IU = 1 μg of alpha-tocopherol equivalents

preformed vitamin is already in a complete state in ingested foods. A **provitamin** requires conversion in the body to be in a complete state. Carotene (provitamin A) is converted to vitamin A in the intestine. The term precursor is often used interchangeably with the term provitamin. A **precursor** is a substance from which another substance is derived.

Absorption, Metabolism, and Excretion

Of preformed vitamin A, 80 to 90 percent is absorbed, whereas only 33 percent of carotene is absorbed. Vitamin A is transported bound to a protein.

This complex is too large for the kidney to filter, so it is retained in the body.

Up to a year's supply of vitamin A is stored in the body, 90 percent of it in the liver. Excessive carotene is stored in adipose tissue, giving fat a yellowish tint, but it is harmless.

Functions of Vitamin A

Several crucial body functions depend on vitamin A. It is necessary for vision, for healthy epithelial tissue, for proper bone growth, and for energy regulation.

CHEMICAL NECESSARY FOR VISION   The eye is like a camera. It has a dark layer to keep out stray light, a lens to focus light, and a light-sensitive layer at the back of the eye, called the **retina.** In the retina, light rays are changed into electrical impulses that travel along the optic nerve to the back of the brain. Vitamin A is part of the molecules of a chemical in the retina that is responsible for this conversion. The body can synthesize this chemical, called **rhodopsin,** or visual purple, only if it has a supply of vitamin A.

When the eye is functioning in dim light, rhodopsin is broken down into a protein, called **opsin,** and vitamin A. In darkness or during sleep, opsin and vitamin A are reunited to become rhodopsin. Figure 7–1 diagrams this reaction. The body can keep reusing the vitamin A, but some of it is depleted during each visual cycle. This explains why a dietary deficiency produces **night blindness.** Clinical Application 7–1 discusses a practical method used to conserve a person's rhodopsin for night vision.

HEALTH OF EPITHELIAL TISSUE   **Epithelial tissue** covers the body and lines the organs and passageways that open to the outside of the body. Skin is epithelial tissue, as is the surface of the eye and the lining

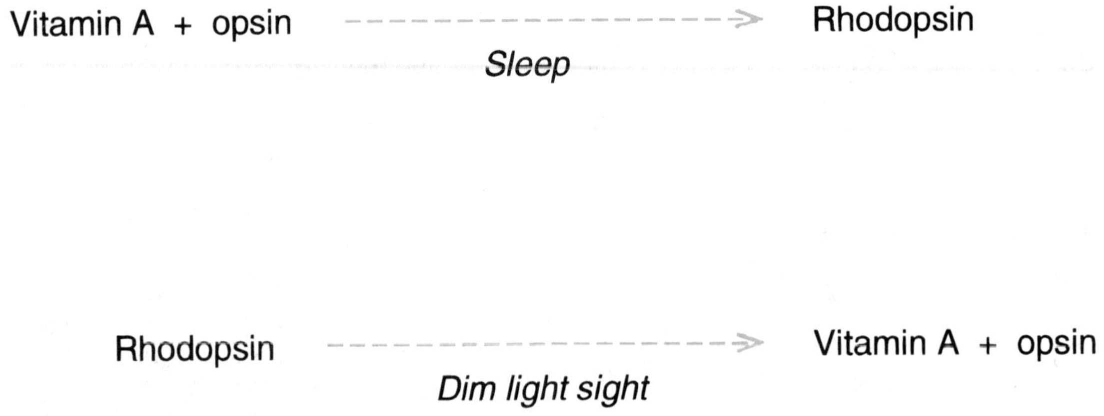

Vitamin A + opsin $- - - - - - - - - - - \longrightarrow$ Rhodopsin
                              Sleep

Rhodopsin $- - - - - - - - - - - \longrightarrow$ Vitamin A + opsin
              Dim light sight

FIGURE 7–1   Vitamin A and the protein opsin combine while we sleep to form rhodopsin. When we need to see in dim light, the rhodopsin breaks down into vitamin A and opsin.

of the alimentary canal. Epithelial tissue has a protective function, often producing mucus to wash out foreign materials. Vitamin A helps to keep epithelial tissue healthy by aiding the differentiation of specialty cells. This function has led some scientists to believe that vitamin A may play a role in cancer prevention. See Clinical Application 7–2 for more information on vitamin A and cancer.

NORMAL BONE GROWTH The mechanism by which vitamin A participates in bone growth and development is unclear. In children with vitamin A deficiency, some bones, such as those in the skull, stop growing, while other bones grow excessively.

ENERGY REGULATION Retinoic acid, a metabolite of vitamin A, has a role in heat production and the regulation of energy balance. Researchers are investigating the implications for obesity control (Wolf, 1995).

Deficiency of Vitamin A

Even though vitamin A is stored in the body, deficiencies can occur. In some parts of the world vitamin A deficiency is widespread. Cases are common in India, south and east Asia, Africa, and Latin America. Vitamin A deficiency is second only to pro-

tein-caloric malnutrition as a nutritional problem affecting young people.

Vitamin A deficiency in the United States is due mostly to disease. For example, patients with long-lasting infectious disease, fat absorption problems, or liver disease are at risk of vitamin A deficiency.

SIGNS AND SYMPTOMS Lack of vitamin A causes night blindness. In this condition the resynthesis of rhodopsin is too slow to allow quick adaptation to dim light.

All epithelial tissue suffers because of vitamin A deficiency. The person may have sinus trouble, a sore throat, and abscesses in the ears, mouth, and salivary glands. The most serious effect is the thickening of the epithelial tissue covering the eye. **Xerophthalmia,** an abnormal thickening and drying of the outer surface of the eye, is a leading cause of blindness in some developing countries. An estimated 500,000 children are blinded each year by this deficiency. The World Health Organization recommends vitamin A supplementation in conjunction with immunization.

Measles still causes 1.5 million deaths worldwide every year. Vitamin A supplementation to children hospitalized with measles reduced the risk of death about 60 percent overall and 90 percent in infants. The World Health Organization recommends vitamin A supplementation to all measles patients in developing countries (Fawzi, et al, 1993).

Vitamin A is related to normal bone growth and development. In the person deficient in vitamin A, the cessation of bone growth produces brain and spinal cord injury.

Recommended Dietary Allowances

The recommended dietary allowance for vitamin A is 800 **retinol equivalents** (RE) for women and 1000 RE for men. One RE corresponds to 1 **microgram** of retinol activity.

Preformed vitamin—A vitamin already in a complete state in ingested foods, as opposed to a provitamin, which requires conversion in the body to be in a complete state.

Rhodopsin—Light-sensitive protein containing vitamin A in the retina; also called visual purple.

Microgram—One millionth of a gram or one thousandth of a milligram; abbreviated mcg or μg.

Food Sources and Preservation of Vitamin A

Preformed vitamin A (retinol) is found in animal foods such as liver, kidney, egg yolk, and fortified milk products. However, two-thirds of the vitamin A in the American diet comes from carotene. Carotene is a yellow pigment found mostly in fruits and vegetables. Its presence can be readily seen in foods such as carrots, sweet potatoes, squash, apricots, and cantaloupe. Although not as noticeable because chlorphyll masks the yellow color, carotene is also present in dark leafy green vegetables, including spinach, collards, broccoli, and cabbage.

Vitamin A is fairly stable to heat, but sunlight, ultraviolet light, air, and oxidation easily destroy it. Carrots that come packaged in plastic bags are better protected from light and air than the "bouquets" secured by a rubber band.

Toxicity of Vitamin A

Most other vitamin toxicities are a result of supplementation. Hypervitaminosis A can be caused by foods. The special hazard to the fetus is discussed in Chapter 11; "Life Cycle Nutrition: Pregnancy and Lactation."

CAROTENEMIA   The condition resulting from ingesting too much carotene is called **carotenemia.** The person's skin becomes yellow, first on the palms of the hands and the soles of the feet. The whites of the eyes do not become yellow, however, as they do in jaundice caused by liver disease.

Carotenemia has occurred in infants fed too many jars of carrots and squash. The skin returns to normal within 2 to 6 weeks after stopping the excessive intake. Carotenemia produces no adverse effects.

HYPERVITAMINOSIS A   Vitamin A toxicity is called **hypervitaminosis A.** Symptoms of vitamin A toxicity are similar to those of a brain tumor. Clients may complain of headaches and blurred vision and display signs of increased pressure within the skull. Other symptoms include pain in the bones and joints, dry skin, and poor appetite. Some clients developed symptoms after consuming beef liver once or twice a week. Self-prescribed vitamin A supplements have produced liver failure. One client died after consuming 25,000 **International Units** (IU) daily for 6 years (Kowalski, et al, 1994). The same intake was judged sufficient to cause cirrhosis in another study (Geubel, et al, 1991).

One hazard is unique to the Arctic. Polar bear liver has made both men and dogs sick. It contains 354,545 micrograms RE per 3-ounce serving. This is 354 times the RDA for men. Other Arctic game poses similar hazards.

Vitamin D

Recently, vitamin D has come to be regarded as a hormone rather than a vitamin because of its functions. Changing its name may be difficult, however.

Absorption, Metabolism, and Excretion

Two forms of vitamin D are metabolically active. Vitamin D_2, **ergocalciferol,** is formed when ergosterol (provitamin) in plants is irradiated by sunlight. Vitamin D_3, **cholecalciferol,** is formed when 7-dehydrocholesterol (another provitamin) in the skin is irradiated by ultraviolet light or sunlight.

Both forms are absorbed into the blood. As with other fat-soluble vitamins, they are transported in the blood bound to protein. The liver alters the vitamin to **calcidiol,** an inactive form of vitamin D. By enzyme action, the kidney converts the calcidiol to **calcitriol,** the active form of vitamin D. Figure 7–2 diagrams the path of these processes.

Functions of Vitamin D

Vitamin D promotes normal bone mineralization in three ways. (1) Vitamin D stimulates DNA to produce transport proteins, which bind calcium and phosphorus, thus increasing intestinal absorption of these minerals. (2) Once these minerals have been absorbed into the blood, vitamin D stimulates bone cells to use them to build and maintain bone tissue. (3) Vitamin D stimulates the kidneys to return calcium to the bloodstream.

Another control mechanism is also at work. **Parathyroid hormone** is secreted in response to a low serum calcium level. Parathyroid hormone causes the catabolism of bone to maintain a correct serum calcium level. The body's priority goal is maintenance of correct serum calcium for blood clotting, nerve function, and muscle contraction. Without this mechanism to sustain vital functions, a person would not live long enough to develop rickets.

Deficiency of Vitamin D

Lack of sunshine or vitamin D, chronic liver or kidney disease, or rare genetic disorders are causes of vitamin D deficiency. Of particular concern are children whose bones are still growing.

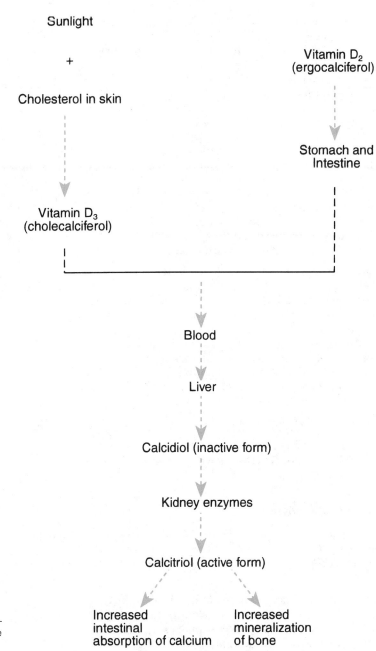

FIGURE 7–2 Vitamin D, whether from food or synthesis in the skin, is metabolized by the liver and the kidneys to its most active form.

RICKETS Vitamin D deficiency in children is called **rickets.** Twenty-four cases occurred in Philadelphia between 1974 and 1978 (Brown, 1990). These patients were children who belonged to a particular religious sect. They wore long hooded robes and ate vegetarian diets. At greatest risk in the United States are dark-skinned children in northern, smoggy cities or breast-fed infants not exposed to sunlight.

Carotenemia—Excess carotene in body tissues, producing yellow skin but leaving whites of eyes white.

Hypervitaminosis—Condition caused by excessive intake of vitamins.

OSTEOMALACIA Vitamin D deficiency in adults is called **osteomalacia.** This deficiency disease occurs most often in women who have insufficient calcium intake and little sunlight exposure, and who are frequently pregnant or lactating.

Environmental factors involved in osteomalacia are similar to those described for rickets. People with skin exposed to little sunlight have increased risk: cloistered nuns, office workers, institutionalized elderly persons, and residents of smoggy areas. Low serum vitamin D levels were found in free-living elderly Europeans (van der Wielen, et al, 1995).

Because of the complex processes involved in vitamin D metabolism, liver or kidney disease can lead to bone deterioration. Chronic kidney failure has caused osteomalacia due to the inability of the kidneys to convert vitamin D to its active form.

SIGNS AND SYMPTOMS Children with rickets have soft, fragile bones. Classic deformities occur, such as bowlegs, knock knees, and a misshapen skull. Infants may have **tetany** due to low levels of blood calcium.

Adults with osteomalacia also have increasing softness of the bones causing deformities due to loss of calcium. The bones most commonly affected are those of the spine, pelvis, and lower extremities.

Recommended Dietary Allowances

Vitamin D is measured in micrograms of cholecalciferol. The adult RDA for vitamin D is 5 micrograms.

Sources of Vitamin D

Two sources of vitamin D are readily available to most people. Vitamin D is synthesized by the body, and it is added to most dairy products in the United States.

SUNLIGHT A major source of vitamin D is the body itself. Vitamin D is manufactured in the skin. Children with low dietary intakes may escape rickets if they are exposed to sunlight.

Light-skinned adults can obtain the necessary 5 micrograms of cholecalciferol by exposing their hands, arms, and face to sunlight for 15 minutes twice a week. It is not possible to overdose on vitamin D from sunshine.

FOOD If a person is not exposed to sunshine, food sources of vitamin D become important. Few natural foods contain enough vitamin D to meet recommended intakes. Cod liver oil, containing 113 percent of children's RDA in 1 teaspoonful, is the exception.

CLINICAL APPLICATION 7–3

Fortification of Foods: Use and Misuse

Fortification is the addition of nutrients to foods in amounts greater than normally present to prevent deficiencies. Many cereals are fortified with vitamins and minerals not normally found in grains. Fluid milk must be fortified with vitamin D in the United States, but there are no mandates for other dairy products.

Occasionally, intentions are better than practices. Between 1985 and 1991, 56 cases of hypervitaminosis D were identified in Massachusetts. Two individuals died as a result and nine were discharged from the hospital with residual effects. Although state law required an upper limit of 500 IU (12.5 micrograms) of vitamin D per quart, the implicated dairy's milk exceeded this by 70 to 600 times (Blank, et al, 1995).

The major food source of vitamin D in the United States is fortified milk. One quart of fortified milk provides the RDA for children. Milk is the ideal food to link with vitamin D since it also contains calcium and phosphorus, which are necessary for bone anabolism. See Clinical Application 7–3 on the fortification of foods.

Stability and Interfering Factors

Vitamin D is stable to heat and not easily oxidized. Little special handling of foods is necessary. A high-fiber diet interferes with the absorption of vitamin D. Abnormalities of absorption such as diarrhea, fat malabsorption, and biliary obstruction also may lead to vitamin D deficiency.

Toxicity of Vitamin D

Since vitamin D is stored in the body, it is possible to ingest too much. Vitamin D from supplements or even foods can be hazardous to health.

MOST TOXIC OF VITAMINS Ten times the RDA for adults and two times the RDA for children, taken for several months can be toxic. Infants face increased risk from multiple fortified foods. One quart of prepared commercial formula contains 10 micrograms of cholecalciferol, the same as a quart of fortified milk. Infants up to 6 months old require only 7.5 micrograms per day.

SIGNS AND SYMPTOMS Clinical manifestations of hypervitaminosis D include loss of appetite, nausea, vomiting, polyuria, muscular weakness, and constipation. The more serious consequences of vitamin D overdose result from calcium deposits in the heart, kidney, and brain.

Vitamin E

The third fat-soluble vitamin is vitamin E. Much less is known about vitamin E than about vitamins A and D.

Absorption, Metabolism, and Excretion

Most vitamin E is stored in adipose tissue. Maximum transfer of vitamin E across the placenta occurs just before term delivery.

Functions of Vitamin E

The major function of vitamin E is as an **antioxidant. Oxidation** is the process of a substance combining with oxygen. Several substances can be destroyed by oxidation, including vitamin E, vitamin A, and vitamin C. Some molecules become very unstable when they are oxidized. Their accelerated movements can damage nearby molecules. Vitamin E accepts oxygen instead of allowing other molecules to become unstable. In this role, vitamin E protects vitamin A and unsaturated fatty acids from oxidation. Vitamin E in lung cell membranes provides an important barrier against air pollution. It also protects the stability of the polyunsaturated fatty acids in the red blood cell membranes from oxidation in the lungs. Oxidation is suspected of contributing to cataract formation and macular degeneration of the retina, although early research produced inconsistent findings. Three large clinical trials are in progress (Christen, 1994). Two antioxidants not being tested, lutein and zeaxanthin, found in spinach and collard greens, also have been associated with a dose-dependent reduction in age-related macular degeneration (Hankinson and Stampfer, 1994).

Deficiency of Vitamin E

In animals, vitamin E deficiency produces sterility. In several species of animals, a deficiency of vitamin E suppresses the immune system, whereas supplementation stimulates it.

Deficiency of vitamin E in humans is very rare. Muscle weakness and forms of muscular dystrophy are seen in cases of chronic fat malabsorption. Premature infants with inadequate reserves of vitamin E develop anemia. Without sufficient vitamin E the membranes of the red blood cells break down easily when exposed to oxygen or an oxidizing agent.

Recommended Dietary Allowances

Vitamin E is measured in milligrams of **alpha-tocopherol equivalents (α-TE).** The RDA is 8 milligrams for women and 10 milligrams for men.

Food Sources and Preservation of Vitamin E

Vitamin E occurs with polyunsaturated fatty acids. The best source is vegetable oils, but whole grains and wheat germ also provide vitamin E. Other sources include milk, eggs, meats, fish, and leafy vegetables. Vitamin E is fairly stable to heat and acid. Normal cooking temperatures do not destroy it, but frying does. Vitamin E is unstable to light, alkalies, and oxygen.

Toxicity of Vitamin E

Very large supplemental doses of more than 600 milligrams of alpha-tocopherol daily (60 times the RDA) for a year or longer may cause excessive bleeding, impaired wound healing, and depression. Clinical Application 7–4 describes a patient with vitamin E toxicity.

Vitamin K

Nurses should understand the functions of vitamin K because it is often prescribed as a medication. It also can interfere with a commonly prescribed anticoagulant.

Absorption, Metabolism, and Excretion

Three forms of vitamin K can meet the body's needs. Vitamin K_1, or **phylloquinone,** is the one found in foods. Vitamin K_2, or **menaquinone,** is synthesized by intestinal bacteria. Vitamin K_3, or **menadione,** is the synthetic, water-soluble pharmaceutical form of the vitamin. Vitamin K_3 is two to three times more potent than naturally occurring vitamin K.

Tetany—Muscle contractions, especially of the wrists and ankles, resulting from low levels of ionized calcium in the blood; causes include parathyroid deficiency, vitamin D deficiency, and alkalosis.

Antioxidant—Substance that prevents or inhibits the uptake of oxygen; in the body, antioxidants prevent tissue damage from unstable molecules; in food, antioxidants prevent deterioration; vitamins A, C, and E and selenium are antioxidants.

Functions of Vitamin K

The role of vitamin K in blood clotting has been known for a long time. An additional function of vitamin K relates to bone metabolism.

BLOOD CLOTTING   At least 13 different proteins plus the mineral calcium are involved in blood clotting. Vitamin K is necessary for the liver to make factors II (**prothrombin**), VII, IX, and X. These factors are key links in the chain of events producing a blood clot.

BONE METABOLISM   A protein has been identified in bone that depends on vitamin K. Vitamin K participates with vitamin D in synthesizing this bone protein, which helps to regulate serum calcium.

Deficiency of Vitamin K

The intestinal tract of the newborn infant is sterile. For this reason the baby is unable to produce vitamin K until the intestine picks up bacteria from the infant's environment, usually within 24 hours. To prevent bleeding problems, a dose of vitamin K_3 may be administered to the mother late in labor or to the infant immediately after birth.

Deficiencies have been associated with disease and drug therapy. Fat absorption problems may hinder vitamin K absorption, resulting in prolonged blood clotting time. Antibiotics kill the normal bacteria in the intestine as well as the organisms causing an infection. In one study, 31 percent of clients with gastrointestinal disorders given antibiotics for prolonged periods developed vitamin K deficiencies (Krasinski and Russell, 1985).

Recommended Dietary Allowances

The RDAs for vitamin K are 65 micrograms for women and 80 for men. The typical US diet supplies 300 to 500 micrograms.

Sources of Vitamin K

The body is capable of manufacturing some vitamin K. Many common foods also contain adequate amounts.

INTESTINAL SYNTHESIS   Approximately half the body's needed vitamin K is manufactured by intestinal bacteria. This synthesis takes place in the large intestine.

FOOD SOURCES   Liver, green leafy vegetables, vegetables of the cabbage family, and milk are the best sources of vitamin K. Examples of the vegetables include lettuce, spinach, asparagus, kale, cabbage, cauliflower, broccoli, and brussels sprouts.

Stability and Interfering Factors

Vitamin K resists heat but is unstable in the presence of oxygen, light, alkalies, and strong acids. Overconsumption of some vitamins can trigger a deficiency of others. Excessive intakes of vitamins A and E may interfere with vitamin K. The anticoagulant **warfarin sodium** interferes with the liver's use of vitamin K. However, this is the desired effect of the medication.

Toxicity of Vitamin K

The naturally occuring forms, vitamins K_1 and K_2, do not cause toxicity. Vitamin K_3, menadione, can cause liver damage, jaundice, excessive bleeding,

TABLE 7–2 Fat-Soluble Vitamins

Vitamin	Adult RDA and Food Portion Containing RDA	Functions	Deficiency Disease	Signs and Symptoms of Deficiency	Best Sources
A	800 to 1000 RE 0.5 cup frzn. or canned carrots	Dim light vision Differentiation of epithelial cells Normal bone growth	Nightblindness Xerophthalmia	Nightblindness Sore throat, sinus trouble, ear and mouth abscesses Dry and thick outer covering of eye Blindness	Preformed: liver, kidney, egg yolk, fortified milk Provitamin: carrots, sweet potatoes, squash, apricots, cantaloupe, spinach, collards, broccoli, cabbage
D	5 μg	Increases intestinal absorption of calcium	Rickets	Bowlegs, knock-knees, misshapen skull Tetany in infants	Sunlight on skin Fortified milk Cod liver oil
	2 cups fortified milk	Stimulates bone production Decreases urinary excretion of calcium	Osteomalacia	Soft fragile bones, especially of spine, pelvis, lower extremities	
E	8 to 10 mg 1 tbsp corn oil	Antioxidant Protects polyunsaturated fatty acids in red blood cell membranes from oxidation in lungs	No specific term	Animals: sterility, suppression of immune system Humans: Muscle weakness; forms of muscular dystrophy Anemia in premature infants	Vegetable oils Whole grains, wheat germ
K	65 to 80 μg 0.75 cup raw cabbage	Used in manufacture of several clotting factors, including prothrombin Assists vitamin D to synthesize a regulatory bone protein	No specific term	Prolonged clotting time	Synthesis in large intestine Green leafy vegetables Liver

hemolysis of red blood cells, and brain damage. As with all drugs, extra care must be taken when administering vitamin K to infants. Overdose in an infant may cause **hemolytic anemia, hyperbilirubinemia,** and irreversible brain damage.

Table 7–2 summarizes the information on the fat soluble vitamins. Table 7–3 summarizes the stability of vitamins to environmental conditions. See Clinical Application 7–5 for a description of two conditions that mimic deficiencies of fat-soluble vitamins.

Water-Soluble Vitamins

Vitamins that dissolve in water are vitamin C, or **ascorbic acid,** and the B vitamins. The B vitamins include thiamin, riboflavin, niacin, pyridoxine,

> **Prothrombin**—A protein essential to the blood clotting process; manufactured by the liver using vitamin K.

TABLE 7–3 Factors Affecting Stability of Vitamins

Vitamin	Stable to				
	Oxygen	Heat	Light	Acids	Alkalies
Fat Soluble					
A	No	Yes	No	No	*
D	Yes	Yes	Yes	*	*
E	No	Yes	No	Yes	No
K	No	Yes	No	No	No
Water Soluble					
C	No	No	No	Yes	No
Thiamin	No	No	*	*	No
Riboflavin	Yes	Yes	No	Yes	No
Niacin	Yes	Yes	Yes	Yes	Yes
B_6	*	Yes	No	Yes	No
Folic acid	No	No	No	No	Yes
B_{12}	No	Yes	No	No	No

* Data unavailable.

folic acid, vitamin B_{12}, pantothenic acid, and biotin.

Water-soluble vitamins are easily destroyed by cooking. For example, one-third to one-half of the vitamin content is lost in the cooking water of boiled vegetables. However, in spite of the heavy losses of all water-soluble vitamins through cooking, only intakes of vitamin C, vitamin B_6, and folic acid are considered to be potential public health issues (US Department of Health and Human Services, 1989).

Vitamin C

Most animals manufacture vitamin C in their livers. Humans, along with other primates, guinea pigs, some birds, some fish, and fruit-eating bats, cannot synthesize vitamin C.

Absorption, Metabolism, and Excretion

Vitamin C is absorbed from the small intestine. A small amount of vitamin C is stored in the adrenal glands, liver, and spleen. As the amount of vitamin C consumed increases, the proportion of the vitamin that is absorbed decreases. So if 100 milligrams is ingested, 90 percent is absorbed. If 1000 milligrams is ingested, less than 70 percent is absorbed. If 10,000 milligrams is taken, less than 20 percent is absorbed. Whatever is absorbed in excess of body needs is excreted in the urine.

Functions of Vitamin C

Vitamin C has diverse functions in the body. It contributes to wound and fracture healing, serves as an antioxidant, and is necessary for adrenal gland function. It enhances the absorption of iron and converts folic acid, a B vitamin, to an active form.

WOUND AND FRACTURE HEALING   Vitamin C contributes to the healing of wounds, burns, and fractures. It is necessary in the formation of **collagen,** the single most important protein of connective tissue. Both bone and scar tissue contain collagen.

ANTIOXIDANT   Vitamin C is a powerful antioxidant. By preventing the uptake of oxygen by other molecules, it deters the destruction of tissue by unstable molecules. Vitamin C is more susceptible to oxidation than either vitamin E or vitamin A; thus it is called the antioxidants' antioxidant.

ADRENAL GLAND FUNCTION   High concentrations of vitamin C are found in the **adrenal glands.** These are the organs that secrete adrenalin, the "fight or flight" hormone, in times of stress. Vitamin C aids in the release of adrenalin from the adrenal glands. Emotional and physical stress increase the body's need for vitamin C by three to four times.

IRON ABSORPTION   Vitamin C facilitates iron absorption. It acts with hydrochloric acid to keep iron in the more absorbable ferrous (2^+) form. Four ounces of orange juice nearly quadruples the iron absorbed from plant foods consumed with it.

FOLIC ACID CONVERSION   Vitamin C converts folic acid to an active form. For this reason deficiency of vitamin C can lead to **anemia** due to inefficient use of iron and folic acid.

CLINICAL APPLICATION 7–5

Conditions Mimicking Deficiencies of Fat-Soluble Vitamins

Protein Deficiency

Water and fat do not mix. To circulate fats in the water-based blood, the liver attaches fat-soluble vitamins to protein carriers. Sometimes a protein deficiency hinders the use of the fat-soluble vitamins.

Zinc Deficiency

Vitamin A is carried from storage in the liver to the tissues by a zinc-containing protein. For this reason zinc deficiency can mimic vitamin A deficiency.

Deficiency of Vitamin C

Until the 17th century, sailors on long voyages often died of **scurvy** due to lack of vitamin C. The disease develops within 3 months after vitamin C is eliminated from the diet.

SIGNS AND SYMPTOMS   Early signs of scurvy are tender, sore gums that bleed easily and small skin hemorrhages due to weakened blood vessels. The late manifestations of scurvy relate to the break down of collagen. Wound healing is delayed; even healed scars may separate. The ends of long bones soften, become malformed and painful, and fractures appear. The teeth loosen in their sockets and fall out. Hemorrhages occur about the joints, stomach, and heart. Untreated, scurvy progresses to often sudden death, probably from internal bleeding.

TREATMENT   Moderate doses of vitamin C will cure scurvy. A daily dose of 300 milligrams (5 times the RDA) replenishes the body tissues in 5 days.

PREVALENCE OF VITAMIN C DEFICIENCY   As many as 25 percent of persons surveyed have a vitamin C intake well below the RDA. Intake may be less than half the RDA for infants, teens, and the elderly. At particular risk are elderly persons living alone, persons avoiding acidic foods, and patients receiving peritoneal or hemodialysis.

Recommended Dietary Allowances

The RDA for adults is 60 milligrams. As little as 10 milligrams per day prevents scurvy. A daily intake of 200 milligrams completely saturates the tissues. Data from a depletion-repletion study and criteria from the Institute of Medicine suggest an RDA of 200 milligrams is appropriate, which still could be achieved by ingestion of five servings of fruits and vegetables (Levine, et al, 1996). After major surgery or extensive burns, a client may need up to 1000 milligrams of vitamin C per day.

Food Sources of Vitamin C

Citrus fruits are excellent sources. Other good sources of vitamin C include green peppers, tomatoes, white potatoes, cabbage, broccoli, chard, kale, turnip greens, asparagus, berries, melons, pineapple, and guavas. Three vegetables high in vitamins A and C are shown in Figure 7–3.

Stability and Preservation

Vitamin C is destroyed by air, light, heat, or alkalies. Boiling the cooking water for 1 minute before add-

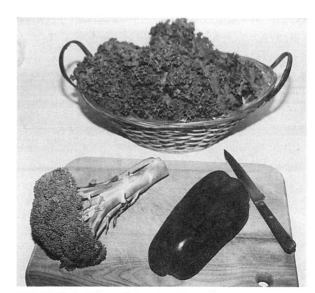

FIGURE 7–3   Broccoli, kale, and red pepper are excellent sources of vitamins A and C.

ing the food eliminates the dissolved oxygen that would oxidize the vitamin C. Orange juice should be stored in an opaque container which holds only an amount that can be consumed in a short time.

Vegetables should be cooked as quickly as possible. Crisp-cooked is better than limp-cooked for retaining the vitamin C content. In years past many food establishments routinely added baking soda to vegetables to enhance their color but the alkali also destroyed the vitamin C. Fortunately this practice is now illegal.

Interfering Factor

Smokers deplete vitamin C faster than nonsmokers. At least 100 milligrams per day are required by smokers to achieve the same tissue saturation as nonsmokers do with 60 milligrams (Levine, et al, 1995). Unfortunately, many smokers do not consume even the RDA.

Collagen—Fibrous insoluble protein found in connective tissue.

Anemia—Condition of less than normal values for red blood cells or hemoglobin or both.

Scurvy—Disease due to deficiency of vitamin C, marked by bleeding problems and, later, by bony skeleton changes.

Toxicity of Vitamin C

Rebound scurvy occurs when a person suddenly stops taking **megadoses** of vitamin C. The body cannot adjust quickly enough and continues to absorb a meager proportion of the now smaller dose. A similar condition occurs in newborns whose mothers took megadoses of vitamin C during pregnancy. Scurvy can occur under these circumstances.

Excessive vitamin C causes false readings in two common laboratory tests. Some urine glucose tests will read falsely positive. Stool guaiac for occult blood will read falsely negative.

B-Complex Vitamins

Eight vitamins belong to the B-complex group: thiamin, riboflavin, niacin, pyridoxine (B_6), folic acid, cyanocobalamin (B_{12}), pantothenic acid, and biotin. They all function as coenzymes. A coenzyme joins with an enzyme to activate it. If a person lacks the coenzyme, the effect is the same as lacking the enzyme itself. Many of the actions of the B-complex vitamins are interrelated giving rise to a theory that combinations of low vitamin intakes may have a greater impact on health than the sum of their individual effects (Lowik, et al, 1994). In 1992 to 1993 an epidemic of peripheral neuropathy in Cuba was attributed to deficiencies of thiamin, folate, cobalamine, and sulfur-containing amino acids. Increased risk was found among those who smoked, missed meals, drank alcohol, lost weight, or consumed excessive sugar (Roman, 1994). However, some diseases, including beriberi and pellagra, are associated with single B-vitamin deficiencies.

Thiamin

Beriberi is the deficiency disease due to the lack of **thiamin,** a vitamin originally named B_1. The neurological symptoms of beriberi were recognized in China in 2600 BC, but it was not until 1937 that thiamin was chemically identified as the causative agent. The enrichment of food products has almost eliminated this disease, but it is still seen in alcoholics in the West and in persons in developing countries where enrichment may not be a standard practice.

ABSORPTION, METABOLISM, AND EXCRETION   Thiamin is absorbed in the small intestine. The need for thiamin increases proportionately with carbohydrate intake. Excess thiamin is excreted in the urine.

FUNCTIONS OF THIAMIN   Thiamin is a coenzyme in carbohydrate metabolism. It is involved in the production of energy from glucose and helps oxidize glucose to form a compound which stores energy. Thiamin is required to convert **tryptophan** to niacin, another B-vitamin.

DEFICIENCY   The deficiency disease beriberi is characterized by neurological, cerebral, and cardiovascular abnormalities. Initially, symptoms such as anorexia, indigestion, and constipation occur because the digestive process is disrupted due to interrupted glucose metabolism. Without a continual supply of glucose for the central nervous system (CNS), apathy, fatigue, and muscle weakness set in. The **myelin sheaths** covering peripheral nerves eventually degenerate, resulting in paralysis and muscle atrophy. If the thiamin deficiency continues, cardiac failure and then death is the result.

Wernicke-Korsakoff syndrome, a neurological disorder associated with chronic alcoholism, results from thiamin deficiency. Thiamin is used to convert alcohol to energy. Clients with **Wernicke's encephalopathy** display many motor and sensory deficits. The person with **Korsakoff's psychosis** has short-term memory deficits.

RECOMMENDED DIETARY ALLOWANCES   The RDAs for thiamine are 1 to 1.5 milligrams for adults. The need for thiamin increases as kilocaloric consumption increases. An athlete consuming 4000 kilocalories needs twice as much as an office worker consuming 1800 kilocalories. Fasting does not decrease the need for thiamin, however. The need is proportional to energy expenditure, not simply food intake.

FOOD SOURCES   Pork, wheat germ, yeast, black beans, black-eyed peas, sunflower seeds, and fortified cereals are the best sources. Many other commonly consumed foods contain lesser amounts. A person who chooses enriched grains and eats a balanced diet should have no problems with lack of thiamin.

STABILITY AND INTERFERING FACTORS   Thiamin is destroyed by air and heat. The destruction is especially pronounced in the presence of alkalies. An enzyme in raw fish, **thiaminase,** destroys up to 50 percent of thiamin. Tea contains an **antagonist** to thiamin.

Riboflavin

Riboflavin, or B_2, was discovered when laboratory workers observed a yellow-green fluorescent pigment that formed crystals.

ABSORPTION, METABOLISM, AND EXCRETION   Absorption of riboflavin occurs in the small intestine. Only small amounts are stored in the liver and kidneys, so daily needs must be supplied in the diet.

FUNCTIONS   Riboflavin is a coenzyme in the metabolism of protein. Thyroid and adrenal hormones control the conversion of riboflavin to the active coenzyme, which is involved in deamination and tissue building.

DEFICIENCY   Riboflavin deficiency often occurs with thiamine and niacin deficiencies. A person who avoids all dairy products, however, may be deficient in riboflavin alone, termed **ariboflavinosis.** Signs of this deficiency include lesions on the lips and in the oral cavity, seborrheic dermatitis, scrotal or vulval skin changes, and normocytic anemia.

RECOMMENDED DIETARY ALLOWANCES   The RDAs for riboflavin are 1.2 to 1.7 milligrams for adults.

Riboflavin needs increase as protein needs increase. Clients facing major healing processes, such as those with extensive burns, require more riboflavin than the average person.

FOOD SOURCES   Good sources are organ meats, milk, whole or enriched grains, legumes, and vegetables.

STABILITY   Riboflavin is relatively stable to heat but is sensitive to ultraviolet light. Cardboard milk cartons or opaque plastic bottles filter out more light than clear glass bottles.

Niacin

Niacin, or nicotinic acid, is vitamin B_3. Lack of niacin causes a specific disease, pellagra.

ABSORPTION, METABOLISM, AND EXCRETION   Not all nutrients present in a food are available to the body. Niacin is found in corn but in a bound form that cannot be absorbed. Treating the corn with lye, as is done in some Latin American cultures, frees the niacin for the body's use. See Figure 7–3.

Not all the body's niacin has to come from preformed niacin in food. The body can convert the amino acid tryptophan to niacin. This is the only known vitamin with an amino acid for a provitamin.

FUNCTIONS OF NIACIN   Niacin is a coenzyme in the production of energy from glucose. Niacin also participates in the synthesis of fatty acids.

DEFICIENCY   **Pellagra** is the deficiency disease caused by the lack of niacin. To have a deficiency, a person must have a diet lacking in both niacin and tryptophan. Adults can get up to 67 percent of their niacin from foods containing complete proteins.

Pellagra has serious effects. The "three Ds" are its major symptoms: dermatitis, diarrhea, and dementia. The dermatitis is a red rash on the face, neck, hands, and feet. The rash is bilaterally symmetrical; on the hands and arms it sometimes resembles gloves.

RECOMMENDED DIETARY ALLOWANCES   The RDAs for adults are 13 to 19 milligrams NE. Niacin is measured in **niacin equivalents (NE).** One milligram of niacin equivalent is the same as 1 milligram of preformed niacin or 60 milligrams of tryptophan.

FOOD SOURCES   Preformed niacin occurs in significant amounts of meat. Other sources include peanuts and legumes. Coffee also contains niacin and prevents pellagra in cultures with low protein and high coffee intakes.

STABILITY   Niacin is a water-soluble vitamin. Small amounts are lost in cooking water. Niacin is stable to heat, light, air, acid, and alkalies. It is the most environmentally stable vitamin.

TOXICITY   Pharmacological doses of niacin cause flushing. The large doses prescribed to lower blood lipid levels over the long term can cause liver damage (Committee on Diet and Health, 1989). A case of niacin toxicity from food is reported in

---

Rebound scurvy—Vitamin C deficiency produced in a person following cessation of megadosing due to a habitually lessened rate of absorption.

Megadose—Dose ten times the RDA.

Wernicke's encephalopathy—Inflammatory, hemorrhagic, degenerative lesions in several areas of the brain resulting in double vision, involuntary eye movements, lack of muscle coordination, and mental deficits; caused by thiamin deficiency often in chronic alcoholism but also in gastrointestinal tract disease and hyperemesis gravidarum.

Korsakoff's psychosis—Amnesia, often seen in chronic alcoholism, caused by degeneration of the thalamus due to thiamin deficiency; characterized by loss of short-term memory and inability to learn new skills.

Antagonist—A substance that counteracts the action of another substance.

Pellagra—Deficiency disease due to lack of niacin and tryptophan; characterized by the 3 Ds: dermatitis, diarrhea, and dementia.

CLINICAL APPLICATION 7–6

Niacin Toxicity

In late 1980, almost half the clients in a small nursing home in Illinois became ill after breakfast. Their faces became flushed, or they developed a rash 15 to 30 minutes after the meal. As in suspected food poisoning epidemics, the foods consumed were compared. Which food was eaten by all those who became ill, but by none of those who did not become ill? In this case, it was cornmeal mush.

Careful observation and documentation is important in food poisoning cases. The sequence of signs and symptoms may steer the investigators in the right direction. Often the signs and symptoms have disappeared by the time the physician arrives. In this nursing home, the signs and symptoms lasted only an average of 50 minutes.

If food poisoning is suspected, health authorities take samples of the food to examine in the laboratory. None of the leftover food should be discarded before health authorities arrive. The Food and Drug Administration tested the cornmeal from the nursing home's kitchen. It contained more than 1000 mg of niacin per pound. The recommended amount for cornmeal is 16 to 24 mg/lb.

Often a food poisoning epidemic has run its course by the time the source of the outbreak is known. In this case, the offending food was identified, but the method of contamination never was positively determined.

Clinical Application 7–6. It explains how food poisoning epidemics are investigated and what the nurse's responsibilities are when assisting with the investigation.

Vitamin B_6

This vitamin serves in many roles, but its lack is not described as a specific disease. The name for the pharmaceutical preparation of vitamin B_6 is **pyridoxine.**

ABSORPTION, METABOLISM, AND EXCRETION   Vitamin B_6 is absorbed in the small intestine and is found throughout the body (tissue saturation). Conversion of most naturally available vitamin B_6 to its functional coenzyme depends on riboflavin (Lowik, et al, 1994).

FUNCTIONS   Vitamin B_6 is a coenzyme in the synthesis and catabolism of amino acids. It is involved in the metabolism of more than 60 enzymes. Vitamin B_6 functions as a coenzyme in the conversion of tryptophan into niacin. It helps to manufacture antibodies. The hormone epinephrine and the neurotransmitters **dopamine** and **serotonin** all require vitamin B_6 as a coenzyme. It also participates in amino acid transport and the transfer of sulfur and nitrogen to form other compounds.

DEFICIENCY   A deficiency of B_6 is unlikely due to the large amounts present in the general diet. However, factors such as drug interactions or errors in food processing may cause a deficiency. In the past, improperly processed commercial infant formula produced vitamin B_6 deficiencies.

Vitamin B_6 deficiency risk is increased by the use of oral contraceptives. Women using oral contraceptives for more than 2 or 3 years require additional vitamin B_6 due to an abnormal tryptophan metabolism. Infants of mothers who took oral contraceptives for more than 30 months before pregnancy should also be monitored for deficiency.

RECOMMENDED DIETARY ALLOWANCES   The RDAs for vitamin B_6 are 1.6 to 2 milligrams for adults. An increase in protein metabolism increases the need for vitamin B_6.

FOOD SOURCES   Vitamin B_6 is widely distributed in foods. Pork and organ meats are the best animal sources. Whole grains and wheat germ are the best plant sources. Vitamin B_6 is not included in the enrichment of breads so whole wheat bread contains more of this vitamin than white bread. Other good sources include legumes, potatoes, oatmeal, and bananas.

STABILITY   As with other water-soluble vitamins, vitamin B_6 is preserved when vegetables are cooked as quickly as possible. Vitamin B_6 is relatively stable to heat and acids, but very sensitive to light and easily destroyed by alkalies.

TOXICITY   Pyridoxine toxicity has resulted from taking 2 to 6 grams per day for 2 to 40 months. These megadoses, 1000 to 2700 times the RDA, were self-prescribed. Signs and symptoms include sensory loss and numbness of the hands and feet, resulting in clumsiness and severe ataxia. Cessation of the drug permitted some, but not all, functions to return.

Folic Acid

Also known as its salt, folate, **folic acid** affects many different tissues in the body. Inadequate supplies, understandably, produce extensive symptoms.

ABSORPTION, METABOLISM, AND EXCRETION   The folic acid in food usually is bound to amino acids. The enzyme to split off the folic acid is called *folate conjugase.* It is found in salivary, gastric, pancreatic, and jejunal secretions. The unbound folate is absorbed through the intestinal wall and transported to the liver. In the liver some of the folate is processed for storage in the tissues and the liver. Some folate is secreted into bile. When the gallbladder releases bile into the duodenum, the folate may again be split off and absorbed. The recycling process is important because folate stores are adequate for only 2 to 4 months.

FUNCTIONS   Folic acid is necessary for the formation of DNA. Thus, folate participates in the reproduction of every cell, not just the ovum and sperm. Folic acid is active in cell renewal and is necessary for rapidly growing cells, including those in the gastrointestinal (GI) tract, blood, and fetal tissue. It also functions in the formation of **heme.**

DEFICIENCY   Folic acid deficiency is probably the most common vitamin deficiency due to inadequate food intake. At risk are poorly nourished children and poverty-stricken people. Pregnant women, infants, and young children are also at risk because increased folic acid is needed during periods of rapid growth. The link between folic acid and neural tube defects is discussed in Chapter 11, "Life Cycle Nutrition: Pregnancy and Lactation."

A deficiency may also occur as a consequence of malabsorption disorders, or of conditions that increase the metabolic rate and hence the need for folic acid. Examples of such conditions include infections, cancer, and hyperthyroidism. For the same reason, serious burns, excessive blood loss, and gastrointestinal damage may lead to a deficiency.

Folic acid deficiency results in impaired cell division and protein synthesis (processes necessary to tissue growth) and the faulty synthesis of heme. Signs and symptoms include a red, smooth, and swollen tongue; heartburn, diarrhea, fainting, and fatigue. In addition, since folic acid functions in the production of heme, the person deficient in this vitamin develops **megaloblastic anemia.**

RECOMMENDED DIETARY ALLOWANCES   The RDAs for folic acid are 180 to 200 micrograms for adults. Pregnant women have an RDA of 400 micrograms.

FOOD SOURCES   From the meat group, liver is a good source of folic acid. Green, leafy vegetables such as spinach, asparagus, and broccoli provide folic acid. Other vegetables containing appreciable folic acid are kidney beans, beets, and vegetables of the cabbage family. Fruits providing folic acid are oranges and cantaloupe.

STABILITY   Folic acid is stable to alkalies but easily oxidized by light and acids. Some forms are easily destroyed by heat, so that cooking losses may be as high as 80 to 90 percent. To minimize losses, vegetables should be cooked as quickly as possible.

INTERFERING FACTORS   Alcohol or oral contraceptives may interfere with the absorption of folic acid. *Methotrexate,* an anticancer drug, is a folic acid antagonist. Its purpose is to interfere with DNA in cancer cells, but it simultaneously affects normal cells. Aspirin displaces folic acid from its carrier protein; the displaced folic acid is excreted.

TOXICITY   Folic acid toxicity is rare. Dose levels of over-the-counter vitamins are limited to 400 micrograms to make it inconvenient to overdose. This is done not to prevent toxicity from folic acid but to avoid masking signs of pernicious anemia, which will be discussed in the next section.

Vitamin B$_{12}$

Vitamin B$_{12}$ is stored to a greater extent than the other B vitamins. Diverse causes can precipitate vitamin B$_{12}$ deficiency, leading to serious consequences.

ABSORPTION, METABOLISM, AND EXCRETION   Absorption of vitamin B$_{12}$ requires a highly specific protein-binding factor called **intrinsic factor,** secreted by the gastric mucosal cells in the stomach. Vitamin B$_{12}$, also called **extrinsic factor,** and intrinsic factor combine in the stomach. The two factors form a complex that permits vitamin B$_{12}$ to be absorbed in the only section of intestine possible, the ileum.

Vitamin B$_{12}$ is not freely absorbed. The amount absorbed depends upon the body's storage levels.

Heme—The iron-containing portion of the hemoglobin molecule.

Megaloblastic anemia—Anemia characterized by the formation of large, immature red cells that cannot carry oxygen properly; caused by folic acid deficiency.

Intrinsic factor—Specific protein-binding factor secreted by the stomach; necessary for the absorption of vitamin B$_{12}$.

Extrinsic factor—Vitamin B$_{12}$ necessary for proper red blood cell development.

Vitamin B_{12} has a long half-life, so that a person's stores last from 3 to 5 years. The principal storage site is the liver.

FUNCTIONS   Vitamin B_{12} is required in a series of reactions that precede the use of folic acid in DNA replication. In fact, without vitamin B_{12}, folic acid is unable to assist in the manufacture of red blood cells. It is also essential for the synthesis and maintenance of myelin, the fatty insulation which speeds transmission of nervous impulses.

DEFICIENCY   Persons may be at increased risk of vitamin B_{12} deficiency because of stomach pathology, intestinal disease, or diet. When a person lacks intrinsic factor, the result is a condition called **pernicious anemia.** It can also occur following the surgical removal of the stomach or a large portion of the stomach.

In those cases vitamin B_{12} is not absorbed because intrinsic factor is missing. A person with Crohn's disease involving the ileum, or a patient whose ileum was removed, will not absorb vitamin B_{12}. Dietary treatment will be ineffective in these cases, so vitamin B_{12} traditionally has been given by injection. The pharmaceutical name for vitamin B_{12} is **cyanocobalamin.** In several studies, large doses administered orally have been effective (Hathcock and Troendle, 1991; Lederle, 1991).

Symptoms of vitamin B_{12} deficiency are, in usual order of appearance, numbness and tingling in the hands and feet, red blood cell changes, moodiness, confusion, depression, delusions, and overt **psychosis.** Eventually, irreparable nerve damage occurs, and finally, death. One study reported 28 percent of clients with neuropsychiatric disorders caused by vitamin B_{12} deficiency displayed no red blood cell pathology, suggesting cobalamin deficiency should be ruled out in clients with unexplained neuropsychiatric disorders (Lindenbaum, et al, 1988).

Diagnosis of vitamin B_{12} deficiency is difficult if the person consumes ample folic acid. The folic acid enables the body to continue manufacturing red blood cells in the correct size and number. In this way folic acid masks vitamin B_{12} deficiency. However, the neurological deterioration continues unabated. This is the reason folic acid in over-the-counter vitamins is limited to 400 micrograms.

Strict vegetarians are at risk of vitamin B_{12} deficiency because animal products are the best sources of vitamin B_{12}. In this case, additional vitamin B_{12}, from either food or supplements, is the treatment.

RECOMMENDED DIETARY ALLOWANCES   The adult RDA for vitamin B_{12} is 2 micrograms. One ounce of beef liver contains 10 times this amount.

FOOD SOURCES   Vitamin B_{12} is synonymous with animal products. Healthy people who regularly eat meat, milk, cheese, or eggs are not at risk of vitamin B_{12} deficiency. Nutritional yeast and vitamin B_{12} fortified soy milk are food sources available to strict vegetarians.

STABILITY AND INTERFERING FACTORS   Vitamin B_{12} is stable to heat. However, light, acids, and alkalies inactivate it. Megadoses of vitamin C interfere with vitamin B_{12} absorption and utilization. The body's use of vitamin B_{12} is also impaired by a deficiency of vitamin B_6 and gastritis.

Recently Emphasized Vitamins

Two B vitamins are so widely distributed in foods that only special circumstances have produced deficiencies. Long-term total parenteral nutrition is one such situation.

PANTOTHENIC ACID   This vitamin plays a role in the metabolism of carbohydrates, fats, and proteins and in the synthesis of the neurotransmitter **acetylcholine.** No cases of deficiency of **pantothenic acid** have been documented in persons consuming a variety of foods, but deficiencies have been produced experimentally. There are no RDAs for pantothenic acid. Instead, an ESADDI of 4 to 7 milligrams has been set for adults. The average US diet supplies 7 milligrams. Rich food sources include liver, egg yolk, milk, brussels sprouts, sweet potato, and dried beans. Intestinal bacteria are believed to synthesize small amounts of pantothenic acid.

BIOTIN   **Biotin,** closely related to folic acid and vitamin B_{12}, is a coenzyme in the synthesis of fatty acids and amino acids. It is required to form purines, which are essential components of DNA and RNA. Deficiencies have been seen in children displaying the chief sign of skin rash. Deficiencies may occur in clients fed intravenously who also receive antibiotics. Antibiotics kill the intestinal bacteria that synthesize biotin. The ESADDI for biotin is 30 to 100 micrograms. **Avidin,** a protein in raw egg white, binds with biotin. Humans given six raw egg whites per day developed dermatitis in 3 to 4 weeks. A week or two later they displayed mental changes, muscle pain, nausea, and loss of appetite. Five days of biotin therapy cured the symptoms. Good food sources of biotin include liver, kidney, meat, egg yolk, and tomatoes.

Of the water-soluble vitamins, ascorbic acid is the most vulnerable to loss and niacin the most resistant. Table 7–4 summarizes information on vita-

TABLE 7–4 Water-Soluble Vitamins

Vitamin	Adult RDA and Food Portion Containing RDA	Functions	Deficiency Disease	Signs and Symptoms of Deficiency	Best Sources
C Ascorbic acid	60 mg 0.5 cup orange juice	Antioxidant Formation of collagen Function of adrenal glands Facilitates iron absorption Converts folic acid to active form	Scurvy	Bleeding mucous membranes Poor wound healing or reopening of scars Softened ends of long bones Teeth loosen, may fall out Death due to internal hemorrhage	Orange juice, grapefruit juice, cantaloupe, strawberries Green peppers, brussels sprouts, broccoli
B$_1$ Thiamin	1 to 1.5 mg 4.5 oz pork chop, lean only	Coenzyme in CHO metabolism Necessary to convert alcohol to energy	Beriberi	Anorexia, indigestion, constipation Apathy, fatigue, muscle weakness Deterioration of myelin sheaths—paralysis, muscle atrophy Wernicke-Korsakoff syndrome Death due to cardiac failure	Pork Black beans, black-eyed peas Sunflower seeds Fortified cereals
B$_2$ Riboflavin	1.2 to 1.7 mg 1.5 oz beef liver, fried	Coenzyme in protein metabolism	Aribino-flavinosis	Lesions on lips and in mouth Seborrheic dermatitis Skin changes on scrotum or vulva Normocytic anemia	Beef liver Milk Fortified cereals Raw or cooked (not canned) mushrooms
B$_3$ Niacin	13 to 19 mg niacin equivalents 4.3 oz water-packed tuna	Coenzyme in production of energy from glucose Assist in synthesis of fatty acids	Pellagra	Bilaterally symmetrical dermatitis on face, neck, hands, and feet Diarrhea Dementia	Tuna Chicken breast Beef liver
B$_6$ Pyridoxine	1.6 to 2 mg 3 bananas	Coenzyme in synthesis and catabolism of amino acids	No specific term	Dermatitis Glossitis Convulsions	Beef liver Bananas Baked potatoes Baked chicken breast
Folate Folic acid	180 to 200 μg 3.3 oz beef liver	Essential to the formation of DNA Functions in formation of heme	No specific term	Red, smooth, swollen tongue Heartburn, diarrhea Fatigue, fainting Confusion, depression Macrocytic anemia	Beef liver Pinto beans Cooked asparagus Cooked spinach
B$_{12}$ Cyanoco-balamin	2 μg 2.7 oz cooked lean beef	Necessary for folic acid use in DNA replication Synthesis and maintenance of myelin	Pernicious anemia (lack of intrinsic factor, not dietary)	Sore tongue Numbness and tingling of hands and feet Macrocytic anemia Moodiness, confusion Depression Delusions, psychosis	Meat Fish Shellfish Poultry Milk

Pernicious anemia—Inadequate red blood cell formation due to lack of intrinsic factor from the stomach, which is required for the absorption of vitamin B$_{12}$, leads to neural deterioration.

Avidin—Protein in raw egg white that inhibits the B-vitamin biotin.

TABLE 7–5   Sources of Vitamins by Food Groups

Vitamin	Synthesis/ Miscellaneous	Meats	Milk	Fruits/Vegetables	Grains
A		Liver	Fortified	Deep yellow, dark green leafy	
D	In skin	Liver, eggs, some fish	Fortified		
E				Vegetable oil	Wheat germ, whole grains
K	In intestine	Liver, eggs	Milk	Green leafy	
C				Fresh fruit, especially citrus	
Thiamin		Pork			Brewer's yeast
Riboflavin		Organ meats	Milk	Green vegetables	Brewer's yeast
Niacin	Coffee	Meat, tuna, eggs	Milk	Legumes	Brewer's yeast, whole grains
B$_6$		Pork, organ meats, chicken, fish		Potatoes, bananas, legumes	Whole grains, wheat germ, oatmeal
Folic acid		Liver		Cabbage family, dark green leafy, beets, kidney beans, cantaloupe, oranges	Whole grains
B$_{12}$		Meat, eggs	Milk		
Pantothenic acid	In intestine	Liver, kidney, egg yolk	Milk	Dried beans, brussels sprouts, sweet potato	
Biotin	In intestine	Meat, liver, kidney, egg yolk		Tomatoes	

min C and six of the B-complex vitamins. Table 7–5 summarizes sources of vitamins by food groups. A large percentage of Americans report consuming no fruit or fruit juice or vegetables on an average day, indicating a high risk for vitamin deficiencies.

Vitamins as Medicine

Supplements

Ordinarily, healthy persons consuming normal foods in variety, balance, and moderation should not need vitamin supplements. If vitamins are taken as supplements, it is best not to exceed 100 percent of the RDA for each vitamin. This will prevent deficiency in the well individual and toxicity is unlikely.

Americans spend an estimated 2 billion dollars per year on vitamin and mineral supplements. The price of vitamin supplements varies widely. The average markup on vitamins is 43 percent. In some health food stores it is 500 percent.

Pharmacological Uses

Vitamin supplements can be used to offset dietary deficiencies or to compensate for diseases causing malabsorption. They also have been given for some conditions unrelated to diet.

Treatment of Deficiencies

The obvious use of vitamins is to treat vitamin deficiencies. Vitamin C is the treatment for scurvy, vitamin D for rickets, and niacin for pellagra. Initially, the treatment of pernicious anemia involves frequent injections of vitamin B$_{12}$. Later, monthly doses are sufficient to control this condition.

Other Uses

MEGADOSES   A dose ten times the RDA is called a megadose. Some individuals take huge doses of vitamin C to prevent the common cold. Evidence of effectiveness has not been proven to the satisfaction of many scientists. Rebound scurvy is possible when megadoses of vitamin C are discontinued abruptly.

Vitamin C and Smoked Meat

Vitamin C blocks the formation of nitrosamines from nitrates. *Nitrates* are chemicals added to smoked and cured meats to preserve them and enhance their flavor. In the small intestine, however, nitrates combine with amino acids to form nitrosamines, which have been linked to some cancers. For this reason meat packers have begun adding vitamin C to protect against nitrosamine formation.

TREATING NONNUTRITIONAL DISORDERS   Many vitamins have uses unrelated to prevention or treatment of deficiencies. Vitamins A, E, C, and niacin are examples. Vitamin A derivatives are often prescribed to control acne and the wrinkles of aging. Clinical Application 7–7 discusses Vitamin C as a food additive intended to reduce the formation of cancer-causing compounds. High doses of niacin, usually 3 to 6 grams per day, have been used to lower serum cholesterol.

Summary

Vitamins are organic substances required in minute quantities that are necessary for many bodily processes. They do not become part of the structure of the body.

Vitamins were first recognized by the respective effects of their absence. Some deficiency diseases have been known for centuries. However, only in this century have each of the known vitamins been isolated in the laboratory. Even so, correct treatments were prescribed based on primitive and incomplete knowledge. Only low intakes of vitamins A, C, B_6, and folic acid are currently regarded as public health problems in the United States.

Vitamins A, D, E, and K are fat soluble and stable to heat. Sufficient dietary fat intake and adequate fat digestion and absorption are required for the proper utilization of these vitamins. Fat-soluble vitamins, especially A and D, can be stored by the body and hence can be sources of toxicity. Both vitamins A and D have clear-cut deficiency diseases: xerophthalmia and night blindness for vitamin A and rickets for vitamin D.

The water-soluble vitamins, C and the B-complexes, are not stored in the body in appreciable amounts. Vitamins C, B_{12}, thiain, and niacin have specific diseases associated with deficiency: scurvy, pernicious anemia, beriberi, and pellagra, respectively.

Because of the interdependent functions of vitamins, people without special needs are advised to rely on a balanced diet for vitamins. If a vitamin supplement is desired, it should be taken at the RDA levels only.

Case Study 7–1

Mr. J, a 79-year-old widower, prides himself on caring for himself in the past year since his wife died. His typical meal pattern is:

- Breakfast—egg, toast, jam, coffee
- Lunch—cheese or lunch meat sandwich, tea
- Dinner—canned stew or hash

Although Mr. J has a refrigerator, he avoids buying fresh fruit or vegetables. He says he has difficulty consuming produce before it spoils. He seldom goes out to eat.

For the past few months Mr. J has noticed that his gums are tender. He stopped wearing his dentures when his gums began to bleed.

The visiting nurse confirmed the inflammation of the gums. When the nurse took Mr. J's blood pressure, she noted a red, flat rash where the blood pressure cuff had been.

NURSING CARE PLAN FOR MR. J

Assessment

Subjective Data	Sore gums
	Diet lacks fresh fruits and vegetables
Objective Data	Erythematous petechiae under blood pressure cuff

Nursing Diagnosis   Nutrition, altered: possible vitamin C deficiency related to lack of fresh fruit and vegetables as evidenced by sore bleeding gums and pressure petechiae after minor pressure.

Desired Outcome/ Evaluation Criteria	Nursing Actions	Rationale
Will consume foods containing 60 mg of vitamin C every day within 3 days.	Teach importance of daily vitamin C.	Little vitamin C is stored in the body; must be consumed every day.
	Explore acceptability of good sources of vitamin C, list amounts necessary to obtain 60 mg.	Foods would be better sources than vitamin supplements because other nutrients supplied also.
	If client selects frozen vegetables, teach to boil water 1 minute before adding vegetables and to cook quickly until crisp-tender.	Heat and oxygen destroy vitamin C.

Study Aids

Chapter Review

1. Which of the following vitamins are water soluble?
   a. A and C
   b. A, D, E, and K
   c. B and C
   d. B, D, E, and K

2. The vitamin that is essential to the synthesis of several blood clotting factors is:
   a. Vitamin A
   b. Vitamin B_6
   c. Vitamin C
   d. Vitamin K

3. Which of the following groups of foods would be the best sources of carotene?
   a. Bananas, cantaloupe, and pears
   b. Broccoli, lettuce, and lima beans
   c. Collards, spinach, and sweet potatoes
   d. Lemons, oranges, and strawberries

4. Deficiency of vitamin A causes:
   a. Nightblindness
   b. Pellagra
   c. Rickets
   d. Scurvy

5. Individuals who elect to take a vitamin supplement should:
   a. Buy the most economical product
   b. Limit the amounts to RDA levels
   c. Obtain a physician's prescription
   d. Select the most expensive product

Clinical Analysis

1. Ms. C is being seen in the well-baby clinic with her 3-month-old baby girl. Ms. C states that the baby is taking 6 ounces of a commercial baby formula every 4 hours. Ms. C has not added solid

foods to the baby's diet. She was told to wait until the baby is 4 months old before adding cereal. Ms. C is giving the baby the multivitamin preparation prescribed. She also has added cod liver oil to the infant's diet. "It's only a teaspoonful," she said. Ms. C's grandmother gave Ms. C cod liver oil as a child. Ms. C credits her grandmother's care during her own childhood for her strong bones and teeth. She admires her grandmother, who at age 75 still stands straight and tall. Which of the following pieces of information should the nurse gather first to focus on the situation presented?

a. The amount of vitamin C in the multivitamin supplement
b. The conditions under which the vitamins are stored
c. Ms. C's technique for measuring the vitamins
d. The total amount of vitamin D the infant receives each day

2. Mr. S has expressed interest in improving his diet. The nurse assessed Mr. S's usual intake, noting the absence of citrus fruit. He stated the acids upset his stomach. Which of the following suggestions to maximize vitamin C content is appropriate?

a. Adding baking soda to the cooking water
b. Cooking thoroughly to kill any bacteria
c. Eating good sources raw when possible
d. Keeping food in a mesh bag to allow air to circulate

3. Ms. P has been taking oral contraceptives for three years. The nurse should assess her vitamin _____ intake and signs of deficiency

a. A
b. B_6
c. C
d. D

Bibliography

Berger, RA, Courtright, P, and Barrows, J: Vitamin A capsule supplementation in Malawi villages: Missed opportunities and possible interventions. Am J Public Health 85:718, 1995.

Blank, S, et al: An outbreak of hypervitaminosis D associated with the overfortification of milk from a home-delivery dairy. Am J Public Health 85:656, 1995.

Brensilver, JM, and Goldberger, E: A Primer of Water, Electrolyte, and Acid-Base Syndromes, ed 8. FA Davis, Philadelphia, 1996.

Brown, JE: The Science of Human Nutrition, Harcourt, Brace, Jovanovich, San Diego, 1990.

Christen, WG: Antioxidants and eye disease. Am J Med (suppl 3A) 97:3A, 1994.

Committee on Diet and Health. Food and Nutrition Board. Commission on Life Sciences. National Research Council: Diet and Health: Implications for Reducing Chronic Disease Risk. National Academy Press, Washington, DC, 1989.

Davis, JR, and Sherer, K: Applied Nutrition and Diet Therapy for Nurses, ed 2. WB Saunders, Philadelphia, 1994.

Deglin, JH, and Vallerand, JA: Davis's Drug Guide for Nurses, ed 4. FA Davis, Philadelphia, 1995.

Eye Disease Case-Control Study Group: Antioxidant status and neovascular age-related macular degeneration. Arch Ophthalmol 111:104, 1993.

Fawzi, WW, et al: Vitamin A supplementation and child mortality. JAMA 269:898, 1993.

Geubel, AP, De Galocsy, C, Alves, N, et al: Liver damage caused by therapeutic vitamin A administration: Estimate of dose-related toxicity in 41 cases. Gastroenterology 100:1710, 1991.

Glasziou, PP, and Mackerras, DEM: Vitamin A supplementation in infectious diseases: A meta-analysis. BMJ 306:366, 1993.

Grimes, MR, Scardino, MA, and Martone, JF: Worldwide blindness. Nurs Clin North Am 27:807, 1992.

Groff, JL, Gropper, SS, and Hunt, SM: Advanced Nutrition and Human Metabolism, ed 2. West Publishing Co., Minneapolis, 1995.

Hankinson, SE, and Stampfer, MJ: All that glitters is not beta-carotene. JAMA 272:1455, 1994.

Hathcock, JN, and Troendle, GJ: Oral cobalamin for treatment of pernicious anemia. JAMA 265:96, 1991.

Kowalski, TE, Falestiny, M, Furth, E, et al: Vitamin A hepatotoxicity: A cautionary note regarding 25,000 IU supplements. Am J Med 97:523, 1994.

Krasinski, SD, and Russell, RM: The prevalence of vitamin K deficiency in chronic gastrointestinal disorders. Am J Clin Nutr 41:639, 1985.

Lederle, FA: Oral cobalamin for pernicious anemia. JAMA 265:94, 1991.

Levine, M, et al: Determination of optimal vitamin C requirements in humans. Am J Clin Nutr 62(suppl):1347S, 1995.

Levine, M, et al: Vitamin C pharmacokinetics in healthy volunteers: Evidence for a recommended dietary allowance. Proc Nat Acad Sci USA 93:3704, 1996.

Lindebaum, J, Healton, EB, Savage, DG, et al: Neuropsychiatric disorders caused by cobalamin deficiency in the absence of anemia or macrocytosis. N Engl J Med 318:1720, 1988.

Lowik, MRH, et al: Interrelationships between riboflavin and vitamin B_6 among elderly people (Dutch Nutrition Surveillance System). Internat J Vit Nutr Res 64:198, 1994.

Mares-Perlman, JA, et al: Dietary fat and age-related maculopathy. Arch Ophthalmol 113:743, 1995.

Roman, GC: An epidemic in Cuba of optic neuropathy, sensorineural deafness, peripheral sensory neuropathy and dorsolateral myeloneuropathy. J Neurol Sci 127:11, 1994.

Seddon, JM, et al: Dietary carotenoids, vitamins A, C, and E, and advanced age-related macular degeneration. JAMA 272:1413, 1994.

Seddon, JM, and Hennekens, CH: Vitamins, minerals, and macular degeneration. Arch Ophthalmol 112:176, 1994.

Sirota, LH: Vitamin and mineral toxicities: Issues related to supplementation practices of athletes. Journal of Health Education 25:82, 1994.

Subcommittee on the 10th Edition of the RDAs. Food and Nutrition Board. Commission on Life Sciences. National Research Council: Recommended Dietary Allowances, ed 10. National Academy Press, Washington, DC, 1989.

US Department of Health and Human Services: Nutrition Monitoring in the United States. US Government Printing Office, Washington, DC, 1989.

van der Wielen, RPJ, et al: Serum vitamin D concentrations among elderly people in Europe. Lancet 346:207, 1995.

West, S, et al: Are antioxidants or supplements protective for age-related macular degeneration? Arch Ophthalmol 112:222, 1994.

Willett, WC: Folic acid and neural tube defect: Can't we come to closure? Am J Public Health 82:666, 1992.

Wolf, G: A regulatory pathway of thermogenesis in brown fat through retinoic acid. Nutrition Reviews 53:230, 1995.

CHAPTER 8

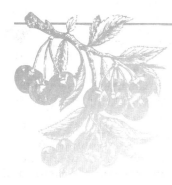

Minerals

LEARNING OBJECTIVES

After completing this chapter, the student should be able to:

1 Discuss the differences and similarities between minerals and vitamins.
2 Describe one or more functions of each mineral.
3 List at least two food sources for each mineral and identify any nonfood sources.
4 Describe individuals at increased risk for mineral deficiencies.
5 Identify the five minerals that are actual or potential public health problems in the United States due to low intake levels; identify the mineral that is a health risk because of overconsumption.

In a broad sense, minerals are obtained from the earth's crust. Through the effects of the weather, rocks that contain minerals are ground into smaller particles, which then become part of the soil. The mineral content in the soil is absorbed by growing plants. Animals eat the plants, and humans eat both the plants and the animals. In this way, minerals become part of the food chain.

Minerals in Human Nutrition

In nutrition, minerals make vital contributions toward promoting growth and maintaining health in the body. In this chapter we will discuss the minerals important in human nutrition and the role each plays in the body.

In this section we will first compare minerals with vitamins. Then we will discuss some of the general functions of minerals and explain how minerals are classified in nutrition.

Functions of Minerals

Minerals are similar to vitamins because they help regulate bodily functions without providing energy and are essential to good health. Minerals differ from vitamins not only because minerals are inorganic substances but also because minerals become part of the structure of the body. Minerals represent 4 percent of total body weight.

Structural Components of Body Systems

Minerals become part of the body's structure and part of the body's enzymes. For instance, calcium and phosphorus combine to give bones and teeth their hardness. Iron becomes attached to the protein globin to form hemoglobin. Iodine becomes part of the thyroid hormones.

Regulators of Bodily Functions

Most minerals serve a variety of functions in the body's regulatory and metabolic processes. Sodium is essential for maintaining fluid balance. Sodium, potassium, and calcium have critical functions in nerve and muscle activity. Potassium and phosphorus play significant roles in acid-base balance. A disruption of the body's balance of any one of these minerals can be life threatening.

Classification of Minerals

In nutrition, minerals are classified into two groups: major and trace. Major minerals, also called macrominerals, are present in the body in quantities greater than 5 grams (approximately 1 teaspoonful). The body needs a daily intake of 100 milligrams (approximately 1/50 teaspoonful) or more of each of the major minerals.

Trace minerals, often called microminerals or trace elements, are present in the body in amounts less than 5 grams. Humans need a daily intake of less than 100 milligrams of each of the trace minerals. The term *trace* does not mean unimportant. Trace minerals make vital and often unique contributions to the body's functioning.

Major Minerals

The seven major minerals include calcium, sodium, and potassium, which are familiar to many people. The other four major minerals are phosphorus, magnesium, sulfur, and chloride.

Calcium

The body of a 150-pound adult contains approximately 3 pounds of calcium. Ninety-nine percent of this amount is in the bones and teeth. The remaining 1 percent of the calcium circulates in the body fluids. Of this 1 percent, one-quarter to one-half is bound to plasma proteins, while the rest travels as free particles that carry an electrical charge (ions). The ionized calcium moves freely from one fluid compartment to another and serves several important functions in the body.

Functions of Calcium

Calcium, with phosphorus, forms the hard substance that characterizes bones and teeth. Bones continue to add minerals until age 30. Ample calcium and phosphorus alone will not guarantee strong bones and teeth, however. Vitamin D is necessary for calcium absorption. Exercise, particularly weight-bearing exercise, is also essential for strong bones. Very little calcium is deposited in fully formed teeth. Consequently, if calcium is lost from the teeth, it cannot be replaced. This is the reason dental cavities or caries cannot heal themselves.

Calcium also performs several vital metabolic

functions in the nervous, muscular, and cardiovascular systems. (1) Calcium assists in the manufacturing of **acetylcholine,** a neurotransmitter, or chemical that enhances transmission of nerve impulses. (2) Calcium acts as a catalyst in initiating and controlling muscle contraction and relaxation. At the beginning of a muscle contraction, calcium is released from its storage area inside the muscle cell. At the end of a contraction, the calcium is again gathered into its storage area. (This function is vital to the heart muscle.) (3) Calcium is a catalyst in two steps of the clotting process: it aids in the conversion of platelets to thromboplastin and in the conversion of fibrinogen to fibrin. (4) Calcium controls the passage of substances across cell membranes by affecting membrane permeability. (5) Calcium activates certain enzymes such as pancreatic lipase and is necessary for absorption of vitamin B_{12}.

Control Mechanisms

Bone is the body's bank account or storage depot for calcium. As much as 700 milligrams of calcium is moved in and out of the bones each day. One reason for this is to maintain the adult serum calcium concentration within the normal limits of 8.5 to 10.5 milligrams per 100 milliliters of serum. Another reason for the movement of calcium in and out of the bones is to renew the bone tissue. In this process bone cells called **osteoclasts** produce enzymes to destroy the protein matrix that holds the calcium phosphate in place. Other bone cells, called **osteoblasts** produce new matrix protein, which chemically attracts calcium and other nutrients to rebuild the bone.

Several hormones work together to accomplish these activities. Vitamin D is one of these hormones. Parathyroid hormone and calcitonin are the other two. Vitamin D is actually a hormone because it regulates tissue functions. It increases calcium absorption by the intestine and increases calcium deposition in the bones and teeth.

Parathyroid hormone is secreted by tiny glands behind the thyroid gland in the neck. When the serum calcium level falls, the parathyroid glands secrete the hormone, which increases the withdrawal of calcium from the bone, thereby raising the serum calcium level. Additionally, parathyroid hormone increases the serum calcium level by stimulating the kidneys to return more calcium to the bloodstream instead of excreting it in the urine.

To balance the action of parathyroid hormone, **calcitonin,** another hormone is secreted by the thyroid gland. Calcitonin is released when the serum calcium level is high. It inhibits the release of calcium from bone.

Other hormones affect calcium utilization by the body. One prominent one is estrogen. Its exact mechanism of action in bone metabolism is unknown.

Recommended Dietary Allowances

The RDA for calcium for adult men and women older than 25 years is 800 milligrams. Nineteen- to 24-year-old women have an RDA of 1200 milligrams.

An independent panel convened by the National Institutes of Health issued a consensus statement on optimal calcium intake. These optimal amounts are listed in Table 8–1. Only for children up to age 5 and for pregnant or lactating women do the amounts correspond to the RDAs.

Sources of Calcium

Even with the bones as a reservoir, daily intake of calcium is important. Calcium can be obtained from animal or vegetable sources, but animal sources are more readily absorbed.

ANIMAL SOURCES   Milk and milk products are the best animal sources of calcium, followed by sardines, clams, oysters, and salmon. In milk, calcium is combined with lactose, which increases absorption. Even so, only 28 percent of the available calcium in milk is absorbed. Another advantageous component in milk is the protein the osteoblasts need to rebuild the bone matrix. In sum, milk is such an important source of calcium that it is virtually impossible to obtain adequate calcium without milk or dairy products. Figure 8–1 shows a child drinking milk with his meal.

Osteoclasts—Bone cells that break down bone.

Osteoblasts—Bone cells that build bone.

Parathyroid hormone—Hormone secreted by the parathyroid glands; regulates calcium and phosphorus metabolism in the body.

Calcitonin—Hormone produced by the C cells of the thyroid gland; it slows bone resorption when serum calcium levels are high.

TABLE 8–1   NIH Consensus Conference—Optimal Calcium Intake Compared to Recommended Dietary Allowances

	Milligrams of Calcium			
	Female		Male	
Age in Years	NIH	RDA	NIH	RDA
0.0–0.5	400	400	400	400
0.5–1.0	600	600	600	600
1–5	800	800	800	800
6–10	800–1200	800	800–1200	800
11–24	1200–1500	1200	1200–1500	1200
25–50	1000	800		
25–65			1000	800
Pregnant	1200	1200		
Lactating	1200	1200		
Postmenopausal				
On estrogen	1000	800		
Not on estrogen	1500	800		
>65	1500	800	1500	800

Table 8–2 lists the quantity of foods containing approximately 300 milligrams of calcium, the amount in 1 cup of milk. "Bargain" foods listed that are high in calcium but low in kilocalories include skim milk and plain yogurt. The "most expensive" sources of calcium, considering kilocalories, are hard and soft ice cream and large-curd, creamed cottage cheese. This table reveals that not all dairy products are equally beneficial as sources of calcium, but it is not a call to abandon all fat intake. Consuming some fat with calcium increases the absorption of the mineral by slowing peristalsis.

Obtaining calcium from supplements is less desirable than obtaining it from foods. Milk products supply other nutrients, such as vitamin D and lactose, that assist in calcium absorption. Milk is also a major source of riboflavin and protein. Figure 8–2 shows the percentages of the RDAs for vitamins A and D, protein, thiamine, and riboflavin an adult woman could obtain from 3 cups of skim milk. Clinical Application 8–1 describes some of the contaminants in "natural" calcium supplements.

PLANT SOURCES   Good plant sources of calcium include rhubarb, spinach, greens (turnip, beet), broccoli, kale, tofu, and legumes. In all cases vegetable yields more calcium when it is cooked. Some experts question the amount that is absorbed due to multiple interfering factors. Another good source is calcium-fortified orange juice.

TABLE 8–2   Quantities of Food Containing Approximately 300 Milligrams of Calcium, Equal to One Cup of Milk, in Order of Energy Content

Food	Amount	Kilocalories
Skim milk	1.0 cup	86
Grated Parmesan cheese	4.3 tbsp	99
Plain low-fat yogurt	0.7 cup	101
Swiss cheese	1.1 oz	118
2 percent milk	1.0 cup	121
Whole milk	1.0 cup	150
Cheddar cheese	1.5 oz	171
Processed American cheese	1.7 oz	180
Low-fat yogurt with fruit	0.9 cup	199
Blue cheese	2.0 oz	200
Vanilla milkshake	0.9 cup	273
2 percent low-fat cottage cheese	2.0 cups	410
Hard ice cream, vanilla	1.7 cups	459
Soft ice cream	1.3 cups	479
Cottage cheese, creamed, large curd	2.25 cups	529
Sherbet	2.9 cups	786

Factors Interfering with Absorption and Excretion

Only 30 percent of the calcium in food is absorbed. In general, the percentage of available calcium absorbed from vegetables is considerably less than that absorbed from milk. For example, only 5 percent of

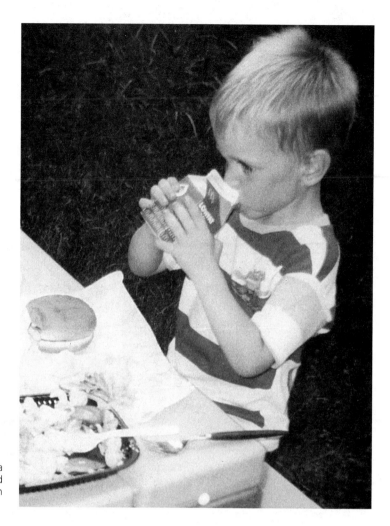

FIGURE 8–1 This child has a balanced meal from a fast food restaurant: a small hamburger, a salad, and milk. Growing bones and teeth need calcium from milk products.

CLINICAL APPLICATION 8-1

Contents of Natural Calcium Supplements

Shells, bones, and dolomite are natural sources of calcium that are used as dietary supplements. Much of the calcium found in shells and bones is in the form of calcium phosphate, one of the most difficult calcium compounds to absorb. In addition, shells and bones often contain excessive amounts of mercury and lead.

Dolomite is a limestone that is rich in both calcium and magnesium. It also may contain lead, mercury, arsenic, and aluminum. Because of the possibility of contamination, it is best to obtain calcium from food sources whenever possible. When this is not possible, pharmaceutical products are preferable to natural supplements.

the total calcium found in spinach is absorbed. Several factors can interfere with the absorption and retention of calcium: oxalates, phytic acid, and excessive intakes of protein or dietary fiber (see Table 8–3).

Some vegetables contain salts of oxalic acid called oxalates. **Oxalates** bind with the calcium present in the vegetable to produce calcium oxalate, an insoluble form of calcium that is excreted in the feces. The calcium content not bound to oxalates is available for absorption, however, and oxalates do not interfere with the absorption of calcium from other

Oxalates—Salts of oxalic acid found in some plant foods; binds with the calcium in the plant, making it unavailable to the body.

% RDA

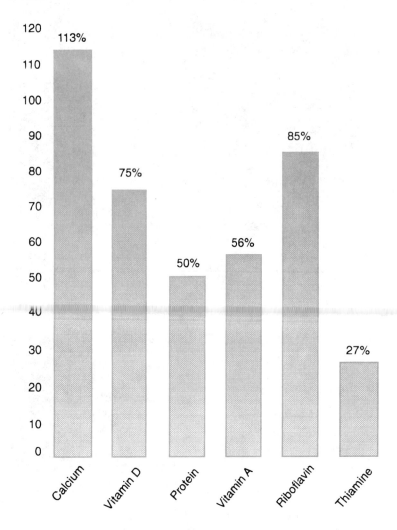

FIGURE 8–2   Milk supplies many nutrients in addition to calcium. Three cups of skim milk give a woman more than 25 years of age 50 percent of her RDAs for vitamin D, protein, vitamin A, and riboflavin, as well as 27 percent of her RDA for thiamine. The caloric cost for all these nutrients is a minuscule 258 kilocalories.

TABLE 8–3   Factors Affecting Calcium Absorption and Excretion

Increase Absorption	Decrease Absorption	Increase Excretion
Acidity	Alkalinity	Excessive animal protein
Estrogen	Insoluble dietary fiber	Excessive sodium
Lactose or sucrose	Oxalic acid	
Protein	Phytic acid	
Vitamin D	Vitamin D deficiency	

foods. Chard, spinach, beet leaves, rhubarb, cranberries, and gooseberries all contain oxalic acid. Unusually high intake of these foods may cause oxalic acid poisoning (see Clinical Application 8–2).

Cereals contain a substance that forms an insoluble complex with calcium. This interfering substance is **phytic acid.** The overall effect of oxalic and phytic acids on calcium availability in most diets usually is not significant. Persons who avoid dairy products, however, may need careful attention to meal planning.

Adequate protein intake facilitates calcium absorption. Eating 100 grams or more of protein a day, not unusual for many Americans, increases urinary excretion of calcium. If protein intake is dou-

It is possible to be poisoned by ingesting too much of one or more foods that contain oxalic acid. Cranberries, gooseberries, chard, spinach, beet leaves, and rhubarb are high in oxalic acid. For example, one normal serving of rhubarb contains one-fifth the toxic dose. Rhubarb leaves contain three or four times as much as the stalks. A fairly small amount of leaves, then, can poison a child.

One way to minimize the chance of oxalic acid poisoning is to consume foods that contain calcium with foods high in oxalic acid. The calcium combines with the oxalate, which then passes through the intestine harmlessly. However, calcium absorption will be decreased.

bled without changing other nutrients, urinary calcium increases by 50 percent (Heaney, 1993). When protein is accompanied by a high phosphorus intake, the calcium loss is lessened considerably. Fortunately, in the American diet, foods high in protein usually are high in phosphorus as well.

Calcium absorption is hindered by excessive intake of insoluble dietary fiber. It passes through the alimentary canal undigested. Any calcium that binds with dietary fiber suffers the same fate.

An alkaline environment decreases calcium solubility. Because the intestine is alkaline, any exaggeration of this quality will impair calcium absorption.

Calcium Deficiencies

Calcium deficiency in children can contribute to poor bone and tooth development. Rickets is more directly related to vitamin D deficiency than calcium deficiency except in premature infants, whose skeletons still need much added mineral. Two other conditions related to calcium balance are osteoporosis and tetany.

OSTEOPOROSIS   *Osteopenia* is a decreased bone mass per unit of volume. In **osteoporosis** the osteopenia is sufficient to allow fracture to occur after minimal trauma. Osteoporosis is most common in postmenopausal, fair-complected white women. A woman loses 2 to 5 percent of bone tissue per year immediately before and for about 8 years after menopause. The most rapid loss of bone occurs in the first five years after menopause. Black women and men lose bone mass also, but because their skeletons are generally heavier, the loss is less conspicuous.

The exact cause of osteoporosis is unknown, but it is more closely associated with a deficiency of calcium than with a deficiency of vitamin D. Furthermore, population studies have not demonstrated a relationship between calcium intake and osteoporosis in all countries. Clinical Application 8–3 discusses some of the research on osteoporosis.

TETANY   Despite the hormonal control of serum calcium and the large reservoir in the bones, serum calcium sometimes falls below normal. It may be caused by an actual lack of calcium or a lack of ionized calcium. A serum calcium level that is too low is called **hypocalcemia.** If the signs and symptoms described below appear, the condition is called tetany. Causes include parathyroid deficiency, vitamin D deficiency, and alkalosis.

Parathyroid deficiency can be caused by disease of the gland or accidental removal of the parathyroid glands during thyroidectomy. Tetany related to vitamin D deficiency can result from inadequate sunlight, malnutrition, or impaired kidney function.

In **alkalosis,** the excessive alkalinity of body fluids, a greater number of calcium ions are bound to serum proteins, effectively inactivating the calcium. Therefore, nerve and muscle function is impaired. Alkalosis may be caused by the loss of acid (due to vomiting or gastric suction) or by the ingestion of alkalies (for example, sodium bicarbonate). Alkalosis can even be caused by breathing too rapidly, either in response to fear or through mechanical ventilation. The result is excessive loss of carbon dioxide. In the blood, carbon dioxide is transported as carbonic acid. Thus, when too much carbon dioxide is exhaled, the blood becomes more alkaline and produces tetany.

Early symptoms of tetany are nervousness, irritability, numbness and tingling of the extremities and around the mouth, and muscle cramps. Diagnostic signs are **Trousseau's sign** and **Chvostek's sign.** In Trousseau's sign, inflation of the blood pressure cuff above systolic pressure for 3 minutes causes ischemia of the peripheral nerves, increasing their excitability. What the examiner sees is muscle spasms of the forearm and hand. In Chvostek's sign, a tap over the facial nerve in front of the ear causes a twitch of the facial muscles on that side. Figure 8–3 depicts these diagnostic signs.

┌───┐
│ **Osteoporosis**—A loss of bone mass.   │
└───┘

Research on Osteoporosis

More than 25 million people in the United States have osteoporosis, which is the major factor in fractures in the elderly. Hip fractures alone cost $7 billion in the United States and have a mortality rate of 12 to 25 percent. Most hip fractures occur in women over 80 years of age.

Two major factors in the development of osteoporosis are the bone mass developed from birth to age 30 and rate of loss of bone mass in later life. Contributing to both of these factors are estrogen levels, calcium intake, vitamin D supply, and exercise. Researchers have investigated all of these topics.

Bone Mass Development

Children given calcium supplements increased their bone mass faster than their identical twins (Johnston, et al, 1992). The effect was lost when supplementation stopped, however. Recollection of milk consumption before age 25 was a significant independent predictor of bone mineral density (Murphy, 1994).

Rate of Bone Loss

The rate of bone loss in women is greatest in the five years immediately after menopause. Until 30 to 40 percent of bone mass is lost, it is not detectable on X ray. More sophisticated detection methods are used for research. In a study of female twins, the one who smoked more had less bone mass than the one who smoked less. Women who smoke one pack of cigarettes daily through adulthood will reach menopause with an average deficit of 5 to 10 percent in bone density, sufficient to increase the risk of fracture (Hopper and Seeman, 1994). Alcohol is toxic to osteoblasts and suppresses bone formation (Blaauw, 1994).

Hormone Therapy

Healthy white women, 3- to 6-years post menopause, who received estrogen and progesterone with calcium and vitamin D lost less bone mineral than women who received only calcium and vitamin D. The latter group lost less than the placebo group receiving only vitamin D (Aloia, 1994).

Calcium Intake

Hip fracture risk in men is inversely correlated with calcium intake (NIH Consensus Conference, 1994). Four years of calcium supplementation of postmenopausal women, with an average age of 58 years, reduced the rate of loss of bone mineral density and the number of fractures compared to a control group (Reid, et al, 1995). Patients diagnosed with osteoporosis who were given cyclical slow-release fluoride and calcium for four years suffered significantly fewer new vertebral fractures than the control group receiving just calcium (Pak, et al, 1995).

Vitamin D Supply

Average dietary intake of vitamin D in community-living elderly in North America and Europe is about 2.5 micrograms (Krall, et al, 1989). Hip fracture patients have lower serum vitamin D concentrations than age-matched healthy persons (Lips, et al, 1987). Healthy ambulatory women, with an average age of 84 years, who received vitamin D and calcium supplements suffered 43 percent fewer hip fractures than women receiving placebo (Chapuy, et al, 1992). Because of the skin's synthesis of vitamin D, researchers have investigated the effects of vitamin D in northern climates where winter sun exposure is minimal. Postmenopausal women supplemented with 10 μg of vitamin D and calcium showed a modest increase in spinal bone mineral density compared to women receiving only equal amounts of calcium (Dawson-Hughes, 1991). Healthy postmenopausal women supplemented to 20 μg of vitamin D showed less bone loss from the femoral neck than women supplemented to 5 μg, the current RDA. All the women received equal amounts of calcium (Dawson-Hughes, et al, 1995).

Exercise

Weight-bearing exercise stimulates osteoblastic activity. Loss of bone mass in immobile patients is well known. Postmenopausal women in a one-year walking program maintained spinal bone mineral density whereas the control group did not (Nelson, et al, 1991). Women coached in two 45-minute high-intensity strength training sessions per week for 1 year showed some improvement in bone density, muscle mass and strength, and balance compared to a control group (Nelson, et al, 1994). Increased muscle mass, strength, and balance lessen the risk of falling, bone density aside.

Recommendations

Because osteoporosis develops in response to multiple factors, no "one size fits all" plan to stave off the disease is advocated. Lifetime adequate intakes of calcium and vitamin D, preferably from dietary sources, along with sufficient exercise will increase bone mass. Estrogen supplementation at menopause is appropriate for some women. A total program should be discussed with the physician.

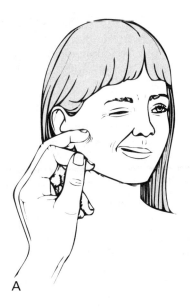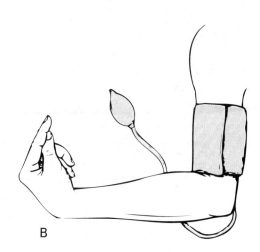

FIGURE 8–3 Indications of hypocalcemia: (A) a positive Chvostek's sign and (B) a positive Trousseau's sign.

A

B

Because of the many functions of calcium, tetany is a medical emergency. Untreated, it can progress to respiratory paralysis, seizures or coma, heart dilatation, and blood clotting problems.

Toxicity of Calcium

A serum calcium level that is too high, above 10.5 milligrams per 100 milliliters of serum in adults, is called **hypercalcemia.**

Hypercalcemia can be caused by **hyperparathyroidism** and other diseases, by vitamin D poisoning, by antacids, and by excessive intake of milk. Idiopathic hypercalcemia associated with vitamin D toxicity is seen most frequently in infants.

In a series of 100 clients with hypercalcemia, the most common causes were malignancy and hyperparathyroidism. The third most common cause was milk-alkali syndrome, including three persons operated for parathyroid disease before the diagnosis was established (Beall and Scofield, 1995). Milk-alkali syndrome was first related to the milk and cream and antacid treatment of peptic ulcers. Recent cases, some of which required hemodialysis for renal failure, resulted from self-prescribed calcium carbonate tablets (Abreo, et al, 1993; Beall and Scofield, 1995). Individuals reported taking 2 to 18 grams daily, usually for indigestion. (Package instructions caution not to take more than 8 grams per day or to use that dose for more than 2 weeks without consulting a physician.) Some concern is raised about the use of calcium carbonate to prevent osteoporosis. These cases emphasize the importance of a careful dietary and medication history and of patient teaching regarding over-the-counter as well as prescription medications.

Phosphorus

An adult has about 2 pounds of phosphorus in the body. Eighty-five percent of this is in the bones, and the remaining 15 percent is in cells and body fluids. Phosphorus is closely associated with calcium both in interrelated metabolic functions in the body and in foods. See Clinical Application 8–4 for information on phosphorus intake and calcium balance.

Functions of Phosphorus

Phosphorus occurs in bones and teeth as calcium phosphate. Phosphorus is also a component of DNA and RNA. The storage forms of energy **adenosine diphosphate (ADP)** and **adenosine triphosphate (ATP)**, contain phosphorus. Phosphorus is an essential mineral in **phospholipids,** which are structural components of cells. Phospholipids contain glycerol, fatty acids, and phosphorus. Examples include lecithin, a part of cell membranes, and myelin, the insulating covering of many nerves. Phosphorus assists with the absorption of glucose and glycerol.

> **Hyperparathyroidism**—Excessive secretion of parathyroid hormone, causing changes in the bones, kidneys, and gastrointestinal tract.

Phosphorus compounds are used as a buffer system to maintain the pH of the blood between 7.35 and 7.45.

Control Mechanism for Phosphorus

A higher proportion of dietary phosphorus is absorbed than calcium. Seventy percent of dietary phosphorus is absorbed while the remaining 30 percent is excreted in the feces. Absorption occurs in the **jejunum,** the middle portion of the small intestine. The same factors affecting absorption of calcium are also at work for phosphorus.

Low levels of serum phosphorus stimulate the kidney to produce more active vitamin D. The vitamin D then increases the absorption of phosphorus from the intestinal tract. Excess phosphorus is excreted by the kidney in response to parathyroid hormone.

Recommended Dietary Allowances and Sources of Phosphorus

The RDAs for phosphorus are: 800 milligrams for men and women aged 25 and older. Phosphorus is widespread in foods because it is essential in plant and animal cells. Animal protein is the best source of phosphorus. Since ATP is an energy source in muscle, lean meat is a good source of phosphorus. Good plant sources include nuts and legumes.

Deficiency of Phosphorus

Dietary deficiency of phosphorus is unlikely. Certain diseases or medications, however, will produce **hypophosphatemia.**

Hyperparathyroidism causes excess excretion of phosphorus. In this disease, parathyroid hormone causes withdrawal of calcium from the bones. Since, in the bones, the two are combined, phosphorus is lost along with calcium. Chronic kidney disease often produces the same result.

Toxicity from Phosphorus

Hyperphosphatemia caused by dietary overload is unusual. Cases have occurred in infants given only cow's milk during the first few weeks of life. Cow's milk has twice the phosphorus content of human milk and infant formula. That, coupled with an infant's immature kidneys, overtaxes the infant's ability to maintain homeostasis.

Sodium

The adult body contains about 90 grams of sodium, approximately 3 ounces. Two-thirds of the sodium in the body is in the blood and other extracellular fluids. The other one-third is in the bones.

Functions and Control of Sodium

Sodium has a major role in maintaining fluid balance in the body. Sodium is also necessary for the transmission of electrochemical impulses along nerve and muscle membranes and is a component of two phosphate buffers.

The intestine readily absorbs sodium. Only about 5 percent of dietary sodium travels within the intestine to remain in the feces. To maintain a normal level of sodium in the blood, the kidney either reabsorbs sodium back into the bloodstream or allows it to be spilled in the urine. A hormone from the adrenal cortex, *aldosterone,* stimulates the kidney to return sodium to the bloodstream.

Recommended Intake and Sources of Sodium

A chief concern is an excess of sodium in the diet. A safe minimum intake for infants and young children is considered to be 23 milligrams per kilogram of body weight. For adults, a safe minimum is regarded as 500 milligrams per day. Additional needs for pregnancy and lactation are estimated to be 69 milligrams and 139 milligrams, respectively, over the adult minimum (Subcommittee on the 10th Edition of the RDAs, 1989).

The average American intake is 4 to 6 grams of sodium per day. The maximum daily intake recommended is 2400 milligrams (Committee on Diet and Health, 1989).

Table salt, which is sodium chloride, is the major

TABLE 8–4   Comparison of Sodium Content in Fresh and Processed Foods

Fresh Food	Sodium (mg)	Processed Food	Sodium (mg)
Natural Swiss cheese 1 oz	74	Pasteurized, processed Swiss cheese, 1 oz	388
Lean roast pork, 3 oz.	65	Lean ham, 3 oz	930
Whole raw carrot, 1	25	Canned carrots, 1/2 cup	176
Tomato juice, canned without salt, 1 cup	24	Tomato juice, canned with salt, 1 cup	881

dietary source of sodium. Table salt is 40 percent sodium and 60 percent chloride. One teaspoonful (5 grams) of salt contains over 2 grams of sodium.

Many foods, such as milk, milk products, and several vegetables, are naturally high in sodium. More often than not, the sodium we consume is from the salt in processed foods. Table 8–4 compares the sodium content of relatively unprocessed foods with processed versions.

Deficiency of Sodium

Deficiency of sodium is associated primarily with increased sodium loss. Conditions such as diarrhea, vomiting, heavy sweating, or kidney disease may cause low serum sodium. The technical name for low serum sodium, less than 135 milliequivalents per liter in adults, is **hyponatremia.** A serum sodium that is low, not because of an absolute lack of sodium, but because of an excess of water is called *dilutional hyponatremia.* One condition producing this effect, the Syndrome of Inappropriate Secretion of Antidiuretic Hormone (SIADH), is discussed in Chapter 9, "Water and Body Fluids."

Toxicity from Sodium

The reported 4 to 6 grams of sodium in the average American diet probably is underestimated. Frequently such surveys do not account for all sources of sodium. Healthy persons excrete excess sodium without adverse effects. For persons with hypertension, heart disease, or kidney disease, the control of sodium balance becomes an important issue. An excess of sodium in the blood, greater than 145 milliequivalents per liter in adults, is called **hypernatremia.**

Potassium

The adult body contains about 270 grams of potassium, approximately 9 ounces. Ninety-eight percent of this amount of potassium is inside the cells, where it helps to control fluid balance.

Functions and Control of Potassium

In addition to fluid balance, potassium is essential for the conduction of nerve impulses and the contraction of muscles, including one vital muscle, the heart. Potassium helps to maintain acid-base balance and is required for the conversion of glucose to glycogen.

The kidney responds to systemic alkalosis by excreting potassium to conserve hydrogen. Retaining the hydrogen will make the blood more acidic and help to correct the alkalosis. Conversely, in acidosis, the body responds by excreting hydrogen and retaining potassium.

Estimated Minimum Intake and Sources of Potassium

There are no RDAs established for potassium. The estimated minimum amount for healthy adults is 2000 milligrams per day. The average American diet contains from 2000 to 4000 milligrams of potassium.

Sources of Potassium

Potassium is present in all plant and animal cells. Only fats, oils, and white sugar have negligible potassium. One cup of cooked, dry lima beans contains 1163 milligrams. Foods that supply almost half the minimum amount include: 1 cup of winter squash, 1 cup of cooked pinto beans, or 1 baked

---

Hypophosphatemia—Too little phosphate per volume of blood; in adults, less than 2.4 mg per 100 mL of serum.

Hyperphosphatemia—Abnormal amount of phosphate in the blood; in adults, greater than 4.7 mg per 100 mL of serum.

Hyponatremia—Too little sodium per volume of blood; less than 135 mEq/L of serum in adults.

potato with skin. Fruits are good sources of potassium. Over 500 milligrams are contained in 1 cup of sliced banana, 1/3 cup of dried apricots or peaches, 1/3 cantaloupe, or 3/4 cup of prune juice.

Deficiency of Potassium

A deficiency of potassium is related to diet only in cases of severe protein-calorie malnutrition. **Hypokalemia,** a serum potassium less than 3.5 milliequivalents per liter, can be fatal if prolonged or severe. Hypokalemia may be caused by diarrhea, vomiting, laxative abuse, alkalosis, and protein-calorie malnutrition. Deficiency symptoms include fatigue, muscle weakness, irregular pulse, nausea, vomiting, and decreased reflexes.

Toxicity from Potassium

Potassium levels greater than 5.0 milliequivalents per liter is **hyperkalemia.** Levels of 10–12 milliequivalents per liter usually produce cardiac arrest (Brensilver and Goldberger, 1996). Potassium toxicity is usually the result of diabetic acidosis, kidney failure, adrenal insufficiency, or severe dehydration. Hyperkalemia may also be caused by excessive destruction of cells in burns, crushing injuries, or severe infections. Vague muscle weakness usually appears first, followed by flaccid paralysis beginning in the legs and moving up the body. The muscles supplied by the cranial nerves are usually spared. The client remains alert and apprehensive (Brensilver and Goldberger, 1996).

Magnesium

The body contains about 1 ounce of magnesium. Up to 70 percent of this amount is combined with calcium and phosphorus in the bones. The remaining 30 percent is found in tissues and body fluids.

Functions and Control of Magnesium

Magnesium is necessary for the transmission of nerve impulses and the relaxation of skeletal muscles after contraction. It activates enzymes for the metabolism of carbohydrates, fats, and proteins, including protein synthesis. Magnesium activates the enzymes that add the third phosphate group to ADP to form ATP. It also aids in the release of energy from muscle glycogen. As a cofactor in calcium utilization, magnesium not only aids bone formation but also helps to hold calcium in tooth enamel, thus preventing tooth decay.

Magnesium competes with calcium for absorption in the upper small intestine. As magnesium intake increases, the percentage absorbed decreases. The kidney selectively excretes excess magnesium.

Recommended Dietary Allowances and Sources of Magnesium

The RDAs for magnesium are 280 to 350 milligrams for adults, or 4.5 milligrams per kilogram of body weight. The US diet usually provides an estimated 120 milligrams per 1000 kilocalories.

Magnesium is widely distributed in foods, especially plant foods, because it is part of the chlorophyll molecule. Green vegetables are good sources of magnesium. For example, one cup of cooked spinach contains 150 milligrams. Other good sources are seeds, legumes, shrimp, and some bran cereals.

Interfering Factors and Deficiency of Magnesium

High intakes of some nutrients may interfere with the absorption of magnesium. Phosphorus, calcium, fat, and protein are four such nutrients.

Magnesium deficiency may occur with protein-calorie malnutrition, but deficiency usually is the result of increased magnesium excretion or decreased magnesium absorption. Excessive excretion of magnesium can result from major surgery, vomiting, diarrhea, or diuretic therapy. Magnesium absorption is decreased in malabsorption syndromes and chronic alcoholism. Magnesium deficiency may exacerbate the increased neuroirritability in clients in acute alcohol withdrawal.

Magnesium deficiency probably occurs more often than it is diagnosed. In one study, 20 percent of the clients admitted to a medical intensive care unit had a deficiency of magnesium (Reinhart and Desbiens, 1985). Insufficient magnesium impairs central nervous system activity and increases muscular excitability. Because magnesium metabolism is intricately linked to calcium metabolism, magnesium-deficient clients display the signs of tetany. Other signs include disorientation, convulsions, and psychosis. Relief of signs and symptoms may take 60 to 80 hours after treatment begins (Brensilver and Goldberger, 1996).

Toxicity from Magnesium

Ordinarily, magnesium levels do not build up in the blood except as a result of kidney disease. A person with magnesium toxicity shows the following signs:

lethargy, sedation, hypotension, slow pulse, and depressed respirations. Respiratory or cardiac arrest may ensue. Because of its close link to calcium, the effects of magnesium toxicity can be blocked by administering calcium.

Sulfur

Sulfur is a component of the cytoplasm of every cell. It is especially notable in hair, skin, and nails, where the **disulfide linkages** help to hold the amino acids in their distinct shapes. Sulfur is a component of thiamine, biotin, insulin, and heparin. A protective function of sulfur is that of combining with toxins to neutralize them.

Important sources of sulfur are cheese, eggs, poultry, and fish. Cases of deficiency of sulfur are unknown. Only persons with a severe protein deficiency will lack this mineral.

Chloride

Whenever an industrial accident involving chlorine occurs, such as the derailment of a chlorine tanker car, the surrounding area is quickly evacuated because of the chemical's toxic effects. A harmless form of chlorine, *chloride*, far from being poisonous, is a required nutrient. The body contains about 90 grams of chloride. Chloride is found in hydrochloric acid in the stomach, and in fluid outside of the cells. Chloride is involved in the maintenance of normal fluid and proper acid-base balance. The estimated minimum recommended intake for chloride ranges from 180 to 300 milligrams for infants and is 750 milligrams for adults. Table salt, 60 percent chloride, contains 3 grams of chloride in 1 teaspoon (5 grams).

Loss of gastrointestinal fluids through severe vomiting, nasogastric suctioning, or diarrhea is a common cause of chloride deficiency. In 1979, an outbreak of chloride deficiency occurred in infants because chloride was omitted from the formula they received.

See Table 8–5 for a summary of the major minerals.

Trace Minerals

Trace minerals are present in the body in amounts less than 5 grams and have a recommended intake of less than 100 milligrams per day. Many trace minerals occur in such small amounts that they are difficult to measure and analyze; thus their physiological functions and possible roles in nutrition are not completely understood. For example, lead, gold, and mercury are found in body tissue but only, as far as is known, as the result of environmental contamination. See Clinical Application 8–5 for a discussion on lead poisoning.

Eight trace minerals have probable, but as yet undetermined, functions in human nutrition. This group includes aluminum, arsenic, boron, cadmium, nickel, tin, silicon, and vanadium.

Of the other trace minerals, only ten have known bodily functions and have been assigned RDAs or Estimated Safe and Adequate Daily Dietary Intakes (ESADDIs). Four of them are commonly recognized as being health related: iron, iodine, fluoride, and zinc. The other six include chromium, copper, cobalt, manganese, selenium, and molybdenum. These ten minerals are discussed individually in the sections below, starting with iron.

Iron

For a nutrient with functions as vital as those of iron, the amount in the body is very slight—about 4 grams. This is approximately the weight of a penny.

Function of Iron

Iron is essential to **hemoglobin** formation. Hemoglobin is composed of heme, the nonprotein portion that contains iron, and globin, a simple protein. Iron is also a component of **myoglobin,** a protein located in muscle tissue. Myoglobin stores oxygen within the muscle cells. When the body needs an immediate supply of oxygen, as during strenuous exercise, myoglobin releases its stored oxygen. Iron is also present in enzymes that permit the oxidation of glucose to produce energy.

About 80 percent of the iron in a healthy body is available for carrying oxygen: 65 percent is contained in the hemoglobin, 10 percent in the myoglobin, and 3 percent in iron-containing enzymes. The remainder is stored.

The main storage form of iron in the body is a protein-iron compound called **ferritin.** It is kept in

---

Hemoglobin—The iron-carrying pigment of the red blood cells; carries oxygen from the lungs to the tissues.

Myoglobin—A protein located in muscle tissue that contains iron and stores oxygen.

Ferritin—Form in which iron is stored in the tissues, mainly in liver, spleen, and bone marrow cells.

TABLE 8–5   Major Minerals

Mineral	Adult RDA and Food Portion Containing RDA	Functions	Signs and Symptoms of Deficiency	Signs and Symptoms of Excess	Best Sources
Calcium	800 mg 2.7 cups milk	Structure of bones and teeth Nerve conduction Muscle contraction Blood clotting	Tetany Osteoporosis Rickets	Renal calculi Calcification of soft tissue	Milk Sardines, oysters, clams, salmon
Phosphorus	800 mg 2.5 cups chili with beans	Structure of bones and teeth Component of DNA and RNA Component of ADP and ATP Component of phospholipids (i.e., myelin) Buffer	Increased calcium excretion Bone loss Muscle weakness	Tetany Convulsions Renal insufficiency	Lean meat Milk
Sodium	None*	Fluid balance Transmission of electrochemical impulses along nerve and muscle membranes	Hyponatremia	Hypernatremia	Table salt Processed foods Milk and milk products
Potassium	None*	Conduction of nerve impulses Muscle contraction	Hypokalemia (not usually dietary)	Hyperkalemia (not ususaly dietary)	Cooked dry lima beans Pinto beans Winter squash Baked potato Banana Dried apricots or peaches Cantaloupe Prune juice
Magnesium	280 mg (female) 350 mg (male) 0.5 to 0.7 cup sunflower seeds	Transmission of nerve impulses Relaxation of skeletal muscle Aids bone formation Helps hold calcium in teeth	Impaired CNS function Tetany	Weakness Depressed respirations Cardiac arrest	Sunflower seeds Sesame seeds Cashews Spinach Wheat germ
Sulfur	None	Component of some amino acids Gives shape to hair, skin, and nails	None known	None known	Protein foods
Chloride	None*	Component of hydrochloric acid Maintains fluid and acid base balance	In infants: failure to thrive, lethargy, muscle weakness	None known	Table salt Seafood Milk Meat Eggs

* See Table of Estimated Sodium, Chloride, and Potassium Minimum Requirements of Healthy Persons (Appendix H).

Lead Poisoning (**Plumbism**)

Lead is a contaminant in the human body. The effects of lead toxicity, such as neurological damage and retardation, can be devastating and permanent.

Food is not the chief source of lead. Years ago, "painters' colic" or chronic lead poisoning was a fairly common occupational hazard. Today, sweet-tasting, lead-based paint in older homes is the primary source of poisoning in inner-city children. A paint chip the size of a penny may contain from 50 to 100 micrograms of lead. This amount, ingested daily for 3 months, could accumulate to 100 times the tolerable level for adults. Recent childhood cases have been discovered after the family pets were affected. In both situations the source of lead was exterior renovation in the neighborhood (Dowsett and Shannon, 1994).

Other sources of lead are automobile emissions from leaded gasoline, lead or lead glazes on serving utensils, and solder in metal cans. Decreasing blood levels of lead in children have been correlated with diminishing amounts of lead in gasoline (Stromberg, Schutz, and Skerfuing, 1995). Two cases of plumbism in toddlers were traced to pool cue chalk (Miller, et al, 1996). A possible source of lead contamination is the ink used on bread wrappers. Turning the bags inside out and then using them for food storage could create a problem.

Hyperactivity has been linked to both lead poisoning and iron deficiency. There is evidence that suggests that these two conditions, not additives, allergens, or sugar, are the causes of hyperactivity.

Early diagnosis and treatment of lead poisoning are essential. Several chelating agents are available that will bind with lead. Even children successfully treated and kept away from further intake showed lasting brain damage in 25 percent of the cases.

Recently, concern about the lead content in aging municipal water pipes contaminating the water supply has resulted in action by the Environmental Protection Agency (EPA). The permissible lead level has been lowered from 50 parts per billion to 15 parts per billion. Many older homes also have plumbing that may contaminate the water. Ten infants were poisoned from formula reconstituted with lead-contaminated water (Shannon and Graef, 1992). To decrease the chance of lead leaching into drinking or cooking water, (1) flush the system before drawing water and (2) use cold water. Local health departments should be able to direct people to appropriate laboratories if they wish to have their water tested.

---

the liver, spleen, and bone marrow for future use. When surplus iron accumulates in the blood due to the rapid destruction of red blood cells, the excess is stored in the liver in another compound, **hemosiderin.**

Absorption of Iron

The body tightly conserves its supply of iron. Most dietary iron is absorbed in the duodenum. When red blood cells are destroyed after their life span of 120 days, the iron is stored for reuse. Once iron is absorbed, there is no mechanism for excreting excess. Fortunately, the body is selective about absorbing iron.

FACTORS AFFECTING AMOUNTS OF ABSORPTION   As the body's need for iron increases, so does the proportion absorbed. In a healthy person, 5 to 15 percent of the iron in foods is absorbed. The anemic person, however, absorbs as much as 50 percent.

The amount of iron that is absorbed is determined by the amount of ferritin already present in the intestinal mucosa (where ferritin is formed). The iron obtained from ingested food is bound to a protein called **apoferritin** to form ferritin. When the total supply of apoferritin has been bound to iron, any additional iron in the gut is rejected and eliminated in the feces.

Absorbed iron combines with a protein in the blood, **transferrin,** which transports iron to the bone marrow for hemoglobin synthesis, to the liver for storage, or to the body cells. Hemoglobin synthesis requires adequate protein and traces of copper, in addition to iron.

FACTORS AFFECTING RATES OF ABSORPTION   Two types of iron are found naturally in food: heme iron and nonheme iron. **Heme iron** is bound to the hemoglobin and myoglobin in meat, fish, and poultry. Forty percent of the total iron in these animal sources is heme iron. Because heme iron is com-

Hemosiderin—An iron oxide-protein compound derived from hemoglobin; a secondary storage form of iron.

Apoferritin—A protein found in intestinal mucosal cells that combines with iron to form ferritin; it is always found in the body attached to iron.

Transferrin—A protein in the blood that binds and transports iron.

Heme iron—Iron bound to hemoglobin and myoglobin in meat, fish, and poultry; 10 to 30 percent of the iron in these foods is absorbed.

posed of ferrous iron, (Fe^{2+}), it is rapidly transported and absorbed intact. The other 60 percent of the total iron in meat, fish, and poultry, and all the iron in plant sources, is **nonheme iron.**

The absorption of nonheme iron is slow because it is closely bound to organic molecules in foods as **fer-** **ric iron** (Fe^{3+}). In the acidic medium of the stomach, the oxygen is removed from ferric iron during a chemical reaction called *reduction.* The end product is **ferrous iron,** which is more soluble. See Figure 8–4 for an overview of the steps involved in the process of iron absorption.

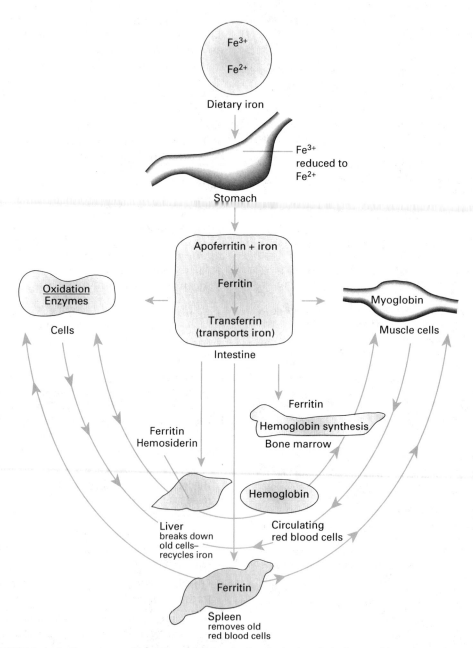

FIGURE 8–4   In the process of iron absorption, iron is absorbed primarily in the small intestine and may be transported or stored to meet the body's needs.

FACTORS ENHANCING THE ABSORPITON OF IRON Several factors increase the absorption of iron through very different mechanisms. Consumption of large amounts of alcohol damages the intestine, which then permits absorption of increased amounts of iron. A high calcium intake increases iron absorption because the calcium combines with phosphates and phytates so that they are not available to inhibit iron absorption. Vitamin C forms a soluble compound with iron, increasing its absorption. Lastly, an MFP (meat, fish, poultry) factor increases the absorption of iron. Nonheme iron absorption is increased when meat, fish, or poultry is consumed at the same time.

FACTORS INTERFERING WITH ABSORPTION OF IRON When less gastric acid is present, whether because of antacids or gastric resection, less iron is absorbed. Both phytic acid from cereals and oxalic acid from certain vegetables combine with iron, reducing its availability. Other minerals compete with iron for binding sites. Excesses of copper, zinc, or manganese decrease absorption of each other and of iron.

Nonheme iron can be locked out of the absorption process by substances called **tannates,** which are found in tea and coffee. Tea may reduce iron absorption by 60 percent; coffee by 40 percent, Table 8–6 summarizes the factors that affect iron absorption.

Excretion of Iron

No known mechanism exists to regulate the excretion of iron. Small amounts of iron are lost daily in sweat, hair, shed skin cells, and urine. Men lose 1 milligram per day, whereas women of reproductive age lose an average 1.5 to 2.4 milligrams per day, depending upon menstrual flow.

Recommended Dietary Allowance

The values set for the RDA are based on the assumption that only 10 to 15 percent of the iron in in-

TABLE 8–6 Factors Affecting Iron Absorption

Increase	Decrease
Large alcohol intake	Less gastric acid
High calcium intake	Coffee or tea (tannates)
Vitamin C	Phytic or oxalic acids
Meat, fish, or poultry	Excessive copper, manganese, or zinc intake

---

CLINICAL APPLICATION 8–6

Contamination Iron

It is possible to increase the iron content of foods by using iron cookware. Iron absorbed into food in this way is referred to as **contamination iron.** Significant transfer occurs during the simmering of acidic foods, especially tomatoes. For instance, 3 1/2 oz of spaghetti sauce cooked for 3 hours in a cast iron pot contains almost 90 mg of iron, compared to less than 5 mg of iron when cooked in a glass container. All foods tested significantly increased in iron content when cooked in a steel wok compared to a glass utensil (Zhou, 1994). The absorption rate of contamination iron is the same as that of iron supplements, 2 percent at best.

---

gested foods is absorbed. The RDAs for iron are: 10 milligrams for men, 15 milligrams for women of reproductive age and lactating women, and 30 milligrams for pregnant women.

Sources of Iron

The western diet contains an estimated 5 to 7 milligrams of iron per 1000 kilocalories. In the United States, one-third of dietary iron is supplied by grains, one-third by meats, and one-third by other sources. Absorption varies among the sources of iron also. Ten to thirty percent of iron is absorbed from liver and other meats; less than 10 percent is absorbed from eggs; and less than 5 percent is absorbed from grains and most vegetables. Spinach, iron supplements, and contamination iron are absorbed at a 2-percent rate. Clinical Application 8–6 describes one way iron is absorbed from nonfood sources. Of the commercial cereals directed toward children, only Cap'n Crunch comes close to the 10-milligram RDA for children aged 1 through 10. Selected cereal products containing significant amounts of iron are listed in Table 8–7. Manufacturers sometimes change these amounts. It is imperative to read labels. Although cereals and grains are nonheme sources, iron from grains is absorbed at a better rate than iron from supplements.

Nonheme iron—Iron that is not bound to hemoglobin or myoglobin; all the iron in plant sources.

TABLE 8–7   Comparison of Iron Content of Cereal Products

Cereal	Iron per Ounce (mg)
Product 19	18
Total	18
Regular Cream of Wheat	11
Kellogg's 40% Bran Flakes	8
Cap'n Crunch	7.5

Deficiency of Iron

Insufficient intake of iron, excessive blood loss, malabsorption, or lack of gastric hydrochloric acid can lead to **iron deficiency anemia.** The most common nutrient deficiency in the United States is iron. Even before the person becomes anemic, his cognitive performance can be impaired (Scrimshaw, 1991).

OCCURRENCE   Iron deficiency anemia affects about 15 percent of the world population. Iron deficiency is seen in 9.3 percent of 1- to 2-year-old children. Women 15 to 19 years old have a prevalence of 7.2 percent and those 20 to 44 years old, 6.3 percent. In sharp contrast, iron deficiency occurred in less than 1 percent of men aged 15 to 64.

RISK OF IRON DEFICIENCY   Individuals at greatest risk of iron deficiency are women of childbearing age and young children. Children 4 months to 3 years old, adolescents, and pregnant women should be monitored carefully for signs of iron deficiency because of increased needs. People with low incomes also are likely to be iron deficient. All women in their menstrual years are at risk, a risk that is increased if an intrauterine contraceptive device is being used. This device increases blood loss.

ASSESSMENT DATA   A common test to determine the hemoglobin level of the blood delivers valuable assessment data. The normal level for men is 14 to 18 grams per 100 milliliters of blood; for women it is 12 to 16 grams.

A second common laboratory test is the **hematocrit.** This test measures the percentage of red blood cells in a volume of blood. Normal hematocrit levels are 40 to 54 percent for men and 36 to 46 percent for women.

In early iron deficiency, before hemoglobin and hematocrit readings drop, serum transferrin levels rise. The person with early iron deficiency will, providing the body is attempting to compensate, manufacture more transferrin to increase iron-carrying capacity. For this reason, serum transferrin is the most reliable indicator of iron status.

After a person has been treated for iron deficiency, iron therapy should be continued for several months after hemoglobin and hematocrit levels return to normal. This prolonged therapy will enable the body to rebuild iron stores.

Toxicity from Iron

Iron toxicity can result from an oversupply of hemosiderin, iron metabolism disorders, chronic alcoholism, or iron poisoning. Surplus iron is stored in the liver as hemosiderin. When large amounts of hemosiderin are deposited in the liver and spleen, a condition called **hemosiderosis** results. If prolonged, it can lead to **hemochromatosis,** a disease of iron metabolism in which iron accumulates in the tissues. The person with this disease suffers from impaired liver function, blood sugar disturbances, joint pain, and skin discoloration. Cardiac failure and death may follow. The incidence of iron overload in parts of Africa is the highest in the world where some autopsy studies reported hepatic iron sufficient to cause cirrhosis at a prevalence of more than 10 percent (Gordeuk, 1992).

Chronic alcoholics have increased absorption of iron because of intestinal damage. Toxicity can occur if 75 milligrams of iron per day is ingested along with a regular intake of alcohol. Some alcoholic beverages themselves contain a significant amount of iron. For example, inexpensive red wines contain 10 to 350 milligrams of iron per liter. Thus, although the use of wine as a tonic may have certain merit, this is not the case when the user is an alcoholic.

Iron supplements present a significant hazard to children. In 1988, 19,676 iron ingestions were reported, 84 percent in children under 6 years of age (Litovitz, Schmitz, and Holm, 1989). As few as six to twelve tablets of ferrous sulfate have been known to cause the death of a child. All health care providers should teach safe storage of nutritional supplements.

Iodine

Iodine can be found in the muscles, thyroid gland, skin, and skeleton. The greatest concentration is in the thyroid gland in the neck. The body of the average adult contains 20 to 50 milligrams of iodine.

Function of Iodine and Control of the Thyroid Gland

The thyroid gland secretes **thyroxine** (T_4) and **triiodothyronine** (T_3) in response to the **thyroid stim-**

ulating hormone (TSH) from the anterior pituitary gland. Both T_3 and T_4 increase the rate of oxidation in cells, thereby increasing the rate of metabolism. The only known function of iodine is its participation in the synthesis of T_4 and T_3. When serum levels of T_3 and T_4 are adequate, secretion of TSH ceases.

Absorption and Excretion of Iodine

Iodine is easily absorbed from all portions of the intestinal tract. Of the absorbed iodine, 33 percent is used by the thyroid cells for the synthesis of T_4 and T_3, and the remaining 67 percent is excreted in the urine. After performing their functions, T_4 and T_3 are degraded by the liver, and the iodine content is excreted in bile.

Recommended Dietary Allowance and Sources of Iodine

The RDA for iodine is 150 micrograms for adult men and women. Iodine can come from foods, either naturally present or fortified, or from incidental sources.

IODINE IN FOODS   Foods that are naturally high in iodine include saltwater fish, shellfish, and seaweed. The iodine content in plants varies with the mineral content of the soil in which they are grown. The amount of iodine present in eggs and dairy products depends on the animals' diets.

Table salt fortified with iodine (1 milligram of iodine in 10 grams of salt) has been available in the United States since 1924. Sea salt is touted as superior to regular table salt. Because sea salt loses iodine during the evaporating (drying) process, it actually contains less iodine than fortified table salt.

INCIDENTAL IODINE   Sometimes iodine is present as a side effect of processing. For example, iodine solutions are used to sterilize milk pasteurization vats; some iodine may remain on the vat and be mixed into the next batch of milk to be processed. Iodine is also used to improve the texture of bread dough. A third source of incidental iodine is FDA Red Dye #3.

Deficiency of Iodine

Because the normal function of the thyroid gland depends on an adequate supply of iodine, a deficiency may result in goiter, cretinism, or myxedema. Fortunately, thyroid function can be readily evaluated by measuring protein-bound iodine and the serum levels of T_4 and T_3.

GOITER   When the thyroid gland does not receive sufficient iodine, it increases in size, attempting to increase production. The gland may reach 1 to 1.5 pounds (500 to 700 grams). This enlargement of the thyroid is called **goiter.** Unfortunately, replacement of iodine does not always reduce the goiter after the thyroid has enlarged. In some cases, prolonged deficiency results in thyroid tissue which produces T_3 and T_4 in response to dietary iodine rather than TSH. Iodine given to these people may cause hyperthyroidism (Medeiros-Neto, 1995; Pennington, 1990).

Goiter has been known as a disease entity since 3000 BC. In Asia alone, 400 million people have goiter. Because of iodine-poor soil, the Great Lakes states and the Rocky Mountain states once were considered the "goiter belt." Now that food supplies are nationwide and iodized salt is readily available, goiter is less common in this country.

CRETINISM   Severe **hypothyroidism** during pregnancy results in cretinism in the newborn. As a consequence of the mother's thyroid deficiency, the infant exhibits mental and physical retardation. Cretinism is a congenital condition (present at birth). The acquired form of this disease, which occurs in older children and adults, is called **myxedema.**

Factors Interfering with Iodine

Substances called **goitrogens** may block the body's absorption or utilization of iodine. Goitrogens are found in vegetables belonging to the cabbage family, including cauliflower, broccoli, brussels sprouts, rutabaga, and turnips. The only food linked to goiter is cassava, a starchy root eaten in developing countries.

Hemosiderosis—Condition resulting from excess deposits of hemosiderin, especially in the liver and spleen; caused by the rapid destruction of red blood cells, which occurs in diseases such as hemolytic anemia, pernicious anemia, and chronic infection.

Goiter—Enlargement of the thyroid gland caused by lack of sufficient iodine, thyroiditis due to infection or tumors, or hypofunction or hyperfunction of the thyroid gland.

Hypothyroidism—Undersecretion of thyroid hormones; reduces the metabolic rate.

Toxicity from Iodine

Toxicity from iodine has occurred in Japan from the ingestion of seaweed. Some nutritionists have expressed concern that there is too much iodine in the American diet, which contains 4 to 13 times the adult RDA. Strangely, too much iodine causes an "iodine goiter" and may also cause skin lesions similar to acne.

Fluoride

Fluoride, an ionized form of the element fluorine, accumulates mostly in the bones and teeth. It seems to make bone mineral less soluble and hence less likely to be reabsorbed. As such, fluoride inhibits dental caries and has been investigated as possibly helping to prevent osteoporosis.

Function of Fluoride

Teeth are strengthened by the incorporation of fluoride into their structure and are thus better able to resist the bacterial acids that cause dental caries. For this reason, fluoride is often added to water supplies, mouthwashes, and toothpastes, or taken as a prescription supplement. In the past 20 years, the use of fluoridated water and fluoride supplements has resulted in a 30 to 50 percent decrease in children's caries. In addition, fluoridated mouth rinses and toothpastes have reduced the incidence of caries in children by about 40 percent.

Estimated Safe and Adequate Daily Dietary Intake and Sources of Fluoride

The ESADDI that has been set for fluoride in adults is 1.5 to 4 milligrams.

One of the main sources of fluoride is fluoridated water. About 50 percent of the community water supply in the United States is fluoridated, to a concentration of one part per million. This amount equals 1 milligram per liter of water. Fluoridation costs only 30 cents per person per year. In Great Britain milk is fluoridated rather than water. Food sources of fluoride include fish, fish products, and tea. Also, foods prepared in fluoridated water will have increased levels of fluoride.

Toxicity from Fluoride

The excessive, prolonged ingestion of fluoride results in **fluorosis,** a condition that can cause mottled discoloration of the teeth in children (from birth to 8 or 10 years old). Fluorosis has been observed when the concentration of fluoride has reached 2 parts per million. The fluorosis produced by this dose may be cosmetically unacceptable, but the teeth are sound. Just as an excess of iodine causes the same symptoms as deficiency (i.e., goiter), a fluoride concentration of 4 parts per million is associated with increased dental caries.

Fluoride intake bears watching: some persons receive too little fluoride; others too much. For example, members of communities that do not have a fluoridated water supply may develop fluoride insufficiency, while the increased availability and excess use of fluoridated products (including water) may lead to toxicity.

Zinc

Estimated content of zinc in adult humans is 1.5 to 2.5 grams. Zinc is a component of all body tissues, including pancreas, liver, kidney, lung, muscle, bone, eye, skin, and sperm. Greater concentrations are found in the eye, bone, and male reproductive organs.

Functions of Zinc

Zinc is essential for the growth and repair of tissues because it is involved in the synthesis of DNA and RNA. Zinc is incorporated into the structure of more than 200 enzymes for protein and DNA synthesis, and it is associated with the hormone insulin. It is also necessary for the metabolism of all the energy nutrients. The production of active vitamin A for the visual pigment rhodopsin requires zinc. It is necessary for the formation of collagen, a requisite material for wound healing. Zinc also protects against disease through its role in providing immunity.

Absorption and Control of Zinc

Zinc is absorbed from the small intestine through the same absorption sites as iron. Up to 40 percent of zinc in animal products is absorbed compared to 15 percent in high phytate diets (Sandstrom, 1995). No storage is available in the body for zinc.

Unabsorbed zinc and the zinc in pancreatic secretions are excreted through intestinal wastes. The liver removes excessive zinc effectively. An abnormal zinc metabolism has been observed in persons with diabetes, but zinc's role in the etiology of diabetes is as yet unknown. The healthy person excretes no zinc in the urine, but in catabolic conditions, zinc (as well as potassium, creatinine, and nitrogen) appears in the urine from the breakdown of muscle tissue.

Recommended Dietary Allowances and Sources of Zinc

The RDAs for zinc are 12 to 15 milligrams for adults. Adolescent boys also have an RDA of 15 milligrams.

The best dietary sources of zinc are shellfish and red meat. Three ounces of shucked Eastern oysters contain 121 milligrams, of Western oysters 17 milligrams. More popular foods high in zinc are canned pork and beans (7.45 milligrams in half cup), canned chili with beans (5.13 milligrams in 1 cup), wheat germ (4.73 milligrams in quarter cup), and beef sirloin steak or rump roast (4.45 and 4.21 milligrams in 3 ounces).

Interfering Factors

Iron and zinc compete for the same absorption sites. Thus, if a person's intake of iron is two to three times that of zinc, the absorption of zinc is reduced. Decreased absorption of zinc has been noted when a 30-milligram supplement of iron is taken. As with iron, excessive copper or manganese decreases the absorption of zinc. Vitamin and mineral supplements with a greater than a 3-to-1 iron-to-zinc ratio inhibit zinc absorption. Calcium, excess folate, fiber, phytates, and **chelating agents** all reduce the absorption of zinc. Zinc itself is a chelating agent protecting the body from poisoning from lead and cadmium. If a person has marginal zinc status, high intakes of coffee, cocoa, tea, or whole grain products (especially if unleavened) may lower zinc levels because of their phytate content.

Deficiency of Zinc

Clinical zinc deficiency is not widespread in the United States. However, the American food supply provides only 12.3 milligrams per person per day. Groups at risk because of limited meat intake include the elderly, the poor, and vegetarians. Zinc supplementation was effective in promoting weight gain in failure to thrive infants, although their laboratory studies were not different from the infants in the placebo group (Walravens, Hambidge, and Koepfer, 1989).

Zinc deficiency in adults can also occur as a result of diseases that either hinder zinc absorption or cause excessive amounts of zinc to be excreted in the urine. Some of the clinical conditions that may precipitate zinc deficiency include acute myocardial infarction, alcoholic cirrhosis, celiac disease, Crohn's disease, and lymphoma.

Symptoms of zinc deficiency include abnormal fatigue, decreased alertness, impaired night vision, anorexia, and diminished sense of taste and smell. Signs include diarrhea and vomiting, retarded growth (dwarfism), delayed sexual maturation (if deficiency occurs during critical growth periods), low sperm counts, and delayed healing of wounds and burns.

Because serum zinc levels greater than 400 milligrams per deciliter may inhibit wound repair, supplemental zinc should not be given to clients who are not deficient. Supplementation speeds the healing process only in the truly deficient client (i.e., serum zinc 100 micrograms per deciliter) (Silane and Oot-Giromini, 1990).

Toxicity from Zinc

Because zinc can be toxic if consumed in excessive amounts, it should be obtained from foods in the diet and not from supplements. Supplemental doses only two to three times the RDA can interfere with copper absorption and lead to copper deficiency. Supplementation at the RDA level blocks the exercise effect of increasing serum levels of high-density lipoproteins (HDLs), the "good cholesterol." Ten times the RDA, 150 milligrams per day, has been shown to impair white blood cells and decrease HDLs (Subcommittee on 10th edition of RDAs, 1989).

Copper

The healthy adult body contains 50 to 120 milligrams of copper. Absorption of copper occurs in the stomach and upper intestine and varies inversely with intake. It is stored in the liver and excreted in feces as a component of bile salts.

Functions of Copper

Copper is a cofactor for enzymes involved in hemoglobin and collagen formation. It helps to incorporate iron into hemoglobin and to transport iron to the bone marrow. As a component of Factor V, copper is necessary for blood clotting. It helps to

> **Chelating agent**—Chemical compound that binds metallic ions into a ring structure, inactivating them; used to remove poisonous metals from the body.

oxidize glucose and release energy. Copper is necessary for melanin pigment formation and for maintaining myelin sheaths.

Estimated Safe and Adequate Daily Dietary Intake and Sources of Copper

The ESADDI for copper is 1.5 to 3 milligrams for adults. In the United States, adult intake averages 1 to 2 milligrams. Unfortunately, data is missing on the copper content of many foods listed or programmed in databases. Also, a food's copper content varies with its handling. The best sources of copper are organ meats, shellfish, nuts, and legumes. Three ounces of liver contains 3 milligrams of copper.

Interfering Factors and Deficiency of Copper

High intakes of zinc, iron, calcium, and manganese interfere with copper absorption. Only 18.5 milligrams of zinc per day impaired copper absorption. Phytates hinder absorption by forming more stable complexes with copper than with calcium or iron. An alkaline medium inhibits copper absorption. A dose of 15 antacid tablets per day may precipitate copper and induce deficiency.

Copper deficiency is not known in adults under normal conditions, but it has occurred as a result of the administration of **total parenteral nutrition** (TPN) for prolonged periods. Total parenteral nutrition is an intravenous feeding designed to meet all a person's nutritional needs. Copper deficiency also has occurred in premature infants fed exclusively on cow's milk.

Because of its link with iron utilization, copper deficiency produces a hypochromic, microcytic anemia. Other manifestations of copper deficiency are skeletal demineralization, impaired immune function, and depigmentation of the skin and hair.

Toxicity from Copper

Clients treated with the artificial kidney and infants fed water high in copper have become toxic. A genetic defect in copper excretion causes **Wilson's Disease.** Copper then accumulates in various organs, particularly the liver, kidneys, and brain. Part of the treatment regimen is avoiding foods high in copper.

Selenium

The mineral selenium is part of an enzyme, *glutathione peroxidase*, which works with vitamin E to protect cellular compounds from oxidation. In this role, selenium functions as an antioxidant. Selenium and vitamin E have a reciprocal sparing relationship (each spares the other). Selenium forms part of the protein matrix of the teeth, appears necessary for iodine metabolism, and helps to protect the liver from cirrhosis. The highest concentrations of this mineral occur in the liver, kidneys, and heart.

The RDA for selenium for adults is 55 to 70 micrograms. Adolescence, pregnancy, and lactation increase the need for selenium while a high vitamin E intake reduces it.

The amount of selenium present in plant foods depends on the selenium content of the soil and water where the foods are grown. In Finland it is necessary to add selenium to the soil. Seafood, low-fat meats, whole grains, dairy products, and legumes are the best dietary sources of selenium.

Deficiencies of selenium have been produced in animals but are unlikely in humans if meat is consumed on a regular basis. Nevertheless, there are some exceptions. Several clients being maintained on TPN have developed heart disease that responded to selenium treatment. A deterioration of the heart due to selenium deficiency has occurred in residents of the province of Keshan, China. The fatality rate in what is called *Keshan disease* is as high as 80 percent. Researchers have linked selenium deficiency in mice to mutation of an avirulent virus to a virulent one producing myocardial disease. Significantly, the virulent strain then caused heart disease in mice not selenium-deficient (Beck, et al, 1995).

Toxicity from selenium occurs in animals grazing on selenium-rich land. In humans, selenium toxicity occurred when the amount in a supplement was 125 times the correct dose. Signs and symptoms of selenium toxicity include fatigue, nausea and vomiting, garlic or sour-milk breath odor, and nail and hair loss. Animals who consume excessive selenium exhibit nervous system impairment and die of respiratory failure.

Chromium

The adult body contains 4 to 6 milligrams of chromium. High concentrations are found in the kidneys, liver, muscle, spleen, and pancreas.

Chromium is associated with RNA and DNA and is a cofactor in the activation of enzymes involved in fat and cholesterol metabolism. Chromium increases the cellular uptake of glucose by helping to bind insulin to its receptor sites on the cell membranes. Chromium is a component of **glucose toler-**

ance factor (GTF), which stimulates the action of insulin.

The ESADDI for chromium for adults ranges from 50 to 200 micrograms. Less than 5 percent of the dietary chromium is absorbed. The chief organ of excretion is the kidney.

Brewer's yeast and whole grains are good sources of chromium. Unprocessed foods are better sources than refined foods. Other sources are meats, especially organ meats, cheese, and seasonings such as thyme and black pepper. Chromium is leached from stainless steel, particularly with acid foods.

Chromium deficiency impairs the effectiveness of insulin and usually results in an elevated blood glucose or glucose intolerance. In some clients receiving TPN, chromium, not insulin, successfully lowered their blood sugar levels. Lack of sufficient chromium intake is also associated with coronary artery disease. Supplementation with chromium has improved blood lipid levels.

Dietary toxicity from chromium usually occurs from eating contaminated foods. The characteristic symptom is a disagreeable metallic taste in the mouth. A more common cause is absorption through the skin or lungs in an industrial setting.

Manganese

The body contains only 10 to 20 milligrams of manganese, found in highest concentrations in the bones and glands. Manganese is a cofactor of enzymes involved in energy metabolism and is required for bone formation. Unlike nutrients that fulfill unique functions, other minerals sometimes can substitute for manganese. One such mineral is magnesium.

The ESADDI for manganese is 2 to 5 milligrams for adults. About 40 percent of the manganese ingested is absorbed. It is excreted in bile and pancreatic secretions.

The best sources of manganese are wheat bran, legumes, nuts, and leafy green vegetables. Other good sources are cereal grains, coffee, and tea. Excessive intakes of iron, zinc, or copper cause decreased manganese absorption.

Low serum manganese levels have been reported in diabetes, pancreatic insufficiency, protein-calorie malnutrition, and some types of epilepsy. The patient displays weight loss, hypocholesterolemia, nausea, vomiting, dermatitis, and color changes of the hair.

Toxicity due to dietary intake has not been reported. However, miners exposed to manganese dust over prolonged periods have suffered liver and CNS damage, muscle spasms, and monotone voice. The clinical picture of manganese toxicity resembles Parkinson's disease.

Cobalt

As an essential component of the vitamin B_{12} molecule, cobalt is necessary for red blood cell formation. An RDA for cobalt has not been established. Foods that provide vitamin B_{12} are also good sources of cobalt; these foods are meats, poultry, fish, shellfish, and milk.

Cobalt deficiency has not been reported in humans or animals. Very large pharmaceutical doses have produced an excess of red blood cells (polycythemia) in humans, and chronic high doses over time can produce goiter (Lindeman, 1987).

Molybdenum

Molybdenum, a cofactor for enzymes involved in protein synthesis, is found primarily in the liver, kidneys, bone, and adrenal glands. It is equally excreted in the urine and the feces.

The ESADDI for adults is 75 to 250 micrograms. Daily intake from the average diet provides from 200 to 500 micrograms. Sources of molybdenum are organ meats, legumes, and grains. Because molybdenum is a copper antagonist, high levels of copper decrease the absorption of molybdenum.

One client on TPN was treated as molybdenum deficient. His signs and symptoms were caused by an inability to process sulfur-containing amino acids. His clinical picture was of increased pulse rate and respiratory rate, visual defects, night blindness, irritability, and coma. After discontinuation of sulfur-containing amino acid intake and supplementation with molybdenum, the symptoms disappeared (Committee on Diet and Health, 1989).

In Russia, intakes of 10 to 15 milligrams of molybdenum per day (40 times the US ESADDI) are associated with hyperuricemia and gout. No definite toxicity has been documented in humans.

A summary of the main food sources of each of the trace minerals discussed in this chapter appears in Table 8–8.

Glucose tolerance factor (GTF)—Organic compound containing chromium, which enhances the action of insulin, facilitating the uptake of glucose by the body's cells.

TABLE 8–8   Trace Minerals

Mineral	Adult RDA and Food Portion Containing RDA	Functions	Signs and Symptoms of Deficiency	Signs and Symptoms of Excess	Best Sources
Iron	15 mg (female) 10 mg (male) 2–3 tbsp Blackstrap molasses	Component of hemoglobin	Fatigue, listlessness Impaired cognition Hypochromic, microcytic anemia	Hemosiderosis Hemochromatosis	Liver, other organ meats Blackstrap molasses Oysters Red meat
Iodine	150 mcg 0.3 tsp iodized salt	Component of thyroid hormones	Goiter Cretinism Myxedema	Acne-like lesions Goiter	Iodized salt Saltwater seafood
Fluoride	None*	Hardens teeth	Dental caries	Mottled teeth Increased caries	Fluoridated water Seafood
Zinc	12 mg (female) 15 mg (male) 0.8 to 1 cup canned pork and beans	Involved in DNA and RNA synthesis Component of >200 enzymes Associated with insulin Required for production of active vitamin A Necessary for formation of collagen Serves role in immunity Essential role in sexual maturation Integral role in energy metabolism, including alcohol detoxification	Growth failure Hypogonadism Poor wound healing Impaired night vision Abnormal taste and smell	Copper deficiency Cancellation of effect of exercise on HDLs Impaired white blood cells	Oysters Canned pork and beans Canned chili with beans Wheat germ Beef sirloin steak or rump roast
Copper	None*	Cofactor for enzymes involved in hemoglobin and collagen formation Component of Factor V in clotting sequence Necessary for melanin formation Required to maintain myelin	Anemia Demineralization of skeleton Depigmentation of skin and hair Impaired immune function	Copper deposits in liver, kidneys, and brain	Oysters Liver Fortified cereal
Selenium	55 mcg (female) 70 mcg (male) Amount in food varies with region	Antioxidant Interchangable with vitamin E for some functions	Keshan cardiomyopathy	Nail and hair loss Nervous system impairment	Seafood Liver Meats Dairy products
Chromium	None*	Cofactor in enzymes used in fat and cholesterol metabolism Component of glucose tolerance factor	Glucose intolerance Elevated blood lipids	Rare related to food Metallic taste	Brewer's yeast Whole grains Meats

TABLE 8–8 Trace Minerals (Continued)

Mineral	Adult RDA and Food Portion Containing RDA	Functions	Signs and Symptoms of Deficiency	Signs and Symptoms of Excess	Best Sources
Manganese	None*	Cofactor of enzymes involved in energy metabolism Required for bone formation Essential for normal brain function Magnesium may substitute for manganese in some functions	In animals: Impaired growth Skeletal abnormalities CNS malfunction	Not reported due to diet Miners: liver damage Parkinson-like syndrome—monotone voice, CNS impairment	Wheat bran Legumes Nuts Leafy vegetables
Cobalt	None	Component of vitamin B_{12}	Not reported	Polycythemia Goiter	Meat, poultry Fish, shellfish Milk
Molybdenum	None*	Cofactor for enzymes involved in protein synthesis	TPN patient: Inability to process sulfur-containing amino acids	Hyperuricemia Gout	Organ meats Legumes Grains

* See Table of Estimated Safe and Adequate Daily Dietary Intakes (ESADDI) of Selected Vitamins and Minerals (Appendix G).

Supplementation

Excessive intake of nutrients can be as harmful as insufficient intake. For healthy people, obtaining minerals from food is preferred over medicinal supplementation. If supplements are elected by healthy people, the dose should not exceed the RDAs or ESADDIs for each mineral. For some minerals, toxicity is possible at levels slightly above the recommended or estimated intake amounts. In addition, an excess of one mineral may cause a deficiency of another.

Summary

Minerals are inorganic substances that are necessary for good health. Like vitamins, they help to regulate body functions without providing energy. Unlike vitamins, minerals become part of the body's structure and enzymes.

In human nutrition, minerals are classified as major or trace. Major minerals are present in the body in amounts of 5 grams (1 teaspoonful) or more and have a daily recommended intake of 100 milligrams

or more. Of the seven major minerals, inadequate calcium intake and excessive sodium intake are considered actual public health problems, and inadequate potassium intake is considered a potential public health problem.

Trace minerals are those present in amounts smaller than 5 grams and have a daily recommended intake of less than 100 milligrams. Of the 10 trace minerals discussed in this chapter, only lack of iron intake is considered a public health issue in the United States. Intakes of fluoride and zinc are being monitored as potential problems by the federal government.

As is the case with vitamins, people can be adversely affected by either insufficient or excessive intakes of minerals. Strangely, some minerals produce the same symptoms in both cases. When a client is nourished only by intravenous feedings for a long time, deficiencies of trace minerals may become apparent.

Food is the safest source for nutrients. To prevent possible toxicity, people who take supplements should limit intake to RDA or ESADDI levels. Pharmaceutical preparations are preferred to "natural" ones, which may have uncertain strengths and possible contaminants.

Case Study 8–1

Mrs. B is a 34-year-old woman who has related her fear of osteoporosis to the nurse. A recent visit to a 75-year-old aunt crystallized this fear. The aunt has become stooped and recently broke her hip. Mrs. B is especially concerned because she has often been told she resembles this aunt. Mrs. B asks, "Is there anything I can do to prevent this from happening to me?"

A 24-hour recall of dietary intake revealed a total of 1 cup of milk and no other dairy products. She did consume two 3 oz servings of meat. Mrs. B has three small children and stated that they are exercise enough for her. She sits outside and watches them play on every nice day.

Mrs. B is 5 ft, 3 in tall and weighs 110 lb. She is Caucasian with fair skin.

NURSING CARE PLAN

Assessment

Subjective Data Fear of osteoporosis

Family history positive for osteoporosis

Less than RDA for calcium previous 24 hours

Meeting Food Pyramid guideline for meat group

No planned exercise program

Objective Data Height: 5 ft, 3 in

Weight: 110 lb

Caucasian, fair, slight build

Nursing Diagnosis Health-seeking behavior regarding preventive measures for osteoporosis related to fear of repeating aunt's experience as evidenced by request for information.

Desired Outcome/ Evaluation Criteria	Nursing Actions	Rationale
Client will list appropriate actions to build a strong skeleton after teaching session.	Teach client how to consume 800 mg of calcium daily: 3 cups of milk or equivalent.	One cup of milk contains approximately 300 mg of calcium.
	Teach client factors favoring calcium absorption: moderate protein intake.	High protein intake causes increased calcium excretion by the kidneys.
	Teach client role of exercise in making bones strong.	Weight-bearing exercise stimulates the osteoblasts to build bone.

Study Aids

Chapter Review

1. Like vitamins, minerals give no energy to the body. Unlike vitamins, minerals:
   a. Are completely absorbed from the intestinal tract
   b. Become part of the structure of the body
   c. Cause few clinical problems because of their great abundance in foods
   d. Cannot accumulate to such an extent to cause problems

2. Calcium is necessary for strong bones and teeth. It is also necessary for:
   a. Keeping the stomach acid
   b. Muscle contraction
   c. Preventing blood clots
   d. The production of insulin

3. From which of the following sources of iron is the greatest percentage of iron absorbed by the average person?
   a. Eggs
   b. Ferrous sulfate tablets
   c. Meat
   d. Vegetables

4. Which of the following individuals would be at greatest risk for a mineral deficiency?
   a. Someone who consumes no dairy products.
   b. Someone who consumes no shellfish.
   c. Someone who consumes no red meat.
   d. Someone who drinks tea or coffee with every meal.

5. The most common nutrient deficiency in the United States is that of:
   a. Calcium
   b. Iodine
   c. Iron
   d. Zinc

Clinical Analysis

Mrs. H is a 30-year-old mother of three children all under 5 years of age. On her 6-week postpartum visit, her hemoglobin level was 10 grams per 100 milliliters of blood. She is given a prescription for ferrous sulfate and referred to the office nurse for nutrition counseling regarding her iron intake.

Mrs. H tells the nurse that she eats what the children eat; cold cereal and milk for breakfast, peanut butter and jelly sandwiches and maybe a banana for lunch, and casseroles of tuna or hamburger for din-

ner. Mrs. H is a heavy coffee drinker, consuming 10 cups per day, two with each meal and a total of four others during "coffee breaks."

The H family is lower middle-class. Mr. H is a long-distance truck driver and is away from home for long intervals. Mrs. H has some knowledge of iron needs and sources because of her three pregnancies. She is reluctant to continue the ferrous sulfate she has been taking throughout her pregnancy. "It binds me up," she tells the nurse. Also, Mrs. H maintains she cannot eat liver: "It gags me."

1. To maximize Mrs. H's iron intake with as little change in her habits as possible, the nurse would want to know:
   a. Whether Mrs. H drinks regular or decaffeinated coffee
   b. What kinds of cereal Mrs. H consumes
   c. At what time of day the H family eats
   d. Whether or not Mrs. H has tried veal liver

2. Which of the following statements by Mrs. H would indicate she understood the nurse's instructions correctly?
   a. "I should eat a little meat, fish, or poultry with every meal containing grain and fruit and vegetable sources of iron."
   b. "I should increase the fiber in my diet because it will increase the absorption of iron."
   c. "If I want an alcoholic beverage, beer contains the most iron in a readily absorbable form."
   d. "Since I am taking an iron supplement, it is not important how I eat."

3. To meet the safety needs of the H children, the nurse instructs Mrs. H to keep her ferrous sulfate in a locked cupboard. The reason for this is:
   a. Oral pharmaceutical iron preparations are absorbed better than the iron in foods.
   b. The human body has no effective means of excreting an overload of iron.
   c. Iron poisoning, although rare, can occur if a child ingests more than 30 tablets of ferrous sulfate.
   d. Because iron binds with calcium, an overdose of iron would cause rickets.

Bibliography

Abreo, K, Adlakha, A, Kilpatrick, S, et al: The milk-alkali syndrome. Arch Intern Med 153:1005, 1993.

Aloia, JF, et al: Calcium supplementation with and without hormone replacement therapy to prevent postmenopausal bone loss. Ann Inter Med 120:97, 1994.

Beall, DP, and Scofield, RH: Milk-alkali syndrome associated with calcium carbonate consumption. Medicine 74:89, 1995.

Beck, MA, et al: Rapid genomic evolution of a non-virulent Coxsackievirus B_3 in selenium-deficient mice results in selection of identical virulent isolates. Nature Medicine 1:433, 1995.

Blaauw, R, et al: Risk factors for the development of osteoporosis in a South African population. South African Med J 84:328, 1994.

Black, DM: Why elderly women should be screened and treated to prevent osteoporosis. Am J Med (suppl 2A) 98:2A–67S, 1995.

Brensilver, JM, and Goldberger, E: A Primer of Water, Electrolyte, and Acid-Base Syndromes, ed 8. FA Davis, Philadelphia 1996.

Brussaard, JH, Hulshof, KFAM, and Lowik, MRH: Calculated iodine intake before and after simulated iodization (Dutch Nutrition Surveillance System). Ann Nutr Metab 39:85, 1995.

Chapuy, MC, et al: Vitamin D_3 and calcium to prevent hip fractures in elderly women. N Engl J Med 327:1637, 1992.

Committee on Diet and Health, Food and Nutrition Board, Commission on Life Sciences, National Research Council: Diet and Health: Implications for Reducing Chronic Disease Risk. National Academy Press, Washington, DC, 1989.

Cook, JD, Skikne, BS, and Baynes, RD: Iron deficiency: The global perspective. In Hershko, C, et al, (eds): Progress in Iron Research. Plenum Press, New York, 1994.

Cooper, C, and Barker, DJP: Risk factors for hip fracture. N Engl J Med 332:814, 1995.

Cory-Slechta, DA: Bridging human and experimental animal studies of lead neurotoxicity: Moving beyond IQ. Neurotoxicology and Teratology 17:219, 1995.

Cummings, SR, et al: Risk factors for hip farctures in white women. N Engl J Med 332:767,1995.

Davis, JR, and Sherer, K: Applied Nutrition and Diet Therapy for Nurses, ed 2. WB Saunders, Philadelphia, 1994.

Dawson-Hughes, B, et al: Effect of vitamin D supplementation on wintertime and overall bone loss in healthy postmenopausal women. Ann Intern Med 115:505, 1991.

Dawson-Hughes, B, et al: Rates of bone loss in postmenopausal women randomly assigned to one of two dosages of vitamin D. Am J Clin Nutr 61:1140, 1995.

Diamond, T, et al: Ethanol reduces bone formation and may cause osteoporosis. Am J Med 86:282,1989.

Dowsett, R, and Shannon, M: Letter to the Editor. N Engl J Med 331:1661, 1994.

Eaton-Evans, J: Osteoporosis and the role of diet. Br J Biomed Sci 51:358, 1994.

ESHA Research: Food Processor Plus. Salem, OR, 1994.

Gordeuk, VR: Dietary iron overload [letter]. N Engl J Med 326:1705, 1992.

Gordeuk, VR: Hereditary and nutritional iron overload. Baillieres Clin Haematol 5:169, 1992.

Gordeuk, VR, et al: Iron overload in Africa—Interaction between a gene and dietary iron content. N Engl J Med 326:95, 1992.

Groff, JL, Gropper, SS, and Hunt, SM: Advanced Nutrition and Human Metabolism, ed 2. West, Minneapolis, 1995.

Haan, MN, Gerson, M, and Zishka, BA: Identification of children at risk for lead poisoning: An evaluation of routine pediatric blood lead screening in an HMO-insured population. Pediatrics 97:79, 1996.

Harris, P, Clark, M, and Karp, RJ: Prevention and treatment of lead poisoning. In Karp, RJ (ed): Malnourished Children in the United States. Springer, New York, 1993.

Heaney, RP: Protein intake and the calcium economy. J Am Diet Assoc 93:1259, 1993.

Hopper, JL, and Seeman, E: The bone density of female twins discordant for tobacco use. N Engl J Med 330:387, 1994.

Johnston, CO, et al: Calcium supplementation and increases in bone mineral density in children. N Engl J Med 327:82, 1992.

Kinsbourne, M: Sugar and the hyperactive child. N Engl J Med 330:355, 1994.

Krall, EA, et al: Effect of vitamin D intake on seasonal variations in parathyroid hormone secretion in postmenopausal women. N Engl J Med 321:1777, 1989.

Lindeman, RD: Minerals in medical practice. In Halpern, SL (ed): Quick Reference to Clinical Nutrition ed 2. JB Lippincott, Philadelphia, 1987.

Lindsay, R and Nieves, J: Milk and bones. Br Med J 308:930, 1994.

Lips, P, et al: Determinants of vitamin D status in patients with hip fracture and in elderly control subjects. Am J Clin Nutr 46:1005, 1987.

Litovitz, TL, Schmitz, BF, and Holm, KC: 1988 annual report of the American Association of Poison Control Centers National Data Collection System. Am J Emerg Med 7:495, 1989.

Lucas, SR, Sexton, M, and Langenberg, P: Relationship between blood lead and nutritional factors in preschool children: A cross-sectional study. Pediatrics 97:74, 1996.

Medeiros-Neto, G: Iodide deficiency disorders. In DeGroot, LJ (ed): Endocrinology ed 3 vol I. WB Saunders, Philadelphia, 1995.

Mertz, W: Chromium in human nutrition: A review. J Nutr 123:626, 1993.

Meyer, HE, et al: Risk factors for hip fracture in a high incidence area: A case-control study from Oslo, Norway. Osteoporosis Int 5:239, 1995.

Miller, MB, et al: Pool cue chalk: A source of environmental lead. Pediatrics 97:916, 1996.

Murphy, S, et al: Milk consumption and bone mineral density in middle aged and elderly women. Br Med J 308:939, 1994.

National Institutes of Health Consensus Development Panel on Optimal Calcium Intake: Optimal calcium intake. JAMA 272:1942, 1994.

Nelson, M, et al: A 1 year walking program and increased dietary calcium in postmenopausal women: Effects on bone. Am J Clin Nutr 53:1304, 1991.

Nelson, ME, et al: Effects of high-intensity strength training on multiple risk factors for osteoporotic fractures. JAMA 272:1909, 1994.

Pac, CYC, et al: Treatment of postmenopausal osteoporosis with slow-release sodium fluoride. Ann Intern Med 123:401, 1995.

Pennington, JAT: A review of iodine toxicity reports. J Am Diet Assoc 90:1571, 1990.

Reid, IR, et al: Long-term effects of calcium supplementation on bone loss and fractures in postmenopausal women: A randomized controlled trial. Am J Med 98:331, 1995.

Reinhart, RA, and Desbiens, NA: Hypomagnesemia in patients entering the ICU. Crit Care Med 13:506, 1985.

Sandstrom, B: Considerations in estimates of requirements and critical intake of zinc: Adaption, availability and interactions. Analyst 120:913, 1995.

Schaffer, SJ, et al: Lead poisoning risk determination in a rural setting. Pediatrics 97:84, 1996.

Scrimshaw, NS: Iron deficiency. Scientific Am 265:46, 1991.

Shannon, M, and Graef, J: Hazard of lead in infant formula. N Engl J Med 326:137, 1992.

Silane, MF, and Oot-Giromini, B: Systemic and other factors that affect wound healing. In Eaglstein, WH (ed): New Directions in Wound Healing. ER Squibb, Princeton, NJ, 1990.

Stromberg, U, Schutz, A, and Skerfring, S: Substantial decrease in blood lead in Swedish children, 1978–94, associated with petrol lead. Occup Environ Med 52:764, 1995.

Subcommittee on the 10th Edition of the RDAs. Food and Nutrition Board. Commission on Life Sciences. National Research

Council: Recommended Dietary Allowances, cd 10. National Academy Press, Washington, DC, 1989.

Walravens, PA, Hambidge, KM, and Koepfer, DM: Zinc supplementation in infants with a nutritional pattern of failure to thrive: A double-blind, controlled study. Pediatrics 83:532, 1989.

Watson, J, and Jaffe, MS: Nurse's Manual of Laboratory and Diagnostic Tests, ed 2. FA Davis Company, Philadelphia, 1995.

Wolraich, ML, et al: Effects of diets high in sucrose or aspartame on the behavior and cognitive performance of children. N Engl J Med 330:301, 1994.

Wolraich, ML, et al: The effect of sugar on behavior or cognition in children. JAMA 274:1617, 1995.

Zhou, Y, and Brittin, HC: Increased iron content of some Chinese foods due to cooking in steel woks. J Am Diet Assoc 94:1153, 1994.

CHAPTER 9

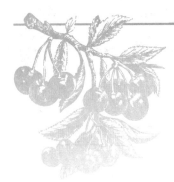

Water and Body Fluids

LEARNING OBJECTIVES

After completing this chapter, the student should be able to:

1 Describe the locations and functions of water in the body.

2 Discuss the body's control mechanisms for maintaining fluid and electrolyte balance.

3 Recognize how acid-base balance is maintained by buffer systems.

4 List amounts of water usually gained and lost by adults in a day.

5 Differentiate insensible from sensible water loss.

6 Distinguish between heat exhaustion and heat stroke with respect to cause and first-aid treatment.

The need for water is more urgent than the need for any other nutrient. Human beings can live a month without food but only 6 days without water. This chapter explains why water is so important in the body and discusses ways in which water balance is achieved. The assessment and treatment of fluid volume deficit and fluid volume excess is also addressed.

The distribution and movement of water in the body is intricately bound to certain elements. Understanding this relationship requires knowledge of the essentials of atomic structure. This chapter begins, then, with a discussion on how atoms interact with one another.

Interactions between Atoms

An element is a substance that ordinary chemical methods cannot divide into smaller units. There are more than 105 known elements. Oxygen is an element, as are sodium, chlorine, and the other minerals discussed in Chapter 8, "Minerals".

Atoms

Elements are composed of smaller parts that make up an **atom.** In the center of an atom is the *nucleus,* which contains protons and neutrons. The nucleus gives an atom its weight and mass. Circling around the nucleus like satellites are *electrons.* These electrons are arranged in a consistent manner: a maximum of two in the orbit or shell closest to the nucleus, and a maximum of eight in each of the outer shells. The ability of an atom to react chemically depends on the number of "empty slots" in the outermost electron shell.

Chemical Bonding

A **compound** is a substance created by the chemical bonding, or joining, of two or more different kinds of atoms (elements). A chemical bond is actually the force that binds atoms together. A compound is formed when atoms either share electrons or when one atom donates one or more electrons to another atom. For example, water (a liquid) is formed when one atom of hydrogen (a colorless, odorless gas) is joined with two atoms of oxygen (another colorless, odorless gas).

Similarly, sodium chloride (table salt) is a compound of sodium (an unstable, silvery white, waxy, soft metal) and chlorine (a greenish yellow poisonous gas). Sodium and chlorine are so chemically active that in nature they are always found bound to each other or to other elements.

A sodium atom has only one electron in its outer shell; a chlorine atom has seven. When placed together, the sodium atom donates the electron in its outer shell to the outer shell of the chlorine atom. With the loss of its electron, the sodium now has a positive electrical charge of $+1$ and is called a sodium **ion** (Na^+). Ions with positive charges are referred to as **cations.** The chlorine atom, which gained an electron, now has a negative charge of -1 and is called a chloride ion (Cl^-). Ions with negative charges are referred to as **anions.**

Because these ions have opposite charges ($+$ and $-$) they are attracted to one another and unite,

---

Ion—An atom or group of atoms carrying an electrical charge; an ion with a positive charge is called a cation; an ion with a negative charge is called an anion.

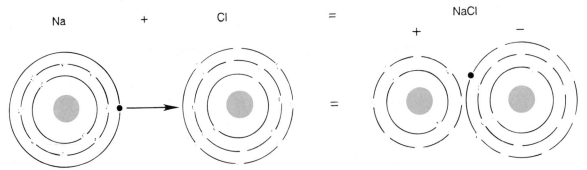

FIGURE 9–1 Formation of an ionic bond. An atom of sodium loses an electron to an atom of chlorine. The two ions formed have unlike charges, are attracted to one another, and form a molecule of sodium chloride. (From Scanlon, VC and Sanders, T: Essentials of Anatomy and Physiology, ed. 2. FA Davis, Philadelphia, 1995, p 25, with permission.)

forming sodium chloride (NaCl). The chemical bond that holds the sodium and chloride ions together is called an **ionic bond.** There are other types of chemical bonds (not discussed here). Sodium can donate its single electron to other elements beside chlorine, and other elements can form ionic bonds as well. See Figure 9–1 for a diagram of the formation of sodium chloride from sodium and chlorine.

An **electrolyte** is an element or compound that when dissolved in water separates (dissociates) into ions that are capable of conducting an electrical current. These electrically charged particles are then available to take part in other chemical reactions in the body. Clinical Application 9–1 discusses examples of uses and hazards related to electrolytes in the body.

Distribution of Water in the Body

More than half the body weight is water, which is found in and around the cells, within the blood and lymph vessels, and in various body cavities.

Body Composition

Some tissues have significantly more water than others: muscle tissue is 70 percent water, fat tissue is 30 percent water, and bone tissue is 10 percent water. A man's body is 60 to 65 percent water and a woman's body is 50 to 54 percent water. Men have a higher water content because of their greater muscle mass.

Age affects the proportion of water in a body. Compared with the 50 to 65 percent for women and men, an infant's body is 75 percent water. Premature infants may be 80 percent water by weight. Infants, especially premature infants, are at high risk

of fluid imbalances. The adult proportion of water to body weight is reached at about 9 to 12 months of age.

Fluid Compartments

Body fluids are held in compartments called *intracellular* and *extracellular* (see Fig. 9–2). These compartments are separated by semipermeable membranes that allow some substances to pass through, while preventing passage of other substances. Water passes

---

CLINICAL APPLICATION 9–1

Diagnostic Uses and Potential Hazards of Electrolytes

Skin sensors attached to an electrocardiograph can trace the electrical activity of the heart. The resulting graphic record is called an **electrocardiogram** (ECG). The machine's sensors on the skin can detect the electric current because the blood is an electrolyte solution and thus capable of conducting electricity. The same principle applies to the use of an electroencephalograph, a device that traces brain-wave activity. The record obtained from this machine is called an **electroencephalogram** (EEG).

The same characteristic of electrolyte solutions that allows these machines to sense electrical activity can also be hazardous. A fluid-filled tube, such as a nasogastric tube or catheter, can conduct stray electricity from faulty electrical devices to the client's heart, which could result in dysrhythmias. The amount of electricity in the shock may be minuscule, but enough to be fatal if it happens at the wrong time in the cardiac cycle.

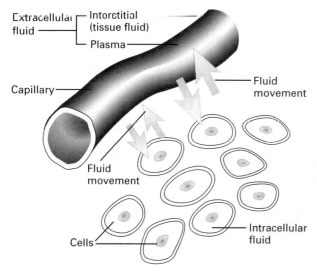

FIGURE 9–2 Three fluid compartments of the body. In distributing nutrients and disposing of waste. Fluid moves from capillaries to interstitial fluid, to the cell, and vice versa. (From Scanlon, VC and Sanders, T: Essentials of Anatomy and Physiology, ed. 2. FA Davis, Philadelphia, 1995, p 438, with permission.)

freely through the membranes. Recently discovered water transport proteins, called aqua porins, explain the speed at which water moves across cell membranes. Promising clinical applications related to aqua porins include cataract formation, hypertension, edema, heart failure, and hydrocephalus (Connolly, Shanahan, and Weissberg, 1996).

Intracellular Compartment

The fluid inside the cells comprises that of the intracellular compartment. In adults, 60 percent of body water is found here. In infants, 46 percent of the body water is intracellular.

Extracellular Compartment

All fluid outside the cells is extracellular. In adults, 40 percent of the body's water is extracellular; in infants, 54 percent. Figure 9–3 illustrates the proportions of intracellular to extracellular fluid in men, women, and infants. The difference is important because extracellular fluid is more easily and rapidly lost to the outside of the body than is intracellular fluid. Extracellular fluid includes interstitial, intravascular, lymph, and transcellular fluids.

INTERSTITIAL FLUID **Interstitial fluid** is located between the cells, or surrounding the cells. It assists in transporting substances between the cells and the blood and lymph vessels.

INTRAVASCULAR FLUID **Intravascular fluid** is found within the blood vessels, arteries, arterioles, capillaries, venules, and veins.

LYMPH FLUID The venous system cannot collect and return all the fluid from the tissues to the heart. The **lymph fluid,** via the lymphatic vessels, assist in returning the fluid part of the blood to the heart.

TRANSCELLULAR FLUID These are fluids in many body cavities. This category includes cerebrospinal fluid, pericardial fluid, pleural fluid, synovial fluid, intraocular fluids, and gastrointestinal secretions. The **transcellular fluids** are constantly being secreted into their spaces and reabsorbed into the vascular system.

Functions of Water

Water has important functions in the body. As a component of cells, water gives the body shape and form. It helps to form the structure of many of the body's large molecules such as protein and glycogen. Some body water also serves as a lubricant, as in mucus secretions and joint fluid.

Water helps to regulate body temperature. It absorbs the heat produced by fever and the heat resulting from metabolic processes. The blood carries excess heat to the skin where it is dissipated by sweating or radiation.

Water serves as a **solvent** for minerals, vitamins, glucose, and other small molecules. The substance that is dissolved in a solvent is called a **solute.** As a solvent, water is able to transport nutrients to the cells and carry waste products away from the cells. In addition, it becomes a medium for chemical reactions. Water also participates in chemical reactions, as may be seen in many of the digestive processes, such as the breakdown of proteins to amino acids. See Table 9–1 for a summary of the functions of water.

Electrolyte—An element or compound that when dissolved in water separates (dissociates) into ions that are capable of conducting an electrical current; acids, bases, and salts are common electrolytes.

Solvent—A liquid holding another substance in solution.

Solute—The substance that is dissolved in a solvent.

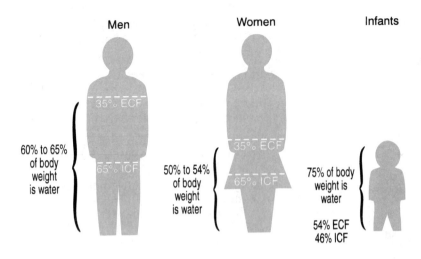

Men

Women

Infants

60% to 65% of body weight is water

35% ECF

65% ICF

50% to 54% of body weight is water

35% ECF

65% ICF

75% of body weight is water

54% ECF
46% ICF

FIGURE 9–3 The relative amounts of body weight that are intracellular and extracellular water in men, women, and infants.

Absorption, Metabolism, and Storage of Water

A small amount of water can be absorbed into the bloodstream from the stomach. A liter of water can be absorbed from the small intestine in an hour.

The metabolism of the energy nutrients produces water. Each energy nutrient produces a different amount of metabolic water: 1 gram of carbohydrate produces 0.60 gram, 1 gram of fat produces 1.07 grams, and 1 gram of protein produces 0.41 gram. One ounce of pure alcohol requires 8 ounces of water for its metabolism. Alcohol, rather than quenching thirst, causes dehydration and increased thirst.

No storage tanks for water exist in the body. Water continually moves from one body compartment to another, and is often reused by the body to perform different tasks.

Under conditions that have disrupted the individual's automatic adaptive mechanisms, water may be retained. The accumulation of excessive amounts of fluid between the cells (in the interstitial fluid compartment) is called **edema.** Hypothyroidism, congestive heart failure, severe protein deficiency, and some kidney conditions may cause such water retention. Excessive water can be dispersed throughout the body, also. This condition is called water intoxication. Many of the symptoms are caused by diluting the concentration of the electrolytes in the body's fluid compartments.

Water Balance

For optimum health, the water lost through the kidneys, skin, lungs, and large intestine must be continually replaced. The electrolyte content of fluids must also be maintained within narrow limits. The body has automatic monitoring and regulating mechanisms to achieve this balance or homeostasis.

The Effect of Electrolytes on Water Balance

All body fluids contain electrolytes. Each fluid compartment has an electrolyte composition that best serves its needs. Each of the fluid compartments has automatic mechanisms that are designed to keep it electrically neutral or balanced. The positive ions within a compartment must equal the negative ones. When shifts and losses occur, compensating shifts and gains take place to reestablish electroneutrality.

Regulation of Fluid Balance

Fluid balance is regulated by electrolytes because cells have no mechanism for holding onto water

TABLE 9–1 **Functions of Water**

- Gives shape and form to cells
- Helps form the structure of large molecules
- Serves as a lubricant
- Helps to regulate body temperature
- Serves as a solvent
- Transports nutrients to cells
- Carries waste products away from cells
- Is a medium for chemical reactions
- Participates in chemical reactions

molecules, which pass freely through all membranes. However, cells can control the movement of electrolytes, and water tends to remain wherever the concentration of electrolytes is highest. In practical terms, this means that water will move to follow high concentrations of electrolytes such as sodium, the ion most closely associated with water balance. The body holds onto its sodium level tenaciously. An abnormal serum sodium level is usually the result of gains or losses of water rather than gains or losses of sodium.

Important Body Electrolytes

Major mineral ions strongly influence not only water balance but also osmotic pressure, blood pressure, and acid-base balance, which will be discussed later in the chapter. Cations of importance in body fluids are sodium, potassium, calcium, and magnesium. Anions of importance include chloride, bicarbonate, phosphate, and sulfate. Sodium (Na^+) is the main electrolyte in extracellular fluid (ECF). Potassium (K^+) is the main electrolyte in intracellular fluid (ICF). Ionized sodium, potassium, and chloride are the solutes that maintain the balance between the intracellular and extracellular compartments. See Table 9–2 for a summary of the major body electrolytes.

Measurement of Electrolytes

Electrolytes are measured according to the total number of particles in solution rather than their total weight. This is because chemical activity is determined by the concentration of electrolytes in any given solution. The unit of measure used is the **milliequivalent** expressed as milliequivalents per liter. The concentration of a pharmaceutical electrolyte in solution is also measured in milliequivalents per liter. Clinical Calculation 9–1 shows the conversion of milligrams of sodium chloride to milliequivalents.

Osmotic Pressure

Osmosis is the movement of water (or another solvent) across a semipermeable membrane from an area with fewer particles to one with more particles. The result, providing the difference is reasonable, is an equalization of concentration on either side of the membrane. Clinical Application 9–2 describes an experiment to demonstrate osmosis.

Osmosis is a passive process. The movement of some substances, however, is active. Some substances require active transport mechanisms to push them through a membrane. Two such transport mechanisms are the *sodium pump* and the *potassium pump*. Located in cell membranes, these pumps are actually proteins that can move ions. Sodium pumps move sodium ions out of the cells (and the water follows). Potassium pumps move potassium ions into the cells. In this manner, the electrolyte concentrations of the intracellular and extracellular fluid compartments are maintained. Unlike osmosis, which is a passive mechanism, active transport requires energy.

DETERMINATION OF OSMOTIC PRESSURE   When two solutions with different concentrations are separated by a semipermeable membrane, pressure develops. This pressure, which is exerted on the semipermeable membrane, is called **osmotic pressure.** Osmotic pressure causes a solvent such as water to cross the membrane, while the solutes (particles) that are outside the membrane cannot go through.

The size of the molecule and its ability to ionize determines the number of particles in a given concentration. Disaccharides and monosaccharides do not ionize. Without the appropriate enzymes to split the disaccharide into its component monosaccharides, the disaccharide molecule remains intact. Just as there are more nails in a pound of tacks than in a pound of spikes, there are more particles in 100 kilocalories of glucose compared with 100 kilocalories of a disaccharide in a given volume. The larger number of particles per unit volume exerts more osmotic pressure.

OSMOLARITY OF BODY FLIUDS   The measure of the osmotic pressure exerted by the number of particles per volume of liquid is referred to as its *osmolarity*. The unit of measure for osmotic activity is the **milliosmole.** Clinically, osmolarity is usually reported in milliosmoles per liter.

Osmolality, in contrast, is the measure of the osmotic pressure exerted by the number of particles

---

Edema—Accumulation of excessive amounts of fluid in interstitial spaces (between the cells).

Osmosis—Movement of water across a semipermeable cell membrane from an area with fewer particles to one with more particles.

Osmotic pressure—Pressure that develops when a concentrated solution is separated from a less concentrated solution by a semipermeable membrane, only water crosses the membrane.

TABLE 9–2 Major Body Electrolytes

Electrolyte	Fluid Compartment*	Functions
Cations		
Sodium (Na^+)	Extracellular	Major cation in ECF. Na^+ concentration in fluids determines the distribution of H_2O by osmosis. With Cl^- and HCO_3^-, Na^+ regulates acid-base balance.
Potassium (K^+)	Intracellular	Major cation in ICF. K^+ with Na^+ maintains water balance. With Na^+ and H^+, K^+ regulates acid-base balance.
Calcium (Ca^{2+})	Extracel-lular†	Participates in permeability of cell membranes, transmission of nerve impulses, muscle action.
Magnesium (Mg^{2+})	Intracellular	Regulates nerve stimulation and normal muscle action.
Anions		
Chloride (Cl^-)	Extracellular	Major anion in ECF. Helps maintain water balance and acid-base balance.
Bicarbonate (HCO_3^-)	Extracellular	Most important ECF buffer.
Phosphate (HPO_4^{2-})	Intracellular	Within the ICF, phosphates and proteins buffer 95 percent of the body's carbonic acid and 50 percent of other acids.

* ECF and ICF both contain all the cations and anions listed in this table, but are labeled as either ECF or ICF according to the concentration. For example, sodium ions make up 142 of the total 155 milliequivalents per liter (of the cations) in the ECF.
† Of the cations, 3 percent in ECF and 1 percent in ICF.

per weight of solvent. Clinically, osmolality is usually reported in milliosmoles per kilogram.

The osmolality of human blood serum is about 300 milliosmoles per kilogram. (Laboratory texts list various ranges between 280 and 310 milliosmoles per kilogram.) Values above 350 milliosmoles per kilogram indicate a grave prognosis (Brensilver and Goldberger, 1996).

Most serum osmolarity is contributed by sodium, potassium, and chloride. In the extracellular fluid, sodium is the primary determinant of osmolality.

OSMOLALITY AND NUTRITION Fluids are designated as **isotonic** if they approximate the osmolality of the blood **plasma.** Fluids exerting less osmotic pressure than plasma are labeled **hypotonic.** Those exerting greater osmotic pressure than plasma serum are called **hypertonic.**

Achieving the correct osmolality of fluids administered intravenously is very important. A solution that is too concentrated pulls water out of the red blood cells and the cells shrivel and die. Too weak a solution allows water to be pulled into the red blood cells until the cells burst.

Examples of isotonic fluids are 5 percent glucose in water and 0.9 percent sodium chloride. Only isotonic sodium chloride is given with red-blood-cell products to avoid shrinking or bursting the red blood cells.

Less concentrated solutions of glucose and sodium chloride and plain water are hypotonic.

Stronger solutions are hypertonic. TPN solutions are so strong that they must be infused into a large vein in the chest so that they are diluted quickly by the liberal volume of blood flowing past the infusion port or catheter.

Oral fluids also can be categorized as to their osmotic pressure. Plain water is hypotonic. Whole milk at 275 milliosmoles per liter is close to isotonic. Two fluids often taken to soothe a digestive upset are ginger ale and 7-Up. Since ginger ale has 510 milliosmoles per liter and 7-Up 640, both are hypertonic.

SERUM ELECTROLYTES The electrolytes in blood are also reported in milliequivalents per liter. Normal **serum** sodium is 135 to 145 milliequivalents per liter. In most cases, because sodium is the most influential extracellular ion, osmolarity of the extracellular fluid can be estimated clinically by doubling the serum sodium value. Normal serum sodium doubled would be 270 to 296 milliosmoles per liter. Normal osmolality of the serum is about 300 milliosmoles per kilogram. This simple method gives a close approximation.

The other ion that is monitored carefully is potassium. Most of the potassium in the body is inside the cells. Potassium concentration is 150 milliequivalents per liter in the intracellular fluid. By contrast, potassium concentration in the blood is only 3.5 to 5.0 milliequivalents per liter. Even slight variations above or below these values can produce severe consequences. The heart muscle is particularly sensitive

CLINICAL CALCULATION 9–1

Converting Milligrams to Milliequivalents

Milligram is a measure of weight. Milliequivalent is a measure of the concentration of electrolytes (number of particles) per volume of solution. The usual amount of solution on which electrolytes are reported is 1 L.

To convert milligrams to milliequivalents, it is necessary to know the number of milligrams per liter, the molecular weight of the substance, and its valence. Valence, a number indicating the combining power of an atom, is found in many dictionaries.

A teaspoonful of table salt in 1 L of water will produce a 0.5 percent solution. (Isotonic sodium chloride is 0.9 percent.) How would the electrolytes be reported in milliequivalents? A teaspoonful is roughly 5 g. Since table salt is 40 percent sodium and 60 percent chloride, the liter of 0.5 percent salt water would contain 2 g (2000 mg) of sodium and 3 g (3000 mg) of chloride.

Two other values are needed: atomic or molecular weights, and valences. The atomic weight for sodium is 22.9898. Sodium has a valence of 1.

The formula for converting milligrams to milliequivalents is:

$$mEq/L = \frac{(mg/L) \times valence}{molecular\ weight}$$

Filling in the sodium values we know for this case, we have:

$$mEq/L = \frac{2000\ (mg/L) \times 1}{22.9898} = 87\ mEq/L\ of\ sodium$$

Continuing, we can use the same formula with different values to calculate the milliequivalents of chloride. The automic weight for chlorine is 35.453. Chlorine has a valence of 1.

Filling in the values for chloride, we have:

$$mEq/L = \frac{3000\ (mg/L) \times 1}{35.453} = 85\ mEq/l\ of\ chloride$$

Then, adding the sodium and chloride, we have:

$$87 + 85 = 172\ mEq/L\ in\ the\ 0.5\ percent\ solution$$

to high or low levels of potassium. Either abnormally high or abnormally low levels can produce cardiac arrest.

Electrolyte Imbalances

Table 9–3 lists the normal values for serum sodium and serum potassium, along with the technical names and some of the signs and symptoms for de-

CLINICAL APPLICATION 9–2

Osmosis in the Kitchen

To make sauerkraut, the cabbage is sliced very fine and placed in the bottom of a crock. Salt is then added to the dry cabbage. This is repeated, layer after layer, until the crock is full. At this point, much liquid will already have gathered, pulled from the cabbage pieces by the concentrated salt. After the cabbage ferments for 5 or 6 weeks, the crock is really full of "extra" juice.

To try a tiny batch of sauerkraut use 2 tsp of canning salt per pound of cabbage.

viations from the normal. Many other signs, including the direct measurement of serum electrolytes and the results of electrocardiograms, assist in the diagnosis. Dire consequences can result from any of the four imbalances. If the nurse recognizes and reports early signs and symptoms, the need for drastic treatment measures may be averted. In the clinical chapters, more information will be presented on electrolyte imbalances commonly accompanying various disease conditions.

The Effect of Plasma Proteins on Water Balance

The body has a highly developed mechanism that maintains the constant flow of water and nutrients to the cells and the flow of water and waste materials from the cells. Water and nutrients in the blood are pushed out through the thin walls of the capillaries into the interstitial fluid by **hydrostatic pressure** (blood pressure) supplied by the heart. From the interstitial compartment, the water and nutrients cross cell membranes to bathe and nourish the cell. Plasma proteins, including **albumin,** remain in the capillaries because they are too large to squeeze through the capillary wall. Inside the blood vessels, the plasma proteins exert **colloidal osmotic pressure** (COP). The COP, now greater than the hydrostatic pressure, pulls water and waste materials from the interstitial fluid back into the blood capillaries.

Hydrostatic pressure—Pressure created by the pumping action of the heart on the fluid in the blood vessels.

Colloidal osmotic pressure (COP)—Pressure produced by plasma and cellular proteins.

TABLE 9–3   Signs and Symptoms of Abnormal Serum Sodium and Potassium Levels

	Low	Normal	High
Sodium			
Lab value	Less than 135 mEq/L	135–148 mEq/L	Greater than 148 mEq/L
Condition	Hyponatremia		Hypernatremia
Symptoms	Irritability		Thirst
	Anxiety		Fatigue
Signs	Muscle twitching		Flushed skin
	Fingerprinting over the sternum		Sticky mucous membranes
	Seizures		Agitation
	Coma		Coma
Potassium			
Lab value	Less than 3.5 mEq/L	3.5–5.0 mEq/L	Greater than 5.0 mEq/L
Condition	Hypokalemia		Hyperkalemia
Symptoms	Nausea and/or vomiting		Irritability
	Paresthesias, esp. lower extremities		Abdominal cramps
			Weakness, esp. lower extremities
Signs	Decreased bowel sounds		Irregular pulse
	Weak, irregular pulse		Cardiac arrest if greater than
	Coma		8.5 mEq/L

However, osmotic pressure within the cell is still being maintained by the balance of fluid and electrolytes as described above. Clinical Application 9–3 describes a condition in which a low serum protein is the cause of water imbalance.

Blood Pressure

Blood pressure is the force exerted against the walls of the arteries by the beating heart. It is reported in two numbers, such as 120/80 (measured in millimeters of mercury). The top number is the pressure when the heart beats, called **systolic pressure.** The bottom number is the pressure between beats, called the **diastolic pressure.** One of the factors necessary to maintain an adequate blood pressure is a sufficient volume of blood in the arteries and veins.

Body Regulation of Water Intake and Excretion

The body has mechanisms that regulate both the intake and the excretion of water. Thirst governs water intake. The excretion of water is controlled mainly by two hormones: antidiuretic hormone causes the body to reabsorb (retain) water; aldosterone causes the body to retain sodium.

Thirst Mechanism

Thirst is the desire for fluids, especially water. Thirst occurs when 10 percent of the intravascular volume is lost or when cellular volume is reduced by 1 to 2 percent. When there is too little water in the blood (or, put another way, when the solutes are too concentrated), there is an increase in the osmotic pressure of the blood. Special sensors in the **hypothalamus** monitor the osmotic pressure of the blood as it circulates in the brain. When the hypothalamus detects an increase in the osmotic pressure, it triggers the desire to drink.

CLINICAL APPLICATION 9–3

Protein-Energy Malnutrition and Water Balance

Starving children often look plump. They are not fat, but edematous. These children are victims of **kwashiorkor,** a disease of protein-energy malnutrition. It occurs most often in children just after weaning when there is not enough protein in their diets to replace their mothers' milk.

Protein plays a crucial role in maintaining the volume of fluid in the blood vessels. These children develop edema because they do not have enough plasma proteins remaining in the capillaries to pull water back into the circulatory system. Thus, it accumulates in the interstitial spaces. Once treatment begins the plasma proteins will pull the retained water into the blood and the children will appear emaciated.

Syndrome of Inappropriate Secretion of Antidiuretic Hormone (SIADH)

Normally, increased osmolality of the blood stimulates the posterior pituitary gland to release ADH. When enough water is returned to the bloodstream by the kidney, the ADH secretion stops.

Several situations cause ADH to be released inappropriately. Certain lung tumors produce an ADH-like substance. Other lung conditions such as pneumonia, tuberculosis, and asthma have caused SIADH. Stress, surgery, some anesthetics, pain, and morphine have been implicated in increased release of ADH. Medications such as chlorpropamide and oxytocin have precipitated SIADH. Conditions directly affecting the brain (including the hypothalamus and the pituitary gland) such as meningitis, brain tumors, and subarachnoid hemorrhage have been linked to SIADH.

The signs and symptoms of SIADH are those of hyponatremia. In this case it is dilutional hyponatremia. The client has enough sodium, but it is diluted in too much retained water. Initially, the client becomes apprehensive. When the serum sodium drops to 120 to 125 mEq per liter, neurological signs appear, owing to edema of the brain cells. The client becomes irritable, apathetic, and displays personality changes. Other signs of hyponatremia include tremors, hyperactive reflexes, muscle spasms, and convulsions. Fingerprints remain over the sternum due to the excess intracellular fluid. Urine osmolality is characteristically higher than serum osmolality (Brensilver and Goldberger, 1996). When the serum sodium drops to less than 115 mEq per liter, seizures, coma, and permanent neurological damage can occur.

Effective treatment of SIADH is based upon discovering and removing the cause of the condition. Beyond that, or in the instance of a postoperative or stress reaction, treatment involves diuretic therapy and fluid restriction. The client is given precisely prescribed amounts of fluids throughout the day. Over a period of several days, through obligatory excretion, the client's body will excrete the extra water.

Antidiuretic Hormone

If thirst is not alleviated, the sensors in the hypothalamus increase the secretion of **antidiuretic hormone** (ADH) from the posterior pituitary gland. ADH causes the kidneys to return more water to the bloodstream rather than spilling it into the urine. Antidiuretic hormone, also named *vasopressin,* has

an additional effect of arterial vasoconstriction. By constricting blood vessels, it increases blood pressure. (When someone places a finger over the end of a garden hose, the amount of water flowing is the same as before, but the smaller outlet increases the pressure.)

Sometimes the ADH mechanism goes awry. In *diabetes insipidus* the hypothalamus does not secrete ADH or the kidneys do not respond appropriately. **Diabetes insipidus** can be caused by brain tumor, surgery, trauma, infection, radiation injury, or congenital conditions. If the hypothalamus is not secreting ADH, a pharmaceutical preparation can be given. Clinical Application 9–4 tells about a condition called *Syndrome of Inappropriate Secretion of Antidiuretic Hormone (SIADH)*.

Aldosterone

The release of **aldosterone,** a hormone secreted by the adrenal glands, is another water-balancing mechanism in the body. It causes sodium ions to be returned to the bloodstream by the kidneys rather than to be spilled into the urine. As the most influential extracellular ion, sodium will pull water along with it.

The trigger for the release of aldosterone is thought to be a decrease in the blood pressure in the **renal** arteries. Aldosterone then stimulates the kidneys to produce **renin.** Renin acts as an enzyme to split angiotensinogen, a serum globulin secreted by the liver, to form angiotensin I. Enzymes in the lungs convert angiotensin I to **angiotensin II.** Angiotensin II constricts blood vessels and stimulates the secretion of aldosterone. Aldosterone then increases sodium retention. Water follows sodium; thus the blood volume is maintained.

Another side of sodium retention is potassium loss. Within fluid compartments, positively charged

Hypothalamus—A portion of the brain that helps to regulate water balance, thirst, body temperature, carbohydrate and fat metabolism, and sleep.

Antidiuretic hormone (ADH)—Hormone formed in hypothalamus and released from posterior pituitary in response to blood that is too concentrated; effect is return of water to the bloodstream by the kidneys.

Aldosterone—An adrenocorticoid hormone that increases sodium and water retention by the kidneys.

Renal—Pertaining to the kidney.

particles must equal negatively charged ones. When sodium is retained, to maintain electroneutrality the kidney excretes more potassium.

Acid-Base Balance

Electrolytes also play an important role in maintaining the acid-base balance of body fluids. Acids are compounds that yield hydrogen ions when dissociated in solution. The more hydrogen ions a solution contains, the more concentrated the acid. Bases, or alkalies, are substances that accept hydrogen ions. The acidity or alkalinity of a substance is measured according to a scale called **pH.** The pH scale ranges from 0 to 14: acids are rated from 0 to 6.999; 7 is neutral; bases are above 7.

The balance between too much and too little acid in body fluids is maintained by the action of the lungs, the kidneys, and the buffer systems of the body. The purpose of buffer systems is to minimize significant changes in the pH of the body fluids by controlling the hydrogen ion (H^+) concentration. **Buffers** are substances that can neutralize both acids and bases. **Bicarbonate** (HCO_3^-) is the most important buffer in the extracellular fluid. Phosphate (HPO_4^{2-}) and proteins are two important buffers in the intracellular fluid.

Extracellular Fluid

The normal pH of the extracellular fluid (including the blood and interstitial fluid) is 7.35 to 7.45. This is slightly alkaline, despite the acidity of the body's waste products. The body is continually working to maintain correct pH. If the serum pH drops below 6.8 or rises above 7.8, death is usually the result.

Extracellular fluid contains both positive sodium ions (Na^+) and negative bicarbonate ions (HCO_3^-). When a strong acid is introduced to the fluid, a chemical reaction takes place. The end products of this reaction are sodium chloride (a salt), which is neutral, and carbonic acid (a weak acid). The carbonic acid breaks down to carbon dioxide and water. The carbon dioxide is excreted by the lungs (exhaled) and the water is excreted by the kidneys.

Another chemical reaction takes place when a strong base (alkali) is introduced into the fluid system. When a strong base enters the system, carbon dioxide and water (the two main waste products of cellular metabolism) react to form carbonic acid to counteract the alkaline effect of the base. The end products of this reaction are water and a weak base that will not drastically affect the pH.

Respiratory System

The lungs help maintain pH by varying the amount of carbon dioxide (CO_2) exhaled. Excess carbon dioxide makes the body fluids more acidic because it reacts to form **carbonic acid,** a source of hydrogen ions. Too much carbonic acid, or any acid, will result in **acidosis.** When this happens, the lungs automatically increase the rate and depth of breathing, eliminating more carbon dioxide and water.

This respiratory response to acidosis begins within minutes of an increase in acidity. Respiratory compensation for acidosis is 50 to 75 percent effective and is an extremely important component in the regulation of pH. Normally, the respiratory system has one or two times the buffering power of all chemical buffers in the body.

Renal System

The respiratory system acts quickly but it can only eliminate carbonic acid. Other acids, as well as excess carbonic acid, must be eliminated in the urine. The kidney spills or retains hydrogen, sodium, and bicarbonate ions as necessary to maintain an acceptable pH in the blood. For example, in response to acidosis, the kidneys excrete hydrogen ions and reabsorb sodium and bicarbonate ions. Conversely, in response to alkalosis, the kidneys conserve hydrogen ions and excrete sodium and bicarbonate ions. The kidneys initiate these actions within 24 hours but require 3 to 4 days to compensate for changes in blood pH.

Intracellular Fluid

The normal pH of the intracellular fluid is 6.8 to 7.0, slightly acid to neutral. Within the intracellular fluid, organic phosphates and proteins are the most important buffers. These substances buffer 95 percent of the body's carbonic acid and 50 percent of other acids. Protein is the most powerful and plentiful buffer system in the body. Of the body's proteins, hemoglobin has the largest buffering capacity. Thus the red blood cells have 70 percent of the buffering power of the blood. This buffering capacity allows large quantities of carbon dioxide to be transported from the tissues to the lungs with only a small change in venous pH compared with arterial pH.

When the blood contains excessive hydrogen ions, they move into the cells to be buffered. Then, to maintain electroneutrality, potassium moves from the intracellular compartment to the extracellular (intravascular), raising serum potassium levels.

Recommended Dietary Allowance

There is no RDA for water. Unless on a high-salt or high protein diet, adults need one milliliter per kilocalorie per day. So a person on a 1500-kilocalorie diet should take in 1½ liters of liquid. Adults require 2 to 4 percent of their body weight as water daily. The 154-pound person would need 3 to 6 pounds of water. A pint is approximately a pound, so 2 to 4 percent of 154 pounds would be 1 1/2 to 3 quarts of liquid. Of this amount, at least 60 percent should be consumed as water and the remainder obtained from foods and metabolic water.

Infants have a greater need for water than adults. Their basal heat production per kilogram is twice that of adults. To rid their bodies of the heat and waste products, 1.5 milliliters of water per kilocalorie are needed. This means that infants must drink 10 to 15 percent of their body weight as water to maintain health.

Sources of Water

Much of our water is consumed disguised as other beverages. Adults consume 6 cups of water per day in beverages. Water may contain other nutrients as well. Hard water has calcium, magnesium, and often iron. Water conditioners used to soften water replace the calcium, magnesium, and iron with sodium. For some people, drinking softened water increases their sodium intake excessively. In fact most experts recommend that the cold water faucet at the kitchen sink be plumbed for unsoftened water.

We obtain about 4 cups of water per day in foods. It is probably not surprising that skim milk is 91 percent water, and whole milk is 88 percent water. Some foods that are solids also have a high water content: head lettuce is 96 percent water, celery is 95 percent water, and raw carrots are 88 percent water. Other foods that contain a large percentage of water include apples (84 percent), grapes (81 percent), bananas (74 percent), hard-cooked eggs (75 percent), drained tuna (61 percent), and chicken breast or thigh (52 percent). Whole wheat bread is 38 percent water, which drops to 29 percent when toasted.

Water is also a product of metabolism. The average person acquires 1 cup of water per day from this process.

Losses of Water

We lose water in obvious ways, such as in perspiration and urine. We also lose water in less obvious ways, such as through breathing. The obvious ways are called **sensible water losses.** The less obvious ways are called **insensible water losses.**

Sensible Water Losses

Sensible water losses include losses of the major extracellular ions, sodium and chloride. Three important routes commonly account for sensible water losses: through the skin as perspiration, through the kidney as urine, and through the gastrointestinal tract in the feces.

Perspiration

To produce 1 liter of perspiration requires 600 kilocalories. In extreme cases, a person may perspire at the rate of 2 liters per hour. For example, during a race, marathon runners may lose 6 to 7 percent of their body weight, primarily as perspiration. For a 150-pound person, this would be a 10 1/2 pound weight loss, or 4.8 liters of fluid.

Sweat is not pure water. It is salty to the taste. Perspiration is hypotonic. One liter of perspiration contains 45 milliequivalents of sodium, 5 milliequiva-

> **pH**—A scale representing the relative acidity or alkalinity of a solution; a value of 7 is neutral, less than 7 is acidic, and greater than 7 is alkaline.
>
> **Buffer**—A substance that can react to offset excess acid or excess alkali (base) in a solution; blood buffers include carbonic acid, bicarbonate, phosphates, and proteins, including hemoglobin.
>
> **Bicarbonate**—Any salt containing the HCO_3 anion; blood bicarbonate is a measure of alkali (base) reserve of the body; bicarbonate of soda is sodium bicarbonate, $NaHCO_3$.
>
> **Acidosis**—Condition that results when the pH of the blood falls below 7.35; may be caused by diarrhea, uremia, diabetes mellitus, and certain drug therapies.
>
> **Sensible water loss**—Visible water loss through sweat, urine, and feces.
>
> **Insensible water loss**—Water that is lost invisibly through the lungs and skin.

lents of potassium, and 58 milliequivalents of chlorine. In this instance, the milliosmole value is the same as the milliequivalent value (because all the ions are monovalent) so the milliequivalents can be added to obtain an osmolarity of 108 milliequivalents per liter of perspiration.

For a sweat loss of less than 5 or 6 liters, rehydration with water suffices. Intense work in a very hot environment (a foundry or mine) may result in "miner's cramps" believed to be caused by sodium depletion. In this case, athletic drinks or salt tablets may be indicated (Groff, Gropper, and Hunt, 1995).

Urine

In the normal, healthy person, urine output is roughly equal to liquid intake. Often this amount equals 1200 to 1500 milliliters per day.

A minimum amount of urine must be excreted each day to carry away the waste products resulting from metabolic processes. This is called **obligatory excretion.** Obligatory excretion of urine amounts to 400 to 600 milliliters per day.

For seriously ill clients, hourly urine output is monitored. These amounts must be interpreted in relation to the client's whole situation. Even if a person is losing massive amounts of fluid through disease, such losses do not rid the body of metabolic wastes as efficiently as the kidney does. Adults should excrete between 40 and 80 milliliters of urine per hour. Clinical Calculation 9–2 shows a method

---

> ### CLINICAL CALCULATION 9–2
> #### Hourly Urine Output in Children
>
> Children should excrete between 0.5 and 2 milliliters of urine per kilogram of body weight per hour. What would be a normal hourly urine output for a child who weighs 50 pounds?
>
> First convert pounds to kilograms. There are 2.2 pounds per kilogram.
>
> $$\frac{50 \text{ lb}}{2.2 \text{ lb/kg}} = 22.7 \text{ kg}$$
>
> To find the desirable range of output, multiply the child's weight in kilograms by the desired factors of 0.5 and 2 mL per kilogram.
>
> $$22.7 \times 0.5 = 11.4 \text{ mL/h}$$
> $$22.7 \times 2 = 45.4 \text{ mL/h}$$
>
> Thus the 50-lb child normally should excrete between 11 and 45 mL/h of urine.

---

of determining a desirable hourly urine output for children.

Gastrointestinal Secretions

Abnormal gastrointestinal function can cause extensive fluid loss. When the secretion lost is high in the gastrointestinal tract, the resulting symptoms differ from those that occur when the secretion is lost from lower in the tract. Gastric juice is acid, while intestinal juices are alkaline. Therefore, conceptually, gastrointestinal losses are divided into those lost above the outlet of the stomach, the pylorus, and those lost below it.

ABOVE THE PYLORUS   The common causes of these losses are vomiting or stomach suctioning. Two organs secrete digestive juices above the pylorus. They are the salivary glands in the mouth and the gastric glands in the stomach. Both of these secretions are isotonic, so their loss threatens electrolyte balance to a greater extent than loss of an equal amount of perspiration would. The ions lost in secretions above the pylorus are sodium, potassium, chloride, and hydrogen.

About 1 liter of saliva per day is mixed with food or just swallowed. The stomach secretes about 1.5 to 2.5 liters of gastric juice per day. If gastric juices are lost, hydrogen ions in the hydrochloric acid are also lost. The person at risk for alkalosis.

BELOW THE PYLORUS   The usual causes of these losses are diarrhea or intestinal suctioning. Gastrointestinal secretions below the pylorus also are isotonic. They contain sodium, potassium, and bicarbonate. About 2 to 3 liters of intestinal secretions per day flow into the bowel to digest the food intake. Normally, bile is released from the gallbladder into the small intestine at the rate of 1 liter per day. The total gastrointestinal secretions amount to 6.5 to 8.5 liters per day. Yet, because water is absorbed back into the blood from the large intestine, normal feces from an adult contain only 100 to 200 milliliters of water.

See Clinical Application 9–5 for a discussion of two conditions resulting from exposure to extreme heat: heat exhaustion and heat stroke.

Insensible Water Losses

An invisible amount of water is lost through the lungs and the skin. These are insensible losses. Between 800 and 1000 milliliters of water is lost each day via the lungs and skin. Breath is visible only in very cold weather. Even in warmer weather and in-

Heat Exhaustion and Heat Stroke

Exposure to extreme heat may overtax the body's adaptive capabilities. Depending on the body's response, two very different clinical conditions appear: heat exhaustion or heat stroke. The client should seek medical attention if either condition occurs.

Heat Exhaustion

In this condition, which is more common, the client suffers the loss of water and sodium chloride in sweat. The client's temperature is normal or below. The pulse is weak, thready, and rapid. Respirations are shallow and quiet. The skin is cool, clammy, and sweaty. First-aid treatment consists of moving the client to a cooler environment. The client should lie down with the feet elevated and clothing should be loosened. If the person can drink it, 1/2 tsp of salt in 1/2 glass of water will begin to replace the water and sodium chloride lost. The salt-in-water treatment should be repeated every 15 minutes until the emergency team arrives.

Heat Stroke

In this condition, the client fails to perspire because the body can no longer regulate body temperature. The client has an extremely elevated temperature, 105°F or above. The pulse is full and bounding. Breathing is difficult and respirations are loud. The skin is flushed, hot, and dry. The client is not sweating. First aid treatment of heat stroke includes complete quiet with the head elevated, removal of clothing, and bathing with cool water. Of the two conditions, heat stroke is more likely to be life threatening.

Insensible Water Loss through the Skin

The rule of thumb for insensible water loss through the skin is 6 mL/kg per 24 hours. Let us look at a 154-lb client to see what his or her amount of water loss would be in a 24-hour period. First, convert pounds to kilograms:

$$\frac{154\ lb}{2.2\ lb/kg} = 70\ kg$$

Then, multiply the client's weight (in kilograms) by the amount of water loss per kilogram:

$$70\ kg \times 6\ mL/kg = 420\ mL$$

Thus, this client's insensible water loss in a 24-hour period is expected to be 420 mL.

Table 9–4 lists average fluid gains and losses for 24 hours.

Assessment of Water Losses

Gathering data on water losses is quite straightforward. Because water is more than 50 percent of body weight, a loss of water will be exhibited in the client's weight. Recording the liquid a client takes in and puts out is a second means of tracking water balance.

Weight

Rapid weight changes usually are a reflection of fluid balance. Daily weight is the single most important indicator of fluid status. An easy way to relate volume to weight is to remember "A pint is a pound the world around." One liter is 1 kilogram or 2.2 pounds. Acute weight loss in adults is rated as follows: mild volume deficit—2 to 5 percent loss; moderate volume deficit—5 to 10 percent loss; and severe volume deficit—10 to 15 percent loss. A loss of greater than 15 percent can be fatal (Horne, Heitz, and Swearingen, 1991).

Fluid balance in the infant is much more precarious. Because a greater proportion of body water is in the extracellular space in infants, they can lose it more rapidly than an adult. Therefore, a loss of 5

doors, 400 milliliters of water per day is lost in exhaled air. Deep respirations or a dry climate increase the amount of water lost.

The insensible loss of water through the skin is evaporative. It is almost pure water and nearly electrolyte-free. This insensible water loss amounts to 6 milliliters per kilogram of body weight in 24 hours.

This is a baseline amount. Clinical Calculation 9–3 gives a client example. Burns, phototherapy, radiant warmers, or fever will increase the amount of insensible water loss. Fever increases evaporative losses by about 12 percent per Celsius degree of temperature elevation. Clinical Calculation 9–4 shows how **evaporative water losses** are calculated.

Obligatory excretion—Minimum amount of urine production necessary to keep waste products in solution, amounting to 400 to 600 milliliters per day.

CLINICAL CALCULATION 9–4

Evaporative Water Loss in Fever

Fever increases the amount of evaporative loss by 12 percent for every degree Celsius of fever. How much of an elevation would this be on the Fahrenheit scale? How much water would be lost by a person with this degree of fever over a 24-hour period?

Let us take 98.6°F as normal. This is equal to 37°C. So an increase of 1°C of fever would give a reading of 38°C. To change Celsius to Fahrenheit add 40 and multiply the result by 9/5:

$$38 + 40 = 78 \times 9/5 = 100.4°F$$

Now, consider the 154-lb client in Clinical Calculation 9–3 whose evaporative losses were 420 mL in 24 hours. If he were feverish, he would lose additional water. We find an increase of 12 percent for the 1°C fever this way:

$$420 \text{ mL} \times 0.12$$
$$= 50.4 \text{ mL additional evaporative loss}$$

$$420 \text{ mL} + 50.4 \text{ mL}$$
$$= 470.4 \text{ total insensible loss through the skin}$$

---

percent of body weight in an infant merits medical attention.

Sudden weight changes are not always due to fluid shifts. If a client receives no oral, enteral, or parenteral nutrition, the loss of body tissue may amount to 0.3 to 0.5 kilogram per day.

Recording Intake and Output

In addition to monitoring weight, recording liquid intake and output is a common nursing action. In the healthy person, liquid intake and output should be approximately equal. Measuring intake is easier than measuring output.

Most institutions post the amounts that food and beverage containers hold. Ice chips should be recorded as one half of their volume. One cup of ice chips yields only 1/2 cup of water.

Fluid that is lost into a dressing or a diaper can be estimated by weighing. The dry material's weight is subtracted from the total. One gram of weight equals 1 milliliter of water. Specific gravity, is the weight of a substance compared with distilled water. Normal specific gravity of urine is 1.010 to 1.025. So, although the diaper weight from urine is not exactly the same as if it were wet with water, this method of recording incontinent urine is adequate in most situations.

In the sick person, intake and output totals may not balance every day. The client's intake and output should be analyzed over a period of several days; a one-day evaluation could prove misleading. Of utmost importance is the ability to see the big picture. See Charting Tips 9–1 for teaching and documentation tips.

Water Imbalances

Because water is being discussed in this chapter, electrolytes are included only to the extent necessary to understand water balance. Two common imbalances are fluid volume deficit and fluid volume excess.

Fluid Volume Deficit

In fluid volume deficit, the individual experiences vascular, interstitial, or cellular dehydration. In the body's effort to compensate, fluid moves from one compartment to another. This means that the client's situation is constantly changing.

Losses of Fluid

Fluid losses can be external or internal. Treatments may differ, but the signs and symptoms of fluid volume deficit are similar regardless of the cause.

TABLE 9–1 Average Fluid Gains and Losses in Adults in 24 Hours

Fluid Gains		Fluid Losses*	
Energy metabolism	300 mL	Kidneys	1200–1500 mL
		Skin	500–600 mL
Oral fluids	1100–1400 mL	Lungs	400 mL
Solid foods	800–1000 mL	Intestines	100–200 mL
Total	2200–2700 mL	Total	2200–2700 mL

* Includes sensible and insensible losses.

CHARTING TIPS 9–1

Be Specific and Document

✓ Be specific when teaching clients.

✓ Record both the content and the client's response to the material.

One client was told to "drink a lot of fluid" when he was discharged from the hospital. He interpreted this to be 3 to 4 gallons per day! His kidneys did their best, but kidneys cannot produce plain water. In a few days, the client was back in the hospital for correction of electrolyte imbalance. This outcome could have been prevented if the client had been taught to drink a specific amount of fluid rather than "a lot."

EXTERNAL LOSSES   Fluids lost to the outside of the body are called **external fluid losses.** Gastrointestinal losses are the most common. Vomiting or diarrhea are just two of the ways in which gastrointestinal fluids are lost. But medical treatments such as gastrointestinal suctioning or surgical rerouting of intestinal contents also produce fluid deficit. Hemorrhage causes not only fluid loss but also the loss of blood cells.

INTERNAL LOSSES   It may be hard to imagine, but fluids can be "lost" inside the body. Excessive fluid accumulation in the interstitial fluid compartment is edema. Although the same amount of fluid is inside the body, any fluid outside the blood vessels is lost to the circulation.

As a result of injury or trauma, capillary permeability increases so that more fluid and cells can travel to the site of the injury to begin repairs or healing. It also causes the swelling, or edema, at the site of an injury. For example, burns can blister. Fluid leaves the vessels and accumulates in the skin. Correct fluid replacement is a high priority for severely burned clients.

There are also several places in the body where vast amounts of fluid can accumulate. These losses are called *third-space* losses. Several liters of fluid can accumulate in the bowel when a person has a bowel obstruction. Certain diseases can cause **ascites**, the accumulation of fluid (often amounting to several liters), not within the bowel but around it in the abdominal cavity. Other third-space losses involve internal bleeding or the collection of fluid in the chest cavity.

An alert nurse can spot an early clue to third-space losses. Decreasing urine output in spite of seemingly adequate fluid intake demands further assessment.

Assessment of Fluid Volume Deficit

Loss of fluid may be mild and corrected easily if the client obeys the body's thirst command to drink. On the other hand, the client's life may be threatened if the fluid loss is severe or sudden.

SYMPTOMS   The thirst response is triggered when 10 percent of intravascular volume is lost or when cellular volume is reduced by 1 to 2 percent. Thus, thirst is a symptom of fluid volume deficit. The client may also suffer a loss of appetite or be nauseated because of decreased blood flow to the intestines.

SIGNS   The individual with fluid volume deficit will be less able to maintain his or her blood pressure immediately after rising from a lying or sitting position. This is called **orthostatic hypotension.** The nurse measures the blood pressure with the client lying or sitting, asks the client to stand, and immediately retakes the blood pressure. A drop of 15 millimeters or mercury in either systolic or diastolic blood pressure upon standing suggests fluid volume deficit. A narrowing of **pulse pressure** (the difference between systolic and diastolic readings) also occurs with fluid volume deficit. In an effort to maintain perfusion of the tissues, the body compensates for a lowered blood pressure by an increase in pulse rate. Taking a pulse when lying or sitting and immediately after rising is another method of assessing fluid volume deficit. An increase of 20 beats per minute upon standing merits further assessment.

Decreased skin **turgor** or elasticity, is a sign of fluid volume deficit associated with sodium loss. To assess skin turgor, pinch the skin on the forearm, over the sternum, or on the back of the hand. If the skin stays pinched, suspect fluid volume deficit. This is a less reliable sign in the elderly person, whose skin has lost much of its elasticity.

Another sign of fluid volume deficit can be found in the client's mouth. Besides dry mouth, many longitudinal furrows of the tongue may be seen to replace the single one in the well hydrated adult.

Turgor—Resilience of skin; when pinched, quickly returns to shape in well-hydrated young individuals; test for fluid deficit that is not accurate for elderly clients.

Delayed filling of hand veins is a sign of fluid volume deficit. To assess vein filling, raise the hand above the heart. Normally, the veins will collapse in 3 to 5 seconds. Then lower the hand below the heart. The veins should refill in 3 to 5 seconds. A person with fluid volume deficit will require more than 5 seconds for the veins to refill.

The symptoms of loss of appetite and nausea may progress to the sign of vomiting. Here, too, the cause is decreased blood flow to the intestines.

Fluid volume deficit produces changes in certain laboratory readings. The client will show increases in hemoglobin and hematocrit levels unless he or she has lost red blood cells through hemorrhage.

Special attention must be given to the assessment of infants. Because 75 percent of the infant's body weight is water and 54 percent of the water is extracellular, dehydration from fluid loss can occur rapidly. Signs to assess in the infant, in addition to poor skin turgor and dry mucous membranes, are depressed fontanel ("soft spot" in skull), sunken eyes, and lack of tears when crying.

SHOCK   If fluid volume deficit continues, the client will go into shock. The loss of 20 to 25 percent of intravascular volume produces shock. Shock is an acute peripheral circulatory failure due to loss of circulatory fluid or derangement of circulatory control. Signs of shock are a decreased blood pressure and an increased pulse. The person's skin is pale, cool, and clammy from perspiration. Urine output is decreased to less than 15 milliliters per hour.

Treatment of Fluid Volume Deficit

When treating fluid volume deficit, it is essential to correct the cause of the fluid depletion. In addition, to replace fluid volume and correct electrolyte imbalances, hypotonic fluids are given. If possible, the oral route is used. See Clinical Application 9–6 for an example of a commonly used oral electrolyte solution. Clinical trials of alternate formulations are being reported (International Study Group, 1995; Lebenthal, et al, 1995).

If hypertonic solutions were given to correct fluid loss, the concentrated solution would remain in the stomach longer than water, providing satiety and restraining water intake (Brensilver and Goldberger, 1996). Additionally, hypertronic solutins draw fluid from the bowel wall into the lumen; the result would be diarrhea. This is called osmotic diarrhea. Some commercial laxatives and enemas are hypertonic solutions that work in this way.

Maximal sodium and water absorption is thought to occur with a glucose concentration of 10 to 25 grams per liter. Higher concentrations allow less sodium and water to be absorbed, in addition to causing osmotic diarrhea. Cola beverages, ginger ale, and apple juice are poor choices for rehydration in prolonged diarrhea, owing to their high glucose and low electrolyte concentrations.

Another electrolyte imbalance is possible if the client in shock requires blood transfusions. Clinical Application 9–7 discusses hyperkalemia following blood transfusion.

Fluid Volume Excess

This situation is the opposite of fluid volume deficit. The individual is retaining fluid intracellularly or

---

CLINICAL APPLICATION 9–6

Oral Electrolyte Solutions

Originally, oral electrolyte solutions were designed to combat diarrheal diseases in developing countries. They proved so useful that they have since been modified for use in Western nations.

One commonly used oral electrolyte solution is Pedialyte. It is available over the counter without a prescription. One liter of Pedialyte contains:

45 mEq sodium
20 mEq potassium
35 mEq chloride
30 mEq citrate, a base

The total osmolarity of Pedialyte is mildly hypotonic, about 243 milliosmoles per liter. Pedialyte also illustrates electroneutrality. The sodium and potassium are cations carrying positive charges. The chloride and citrate are anions carrying negative charges.

45 mEq Na$^+$	35 mEq Cl$^-$
+ 20 mEq K$^+$	+ 30 mEq citrate$^-$
65 cations	65 anions

Pedialyte is designed for maintenance of an infant or child experiencing vomiting or diarrhea. If the client becomes dehydrated, medical attention is needed. Intravenous fluids or an oral rehydration solution of different composition from Pedialyte may be prescribed for the dehydrated client. Loss of 5 percent of body weight indicates dehydration.

Pedialyte also has the ideal concentration of glucose to promote sodium and water absorption, 25 g/L. In contrast, athletic beverages contain concentrated sweeteners to mask the bitter taste of the electrolytes (Brensilver and Goldberger, 1996).

CLINICAL APPLICATION 9-7

Hyperkalemia following Blood Transfusion

A person who has hemorrhaged may need blood replacement. Red blood cells do not live as long in the blood bank as they do in the human body. Potassium is the major cation in red blood cells (intracellular). When the red blood cells die and their cell walls rupture, potassium is spilled into the serum.

Blood that has been stored for a prolonged period may contain up to 30 mEq per liter of potassium due to the destruction of the red blood cells. This may not sound like a lot, but potassium is usually administered intravenously at a concentration of 40 mEq per liter to a person who is potassium depleted. The person receiving a blood transfusion may have a serum potassium level that is nearly normal, and the old blood containing a higher concentration of potassium may push him or her into hyperkalemia.

extracellularly. A fluid compartment does not operate in isolation: if one is out of balance, the other compartments eventually will be affected as the body attempts to equalize osmotic pressure across the compartments.

Gains of Fluid

If the kidney and the hormones from the adrenal and pituitary glands are functioning normally, excess water is excreted from the body in the urine. When a person becomes ill and these control mechanisms stop working, fluids shift from the intravascular and interstitial spaces to the intracellular space so as to equalize osmotic pressure.

Inflammation increases the fluid in interstitial space, causing edema. In most cases, localized edema is not life threatening. However, the accumulation of fluid in the brain (cerebral edema) or in lung tissue (pulmonary edema) are life-threatening conditions. Cerebral edema may result from tumors, toxic chemicals, or infection. Pulmonary edema can be a consequence of a failing heart or irritation of the lung, as when a client inhales toxic gases.

Assessment of Fluid Volume Excess

Many of the presenting signs and symptoms of fluid volume excess are opposite those of fluid volume deficit. One common symptom is loss of appetite.

SYMPTOMS The client with fluid volume excess complains of loss of appetite and nausea. Here the symptoms are due to edema of the gastrointestinal tract, rather than decreased blood flow as in fluid volume deficit.

SIGNS Because the brain cells are so sensitive to changes in the internal environment, the person with fluid volume excess exhibits deteriorating consciousness. The same edema of the gastrointestinal tract causing the anorexia and nausea causes the sign of vomiting.

Because increased fluid in the blood decreases the proportion of red blood cells to total volume, the hematocrit reading is decreased. The increase in blood volume causes an increased pulse pressure. The same technique described under fluid volume deficit is used to assess hand veins. With fluid volume excess the veins will not empty 3 to 5 seconds after raising the hand above the heart.

Increased blood flow to the kidneys causes increased urine output if the kidneys are functioning. The increased systolic blood pressure due to the excessive fluid pushes more fluid into the interstitial space, causing edema. Firm pressure over a bone, the ankle, or the top of the foot, forces some of the fluid aside. If the indentation remains visible for 5 seconds, it is called pitting edema. Table 9–5 lists signs and symptoms for fluid volume deficit and fluid volume excess.

Treatment of Fluid Volume Excess

As with fluid volume deficit, the remedy for fluid volume excess is to treat the cause. Osmotic diuretic drugs such as mannitol remain in the plasma and extracellular spaces. By increasing the osmotic pressure there, these drugs pull excess fluid from the cells to be excreted by the kidney.

Nutritionally, the client may be on a restricted fluid regimen. The physician may prescribe an intake of no more than 1000 milliliters in 24 hours. This amount will compensate for insensible losses through the skin and lungs. It is essential for the nurse to supply fluid as prescribed and to teach the client the reason for the restriction. Over a period of several days, the obligatory urine output and any diuretic therapy will help the client's body to excrete the excess fluid.

Summary

Water is our most essential nutrient. It comprises at least half of everyone's body weight. The amount of water varies with the type of tissue, with gender, and

TABLE 9–5 Signs and Symptoms of Abnormal Fluid Volume

		Fluid Volume Deficit	Fluid Volume Excess
Symptoms			
Gastrointestinal		Thirst	Loss of appetite (edema of the bowel)
		Loss of appetite (decreased blood to intestines)	Nausea
Signs			
General		Weight loss	Weight gain
		Depressed fontanel (infant)	Edema
		Sunken eyes (infant)	
		Lack of tears when crying (infant)	
Skin and mucous membranes		Dry mucous membranse	Skin stretched and shiney
		Decreased skin turgor	
Cardiovascular system		Orthostatic hypotension (pressure decrease of 15 mmHg in systolic or diastolic)	Increased hematocrit values
		Increased pulse rate upon standing	Increasing pulse pressure
		Increased hematocrit values (unless red blood cells also lost)	Emptying of hand veins takes longer than 5 s
		Narrowing pulse pressure	
		Filling of hand veins takes longer than 5 s	
Urinary		Decreased urine output	Polyuria
		Concentrated urine	Dilute urine
Gastrointestinal		Vomiting (decreased blood to intestines)	Vomiting
		Longitudinal furrows on tongue	
Central nervous system		Confusion, disorientation	Deteriorating consciousness

with age. Body fluids are held in two compartments: intracellular fluid is the water within the cells; extracellular fluid is the water outside the cells. The latter includes intravascular fluid, lymph, interstitial, and transcellular fluid.

Water has many vital functions in the body. It gives shape and form to the cells, helps form the structure of large molecules, serves as a lubricant, and helps regulate body temperature. As a solvent, water transports solutes to and from the cells, is a medium for chemical reactions, and participates in chemical reactions.

The human body has no storage tanks for water. When necessary, the body can absorb water rapidly. Although some water can be absorbed from the stomach, 1 liter per hour can be absorbed from the small intestine.

The movement, distribution, and composition of body fluids are influenced and controlled by electrolyte and plasma protein concentrations. In the extracellular fluid, sodium is the major cation and chloride is the major anion. The major cation in the intracellular fluid is potassium. Ionized sodium, potassium, and chloride are the solutes that maintain the balance between the extracellular and intracellular compartments.

A complex system regulates the amount of water retained or excreted by the kidney. Aldosterone and ADH are hormones that cause retention of sodium and water, respectively. The hypothalamus stimulates the thirst mechanism when fluids inside the cells become too concentrated (with solutes).

Acid-base balance is maintained in the body by the action of the lungs, the kidneys, and chemical buffers. Bicarbonate is the most important buffer in the extracellular fluid. Phosphate and protein are two important buffers in the intracellular fluid.

The body's sources of water include beverages, foods, and water from the metabolism of the energy nutrients (except alcohol). Water can be lost through the skin, lungs, kidneys, and intestinal tract. Although still present in the body, fluid can be lost to circulation in "third spaces." The single most important measure of fluid balance is daily weight.

Since most fluid losses are hypotonic, the fluids usually used to correct fluid volume deficits and electrolyte imbalances are hypotonic. The use of hypertonic fluids would have the opposite effect, pulling more water out of the tissues and into the bowel or bloodstream.

Fluid volume excess can be local or generalized. The most dangerous sites for local edema are the brain and the lungs. Generalized fluid volume excess can make exorbitant demands on the heart.

Case Study 9–1 Mr. N, a 75-year-old retired office worker, recently arrived from his summer home in the North to his winter home in Florida. He had anticipated enjoying the 85°F weather. He left temperatures in the forties. Although Mr. N had hired someone to care for his small yard while he was away from Florida, there were still a number of chores to be done, which he tackled with a vengeance.

After an 1 1/2 hours, Mr. N began to get a headache. He felt a bit weak and dizzy, but continued his work. He was nearly finished with the outside tasks.

Half an hour later, Ms. N found her husband lying on the ground. She called their neighbor, who is a retired nurse.

The nurse noted that Mr. N's skin was pale and cool but that he was perspiring profusely. He was conscious and coherent but said he felt weak. The nurse took Mr. N's pulse. It was 90 beats per minute, regular but weak. His respirations were 12 per minute and shallow.

The nurse provided the emergency care described in the following nursing care plan. (Of course, she did not write it all out before helping Mr. N).

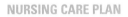

NURSING CARE PLAN

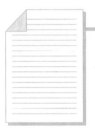

Assessment

Subjective Data	Has worked outside in 85°F heat 2 hours
	Headache, weakness, dizziness
	Recently arrived from colder climate
Objective Data	Conscious, coherent
	Skin pale, cool, wet with perspiration
	Pulse 90, regular and weak
	Respirations 12 and shallow

Nursing Diagnosis Fluid volume deficit related to excessive loss of hypotonic fluid (sweat) as evidenced by wet, pale skin and weak, rapid pulse.

Desired Outcome/ Evaluation Criteria	Nursing Actions	Rationale
Client will remain conscious and oriented, with a pulse no greater than 90, until the emergency team arrives.	Instruct Ms. N to call emergency medical services and return to help.	In an emergency situation, the nurse stays with the client. Potential electrolyte imbalance requires medical care.
	Loosen Mr. N's clothing.	Mr. N is already in a state of shock. Loosening the clothing will allow maximum air exchange and permit relaxation.
	With Ms. N, move client to shade or provide shade where he lies.	Mr. N must get out of the sun. Depending on the situation, he might be moved indoors, but perhaps the two women could not manage to move him.

Table continued on following page

Desired Outcome/ Evaluation Criteria	Nursing Actions	Rationale
	Keep client lying down with legs elevated slightly.	Lying down permits maximum blood circulation to the brain. Raising the legs increases the return of blood to the heart. The head should not be lowered because this causes venous congestion in the brain.
	Send Ms. N to kitchen for 1/2 glass of water with 1/2 teaspoonful of salt in it. Administer salty water to Mr. N.	Although this is a hypertonic solution, sodium is readily absorbed by the intestine, so it is unlikely to cause osmotic diarrhea. Only 5 percent of consumed sodium remains in the feces. Sodium levels in the blood are controlled by the kidneys. This client has lost water and sodium chloride in perspiration.

Study Aids

Chapter Review

1. Which of the following persons would have the greatest percentage of body weight as water?
   a. A 3-pound premature infant
   b. A 154-pound man
   c. A 120-pound woman
   d. All of them would have an equal percentage.

2. Which of the following represents the approximate amount of water contained in oral fluids consumed by the average adult?
   a. 100–200 milliliters
   b. 500–600 milliliters
   c. 800–1000 milliliters
   d. 1100–1400 milliliters

3. Heat exhaustion is caused by:
   a. Insufficient secretion of ADH
   b. Loss of water and salt in sweat
   c. Inability to perspire
   d. Retention of excessive water

4. When aldosterone secretion is increased, _____ is retained by the kidney and _____ is excreted to maintain electroneutrality.

   a. Sodium, potassium
   b. Potassium, sodium
   c. Calcium, hydrogen
   d. Hydrogen, potassium

5. If a person's body is too acid, the automatic response of the body is to:
   a. Increase sweat production
   b. Retain water
   c. Decrease rate and depth of breathing
   d. Increase rate and depth of breathing

Clinical Analysis

Baby I, a 4-month-old boy, has developed diarrheal stools within the past 2 days. At birth he weighed 7 pounds 8 ounces. Since then he has gained steadily to 12 pounds 8 ounces three days ago. Baby I's present weight is 12 pounds 2 ounces.

Mrs. I has been feeding the baby his usual formula. He drinks eagerly but then has an explosive bowel movement with loud crying. Baby I has had six bowel movements per day instead of his usual two.

1. With this history, what physical assessment measures would the nurse include initially?
   a. Skin turgor, fontanel fullness, moisture of mucous membranes

b. Condition of hair, strength of grasp, presence of sucking reflex

c. Heart sounds, lung sounds, blood pressure

d. Urine specific gravity, observation of diaper rash

2. Which of the following recommendations by the nurse would show understanding of supportive care of this client?

a. Give Baby I whole milk to maintain nutrition.

b. Continue, as Mrs. I has been doing, to allow the bowel to empty itself.

c. Substitute orange juice for the formula for 3 days.

d. Start Baby I on an oral electrolyte solution.

3. The nurse instructs Mrs. I to return for additional care for Baby I if one of the following events takes place. Which one would indicate the need for reassessment of Baby I?

a. The baby sleeps soundly and has to be awakened for a night feeding.

b. The baby has three loose bowel movements the day after beginning treatment.

c. The baby continues to lose weight or passes blood in the stool.

d. The baby gains more than 2 ounces per day.

Bibliography

Borowitz, D: Pediatric nutrition. In Feldman, EB (ed): Essentials of Clinical Nutrition. FA Davis, Philadelphia, 1988.

Brensilver, JM, and Goldberger, E: A Primer of Water, Electrolyte, and Acid Base Syndromes, ed 8. FA Davis, Philadelphia, 1996.

Connolly, DL, Shanahan, CM, and Weissberg, PL: Water channels in health and disease. Lancet 347:210, 1996.

Cumming, CM, Brevard, PB, and Pearson, JM: Recreational runners' beliefs and practices concerning water intake. J Nutr Educ 26:195, 1994.

Deglin, JH, and Vallerand, AH: Davis's Drug Guide For Nurses, ed 4. FA Davis, Philadelphia, 1995.

DeSilva, M, and Seghatchian, MJ: Is depletion of potassium in blood before transfusion essential? Lancet 344:136, 1994.

Groff, JL, Gropper, SS, and Hunt, SM: Advanced Nutrition and Human Metabolism, ed 2. West, Minneapolis, 1995.

Horne, MM, Heitz, UE, and Swearingen, PL: Fluid, Electrolyte, and Acid-Base Balance. Mosby Year Book, St Louis, 1991.

Inaba, S, and Shirahama, N: Potassium ion depletion filter for blood transfusion. Lancet 343:1223, 1994.

International Study Group on Reduced-Osmolarity ORS Solutions: Multicentre evaluation of reduced-osmolarity oral rehydration salts solution. Lancet 345:282, 1995.

Lebenthal, E, et al: Thermophilic amylase-digested rice-electrolyte solution in the treatment of acute diarrhea in children. Pediatrics 95:198, 1995.

Lederer, JR, et al: Care Planning Pocket Guide, ed 5. Addison-Wesley Nursing, Redwood City, CA, 1993.

Members of the Research Committee, greater Milwaukee Area chapter of the AAC—CN: Fluid volume deficit: Validating the indicators. Heart Lung 19:152, 1990.

Pagana, KD, and Pagana, TJ: Mosby's Diagnostic and Laboratory Test Reference, ed 2. Mosby Year Book, St Louis, 1995.

Scanlon, VC, and Sanders, T: Essentials of Anatomy and Physiology, ed 2. FA Davis, Philadelphia, 1995.

Thorp, FK, Pierce, P, and Deedwania, C: Nutrition in the infant and young child. In Halpern, SL (ed): Quick Reference to Clinical Nutrition, ed 2. JB Lippincott, Philadelphia, 1987.

Watson, J, and Jaffe, MS: Nurse's Manual of Laboratory and Diagnostic Tests, ed 2. FA Davis, Philadelphia, 1995.

Yucha, C, and Suddaby, P: David could have died of thirst, yet he never felt thirsty. Nursing 91 21:42, 1991.

CHAPTER 10

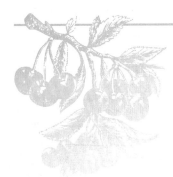

Digestion, Absorption, Metabolism, and Excretion

LEARNING OBJECTIVES

After completing this chapter, the student should be able to:

1 List the anatomic structures which make up the gastrointestinal tract.
2 Describe digestion, absorption, metabolism, and excretion.
3 Discuss how nutrients are used by the cells.
4 Describe appropriate dietary treatments for lactose intolerance, lipid malabsorption, food allergies, and gluten-sensitive enteropathy.
5 List the ways the body eliminates waste.

Every part of the human body requires nutrients for energy, maintenance, and growth. Food supplies the necessary nutrients. However, food is composed of complex substances that must be broken down to simpler forms that can be used by the cells. The **cell** is the ultimate destination for the nutrients found in food. Digestion, absorption, and metabolism are the three interrelated processes that act on food to prepare it for use by the body. A fourth process, excretion, is the elimination of undigestible or unusable substances. In this chapter we will discuss all the bodily activities, organs, and systems involved in these major processes.

Overview of the Major Processes

The first step in preparing food for use by the cells is digestion. Digestion is the process by which food is broken down mechanically and chemically in the gastrointestinal tract into forms small enough for absorption to occur. The end products of digestion move from the gastrointestinal tract into the blood or lymphatic system in a process called *absorption.* After absorption, the nutrients usually are transported to the liver where they may be adjusted to suit the needs of the body. Metabolism, the sum of all physical and chemical changes that take place in the body, determines the final use of the individual nutrients and medications. What the cells have no use for becomes waste that is eliminated through excretion.

Digestion

Digestion takes place in the alimentary canal and the accessory organs.

Alimentary Canal

The **alimentary canal** is a long, hollow, muscular tube passing through the body that extends from the mouth to the anus. It includes the oral cavity, pharynx, esophagus, stomach, small intestine, and large intestine.

Muscle rings, called **sphincters,** separate segments of the alimentary canal. They act as valves to control the passage of food. When the muscles contract, the passageway closes; when the muscles relax, the passageway opens.

Mucosa lines the alimentary canal. It secretes **mucus**, which lubricates the canal and helps facilitate the smooth passage of food. The mucosa se-

cretes digestive enzymes of the stomach and small intestine.

Accessory Organs

Three **organs** located outside of the alimentary canal are considered part of the digestive system. These are the liver, gallbladder, and pancreas. They make important contributions to the digestive process.

Liver

The **liver** is the second largest single organ in the body (skin is the largest). Many functions are performed by the liver, but the only digestive function is the production of **bile.** Bile is important in breaking down dietary fats. Bile is taken out of the liver by the hepatic duct. A **duct** is a narrow tube that permits the movement of fluid from one organ to another. Later in the chapter we will discuss some of the tasks the liver performs after the absorption of nutrients.

Gallbladder

The **gallbladder** is a 3- to 4-inch sac that concentrates and stores bile until it is needed in the small intestine. Bile is delivered to the small intestine through the common bile duct. About 2 to 3 cups of bile are secreted each day into the alimentary canal.

Pancreas

The **pancreas** secretes enzymes that are involved in the digestion of all the energy nutrients. These secretions are collectively known as pancreatic juice.

Digestion—The process by which food is broken down mechanically and chemically in the gastrointestinal tract into forms small enough for cells to use.

Mucus—A thick fluid secreted by the mucous membranes and glands.

Liver—A digestive organ that aids in the metabolism of all the energy nutrients, screens toxic substances from the blood, manufacturers blood proteins, and performs many other important functions.

Bile—Dark yellow secretion of the liver that alkalinizes the intestine and breaks large fat globules into smaller ones to facilitate enzyme digestive action.

Pancreatic juice is carried to the small intestine via the pancreatic and common bile ducts.

Digestive Action

Mechanical and chemical digestion occur simultaneously throughout the alimentary canal. **Mechanical digestion** is the physical breaking down of food into smaller pieces. **Chemical digestion** involves the splitting of complex molecules into simpler forms.

Mechanical Digestion

Examples of mechanical digestion include chewing or **mastication,** swallowing, peristalsis, and emulsification. **Peristalsis** is a wavelike movement that propels food along the entire length of the alimentary canal. This one-way movement is caused by the alternate contraction and relaxation of the circular and longitudinal muscles that make up the external muscle layer of the alimentary canal. Other muscular activity churns the food, which reduces it to successively smaller particles and mixes it with digestive secretions. All of these muscular actions are regulated by a network of nerves within the wall of the alimentary canal. Emulsification is discussed later in the chapter.

Chemical Digestion

Many chemical reactions are involved in digestion. For example, the conversion of starch to maltose, of fat to glycerol and fatty acids, and of protein to amino acids all involve the process of **hydrolysis.** The hydrolysis of nutrients is achieved mostly through the action of digestive enzymes, which are present in saliva, gastric juice, pancreatic juice, and intestinal juice. Each enzyme is specific in its action; it will only act upon a certain substance and no other. Enzymes sometimes require the presence of additional substances such as activators, coenzymes, or hormones to make them active. There are more than 500 enzymes involved in the digestive process. However, only a few of the major ones will be discussed in this chapter.

In addition to enzymes, other secretions and chemicals are used in the chemical digestion of food. These include mucus, electrolytes, and water. Mucus lubricates passages and facilitates the movement of food. It also protects the inside walls of the alimentary canal from acidic solutions. Electrolytes are substances that conduct an electric current in solution. One example of an electrolyte is the **hydrochloric acid** (HCl) secreted by the stomach. It performs many functions necessary to the digestive process. The ways in which HCl aids digestion will be discussed later in this chapter.

Control of Secretions

The amount of mucus, electrolytes, water, and enzymes released during the digestive process depends on several factors. Hormones frequently turn on or turn off a given secretion. For example, the acid content of the food causes a hormone called secretin to be released. The release of secretin in the small intestine causes the pancreas to send pancreatic juices into the small intestine.

A person's feelings can affect the amount of a secretion released. For example, the smell of a roasting turkey on Thanksgiving Day will cause the release of hydrochloric acid in the stomach. Stress and tension can also produce this effect sometimes with deleterious results.

The presence of food in the gastrointestinal tract can influence the release of alimentary canal secretions. For example, coffee causes a hormone to be released into the stomach, which in turn causes the secretion of hydrochloric acid. Another example is the release of bile from the gallbladder caused by the presence of fat in the small intestine. This chain of reactions whereby one event causes another and then another is very common in all biological systems.

End Products of Digestion

Within about four hours after a meal, the body has broken the food into some trillion molecules. Each of the energy nutrients is broken down into simpler molecules. Carbohydrates are digested into monosaccharides. Fats are broken down into molecules of glycerol, fatty acids, and monoglycerides. The end products of protein digestion are amino acids and small peptides. Up to one-third of dietary protein is believed to be absorbed into mucosal cells as di- and tri-peptides. Vitamins, minerals, and water are also released during digestion. In the next section we will follow the pathway of food as it goes through the digestive process. Then, the digestive activities that occur along this pathway (by location in the alimentary canal) will be discussed in detail.

The Food Pathway

Food passes through the mouth into the oral cavity, where it is chewed and exposed to chemicals in the saliva. The tongue voluntarily forces the mass of food, called a **bolus,** into the pharynx, which is responsible for the reflex action of swallowing. When swallowed, the bolus enters the esophagus, a muscular, mucus-lined tube, and is propelled downward by peristalsis to the stomach. Both mechanical and chemical digestion occur in the stomach, reducing the food to a semifluid mass that is then released into the small intestine. Further digestion takes place in the small intestine, and most of the absorption of nutrients occurs here as well. Any food remaining after digestion and absorption passes into the large intestine and is excreted as fecal matter.

Oral Cavity

The **oral cavity** is the hollow space in the skull directly behind the mouth. Its boundaries are the roof of the mouth, the cheeks, and the floor of the mouth. Within the oral cavity are the teeth, tongue, and the openings of the ducts of the salivary glands.

DIGESTIVE ACTION   Food entering the oral cavity is chewed and thus broken into smaller particles. This mechanical action increases the surface area of the food for exposure to saliva, a digestive secretion produced by the **salivary glands.** Saliva moistens and softens the food for swallowing and contains the digestive enzyme known as **salivary amylase.** Salivary amylase converts starch to maltose (a disaccharide) or to shorter chains of glucose. Because they require no digestion, some absorption of simple sugars (monosaccharides) may occur in the mouth. The chemical digestion of carbohydrates (starch) continues until the hydrochloric acid in the stomach halts the action of the salivary amylase. After being chewed, the bolus (food mass) is maneuvered backward by the tongue into the pharynx. Box 10–1 introduces the dietary treatment of dysphagia.

Pharynx

The **pharynx** is a muscular passage between the oral cavity and the esophagus. No digestive action occurs here. The pharynx continues the movement of the bolus by the reflexive action of swallowing. The bolus then enters the esophagus.

Esophagus

The **esophagus** is a muscular tube about 10 inches long that takes food from the pharynx to the stomach. No digestive action occurs here. Peristalsis

forces the bolus into the stomach with the help of mucous secretions. Between the esophagus and the stomach is the **cardiac sphincter** which opens to permit passage of the food. The sphincter closes after the passage of food to prevent the backup of stomach contents.

Stomach

The **stomach** is a J-shaped sac that extends from the esophagus to the small intestine. Folds in the mucous membrane, called **rugae,** smooth out when the stomach is full. They allow the stomach to expand. The need to eat constantly is prevented because the stomach serves as a reservoir for food, which takes from 2 to 6 hours to completely pass through to the small intestine. Gastric juice, the collective secretions of the stomach, consists of hydrochloric acid, mucus, and the enzymes pepsin, rennin, and gastric lipase.

DIGESTIVE ACTION   In the stomach, the chemical digestion of protein begins and further mechanical digestion takes place. Some water and minerals, certain drugs, and alcohol are absorbed in the stomach. Even before food enters the mouth, the sight or smell of food will cause the gastric mucosa to excrete the hormone **gastrin.** This hormone stimulates the secretion of gastric juice so that there is some present in the stomach when the food arrives. The stomach's lining is partially protected from the corrosive effects of gastric juice by mucus.

The hydrolysis of protein is initiated when hydrochloric acid activates and then converts **pepsino-**

Mechanical digestion—The digestive process that involves the physical breaking down of food into smaller pieces.

Chemical digestion—Digestive process that involves the splitting of complex molecules into simpler forms.

Peristalsis—A wavelike movement that propels food along the alimentary canal.

Hydrolysis—A chemical reaction that splits a substance into simpler compounds by the addition of water.

Salivary amylase—An enzyme that initiates the breakdown of starch in the mouth.

Gastrin—A hormone secreted by the gastric mucosa; stimulates the secretion of gastric juice.

BOX 10–1   DIETARY TREATMENT FOR DYSPHAGIA

Approximately 15 million people in the United States have a swallowing disorder called *dysphagia*, literally meaning difficulty swallowing. Many swallowing disorders are undiagnosed. A reported 10,000 to 12,000 Americans choke to death each year because of dysphagia. Recent research about the swallowing process has given health care providers improved measures to feed these clients a safe, enjoyable, and nourishing diet. These are tips for safe swallowing:

Eat slowly.

Avoid distractions while eating.

Do not talk while eating.

Remove loose dentures.

Avoid foods requiring much chewing.

Sit up straight while eating.

Position the head correctly. A speech therapist can help determine the correct position.

Use a regular teaspoon and take only one-half teaspoon of food or liquid at a time.

Swallow completely between bites or sips.

Select foods of appropriate consistency.

    Some clients tolerate liquids best.

    Some clients tolerate only thick purees. A commercial food thickener can help

    Some clients best tolerate a more textured diet consisting of semisolids that form a cohesive bolus.

A dietitian should be consulted regarding the types and consistencies of foods that dysphagic clients can tolerate and will accept.

---

gen to its active form, **pepsin.** A protein molecule is made up of possibly hundreds of amino acids joined together by **peptide bonds.** Such chains of amino acids linked by peptide bonds are called **polypeptides.** What pepsin does is to break down large polypeptides into smaller polypeptides. In infants, the milk protein casein is broken down by the enzyme **rennin.** The action of rennin coagulates (curdles) the milk. In addition to activating pepsin, hydrochloric acid destroys harmful bacteria, makes certain minerals such as iron and calcium more absorbable, and maintains the pH (1 to 2) of the gastric juice.

Some butterfat molecules of milk are also broken down into smaller molecules in the stomach. The enzyme that accomplishes this is **gastric lipase.** This enzyme is most active in infants because the more alkaline environment of the infant's stomach enables gastric lipase to work more effectively.

The mechanical digestion that occurs in the stomach is a result of the churning action of the muscular walls. This muscular activity agitates the contents of the stomach, thoroughly mixing the food with gastric juice. In this way, the food is reduced to a semifluid mass of partially digested material called **chyme.** Peristaltic waves push the chyme toward the **pyloric sphincter,** the valve separating the stomach from the small intestine. With each peristaltic wave, a small amount of chyme is forced through the pyloric sphincter into the small intestine.

Small Intestine

The **small intestine** is the longest portion of the alimentary canal, approximately 20 feet in length. It extends from the pyloric sphincter of the stomach to the large intestine. The small intestine is looped and coiled in the central part of the abdominal cavity, surrounded by the large intestine. It consists of three parts: the **duodenum** is the first 10 inches, the **jejunum** is the middle 8 feet, and the **ileum** is the last 11 feet. Ninety percent of the digestive action in the alimentary canal and nearly all absorption of the end products of digestion occurs in the small intestine. Its anatomy will be discussed further in the section on absorption.

The entry of chyme into the duodenum stimulates the secretion of two hormones, secretin and cholecystokinin. Collectively, these hormones are responsible for the secretion and release of bile and the secrction of pancreatic juice. **Secretin** stimulates the production of bile by the liver and the secretion of sodium bicarbonate juice by the pancreas. The bile salts in bile emulsify fats, and sodium bicarbonate juice (which is alkaline) neutralizes the gastric juice that enters the duodenum. This neutralization is necessary to prevent damage to the lining of the duodenum. Mucus secreted by intestinal glands also provides some measure of protection against such damage. **Cholecystokinin** stimulates the contraction of the gallbladder, an action that forces stored bile into the duodenum. It also stimulates the secretion of pancreatic enzymes, which are essential for the breakdown of carbohydrates, fats, and proteins. Intestinal juice is also secreted in response to the presence of chyme in the duodenum. Peristaltic action of the small intestine mixes the bile, the pancreatic juice, and the intestinal juice together with the chyme as it moves toward the colon. It is the collective action of these juices that yields the final end products of the digestive process.

DIGESTION OF CARBOHYDRATES   Carbohydrate digestion is completed through the action of pancreatic and intestinal enzymes. Pancreatic **amylase** breaks down any remaining starch into maltose. The disaccharides maltose, sucrose, and lactose are reduced to monosaccharides by the action of three enzymes located in the walls of the small intestine. Each of these enzymes is specific for a given disaccharide: **maltase** breaks down maltose to glucose and glucose, **sucrase** breaks down sucrose to glucose and fructose, and **lactase** breaks down lactose to glucose and galactose. Often, low levels of these enzymes can lead to intolerances for the respective disaccharides.

In fact, approximately 70 percent of the world's population has some degree of lact*ose* intolerance. This intolerance is the result of a lack of the intestinal enzyme lact*ase*. Clinical Application 10–1 discusses carbohydrate intolerances, including lactose intolerance. Table 10–1 lists food items that are lactose-free, low in lactose, and high in lactose. Box 10–2 contains a lactose-restricted diet with a sample menu.

DIGESTION OF FATS   Fats are emulsified by bile salts in the small intestine before they are digested further. **Emulsification** is the physical breaking up of fats into tiny droplets. Lingual lipase is an important enzyme in infants, although not in adults. In this way, more surface area of the fat is exposed to the chemical action of the pancreatic enzyme **pancreatic lipase.** Pancreatic lipase completes the digestion of fats by reducing triglycerides to diglycerides and monoglycerides, fatty acids and glycerol.

DIGESTION OF PROTEIN   Although hundreds of enzymes are involved in protein digestion, this text reviews only a few of the major ones. The shorter polypeptides resulting from the digestive action in the stomach are broken down even further by the action of pancreatic and intestinal enzymes. Two of the major enzymes produced by the pancreas that are responsible for this additional protein-splitting are **trypsin** and **chymotrypsin.** Both trypsin and chymotrypsin have inactive precursors that are activated by other enzymes. The intestinal wall also secretes a group of enzymes known as **peptidases.** The peptidases act on the smaller molecules produced by the pancreatic enzymes, reducing them to single amino acids and small peptides, the final end products of protein digestion.

Table 10–2 shows a summary of the digestion of carbohydrates, fats, and proteins by body organ (mouth, stomach, or small intestine). The subcategories in the table identify whether the digestive action is mechanical or chemical. This table includes only the material that is covered in the text.

Absorption

The end products of digestion move from the gastrointestinal tract into the blood or **lymphatic system** in a process called **absorption.** The lymphatic

---

Pepsin—An enzyme secreted in the stomach that begins protein digestion.

Chyme—The mixture of partly digested food and digestive secretions found in the stomach and small intestine during digestion of a meal.

Secretin—A hormone that stimulates the production of bile by the liver and the secretion of sodium bicarbonate juice by the pancreas.

Cholecystokinin—A hormone secreted by the duodenum; stimulates contraction of the gallbladder (releases bile) and the secretion of pancreatic juice.

Pancreatic lipase—An enzyme that splits fats into fatty acids and glycerol; present in pancreatic juices; also known as pancreatic lipase.

Peptidases—Enzymes that assist in the digestion of protein by reducing the smaller molecules to single amino acids.

Absorption—The movement of the end products of digestion from the gastrointestinal tract into the blood and/or lymphatic system.

Carbohydrate Intolerances

Some individuals are deficient in one or more of the enzymes lactase, maltase, or sucrase. They are unable to digest these disaccharides into monosaccharides. The resulting disease is called a *lactose intolerance, maltose intolerance,* or *sucrose intolerance.* Lactose intolerance is the most common of these diseases. Lactose intolerance may occur in 60 percent to 100 percent of Hispanics, blacks, and southeast Asians. The condition can be hereditary or can be secondary to other disease processes involving the small intestine. Symptoms of a lactose intolerance include abdominal cramping and pain, loose stools, and flatulence (gas) after eating or drinking milk products.

Dietary treatment of a lactose intolerance involves three steps: (1) identifying food items that contain lactose; (2) eliminating all sources of lactose from the diet; and (3) establishing an individual tolerance level for the client on a trial-and-error basis. There is a broad range of tolerance levels for lactose in these clients.

The lactose content of cheeses varies. One gallon of milk is required to produce 1 lb of cheese. During cheese making, the whey is separated from the curd. The whey is the liquid and the curd is the solid material (similar to the curd in cottage cheese). Most of the lactose in cheese is contained in the whey. In ripened cheese, the small amount of lactose entrapped in the curd is transformed into lactic acid, which does not require lactase for absorption.

Generally, cheese must age for more than 90 days to be lactose free. The following cheeses are considered hard ripened (low in lactose): blue, brick, Brie, Cambert, Cheddar, Colby, Edam, Gouda, Monterey, Muenster, Parmesan, Provolone, and Swiss. The following cheeses are considered "soft cheeses" and thus contain more lactose: cream cheese, Neufchatel, ricotta, mozzarella, and cottage cheese.

Clients on a lactose-free diet should read all labels carefully to see if milk or milk solids, lactose, or whey have been added to the products. Many toothpastes or over-the-counter medications contain a small amount of lactose. Generally, the amount is very small and is tolerated well.

Lactaid is an over-the-counter product specially designed for individuals with a lactose intolerance. Lactaid is a natural enzyme that is available in liquid or tablet form. The liquid form is typically added to milk, whereas the tablet form is chewed before consumption of a food product containing lactose. Some grocery stores also sell milk that has been pretreated with Lactaid. This product will digest 70 percent of the lactose in a product into glucose and galactose. As a result, most lactose-intolerant persons can drink Lactaid-treated milk or eat foods which contain lactose and digest it comfortably. Milk treated with Lactaid is slightly sweeter than regular milk. The sweeter taste results naturally when lactose is broken down into glucose and galactose.

A lactose-restricted diet may be low in calcium, riboflavin, and vitamin D. Clients should be instructed in alternate sources of these nutrients or advised to take supplements.

---

system transports **lymph** from the tissues to the bloodstream. This **system** is technically part of the circulatory or cardiovascular system. Eventually, all fluid in the lymphatic system enters the blood. It is only after nutrients have been absorbed into either the blood or lymphatic system that they can be utilized by the cells of the body.

The end products of digestion include the monosaccharides from carbohydrate digestion, the fatty acids and glycerol (and often monoglycerides) from fats, and small peptides and amino acids from protein digestion. Absorption occurs primarily in the small intestine.

Small Intestine

The inner surface of the small intestine has mucosal folds, villi, and microvilli to increase the surface area for maximum absorption (see Fig. 10–1). The mucosal folds can be compared to pleats in fabric. On each fold (or pleat) are millions of finger-like projections, called **villi.** Each villus has hundreds of microscopic, hairlike projections (resembling bristles on a brush), called **microvilli,** on its surface. The large surface area resulting from this arrangement fosters the movement of nutrients into the blood or lymphatic system. This is similar to the idea that four lanes of traffic move more quickly than two—the surface area of the highway is larger so more traffic can be accommodated. The structure of the mucosa serves as a unit that accomplishes the absorption of nutrients.

Within each villus is a network of blood **capillaries** and a central lymph vessel called a **lacteal.** The villi absorb nutrients from the chyme by way of these blood and lymph vessels. Monosaccharides, amino

TABLE 10–1   Lactose Content of Foods

Lactose-Free Foods		Low-Lactose Foods (0 to 2 g/serving)	
Broth-based soups		1/2 cup	Milk treated with lactase enzyme
Plain meat, fish, poultry, peanut butter		1/2 cup	Sherbet
Breads that do not contain milk, dry milk solids, or whey		1–2 oz	Aged cheese
Cereal, crackers		1 oz	Processed cheese
Fruit, plain vegetables		Butter or margarine	
Desserts made without milk, dry milk solids, or whey		Commercially prepared foods containing dry milk solids or whey	
Tofu and tofu products, such as tofu-based ice cream substitute		Some medications and vitamin preparations may contain a small amount of lactose. Generally, the amount is very small and is tolerated well.	
Nondairy creamers			

High-Lactose Foods (5 to 8 g/serving)			
1/2 cup	Milk (whole, skim, 1 percent, 2 percent, buttermilk, sweet acidophilus)	1/2 cup	White sauce
1/8 cup	Powdered dry milk (whole, nonfat, buttermilk—before reconstituting)	1/2 cup	Party chip dip or potato topping
		3/4 cup	Creamed or low-fat cottage cheese
		1 cup	Dry cottage cheese
1/4 cup	Evaporated milk	3/4 cup	Ricotta cheese
3 tbsp	Sweetened condensed milk	2 oz	Cheese food or cheese spread*
3/4	Heavy cream	3/4 cup	Ice cream or ice milk
1/2 cup	Half and half	1/2 cup	Yogurt†
1/2 cup	Sour cream		

* Lactose content is higher than that of aged cheese and of processed cheese because of the addition of whey powder and of dry milk solids.

† Yogurt may be tolerated better than foods with similar lactose content because of hydrolysis of lactose by bacterial lactase found in the culture. Tolerance may vary with the brand and the processing method.

SOURCE: Mayo Clinic Diet Manual, 1988, with permission.

BOX 10–2   LACTOSE-RESTRICTED DIET

Description: This diet restricts foods which contain lactose. Soy milk substitutes are used as a milk replacement. Individual tolerances should be taken into consideration as some clients may tolerate foods low in lactose. (See Table 10–1.)

Note: All labels should be read carefully for the addition of milk, lactose, or whey.

Indications: This diet is used for the management of patients exhibiting the signs and symptoms of lactose intolerance, Crohn's Disease, short bowel syndrome, or colitis. Persistent diarrhea and excessive amounts of gas may be lessened by decreasing lactose intake.

Nutritional adequacy: This diet is low in calcium, riboflavin, and vitamin D. Supplementation is recommended.

Continued on following page

Capillary—Minute vessel connecting arteriole and venule; wall acts as semipermeable membrane to exchange substances between blood or lymph and tissue fluid.

Food Group	Allowed	Avoided
Milk	Hard, ripened cheese Ensure Sustacal Ensure Plus Soy milk Lact-aide treated milk Coffee Rich	Unripened cheese Fluid milk Powdered milk Milk chocolate Cream Most chocolate drink mixes Most coffee creamers
Breads and Cereals	Most water-based bread (French, Italian, Jewish) Graham crackers Ritz crackers without cheese	Bread to which milk or lactose has been added (Check label)
Fruits	Any	None
Vegetables	Fresh, frozen, or canned without milk	Creamed, buttered, or breaded vegetables
Meats	Those not listed under avoided Kosher prepared meat or milk products	Breaded or creamed meat, fish, poultry Most luncheon meats Sausage Frankfurters
Desserts and Miscellaneous	Angel food cake Gelatin desserts Milk-free cookies Popcorn (with milk-free margarine) Pretzels Mustard, catsup Pickles	Most commercially made desserts Sherbet Ice cream Cream candies Toffee Caramels Most chewing gums

SAMPLE MENU

Breakfast

1/2 cup orange juice
1/2 cup cream of wheat
2 slices whole grain milk-free bread
2 tsp milk-free margarine
Jelly
Coffee
1/2 cup Coffee Rich

Lunch/Dinner

3 oz baked chicken
Baked potato
1/2 cup carrots
Sliced tomato
1 slice milk-free bread
2 tsp milk-free margarine
Angel food cake with fresh fruit topping
Coffee

TABLE 10–2 Summary of Digestion

Nutrient	Mouth and Esophagus	Stomach	Small Intestine
Carbohydrates yield	*Mechanical* Mastication Swallowing Peristalsis Mucus	*Mechanical* Peristalsis Mucus	*Mechanical* Peristalsis Mucus

	Chemical
	Salivary amylase
		Chemical
		None
			Chemical
			Pancreatic enzymes:
			   Pancreatic amylase
			Intestinal enzymes:
			   Maltase
			   Sucrase
			   Lactase

↓ Monosaccharides			
Fats yield	*Mechanical* Mastication Swallowing Peristalsis Mucus	*Mechanical* Peristalsis Mucus	*Mechanical* Peristalsis Mucus Gallbladder: Bile*

	Chemical
	None
	Lingual lipase in infants
		Chemical
		Gastric lipase†
			Chemical
			Pancreatic enzymes:
			   Pancreatic
			   lipase

↓ Glycerol, fatty acids, and monoglycerides			
Proteins yield	*Mechanical* Mastication Swallowing Peristalsis Mucus	*Mechanical* Peristalsis Mucus	*Mechanical* Peristalsis Mucus

	Chemical
	None
		Chemical
		Rennin
		Pepsin
		Hydrochloric acid
			Chemical
			Pancreatic enzymes:
			   Trypsin
			   Chymotrypsin
			Intestinal enzymes:
			   Peptidases

↓ Amino acids and small peptides			

* Emulsifies fat.
† Digests butterfat only.

acids, glycerol (which is water soluble), minerals, and water-soluble vitamins are absorbed into the blood in the capillary network. Because short- and medium-chain fatty acids have fewer carbons in their chain length, they are more water soluble than long-chain fatty acids. Thus, they are absorbed directly into the blood as well. These water-soluble nutrients, including short- and medium-chain fatty acids, eventually enter into hepatic portal circulation (via the portal vein) and travel to the liver. **Hep-atic portal circulation** is a subdivision of the vascular system by which blood from the digestive organs and spleen circulates through the liver before re-

Hepatic portal circulation—A subdivision of the vascular system by which blood from the digestive organs and spleen circulates through the liver before returning to the heart.

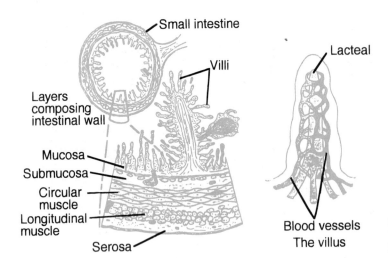

FIGURE 10–1 Cross section of the small intestine. The multiple folds greatly increase the surface area of the small intestine.

turning to the heart. In the liver, the nutrients are modified according to the needs of the body.

Because long-chain fats are not soluble in water and the blood is chiefly water, the fat-soluble nutrients cannot be absorbed directly into the blood. Instead, fat-soluble nutrients—including long-chain fatty acids, any monoglycerides remaining from fat digestion, and fat-soluble vitamins—are first combined with bile salts as a carrier. Then, this complex of fat-soluble materials is absorbed into the cells lining the intestinal wall. Once absorbed, the bile separates from the fat and returns to recirculate. Within the intestinal cells, any remaining monoglycerides are reduced to fatty acids and glycerol by an enzyme. Glycerol, fatty acids, and absorbed long-chain fatty acids are recombined (within the intestinal cells) to form human triglycerides in a process called *triglyceride synthesis.*

After triglyceride synthesis, the newly formed triglycerides and any other fat materials present (such as cholesterol) are covered with special proteins, forming lipoproteins called **chylomicrons.** The chylomicrons are released into the lymphatic system via the lacteals. Remember that the lymphatic system is connected to the blood system. The protein "wrapping" these packages of fat enables the chylomicrons to move into the blood via the **thoracic lymphatic duct** (and hence into portal blood). In the liver, lipids are also modified to suit the needs of the body before distribution to body cells. Table 10–3 describes some of the nutrient modifications that are made in the liver.

After absorption of nutrients in the small intestine, the watery chyme moves into the large intestine, where final absorption and elimination take place. No digestion occurs in the large intestine.

Large Intestine

The **large intestine,** also called the **colon,** extends from the ileum (last part of the small intestine) to the anus. When any remaining chyme leaves the small intestine it enters the first portion of the large intestine, the **cecum.** The appendix, an organ with no known function, is attached to the cecum. Further passage of undigested food is controlled by the **ileocecal valve,** which relaxes and then closes with each peristaltic wave. This valve prevents backflow and ensures that chyme remains in the small intestine long enough for sufficient digestion and absorption. Chyme leaves the cecum and travels slowly through the remaining parts of the large intestine:

TABLE 10–3   Metabolic Modifications in the Liver

Energy Nutrient	Modification
Carbohydrates	Fructose and galactose changed to glucose, excess glucose converted to glycogen
Lipids	Lipoproteins formed, cholesterol synthesized, triglycerides broken down and built
Amino acids	Nonessential amino acids manufactured, excess amino acids deaminated and then changed to carbohydrates or fats, ammonia removed from the blood, plasma proteins made
Other	Alcohol, drugs, and poisons detoxified

the ascending colon, the transverse colon, the descending colon, the sigmoid colon, the **rectum,** and the anal canal.

Water is the main substance absorbed by the large intestine. However, the absorption of some minerals and vitamins also occurs in the colon. Most of the water, up to 80 percent, is extracted in the cecum and the ascending colon. Vitamins synthesized by intestinal bacteria, including vitamin K and some of the B-complexes, are absorbed from the colon. After absorption and digestion have taken place, the remaining waste products are eliminated in the feces by way of the rectum.

Elimination of Unabsorbed Materials

Absorption of water into the bloodstream reduces the water content of the material left inside the large intestine slowly, so in the end a solid consistency remains. This solid material is the feces. Mucus, the only secretion in the large intestine, provides lubrication for the smooth passage of the feces. By the time the feces reach the rectum they consist of 75 percent water and 25 percent solids. The solids include cellular wastes, undigested dietary fiber, undigested food, bile salts, cholesterol, mucus, and bacteria.

Indigestible Carbohydrates

The body cannot digest some forms of carbohydrates because it lacks the necessary enzyme to split the appropriate molecule. Some vegetables and legumes contain these indigestible sugars and fibers. Intestinal gas is formed in the colon by the decomposition of undigested materials. Examples of gas-forming foods are beans, onions, cabbage family vegetables, and radishes.

Factors Interfering with Absorption

Malabsorption is the inadequate movement of digested food from the small intestine into the blood or lymphatic system. Malnutrition can be caused by malabsorption. Table 10–4 lists factors that interfere with the absorption of nutrients. Note from the table that many diseases, medications, and some medical treatments have a negative impact on the absorption of nutrients. Clinical Application 10–2 discusses surgical removal of all or part of the alimentary canal and the effect on absorption. Clinical Application 10–3 discusses inadequate absorption.

Steatorrhea

Some diseases and medications result in the malabsorption of fat. In these conditions, clients have

TABLE 10–4 Factors Decreasing Absorption

Medications	Antacids
	Laxatives
	Birth control pills
	Anticonvulsants
	Antibiotics
Parasites	Tapeworm
	Hookworm
Surgical procedures	Gastric resections
	Any surgery on the small intestine
	Some surgical procedures on the large intestine
Disease states	Infection
	Tropical sprue
	Gluten-sensitive enteropathy
	Hepatic disease
	Pancreatic insufficiency
	Lactase deficiency
	Sucrase deficiency
	Maltase deficiency
	Circulatory disorders
	Cancers involving the alimentary canal
Medical complications	Effects of radiation therapy
	Chemotherapy

Note: Most of these conditions will be discussed in later chapters.

steatorrhea, or fat in the stools. Frequently the condition is caused by the inhibition of pancreatic lipase, an enzyme necessary for the digestion of fats. Clinical Application 10–4 discusses lipid malabsorption and dietary treatment.

Nontropical Sprue

Nontropical **sprue** is a disorder of the small intestine. This disease is commonly referred to as **celiac disease** or **gluten-sensitive enteropathy.** Gluten-sensitive enteropathy results from the toxic effects

---

Chylomicron—A lipoprotein that carries triglycerides in the blood after meals.

Malabsorption—Inadequate movement of digested food from the small intestine into the blood or lymphatic system.

Celiac disease (gluten-sensitive enteropathy)—An intolerance to dietary gluten, which damages the intestine and produces malabsorption and diarrhea.

CLINICAL APPLICATION 10–2

Surgical Removal of All or Part of the Alimentary Canal

Clients may need to have a portion of their small intestine surgically removed for a variety of reasons. These clients are frequently at a nutritional risk because they are either permanently or temporarily unable to absorb essential nutrients. In such cases, a nutritional assessment is indicated. In the past, some clients elected to have a portion of their alimentary canal removed to lose weight. This is discussed in the weight control chapter.

CLINICAL APPLICATION 10–3

Inadequate Absorption

Visually inspecting a client's feces can confirm a suspicion of poor digestion or poor absorption. Large chunks of food indicate a problem with digestion. A large amount of liquid or near-liquid stools suggests poor absorption. A simple question directed to the client, such as "Are your stools formed?" can provide some information. Sometimes, however, client's concept of normal may be different from the healthcare provider's.

The cells lining the inside layer of the small intestine have a very short life. The smallest structures are replaced every 2 to 3 days. Although this rapid cell turnover helps to promote healing after injury, it also allows vulnerability to any nutritional deficiency or process that might interfere with cell reproduction.

"**Gut failure**" is a term used to describe a situation in which the small intestine fails to absorb nutrients properly. Symptoms include diarrhea, malabsorption, and a poor response to oral feedings. A vicious cycle starts when the cells lining the small intestine fail to reproduce because they do not have the necessary nutrients for cell replacement. This in turn leads to chronic diarrhea caused by malabsorption. In turn, the malabsorption leads to malnutrition which prevents cell reproduction. Figure 10–2 diagrams this cycle.

---

that occur from the ingestion of **gluten** a protein present in the following grains: wheat, rye, oats, and barley. Individuals with this disease suffer from a wide variety of nutritional problems.

The result of the toxic effect of gluten is the direct destruction of intestinal cells. This may be related to an allergic reaction and can be either severe or mild. In the severe form, the loss of the intestinal mucosa causes lactose intolerance.

Treatment in this situation would involve the use of medium-chain triglycerides to increase the kilocaloric content of the diet and a lactose-free, gluten-free diet. This is a complex diet for the health care professional to plan and for the client to follow. Usu-

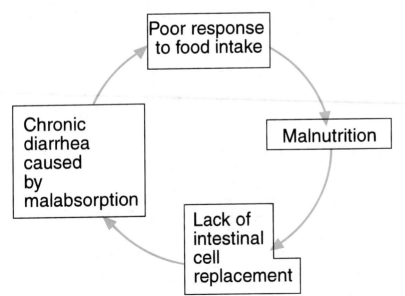

FIGURE 10–2   "Gut failure." Gut failure is a self-perpetuating cycle. Poor response to food intake leads to poor intestinal cell regeneration, which leads to chronic diarrhea caused by malabsorption.

CLINICAL APPLICATION 10–4

Lipid Malabsorption

Some clients for a variety of reasons are unable to digest and absorb long-chain fatty acids. For these clients, the use of MCT (medium-chain triglyceride) oil is indicated. MCT oil can provide a kilocalorie source for patients with a fat malabsorption problem.

Any food that contains fat must be carefully planned into the diet of any client who suffers from a lipid malabsorption. The American Dietetic and Diabetes Associations' Exchange Lists for Menu Planning can be used as a guide in planning this type of diet. Usually the physician will order a specified number of grams of fat high in long-chain fatty acids. A typical low-fat diet order may read: 40-g fat diet. Such as diet may be planned as follows:

Exchange	Number of Exchanges/ Day	Grams of Fat
Skim milk	Unlimited	0
Starches	8	4 (0.5 g of fat/exchange)
Fruits	Unlimited	0
Vegetables	Unlimited	0
Meat, lean	7	21 (7 × 3 g/exchange)
Fat	3	15 (3 × 5 g/exchange) 40 g fat/day

The MCT oil is then added to the diet as necessary to bring the kilocalories up to meet the client's

ally, frequent consultations with the physician regarding the status of the client's intestinal cells are necessary. These clients are often malnourished. As such, the client benefits from being kept on this severe a diet only until intestinal cell regeneration is completed. Once the client is able to tolerate both lactose and long-chain triglycerides they should be included in the diet. This will increase the client's compliance in maintaining a high kilocalorie intake and assist in treating the malnutrition.

In milder forms, only a gluten-restricted diet is indicated (Box 10–3). Gluten is present in a number of prepared foods that contain thickened sauces. Extensive client teaching is necessary for a positive client outcome. Removal of all forms of wheat, rye, oats, and barley from the diet frequently results in remission or improvement within weeks. Table 10–5

lists products that can be substituted for flour in many recipes.

Food Allergies

A **food allergy** is a sensitivity to a food that does not cause a negative reaction in most people. Individuals may be genetically predisposed to a food allergy. Almost any food can cause an allergic reaction, but milk, eggs, wheat, shellfish, chocolate, and oranges are frequent offenders. Some food allergies may be due to an alteration in absorption. The susceptible person absorbs a part of a food before it has been completely digested. The incomplete digestion of protein in particular is responsible for many allergic reactions. The body does not recognize the sequence of amino acids (because the protein was absorbed partly undigested) and therefore treats the protein as a foreign substance and tries to destroy it. This attempt produces the symptoms of food allergy, including skin rash, nausea, vomiting, diarrhea, intestinal cramps, swelling in various parts of the body, and spasm of the small intestine. The treatment for a food allergy is to avoid the offending food.

Metabolism

After digestion and absorption, nutrients are carried by the blood (usually after being modified in the liver cells) to all cells of the body. After entry into the cells, the nutrients from food undergo many chemical changes, which result in either the release of energy or the use of energy. **Metabolism** is the sum of all chemical and physical processes continuously going on in living organisms, comprising both anabolism and catabolism. Catabolic reactions usually result in the release of energy. Anabolic reactions require energy. In the next section we will describe how cells utilize the end products of digestion to meet the energy needs of the body.

Catabolic Reactions

Glucose, glycerol, fatty acids, and amino acids can be broken down even further. These nutrients are

> **Metabolism**—The sum of all the physical and chemical changes that take place in the body; the two fundamental processes involved are anabolism and catabolism.

BOX 10–3   GLUTEN-RESTRICTED DIET

Description: The diet is free of cereals that contain gluten: wheat, oats, rye, and barley.

Indications: This diet is used to treat the primary intestinal malabsorption found in celiac disease.

Adequacy: Unless an effort is made to increase kilocalories, the energy intake may be inadequate to replace previous weight loss. This diet may not meet the RDA for B-complex vitamins, especially thiamin. Iron intake may be inadequate for the premenopausal woman.

Food Groups	Foods That Contain Gluten	Foods That May Contain Gluten	Foods That Do Not Contain Gluten
Beverage	Cereal beverages (e.g., Postum), malt, Ovaltine, beer and ale	Commercial* chocolate milk; cocoa mixes; other beverage mixes; dietary supplements	Coffee; tea; decaffeinated coffee; carbonated beverages; chocolate drinks made with pure cocoa powder; wine; distilled liquor
Meat and meat substitutes		Meat loaf and patties, cold cuts and prepared meats, stuffing, breaded meats, cheese foods and spreads; commercial souffles, omelets, and fondue; soy protein meat substitutes	Pure meat, fish, fowl, egg, cottage cheese, and peanut butter
Fat and oil		Commercial salad dressing and mayo, gravy, white and cream sauces, nondairy creamer	Butter, margarine, vegetable oil
Milk	Milk beverages that contain malt	Commercial chocolate milk	Whole, low-fat, and skim milk; buttermilk
Grains and grain products	Bread, crackers, cereal, and pasta that contain wheat, oats, rye, malt, malt flavoring, graham flour, durham flour, pastry flour, bran, or wheat germ; barley; millet; pretzels; communion wafers	Commercial seasoned rice and potato mixes	Specially prepared breads made with wheat starch,† rice, potato, or soybean flour or cornmeal; pure corn or rice cereals; hominy grits; white, brown, and wild rice; popcorn; low protein pasta made from wheat starch

Food Groups	Foods That Contain Gluten	Foods That May Contain Gluten	Foods That Do Not Contain Gluten
Vegetable		Commercially seasoned vegetable mixes; commercial vegetables with cream or cheese sauce; canned baked beans	All fresh vegetables; plain, commercially frozen or canned vegetables
Fruit		Commercial pie fillings	All plain or sweetened fruits; fruit thickened with tapioca or cornstarch
Soup	Soup that contains wheat pasta; soup thickened with wheat flour or other gluten-containing grains	Commercial soup, broth, and soup mixes	Soup thickened with cornstarch, wheat starch, or potato, rice or soybean flour; pure broth
Desserts	Commercial cakes, cookies and pastries	Commercial ice cream and sherbet	Gelatin; custard; fruit ice; specially prepared cakes, cookies, and pastries made with gluten-free flour or starch; pudding and fruit filling thickened with tapioca, cornstarch, or arrowroot flour
Sweets		Commercial candies, especially chocolates	
Miscellaneous‡		Ketchup; prepared mustard; soy sauce; commercially prepared meat sauces and pickles; vinegar; flavoring syrups (syrups for pancakes or ice cream)	Monosodium glutamate; salt; pepper; pure spices and herbs; yeast; pure baking chocolate or cocoa powder; carob; flavoring extracts; artificial flavoring

Box continued on following page

SAMPLE MENU

Breakfast

>   1/2 cup orange juice
>   Cocoa puffs, sugar pops, puffed rice
>   2 slices gluten-free bread
>   1 poached egg
>   1 cup milk
>   2 tsp margarine
>   Jelly

Lunch/Dinner

>   Chicken breast
>   Baked potato
>   1/2 cup broccoli
>   Lettuce/tomato salad
>   French dressing
>   Sour cream
>   1/2 cup milk
>   Cornstarch pudding

* The terms "commercially prepared" and "commercial" are used to refer to partially prepared foods purchased from a grocery or food market and to prepared foods purchased from a restaurant.

† Wheat starch may contain trace amounts of gluten. Avoid if not tolerated.

‡ Medications may contain trace amounts of gluten. A pharmacist may be able to provide information on the gluten content of medications.

Mayo Clinic Diet Manual, 1988, with permission.

---

held together by bonds that, when broken, release energy. The breakdown of the fuel-producing nutrients yields carbon dioxide, water, heat, and other forms of energy. The carbon dioxide is eventually exhaled and the water becomes part of the body fluids or is eliminated in the urine. Fifty percent or more of the total potential energy usually is lost as heat. The remaining available energy is temporarily stored in the cells as ATP, adenosine triphosphate.

ATP, a high-energy compound that has three phosphate groups in its structure, is thus available in all cells. Practically speaking, ATP is the storage form of energy for the cells since each cell has enzymes that can initiate the hydrolysis (breakdown through the addition of water) of ATP. In this reaction, one or more phosphate groups split off and subsequently release energy. If one phosphate group is removed, the result is ADP (adenosine diphosphate) plus phosphate.

Many steps are involved in the catabolic process responsible for the release of this energy. These steps require one or more of the following agents: enzymes, coenzymes, and/or hormones. Some vitamins and minerals act as coenzymes. Oxygen is also necessary for the full release of any potential energy. This addition of oxygen to the reaction is called **oxidation.** During the many steps that occur, the energy is released little by little and stored as ATP. The breakdown process includes the formation of intermediate chemical compounds such as **pyruvate** (pyruvic acid) and **acetyl CoA.** Acetyl CoA can be broken down further by entering a series of **chemical reactions** known as the **Krebs cycle** or the TCA (tricarboxylic acid) cycle. See Figure 10–3 for a simplified schematic of the steps involved in the release of energy by the cells.

TABLE 10–5   Substitutions for 2 Tablespoons of Wheat Flour

3 tsp cornstarch
3 tsp potato starch
3 tsp arrowroot starch
3 tsp quick-cooking tapioca
3 tbsp white or brown rice flour

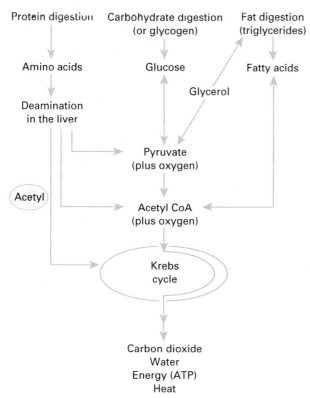

FIGURE 10–3 Energy production in the cells. Energy is released bit by bit during the further breakdown of amino acids, glucose, glycerol, and fatty acids.

Storage of Excess Nutrients

If the cells do not have immediate energy needs, the excess nutrients are stored. Glucose is stored as glycogen in liver and muscle tissue; surplus amounts are converted to fat. Glycerol and fatty acids are reassembled into triglycerides and stored in adipose tissue. Amino acids are used to make body proteins; any excess is deaminated (stripped of nitrogen) and ultimately used for glucose formation or stored as fat. If energy is not available from food, the cells will seek energy in body stores.

Anabolic Reactions

Once immediate energy needs have been met, the cells utilize the nutrients as needed for growth and repair of body tissue. The cellular supply of ATP is used first. When this instant energy source is exhausted, glycogen and fat stores are used. In addition to building up body protein, other anabolic reactions include the recombination of glycerol and fatty acids to form triglycerides and the formation of glycogen from glucose.

Excretion of Waste Products

What the cells have no use for becomes waste that is eliminated through **excretion.** Solid waste is disposed of in the feces. The digestive system needs assistance from other body systems in the disposal of nonsolid waste. The lungs dispose of gaseous waste. Most liquid waste is sent first to the kidneys and then to the **bladder** to be eliminated in the urine. Some liquid waste is disposed of by the skin through perspiration.

Carbon dioxide (CO_2) is a gas that is eliminated through the lungs each time you exhale. The amount of carbon dioxide exhaled depends on the type of fuel (lipid, protein, or carbohydrate) and/or the source of fuel that the body is currently burning for energy. For example, more CO_2 is produced when carbohydrates are being utilized than with protein or fat.

The skin removes some of the liquid waste in the form of perspiration or water and some is excreted in the feces. The kidneys eliminate most of the excess water, sodium, hydrogen, and urea. **Urea** is synthesized in the liver from the nitrogen resulting from the breakdown of amino acids. Some water is also removed from the body each time you exhale.

Summary

The cell is the ultimate destination for the nutrients in food. For food to be of use to the cells, it must first be broken down into many tiny particles and then absorbed into the body. Digestion is the process whereby food is broken down into a form usable by the cell: carbohydrates are broken down to monosaccharides, fats are reduced to glycerol and fatty acids, and proteins are split to yield amino acids. This is accomplished by both mechanical and chemical means. Secretions from the salivary glands, stomach, small intestine, liver, and pancreas assist in chemical digestion. Absorption refers to the movement of food from the gastrointestinal tract into the blood and lymphatic system. Metabolism

---

Chemical reaction—The process of combining or breaking down substances to obtain different substances.

Excretion—The elimination of waste products from the body in feces, urine, exhaled air, and perspiration.

involves the two processes of anabolism and catabolism. The liver plays a major role in metabolism.

After absorption, water-soluble nutrients go directly to the liver for further processing. The liver releases the nutrients into the bloodstream for delivery to the cells. Most of the fat-soluble nutrients are absorbed into the lymphatic system before entering the bloodstream. Short- and medium-chain triglycerides are absorbed differently than long-chain triglycerides. The cells remove the nutrients from the bloodstream as needed for energy and growth. Energy is released little by little from the end products of digestion in a series of chemical reactions. Energy nutrients not needed immediately by the cells are placed in storage as glycogen and adipose tissue.

The metabolism of food produces waste. Waste products are released from the body in the feces, urine, perspiration, and exhaled air.

Many ailments and diseases are related to the structure and function of the gastrointestinal system. Many forms of malabsorption, including disaccharide intolerances and gluten-sensitive enteropathy, are related to structural damage of the small intestine.

Case Study 10–1

Mr. H is a 25-year-old male who is 6 ft tall and weighs 170 lb (dressed without shoes). He has a medium frame, as determined by measuring his wrist circumference. Mr. H has just been admitted to the hospital where you are employed for an elective arthroscopic (surgical procedure) on his right knee. During the nursing admission process, Mr. H complained of gas pains and frequent loose stools. He stated that he does not avoid any particular foods and has a healthy appetite. He claims to drink about three cups of milk each day. The client complained of a loss of 5 lb during the prior month. Mr. H needed to use the restroom twice during the interview to "move his bowels." The second time the nurse inspected the stool. The client's stool was loose and unformed.

The next day the nurse noted that a diagnosis of lactose intolerance had been made. A lactose-restricted diet was ordered.

The following nursing care plan originated on the day the client was admitted. The physician used the information collected from the nurse in making his or her diagnosis. Please note that the client has already met the first desired outcome and part of the second; they have been charted. The client has not met the third desired outcome.

NURSING CARE PLAN FOR MR. H

Assessment

Subjective Data   Client complains of gas pains and loose stools. Client stated that he does not avoid any particular foods.

Objective Data   Client observed to use the restroom twice in 10 minutes to defecate. Visual inspection showed stool to be loose and unformed.

Nursing Diagnosis   Diarrhea related to client's complaints of loose stools as evidenced by the client's need to use the restroom twice in a 10-minute period and by direct observation of one loose and unformed stool.

Desired Outcome/ Evaluation Criteria	Nursing Actions	Rationale
The client will assist in ruling out causes for his loose stools and report his signs and symptoms to the nurse.	Teach the client to observe and record the pattern, onset, frequency, characteristics, amount, time of day, and precipitating events related to occurrence of diarrhea. Refer client to the dietitian to determine usual food intake and nutritional status. Determine exposure to recent environmental contaminants, that is, drinking water; food safety; illness of others; food handling practices. Review drug intake for medications affecting absorption (see Table 10–4, Factors Decreasing Absorption).	Observation and documentation of the client's response to these factors will assist in determining the cause of his loose stools.
The client will eliminate causative factors at once after these factors have been determined.	Follow through with the elimination of causative factors, restrict intake if necessary, note change in drug therapy, if any.	Elimination of the causative factors should decrease the frequency of loose, unformed stools. The client needs to be instructed on the relationship of his diarrhea to causative factors.
The client will have formed stools within 24 hours after the causative factors have been eliminated.	Document the stool consistency.	Whenever possible an objective measure should be used to evaluate the success of any client intervention. Stool consistency is an objective measure for treatment response to diarrhea and malabsorption.

Study Aids

Chapter Review

1. A client on a gluten-free diet can usually tolerate which of the following? (See Box 10–3.)
   a. Rice and granola
   b. Barley and wheat
   c. Oats and bulgur
   d. Corn and potatoes

2. Most of the absorption of food takes place in the _____ .
   a. Large intestine
   b. Gallbladder
   c. Small intestine
   d. Stomach

3. The body eliminates waste through all of the following except one. Identify the exception.
   a. Skin
   b. Hair
   c. Feces
   d. Lungs

4. The smallest functional unit of the human body is a _____ .
   a. Molecule
   b. Cell
   c. Tissue
   d. Organ

5. Which of the following groups of food items should be avoided on a lactose-free diet? (See Table 10–1.)
   a. Oranges, apples, bananas
   b. Green beans, peas, asparagus
   c. Sausage, nondairy creamers, some breads, canned soups
   d. Monosodium glutamate, angel food cake, pure cocoa powder, hard ripened cheeses such as cheddar and Swiss

Clinical Analysis

1. The nurse is visiting Mr. D, who is receiving home health care. His caregiver is concerned that Mr. D "is choking" on his solid food, but swallows liquids well. Which of the following initial actions by the nurse would be most appropriate?
   a. Observe Mr. D's efforts to swallow
   b. Refer Mr. D to the staff speech therapist
   c. Instruct the caregiver to offer only liquids to Mr. D
   d. Recommend that Mr. D watch television at mealtime to decrease anxiety associated with eating

2. Kathy, 24 months old, has been admitted to the pediatric unit. She has a gluten-free diet ordered for celiac disease. Which of the following meals would be permitted?
   a. Tuna noodle casserole, peas, milk, and fruit cocktail
   b. Swiss steak, mashed potatoes, corn, and chocolate pudding
   c. Tomato soup, grilled cheese sandwich, and french fries
   d. Roast turkey, baked potato, milk, green beans, and sour cream

3. Mrs. H has experienced worsening flatulence and loose stools after meals. She has been advised to follow a lactose-free diet. She can eat or drink:
   a. Any type of bread product, any type of cereal
   b. Fruit pies, angel food cake, parmesan cheese
   c. Frankfurters, ricotta cheese, caramels
   d. All fruit drinks, convenience desserts, any form of vegetable

Bibliography

Anatasio, P: Flatulence felled by gas-fighting enzyme. Environmental Nutrition 2:3, 1991.

Christian, JL and Greger, JL: Nutrition for Living, ed 3. Benjamin and Cummings, Redwood City, CA, 1991.

Dobler MC: Gluten Intolerance. The American Dietetic Association, Chicago, 1991.

Logemann, JA: Dysphagia: A Review for the Health Professional. Milanti Foods, Melrose Park, IL, 1991.

Pecora, AA: Lactose Intolerance. Osteopathic Medical News 7:7, 1990.

Pemberton, CM, et al: Mayo Clinic Diet Manual: A Handbook of Dietary Practice, ed 6. BC Decker, Philadelphia, 1988.

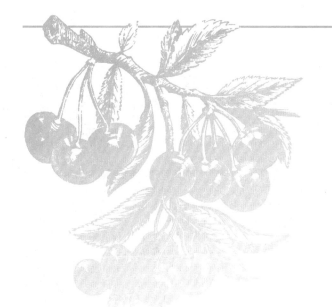

Family and Community Nutrition

CHAPTER 11

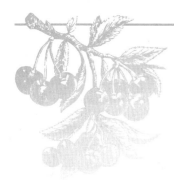

Life Cycle Nutrition: Pregnancy and Lactation

LEARNING OBJECTIVES

After completing this chapter, the student should be able to:

1 Compare the nutritional needs of a pregnant woman with those of a non-pregnant woman of the same age.
2 Contrast the nutritional needs of the pregnant adolescent with those of a pregnant adult.
3 Explain the reasons folic acid intake is critical in pregnancy.
4 Discuss the dietary treatment of common problems of pregnancy.
5 List three advantages that breast-feeding offers to the mother.

The need for many nutrients changes at different stages of our lives. Social, economic, and psychological circumstances all influence nutritional status. Human beings are most vulnerable to the impact of poor nutrition during rapid growth. If the essential nutrients are not present to support growth, permanent damage to tissues and organs can occur. This chapter focuses on the period of most rapid growth, that of the unborn child.

Nutrition during Pregnancy

An expectant mother's nutritional status can affect the outcome of pregnancy. For example, during the first month of **gestation,** it is crucial that the mother be well nourished so that a healthy **placenta** will form. Also, within 2 to 3 months of conception all the major body organs are formed in the **embryo.** From the beginning of the third month until birth, the embryo is called a **fetus.** Because the fetus obtains nutrients from the mother's diet or body stores, its health depends on her nutritional intake.

Poor outcomes of pregnancy include spontaneous abortion (miscarriage), premature delivery, a low-birth-weight (LBW) infant, a small-for-gestational age (SGA) infant, and mental and physical abnormalities in the newborn. The best insurance an expectant mother can provide for her unborn child is to enter the pregnancy with good nutrient stores, to consume a well-balanced diet while pregnant, and to avoid harmful substances, such as alcohol and illicit drugs.

From **implantation** to birth, the fertilized **ovum** (which weighs less than 100 micrograms) develops into an infant that weighs about 3.4 kilograms (7.5 pounds). During this period of rapid growth and development the mother needs additional nutrients, including kilocalories, protein, and certain vitamins and minerals.

Increase in Energy Needs

Increased energy is needed for the development of the mother, the fetus, and the placenta. From the third through the sixth month, much of this energy supports the growth of the uterus (womb) and other maternal tissues. During the seventh through ninth months, the third trimester, much of the energy supports the fetus and the placenta. To meet this increased metabolic workload and to spare protein for tissue building, the pregnant woman needs an additional 300 kilocalories per day.

Increase in Protein Needs

Building fetal **tissue** requires protein. The mother also needs adequate protein for growth of her tissues. Her blood volume increases in anticipation of blood loss at delivery. Her breasts develop in preparation for lactation. The uterus enlarges and fills with **amniotic fluid.** For these reasons, an additional 10 grams of protein per day are needed. Translating this to the exchange system, 1 extra cup of milk (8 grams of protein) and 1 additional ounce of meat (7 grams of protein) would more than meet the increased protein requirement.

A complication arises if a woman with phenylketonuria (PKU) consumes a regular diet during pregnancy. (See Clinical Application 5–4.) The high level of phenylalanine in a woman's bloodstream can cross the placenta and cause fetal malformations and defects. Careful monitoring of blood levels of phenylalanine and provision of a special medical food are begun before conception and continued throughout the pregnancy. Because women of childbearing age with PKU may have been taken off the special diet after age 4 to 6, they may have little memory of this part of their medical history. The health care worker should investigate further when a woman cites a history of troubled pregnancies: congenital abnormalities, a mentally retarded infant, spontaneous abortion, or stillbirth. This is especially true if the woman is intellectually slow or is subject to seizures.

Vitamin Needs

Pregnant women have an increased need for some vitamins. Yet others are to be avoided in excess because of the hazard to the fetus.

Water-Soluble Vitamins

Increased amounts of certain B-vitamins, vitamin C, and folic acid, are needed during pregnancy. Vitamin C is needed to (1) convert folic acid to an active form, (2) enhance the absorption of iron, and (3) help to form connective tissues.

To prevent neural tube defects (NTD), the U.S. Public Health Service recommends that all women who might become pregnant consume 0.4 milligrams (400 micrograms) of folic acid daily. A guideline issued by the Centers for Disease Control recommends 4 milligrams of folic acid per day from conception through the first trimester for women who have borne a child with a neural tube defect (Centers for Disease Control, 1992). A committee opinion of the American College of Obstetricians and Gynecologists recommends offering the latter treatment to women with a history of bearing a child with neural tube defect (Committee on Obstetrics, 1993). A similar recommendation was made in Canada (Van Allen, et al, 1993). Because of the lack of data from large, well-designed, prospective, randomized studies, the American College of Obstetricians and Gynecologists Committee declined to endorse a lessor, prophylactic dose of folic acid for all women of child-bearing age (Committee on Obstetrics, 1993). Obstetricians are advised to offer serum alpha-fetoprotein screening for birth defects, including NTD, to pregnant women, including those taking folic acid supplements (Committee on Obstetrics, 1993).

Box 11–1 reviews research pertinent to these recommendations. None of the studies suggest that folic acid supplementation will prevent all cases of NTD. An interaction of genetics and environment is also suspected. A higher incidence of NTD in Newfoundland, Quebec, parts of China, parts of India, Scotland, and Ireland has stimulated a search for a genetic cause. Women with histories of NTD pregnancies attained lower serum folate levels than control subjects following oral doses of folate (Schoral, et al, 1993). The identification of a gene producing an abnormality in an enzyme necessary to folate metabolism bolsters the argument for genetic susceptibility, but this is only estimated to be responsible for 13 percent of NTDs (Whitehead, et al, 1995). The fact that the abnormal **allele** is thermolabile may help explain the increased occurrence of NTD associated with a history of fever, or use of a hot tub or sauna in the first trimester (Milunsky, et al, 1992). Assembling these pieces of the research puzzle to devise a comprehensive, cost-effective, and harmless public policy is a daunting task. For the first time since 1943, the Food and Drug Administration has issued a fortification order. Beginning January 1, 1998, 43 to 140 micrograms of folic acid per pound will be added to all enriched foods in an attempt to reduce the occurrence of NTDs (Food and Drug Administration, 1996; Kolata, 1996).

Due to increased metabolic demands, some of the other B-vitamins are also required in additional amounts. They include thiamin, riboflavin, niacin, and vitamin B_6. These B-vitamins are all coenzymes involved in the metabolism of carbohydrates, fats, and proteins.

Fat Soluble Vitamins

For the pregnant woman older than 25 years of age, an adequate diet usually provides the needed addi-

tional vitamins D, E, and K. Because of the risk of fetal deformities, vitamin A consumption beyond the RDA is contraindicated during the first trimester. Because vitamin A sometimes is used to treat acne, the fetus of the teenager who did not plan to become pregnant may be in jeopardy. The risk of a major congenital abnormality in a child exposed to isotretinoin, a vitamin A metabolite, in utero during the first trimester appears to be increased about 25 times (Futoryan and Gilchrest, 1994).

A folic acid trial of pregnant women included 4,000 to 6,000 IU of vitamin A in supplement given to the experimental group without teratogenic effects (Cziezel and Dudas, 1992). The increased risk to the fetus involves preformed vitamin A, not carotene. See the RDA table (back cover) for the specific amounts recommended for each vitamin during pregnancy.

Mineral Needs

Minerals differ from vitamins in that minerals become part of the structure of the body whereas vitamins do not. Both the mother and the fetus are building new tissues.

Iron

The mother's volume of red blood cells increases by 21 to 26 percent. Additional iron is needed for the red blood cells in the fetus, placenta, and umbilical cord. Iron is transported to the fetus regardless of the mother's iron status. The total iron need for a single fetus pregnancy is estimated to be 0.8 to 1 gram.

Gestation—The time from the fertilization of the ovum until birth; in humans, the length of gestation is usually 38 to 42 weeks.

Placenta—The organ in the uterus through which the unborn child exchanges carbon dioxide for oxygen and wastes for nourishment; lay term is afterbirth.

Embryo—Developing infant in the prenatal period between the second and eighth weeks inclusive.

Fetus—The human child in utero from the third month until birth.

Implantation—Embedding of the fertilized egg in the lining of the uterus.

Amniotic fluid—Albuminous liquid that surrounds and protects the fetus throughout pregnancy.

BOX 11–1   RESEARCH ON FOLIC ACID'S EFFECT ON NEURAL TUBE DEFECTS

The neural tube is embryonic tissue that develops into the brain and spinal cord. A critical time in the development of this structure is from conception through the fourth week of pregnancy. Interference with normal development produces major congenital defects including anencephaly (fatal within a few weeks), meningoencephalocele, spina bifida, and meningocele. A minority opinion suggests a reopening of the neural tube causes some of the cases (Hook, 1992).

In the United States, about 2500 infants are born with anencephaly or spina bifida each year (Centers for Disease Control, 1992). Only 4 percent of these occur in families with a positive history for NTD. Lifetime cost of one case of spina bifida is estimated to be $349,133, assuming a 4 percent inflation rate (Romano, et al, 1995).

A large randomized trial of folic acid supplementation was conducted in seven countries. Women with a history of a NTD pregnancy were given 4 mg of folic acid per day. Control groups received placebos or other vitamins. The study was stopped early to permit treatment of all participants because the folic acid reduced the risk of a subsequent child with NTD by 70 percent (MRC Vitamin Study Research Group, 1991).

The dose of folic acid just sufficient to prevent NTD in women without a positive history has not been determined. A dose of 0.8 mg of folic acid reduced NTD to zero in 2104 women without prior occurrences. This compares to 6 NTD cases in 2050 control subjects (Czeizel and Dudas, 1992).

Likewise, the best method of prevention for NTD has not been determined. Most experts believe NTD occurs in the first four weeks of gestation when many women are unaware they are pregnant. In the United States more than half of all pregnancies are unplanned and 13.2 million sexually active women of child-bearing age are not using effective contraception (Romano, et al, 1995). Pre-conception health counseling is the ideal, but not the norm.

Dietary intake of folic acid is desirable, but presents implementation difficulties. First, folates obtained from foods are not as well absorbed as folic acid (Centers for Disease Control, 1992). Dietary folates appear to be no more than 50 percent available (Sauberlich, 1987). Second, only 8 percent of adult women obtained 400 μg of dietary folate from 1976 through 1980 (Romano, et al, 1995). Third, two registered dietitians required 30 hours to develop a one-week menu that includes 400 μg of folic acid daily (Bendich, 1994) since bioavailability of dietary folate is about 50 percent (Pérez-Escamilla, 1995).

Supplementation by pharmaceutical folic acid is currently more practical but misses a large proportion of women at risk. In Britain in 1993, only 33 percent of 411 pregnant women were aware of the government folic acid recommendations, and only 37 percent of these received the information before conception (Clark and Fisk, 1994). Nevertheless, counsel congruent with that of the U.S. Public Health Service and the Centers for Disease Control is strongly advised lest health care providers be held liable for its omission (Rush, 1994). Using supplements, consumers would spend an estimated $132,000 to prevent each case of NTD (Romano, et al, 1995).

Fortification of food is another method. It would be much less expensive than pharmaceutical supplementation, an estimated $65,000 to $92,000 per case of NTD prevented (Romano, et al, 1995). One hazard of fortification is the masking of vitamin B_{12} deficiency. Although pernicious anemia is more common in older people, adding folic acid to everyone's food supply would increase the risk of neurologic damage due to undiagnosed pernicious anemia (Rush, 1994). No reports of delayed diagnosis have been published since 1973 (Oakley, Adams, and Dickinson, 1996), however, and neurological signs and symptoms of pernicious anemia do occur without anemia (Dickinson, 1995). An additional concern is that of folic acid interfering with anticonvulsant medications, but numerous controlled trials have demonstrated no effect by oral folic acid at doses up to 20 mg daily (Romano, et al, 1995).

Fortunately, absorption of iron is enhanced in the second and third trimesters. In the woman who is not taking an iron supplement, the percent of iron absorbed increases from 6.5 early in pregnancy to 14.3 percent at term. This rate drops to 8.6 percent with an iron supplement. The body reacts to limited or abundant sources.

Women who receive prenatal care often are given an iron supplement. One common preparation is ferrous sulfate. A 150-milligram dose of ferrous sulfate contains 30 milligrams of iron, the RDA for pregnancy. If iron needs are not met, the pregnant woman may develop **iron-deficiency anemia.** Even when supplements are taken, the woman's hemoglobin and hematocrit should be monitored every 2 to 3 months.

An opposite view is that decreases in hemoglobin and hematocrit values result from physiological hemodilution. Possible consequences of inappropriate iron supplementation are increased blood viscosity and zinc depletion (Long, 1995). Supporting the caution against universal supplementation is research documenting increased absorption of nonheme iron from 7 percent at 12 weeks to 36 percent at 24 weeks to 66 percent at 36 weeks (Barrett, et al, 1994).

For 30 years anemia has been associated with preterm birth, but other causes of low birth weight often were not considered (U.S. Preventive Services Task Force, 1993b). Evidence is insufficient to recommend for or against routine iron supplementation in pregnancy so clinicians are expected to judge individual cases (U.S. Preventive Services Task Force, 1993a).

Calcium

Calcium is the chief mineral in the adult body, with the bones serving as a storage depot. When serum calcium is low, the bones demineralize to restore the serum level. The requirement for calcium during pregnancy is 1.5 times the amount required for the nonpregnant woman. Almost all of the additional amount is used by the fetus, mostly in the third trimester, for the development of skeletal tissue. As with iron, intestinal absorption of calcium increases during pregnancy. Early in the pregnancy, intestinal absorption doubles and remains high. (Normally only 10 to 30 percent of calcium is absorbed.) One reason for this increased absorption is the ability of the placenta to convert inactive vitamin D to the active form.

The RDA and the National Institutes of Health (NIH) recommendation for calcium for pregnant and lactating women is 1200 milligrams. This can be obtained from four servings of milk or milk products equivalent in calcium.

Iodine

As part of thyroid hormones, iodine is essential to the control of metabolism. During the second half of pregnancy resting energy expenditure increases by as much as 23 percent. A pregnant woman's usual need for iodine is met, as with other adults, by the use of iodized salt.

Fluoride

The fetus begins to develop teeth at the 10th to 12th week of pregnancy. Fewer dental caries have been found in infants of mothers whose diets were supplemented with 1 milligram of fluoride daily (Glenn, Glenn, and Duncan, 1982).

Zinc

Zinc is not mobilized from the mother's tissues. To provide for the fetus, the mother needs constant intake. Zinc deficiency has been associated with abnormally long labors and delivery of small and malformed infants. African American women with low plasma-zinc levels who took a zinc supplement delivered heavier infants than the control group. The greatest increase occurred in women with prepregnant BMIs of less than 26 (Goldenberg, et al, 1995). Three servings of meat or meat substitute per day will provide adequate zinc for the pregnant woman.

Other Minerals

In addition to calcium, two other minerals involved in skeletal formation are also in great demand during pregnancy. These are phosphorus and magnesium. For pregnant women 25 years of age and older, the allowance recommended for phosphorus is 1.5 times the amount allowed for nonpregnant women. See the RDA table (Appendix F) for the specific amount recommended for each mineral during pregnancy.

Water and Weight Gain

The average increase in plasma volume during pregnancy is 49 percent (O'Connor, 1994). Increase in total body water is about 7 liters or approximately 15 pounds (Van Loan, et al, 1995). The pregnant woman needs about 6 to 8 cups of water per day. Because some women fear excessive weight gain, the nurse may be obliged to reinforce the concept of adequate fluid intake.

The amount of weight a woman was expected to gain during pregnancy has varied over the years. The current recommendation is made based on a BMI, which incorporates the woman's height and weight before pregnancy.

Clinical Calculation 11–1 shows the procedure to determine a goal for weight gain in pregnancy. For a woman of normal weight, 2 to 4 pounds should be gained during the first trimester, followed by a pound a week for the remainder of the pregnancy. Figure 11–1 is a graph on which the woman can plot her weight gain.

Only among pregnant women who smoked did the amount of weight gain predict SGA infants. To have delivered infants equal in size to those of non-smokers, the smokers would have had to gain 44 pounds rather than the 26 cited as a standard (Muscati, Gray-Donald, and Newson, 1994).

Meal Pattern

Relatively few modifications in the Food Pyramid recommendations for adults are needed for the mature woman who becomes pregnant. She can meet the needs of the fetus and herself by consuming one additional serving of milk, an additional ounce of meat, and one additional source of vitamin C each day.

The pregnant teenager needs nutrients to provide for her own growth as well as that of the fetus. She should have an additional serving from each of the milk and starch/bread groups over and above the number of servings recommended for the mature pregnant woman. Table 11–1 can be used as a food guide for pregnant adult women and adolescents during pregnancy and lactation. Clinical Application 11–1 relates the hazards of teenage pregnancy.

Substances to Avoid

Women are urged to eliminate certain substances from their diets while they are pregnant. Alcohol and caffeine are two such substances that merit special mention.

Alcohol

Fetal alcohol syndrome (FAS), first recognized in 1973, occurs in 30 to 50 percent of alcoholic mothers' offspring. The fetus is most vulnerable to FAS during the first trimester when basic structural development occurs. Often, the woman does not know that she is pregnant until late in the first trimester.

Children with FAS are malformed and suffer from mental retardation (Fig. 11–2). This condition is completely preventable. Because research has not been able to determine how much alcohol is safe to ingest during pregnancy, women who are planning a pregnancy should be encouraged to abstain from alcohol for the good of the fetus.

CLINICAL CALCULATION 11-1

Determining Recommended Weight Gain During Pregnancy

$$\text{Body mass index (BMI)} = \frac{\text{Weight in kilograms}}{\text{Height in meters}^2}$$

Suppose a woman is 5 ft, 4 in tall and weighs 125 lb.

$$5 \text{ ft, } 4 \text{ in} = 64 \text{ in}$$

$$1 \text{ m} = 39.371 \text{ in}$$

$$\frac{64}{39.371} = 1.6 \text{ m}$$

$$\frac{125 \text{ lb}}{2.2 \text{ lb/kg}} = 56.8 \text{ kg}$$

$$\text{BMI} = \frac{56.8}{2.56} = 22.2$$

Looking at the table below, we see that 22.2 is in the normal category. Recommended weight gain for this woman is 25 to 35 lb.

Recommended Weight Gain for Pregnancy

BMI Category	Kilograms	Pounds
<19.8 = Low	12.5–18	28–40
19.8–26 = Normal	11.5–16	25–35
26–29 = High	7–11.5	15–25
>29 = Obese	6	15

Young adolescents and black women should strive for gains at the upper end of the recommended range. Women whose height is less than 157 cm (62 in) should strive for gains at the lower end of the range.

Reprinted with permission from Nutrition During Pregnancy, © 1990 by the National Academy of Sciences. Published by National Academy Press, Washington, DC.

TABLE 11–1   Daily Food Guide in Pregnancy and Lactation

	Pregnant Adult	*Pregnant Adolescent**	*Lactation*
Milk, cups	3–4	4–5	3–4
Meat, oz	6	6	6
Fruit, servings			
High vitamin C	2	2	2
Other	2	2	3
Vegetable, servings			
High vitamin A	1	1	1–2
Other	2–4	2–4	2–4
Starch/Bread, servings	10	11	10
Other foods	To meet kilocaloric needs	To meet kilocaloric needs	To meet kilocaloric needs

* Meets adolescent RDA except for iron and folic acid.

Caffeine

In contrast to the evidence linking alcohol consumption with fetal defects, the connection between caffeine and defects is inconsistent and fragmentary (Subcommittee on Nutritional Status and Weight Gain during Pregnancy and the Subcommittee on Dietary Intake and Nutrient Supplements during Pregnancy, 1990). When alcohol, smoking, maternal age, and pregnancy history are controlled, heavy coffee drinking has minimal, if any, adverse effect on the outcome of pregnancy (Feldman, 1988). However, caffeine intake should be moderated to maximize the mother's rest and to avoid excessive diuresis.

Common Problems and Complications of Pregnancy

The physiological changes that take place in a woman's body during pregnancy may cause a variety of possible medical conditions. Some of the more common problems such as morning sickness and leg cramps are usually annoying but only occasionally require medical intervention. Other conditions, such as pregnancy-induced hypertension and gestational diabetes, are more complicated and must have medical treatment.

Common Problems of Pregnancy

Four of the most common problems of pregnancy are morning sickness, leg cramps, constipation, and heartburn. Pica (discussed later in this section) is a regional complaint that is mainly influenced by culture.

MORNING SICKNESS   Hormonal changes cause the nausea and vomiting of pregnancy. The occurrence and duration of morning sickness vary widely, but it is not confined to mornings. Control of the signs and symptoms without medication is the goal. Eating dry crackers before getting out of bed is the classic treatment. Other suggestions include (1) avoiding fatty foods in favor of fruits and complex carbohydrates taken in small, frequent meals; (2) consuming cold foods rather than hot foods; (3) drinking liquids between rather than with meals; and (4) eating a high-protein snack at bedtime. In most cases, morning sickness subsides after the first trimester.

CLINICAL APPLICATION 11–1

Teenage Pregnancy

One million teenagers in the United States become pregnant every year. Forty percent of these girls are under 18 years of age. Three percent are girls under age 15. Sixty percent of teenagers continue the pregnancy to delivery and 25 percent become pregnant again within a year.

The average girl does not reach her full height or attain gynecologic maturity until age 17. She herself is still growing and now has a fetus to nourish as well.

Nutrients most often lacking in the pregnant teenager's diet are calcium, iron, vitamin A, and niacin. In addition, kilocaloric intake is usually insufficient to meet daily needs. The 11- to 14-year-old expectant mother requires 2700 kcal per day, the 15- to 18-year-old, 2400 kcal. Teenage mothers are at increased risk of complications of pregnancy, such as preeclampsia and premature delivery. The cause is not solely age, however. Complications of pregnancies are more strongly associated with poor nutrition than with maternal age.

The Weighting Game

Here's How It All Adds Up

Baby	7-8 1/2 pounds
Amniotic fluid	2 pounds
Placenta	2-2 1/2 pounds
Increased blood volume	4-5 pounds
Tissue fluid	3-5 pounds
Increased weight of uterus	2 pounds
Body changes for breast feeding	1-4 pounds
Mother's stores*	4-6 pounds
	25-35 pounds

*Mother's stores are reserves of extra fat and probably a little protein. These serve as a source of energy to support the work of pregnancy. These stores also supply energy for labor and delivery and for milk production after birth.

You can record your weight changes on the graph below. The colored areas represent weight gain ranges that can be expected during a normal pregnancy. Ask your health care provider which category you belong in.

If your weight was normal before you became pregnant, try to keep your weight in this range:

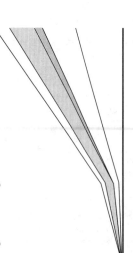

If you were underweight before you became pregnant, your weight gain should be in this range:

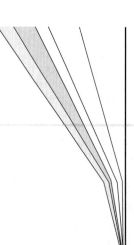

If your weight was much higher than ideal, your weight gain should be in this range:

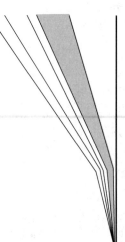

This is not the time to lose weight. Try to gain weight at a steady pace. Report any sudden and/or unexplained weight changes to your health care provider.

The Weighting Game Weight Graph

Your Beginning Weight _____ **lbs.**

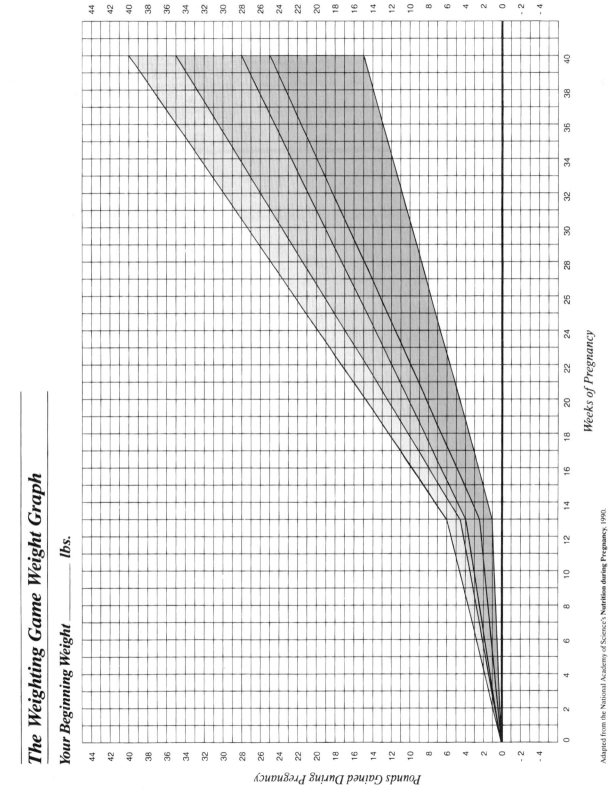

Weeks of Pregnancy

Pounds Gained During Pregnancy

Adapted from the National Academy of Science's **Nutrition during Pregnancy**, 1990.

FIGURE 11–1 The weighting game weight graph. This is an example of a chart on which a woman can plot her weight gain during pregnancy. (From the Great Beginnings Calendar, ed 2. National Dairy Council®, 1991, with permission.)

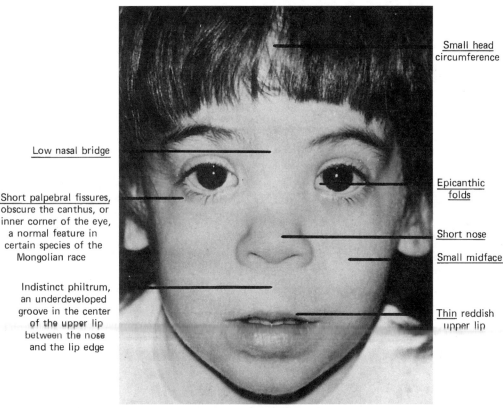

Low nasal bridge

Short palpebral fissures,
obscure the canthus, or
inner corner of the eye,
a normal feature in
certain species of the
Mongolian race

Indistinct philtrum,
an underdeveloped
groove in the center
of the upper lip
between the nose
and the lip edge

Small head
circumference

Epicanthic
folds

Short nose

Small midface

Thin reddish
upper lip

FIGURE 11–2   Characteristic facial features of a child with fetal alcohol syndrome (FAS). Children with FAS also suffer from hampered growth and mental retardation. (From Feldman, 1988, p 164, with permission.)

LEG CRAMPS   Pregnant women often complain of leg cramps. One theory attributes the cause to neuromuscular irritability due to low serum calcium. Increasing calcium intake is the prescribed treatment. Another theory postulates the cause to be a high serum phosphorus level in relation to calcium. Here the treatment prescribed is to substitute a calcium supplement for some of the milk intake, thus decreasing serum phosphorus. Because of its close link to calcium metabolism, magnesium deficiency has been postulated to cause leg cramps. A small study of magnesium supplementation reported positive results (Dahle, et al, 1995).

CONSTIPATION   The increasing size and weight of the uterus presses on the intestines, causing constipation. Adequate fluid intake, regular exercise, and a high-fiber diet should relieve this condition. The suggested amount of fiber intake, 30 grams per day, should be accomplished by consuming food rather than pharmaceutical preparations. Table 11–2 lists foods high in fiber but relatively low in kilocalories.

HEARTBURN   Hormonal changes cause relaxation of the cardiac sphincter, located between the esophagus and the stomach. This, coupled with the upward pressure of the diaphragm from the enlarging uterus causes reflux of gastric contents into the esophagus. *Heartburn* is the characteristic burning sensation beneath the breastbone.

Heartburn can be controlled by avoiding spicy or acidic foods and taking small, frequent meals. Sitting up for an hour after a meal may help. The pregnant woman should not self-medicate with sodium bicarbonate or antacids. The bicarbonate can be absorbed, producing alkalosis. The antacids decrease iron absorption by decreasing gastric acids, thus increasing the risk of anemia.

PICA   **Pica** is the compulsive ingestion of nonfood items, usually dirt, clay, laundry starch, or ice, and is an ancient practice, relayed by tradition. Most notable in some regions of the South, pica occurs in conjunction with inadequate diets due to poverty, but is seen in other socioeconomic levels also. Many women who practice pica do so only during pregnancy, believing it cures the annoyances of pregnancy or ensures a beautiful baby. Others contend that the substances taste good.

Health concerns about pica include inadequate nutrition due to substitution of nonfood items for

TABLE 11 2   Nutrient-Dense Foods High in Fiber

Food	Quantity	Grams of Dietary Fibers	Kilocalories
Grains			
All bran	1/3 cup	10	70
Bran buds	1/2 cup	11.5	109
100% Bran	1/2 cup	10	89
Fruits			
Applesauce, unsweetened	1 cup	4	106
Orange sections, raw	1 cup	4	85
Pear, D'Anjou, raw with skin	one each	6	120
Prunes, ckd. unsweetened	1/2 cup	4.5	114
Strawberries, fresh	1 cup	4	45
Vegetables			
Baked beans, in tomato sauce with pork	1/2 cup	7	129
Lima beans, ckd. from frozen	1/2 cup	8	94
Broccoli, raw	one spear	6	42
Brussels sprouts, ckd. from raw	1 cup	6	60
Kidney beans, canned	1/2 cup	8.5	108
Navy beans, ckd. from dry	1/2 cup	8	130
Black-eyes peas, ckd. from dry	1/2 cup	10.5	99

nutritious foods, iron deficiency anemia, constipation, and lead poisoning. Laundry starch interferes with iron absorption. Ingestion of clay may lead to fecal impaction. If the chosen substance is paint chips, lead poisoning may result.

A caring, nonjudgmental assessment may reveal the practice. Women transplanted to an area where pica is uncommon may continue the custom.

Complications of Pregnancy

This chapter introduces three complications with nutritional ramifications: hyperemesis gravidarum, pregnancy-induced hypertension, and gestational diabetes.

HYPEREMESIS GRAVIDARUM   Severe nausea and vomiting persisting after the fourteenth week of pregnancy is called **hyperemesis gravidarum.** Estimated to occur in 2 percent of pregnancies, it can be life threatening due to dehydration, electrolyte imbalance, and weight loss. It develops most often in Western countries and in first pregnancies. Many approaches have been used to treat it: rehydration, antiemetics without teratogenic effects, bedrest, and psychiatric intervention. Treatments that will not harm the fetus are chosen. In a one year study of all 20 women admitted to the hospital with hyperemesis gravidarum, intravenous saline with multivitamins was an effective treatment. The clients received nothing by mouth until the vomiting subsided, which occurred in all the patients within 24 hours.

The intravenous treatment lasted for ten days. Two women suffered relapses 3 to 4 weeks later. The treatment was repeated and the vomiting stopped. All clients gave birth to healthy babies weighing at least 5.5 pounds without congenital abnormalities (van Stuijvenberg, et al, 1995).

PREGNANCY-INDUCED HYPERTENSION   This pathology, involving edema, proteinuria, and hypertension, occurs in 5 to 7 percent of pregnancies. The signs and symptoms appear after the 20th week of pregnancy, usually in the 2 months before term. **Pregnancy-induced hypertension** (PIH), also called *preeclampsia-eclampsia syndrome,* is potentially life threatening for both the mother and the fetus. The cause is unknown. Excesses or deficiencies of magnesium, calcium, polyunsaturated fatty acids, zinc, cadmium, and sodium have been investigated as contributing factors. The syndrome occurs most frequently in women under 20 or over 35 years old pregnant for the first time, and in women who have had five or more pregnancies. Also increasing the risk of this syndrome are personal or family histories of diabetes, hypertension, or vascular or renal disease.

Pregnancy-induced hypertension may progress

Pregnancy-induced hypertension (PIH)—A potentially life-threatening disorder that may develop after the 20th week of pregnancy; includes preeclampsia and eclampsia.

from mild preeclampsia to severe preeclampsia to eclampsia. The signs of **preeclampsia** are hypertension, edema, and proteinuria (protein in the urine). When the client becomes eclamptic, edema of the brain causes convulsions and coma.

Mild preeclampsia is characterized by a systolic blood pressure increase of 30 millimeters of mercury or a diastolic increase of 15 millimeters of mercury over prepregnancy levels. It is treated with bed rest and possibly a high-protein diet to replace urinary losses. Diuretics are not used; they would aggravate the condition by increasing the permeability of the kidney's filtering system, causing greater losses.

Severe preeclampsia is characterized by a systolic blood pressure greater than 160 millimeters of mercury or a diastolic pressure greater than 110 millimeters of mercury. This client is hospitalized to provide rest and to monitor the mother and the fetus. Sedative drugs may be prescribed to lessen the irritability of the brain.

Eclampsia is an obstetrical emergency, which occurs in 1 of 200 cases of preeclampsia. The mother is in immediate danger of convulsing, if not already doing so. She requires intensive nursing care because she is at high risk of cerebral hemorrhage, circulatory collapse, or kidney failure. The fetus, too, is in grave danger.

The preferable method of dealing with pregnancy-induced hypertension is prevention. Good prenatal care, including weight and blood pressure monitoring and urine testing, and early intervention are the keys to minimizing the hazard of pregnancy-induced hypertension.

GESTATIONAL DIABETES   Pregnancy may precipitate the onset of diabetes in some women. This condition, known as **gestational diabetes,** is detected by glucose tolerance tests. Gestational diabetes is discussed in detail in the chapter on diabetes mellitus.

The Breast-Feeding Mother

In the next chapter, the advantages breast milk confers on the infant will be discussed. Here, the nutritional implications of breast-feeding for the mother are presented.

Nutritional Needs

The concern for proper nutrition for the mother does not end with the birth of the baby. All mothers must replenish their body stores after childbirth. The breast-feeding mother also has to produce the infant's milk.

Energy

Thirty ounces of breast milk a day at 20 kilocalories per ounce equals to 600 kilocalories total. Another 150 kilocalories are needed to make the milk. The RDA allows for 500 of these 750 kilocalories from food. The other 250 kilocalories are expected to be taken from fat stores laid down for this purpose during pregnancy.

Effect of Maternal Deficiencies

Even if a mother lacks some nutrients in her current diet, her milk contains the correct level of nutrients. The lack of nutrients in the mother's diet ultimately will affect her nutrient stores, but while she nurses, she usually will produce good quality milk, but in less quantity. However, if the mother's diet is low in vitamin C, her milk also will be deficient. In an otherwise well-nourished mother, the use of a vitamin supplement does not increase the vitamin content of her milk.

Benefits to the Mother

Several advantages to the mother are associated with breast-feeding. It helps the uterus return to its nonpregnant state more quickly. Breast-feeding is convenient and less costly than bottle feeding, and may be protective against later breast cancer.

Aids Uterine Involution

During breast-feeding, the sucking of the infant stimulates the release of **oxytocin** from the posterior pituitary gland in the brain. Oxytocin causes the uterine muscles to contract. This aids in returning the uterus to its nonpregnant size.

Convenience at Less Cost

Breast milk is always ready at the correct temperature. There is no formula to make or contamination problems to worry about. Recommended additional foods for a breast-feeding woman are two milk exchanges, one meat exchange, and one fruit or vegetable high in vitamin C. An increase in fluid intake of 1 liter per day is also advised.

Lessens Risk of Breast Cancer

Over the long term, breast-feeding has been associated with a decreased risk of breast cancer later in life. In a Japanese study, the risk was lowest among premenopausal women who had ever lactated for 7 to 9 months. (Yeo, et al, 1992). This is a statistical projection for the group, not an individual guarantee.

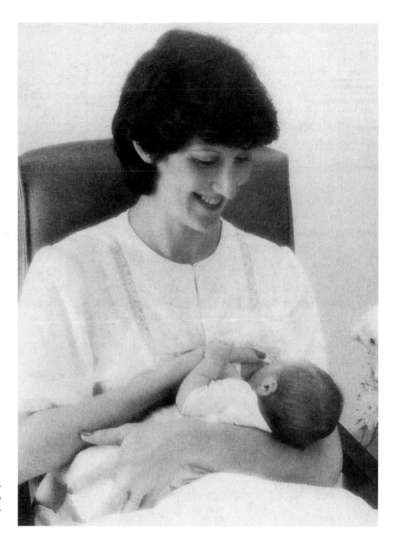

FIGURE 11–3   One correct breast-feeding position, tummy to tummy. The infant takes the entire areola in its mouth. (Used and reprinted with permission of Ross Laboratories, Columbus, OH.)

Techniques of Breast-Feeding

The medical and nursing staff will assist the mother to start breast-feeding her infant. However, some general principles have been established.

The mother and infant should be permitted to spend as much time together as possible during the first 24 hours after birth. This practice permits bonding of infant and mother. Some areas encourage fathers to "room in," also, to bond with the baby.

One correct position for breast-feeding is shown in Figure 11–3. It is tummy to tummy. The infant should face the breast squarely. If the breast is very large, care must be taken not to block the infant's nose, which may otherwise cause the infant to have trouble breathing. When nursing, the infant should grasp the entire areola (the colored portion around the nipple) to prevent the nipples from becoming sore.

Most infants will take 80 to 90 percent of the milk from each breast in the first 4 minutes of nursing. Because nursing stimulates further milk production, the mother should alternate which breast is first offered to the infant. This method allows the infant to empty the first breast offered and to finish feeding

Preeclampsia—Hypertension, edema, and proteinuria, appearing after the 20th week of pregnancy.

Eclampsia—An obstetrical emergency involving hypertension, edema, proteinuria, and convulsions, appearing after the 20th week of pregnancy.

Gestational diabetes—An exaggeration of the natural resistance to insulin that develops in the pregnant woman's tissues late in pregnancy.

Teratogenic—Capable of causing abnormal development of the embryo; results in a malformed fetus.

on the other breast if it is still hungry or is just enjoying the experience. At the next feeding, the mother should start with the breast the infant finished on the time before.

Maternal Contraindications to Breast-Feeding

Several situations make breast-feeding inadvisable. These include the mother's exposure to toxic chemicals, the mother's use of certain medications, and illness in the mother. The physician is the best source of guidance in a particular case. Galactosemia, a contraindication due to a metabolic defect in the infant, is discussed in the next chapter.

Exposure to Toxic Chemicals

Certain chemicals, such as DDT and PCB, have been shown to be **teratogenic.** If the mother has consumed food contaminated with a chemical, she may transmit it to the infant in breast milk. The contaminants are stored in her adipose tissue and the lactating mother's fat stores are mobilized to produce milk.

Some experts believe that the risk to the infant is minimal unless the mobilization of the mother's fat is due to inadequate intake. Others say that there is no hazard unless the woman has had occupational exposure to the chemicals or has consumed a large amount of fish from contaminated waters.

Medication Use

Many medications are secreted in breast milk. The physician should be consulted about both prescription and nonprescription drugs taken by the mother.

Substances that are often not thought of as drugs may also affect the breast-fed infant. These include alcohol and caffeine. Here again, experts offer opposite advice to the breast-feeding mother. While some recommend abstinence, others think that the moderate use of alcohol and caffeine is acceptable. The primary care provider is the best source of advice for the individual client.

Altered Physiology or Pathology

Absolute contraindications to breast-feeding include AIDS and active tuberculosis. Acute or chronic diseases in the mother may preclude breast-feeding. Some of these are heart disease, severe anemia, and nephritis. If the woman becomes pregnant again, she will have to stop breast-feeding. In some parts of the world, breast-feeding is used as a means of birth spacing, but this is not a reliable practice. If a couple wants to delay the birth of another child, they should use more effective methods of birth control.

Summary

To support her own and the fetus's growth, a pregnant woman requires increased intake of kilocalories, protein, B and C vitamins, iron, calcium, iodine, fluoride, and zinc. A major public health issue has been the provision of folic acid with the intention of preventing neural tube defects in the embryo. Substances for the pregnant woman to avoid are alcohol, immoderate or supplemental intake of preformed vitamin A, and excessive caffeine.

The pregnant teenage client is at especially high nutritional risk. Her own body still needs adequate nutrients for growth, and, in addition, she has a fetus to nourish.

Nutritional interventions are sometimes helpful for common complaints of pregnancy: morning sickness, leg cramps, constipation, and heartburn. Tact and diplomacy may be required to counsel women practicing pica. Medical intervention and nutritional support are indicated for clients with hyperemesis gravidarum, pregnancy-induced hypertension (preeclampsia and eclampsia), or gestational diabetes.

Breast-feeding offers benefits to the mother. It aids uterine involution and offers convenience since the milk is constantly read-to-feed. Some maternal contraindications to breast-feeding are exposure to toxic chemicals, ingestion of certain medications, and some illnesses, including AIDS and tuberculosis.

Case Study 11–1 Ms. T is a 21-year-old sexually active female who has been followed in a family planning clinic for three years. She has been faithful about keeping appointments and taking her oral contraceptives and the pyridoxine which was prescribed. She is taking no other medications or vitamin supplements. Now she relates that she is seriously considering becoming pregnant. Her boyfriend proposed at her 21st birthday celebration. She denied knowledge of means to minimize fetal risk and stated she drinks "a beer"

or a glass of wine on Saturdays and Sundays. She does not smoke. She had received the standard measles, mumps, and rubella (MMR) vaccinations as a child.

Ms. T is a 5 ft, 3 in woman and weighs 136 lb. Her wrist measures 5.5 in. Her hemoglobin was 14 g/dL and hematocrit was 42 percent last month.

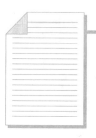

NURSING CARE PLAN

Assessment

Subjective Data	Expressed interest in becoming pregnant
	Regular moderate alcohol intake
	History of compliance with medical regimen
	Immunized against measles, mumps, and rubella
Objective Data	115 percent of healthy body weight
	Hemoglobin 14 g/dL, within normal limits (WNL)
	Hematocrit 42 percent, within normal limits (WNL)

Nursing Diagnosis

Risk for injury (fetal)
Related to lack of knowledge of measures to decrease risk to embryo

Desired Outcome/ Evaluation Criteria	Nursing Actions	Rationale
Will affirm intention to abstain from alcohol when attempting to achieve a pregnancy and throughout gestation.	Teach Ms. T about fetal alcohol syndrome. Use photographs of affected children.	No amount of alcohol is assumed to be safe in pregnancy. "A picture is worth 1,000 words." Photographs introduce visual learning and impact feelings.
Will recognize the unsettled issue relating folic acid intake to the occurrence of neural tube defects. After discussion with the primary health care provider, will make an informed choice.	Advise Ms. T of government guidelines and American College of Obstetricians and Gynecologists (ACOG) positions on prevention and early diagnosis of neural tube defects. Have research findings available if she wishes greater detail.	Informed consent is based on adequate information. Some persons will accept recommendations without questions; others want to weigh the evidence themselves.
Will recount the limits to vitamin A intake during pregnancy.	Inform Ms. T of RDA for vitamin A in pregnancy. Alert Ms. T to the large amounts of preformed vitamin A in liver and liver products. Caution against supplements containing more than 8000 IU (800 mcg RE) of beta carotene. Instruct Ms. T on the safety of carotene.	Large doses of vitamin A are associated with increased risk of birth defects. Supplements containing provitamin A are considered safe for pregnant women at the RDA level.

Study Aids

Chapter Review

1. A pregnant woman should consume one additional ounce of meat and one additional serving of both:
   a. Fruit and vegetable
   b. Milk and a vitamin C source
   c. Starch and/or bread and a fat
   d. Vegetable and milk

2. Which of the following substances is contraindicated during pregnancy?
   a. Alcohol
   b. Cocoa
   c. Coffee
   d. Tea

3. Compared to a pregnant adult, the pregnant teenager should consume 1 additional serving of both:
   a. Fruit and meat
   b. Milk and meat
   c. Milk and starch/ bread
   d. Vegetable and fruit

4. The critical time for folic acid intake to prevent neural tube defects is:
   a. Beginning of last menstrual period through month 2 of gestation
   b. Conception through week 4 of gestation
   c. Weeks 8 through 12 of gestation
   d. Throughout the pregnancy

5. If a pregnant woman complains of heartburn, she should be instructed to:
   a. Increase her intake of milk products
   b. Decrease her overall food intake
   c. Rest in bed after eating
   d. Avoid spicy or acidic foods

Clinical Analysis

Ms. T is a 15-year-old girl who thinks that she is 2 months pregnant. She confides to the school nurse that she is not sure if she should have an abortion. She has not told anyone else of the pregnancy. Her purpose in disclosing the information to the school nurse is to obtain assistance with weight control so she has more time to make up her mind.

1. Based on the above information, which one of the following interventions would be of highest priority at this time?
   a. Designing a weight control program that is high in calcium

   b. Giving information on the desirability of breast-feeding the infant
   c. Instructing the girl regarding substances that are likely to harm the fetus
   d. Scheduling a visit with a social worker to help the girl decide on a course of action

2. Knowing that adolescents are often lacking in certain nutrients, the nurse would want to assess the girl's intake of:
   a. Cola, coffee, and tea
   b. Fruits, vegetables, milk, and red meat
   c. Fried foods and pastries
   d. Poultry, seafood, and white bread

3. Ms. T complains of morning sickness. The nurse instructs her to:
   a. Eat breakfast later in the morning.
   b. Drink at least two glasses of liquid with every meal.
   c. Increase her intake of whole-grain breads and cereals to two servings per meal.
   d. Drink a large glass of skim milk at bedtime.

Bibliography

Acosta, RB, and Wright, L: Nurses' role in preventing birth defects in offspring of women with phenylketonuria. JOGNN 21:270, 1992.

Anderson, AS: Folic acid: The message we're failing to get across. Prof Care Mother Child 5:64, 66, 1995.

Barrett, JFR, et al: Absorption of nonhaem iron from food during normal pregnancy. Brit Med J 309:79, 1994.

Bendich, A: Folic acid and prevention of neural tube defects: Critical assessment of FDA proposals to increase folic acid intakes. J Nutr Educ 26:294, 1994.

Beresford, SAA: Annotation: How do we get enough folic acid to prevent birth defects? Am J Public Health 84:348, 1994.

Borowitz, D: Pediatric nutrition. In Feldman, EB (ed): Essentials of Clinical Nutrition. FA Davis, Philadelphia, 1988.

Centers for Disease Control: Recommendations for the use of folic acid to reduce the number of cases of spina bifida and other neural tube defects. MMWR 41(No. RR-14):1, 1992.

Clark, NAC, and Fisk, NM: Minimal compliance with the Department of Health recommendation for routine folate prophylaxis to prevent neural tube defects. Br J Obstet Gynaecol 101:709, 1994

Committee on Obstetrics: Maternal and Fetal Medicine: Folic acid for the prevention of recurrent neural tube defects. ACOG Committee Opinion No. 120:1, March 1993.

Czeizel, AE: Congenital abnormalities are preventable. Epidemiology 6:205, 1995.

Czeizel, AE, and Dudas, I: Prevention of the first occurrence of neural-tube defects by periconceptional vitamin supplementation. N Engl J Med 327:1832, 1992.

Dahle, LO, et al: The effect of oral magnesium substitution on pregnancy-induced leg cramps. Am J Obstet Gynecol 173:176, 1995.

Daly, LE, et al: Folate levels and neural tube defects. JAMA 274:1698, 1995.

Deglin, JH, and Vallerand, AH: Davis's Drug Guide for Nurses, ed 4. FA Davis, Philadelphia, 1995.

Dickinson, CJ: Does folic acid harm people with vitamin B_{12} deficiency? Q J Med 88:357, 1995.

Feldman, EB: Pregnancy and lactation. In Feldman, EB (ed): Essentials of Clinical Nutrition. FA Davis, Philadelphia, 1988.

Food and Drug Administration: Food standards: amendment of standards of identity for enriched grain products require addition of folic acid. Federal Register 61:8781, 1996.

Futoryan, T, and Gilchrest, BA: Retinoids and the skin. Nutrition Reviews 52:299, 1994.

Gaull, GE, et al: Fortification of the food supply with folic acid to prevent neural tube defects is not yet warranted. J. Nutr (Suppl) 126:773S, 1996.

Glenn, FB, Glenn, WD, and Duncan, RC: Fluoride tablet supplementation during pregnancy for caries immunity: A study of the offspring produced. Am J Obstet Gynecol 143:560, 1982.

Goldenberg, RL, et al: The effect of zinc supplementation on pregnancy outcome. JAMA 274:463, 1995.

Hathcock, JN, et al: Evaluation of vitamin A toxicity. Am J Clin Nutr 52:183, 1990.

Hook, EB: Letter to the Editor. Lancet 339:1000, 1992.

Jack, BW, et al: The negative pregnancy test. Arch Fam Med 4:340, 1995.

Karp, RJ, et al: Fetal alcohol syndrome. In Karp, RJ (ed): Malnourished Children in the United States. Springer, New York, 1993.

Keagy, PM, Shane, B, and Oace, SM: Folate bioavailability in humans: Effects of wheat bran and beans. Am J Clin Nutr 47:80, 1988.

Kirke, PN, et al: Maternal plasma folate and vitamin B_{12} are independent risk factors for neural tube defects. Q J Med 86:703, 1993.

Kolata, G: Vitamin to protect fetuses will be required in goods. New York Times, 1 March 1996, sec. A p. 8 (N), sec. A p. 10 (CL).

Long, PJ: Rethinking iron supplementation during pregnancy. J Nurse Midwife 40:36, 1995.

Milunsky, A, et al: Maternal heat exposure and neural tube defects. JAMA 268:882, 1992.

Morse, JM, et al: The effect of maternal fluid intake on breast milk supply: A Pilot study. Can J Public Health 83:213, 1992.

MRC Vitamin Study Research Group: Prevention of neural tube defects: Results of the Medical Research Council Vitamin Study. Lancet 338:131, 1991.

Muscati, SK, Gray-Donald, K, and Newson, EE: Interaction of smoking and maternal weight status in influencing infant size. Can J Public Health 85:407, 1994.

Newman, V, and Fullerton, JT. Role of nutrition in the prevention of preeclampsia. Journal of Nurse Midwifery 35:282, 1990.

Oakley, GP, Adams, MJ, and Dickinson, CM: More folic acid for everyone, now. J Nutr (Suppl) 126:251 S, 1996.

Oakley, GP, and Erickson, JD: Vitamin A and birth defects. N Engl J Med 333:1414, 1995.

O'Connor, DL: Folate status during pregnancy and lactation. Adv Exp Med Biol 352:157, 1994.

Pérez-Escamilla, R: Periconceptual folic acid and neural tube defects: Public health issues. Bull Pan Am Health Organ 29:250, 1995.

Rieder, MJ: Prevention of neural tube defects with periconceptional folic acid. Clin Perinatol 21:483, 1994.

Romano, PS, et al: Folic acid fortification of grain: An economic analysis. Am J Public Health 85:667, 1995.

Rothman, KJ, et al: Teratogenicity of high vitamin A intake. N Engl J Med 333:1369, 1995.

Rush, D: Periconceptional folate and neural tube defect. Am J Clin Nutr (suppl) 59:511S, 1994.

Sauberlich, HE, et al: Folate requirement and metabolism in nonpregnant women. Am J Clin Nutr 46:1016, 1987.

Scholl, TO, et al. Growth and nutrition during adolescent pregnancy. In Karp, RJ (ed): Malnourished Children in the United States. Springer, New York, 1993.

Schoral, CJ, et al: Possible abnormalities of folate and vitamin B_{12} metabolism associated with neural tube defects. Ann NY Acad Sci 678:81, 1993.

Shaw, GM, et al: Periconceptional vitamin use, dietary folate, and the occurrence of neural tube defects. Epidemiology 6:219, 1995.

Steinmetz, G: Fetal alcohol syndrome. National Geographic 181:36, 1992.

Subcommittee on Nutritional Status and Weight Gain During Pregnancy. Subcommittee on Dietary Intake and Nutrient Supplements During Pregnancy. National Academy of Sciences: Nutrition During Pregnancy. National Academy Press, Washington, DC, 1990.

Thorp, FK, Pierce, P, and Deedwania, C: Nutrition in the infant and young child. In Halpern, SL (ed): Quick Reference to Clinical Nutrition, ed 2. JB Lippincott, Philadelphia, 1987.

US Preventive Services Task Force: Routine iron supplementation during pregnancy policy statement. JAMA 270:2846, 1993.

US Preventive Services Task Force: Routine iron supplementation during pregnancy review article. JAMA 270:2848, 1993.

Van Allen, MI, et al: Recommendations on the use of folic acid supplementation to prevent the recurrence of neural tube defects. Can Med Assoc J 149:1239, 1993.

Van Loan, MD, et al: Fluid changes during pregnancy: Use of bioimpedance spectroscopy. J Appl Physiol 78:1037, 1995.

van Stuijvenberg, ME, et al: The nutritional status and treatment of patients with hyperemesis gravidarum. Am J Obstet Gynecol 172:1585, 1995.

Whitehead, AS, et al: A genetic defect in 5,10 methylenetetrahydrofolate reductase in neural tube defects. Q J Med 88:763, 1995.

Yoo, K-Y, et al: Independent protective effect of lactation against breast cancer: A case–control study in Japan. Am J Epidemiol 135:726, 1992.

CHAPTER 12

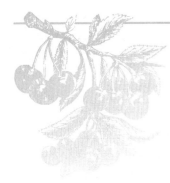

Life Cycle Nutrition:
Infancy, Childhood, Adolescence

CHAPTER OUTLINE

LEARNING OBJECTIVES

After completing this chapter, the student should be able to:

1 Describe the normal growth pattern and corresponding nutritional needs for a full-term infant, a toddler, a school-age child, and an adolescent.

2 Explain why breast milk is uniquely suited to the human infant's capabilities.

3 Compare breast-feeding to formula-feeding as to advantages and disadvantages.

4 Discuss the rationale for the sequence in which semisolid foods are introduced into an infant's diet.

5 List causes and treatments for five common nutritional problems in infancy.

6 Summarize common nutritional problems of the preschool child.

7 Relate ways in which a child can be encouraged to establish good nutritional habits.

8 Identify frequent areas of concern regarding an adolescent's diet.

This chapter focuses on periods of rapid growth: infancy, childhood, and adolescence. In addition to nutritional needs for all periods of rapid growth, we will also discuss the physical and **psychosocial development** that should occur during infancy, childhood, and adolescence.

Psychosocial Development

Psychologists have defined developmental tasks that should be mastered by individuals during their lifetimes. Developmental needs also impact nutritional practices. In this chapter, we discuss the developmental tasks to be achieved by the infant, toddler, preschooler, school-age child, and adolescent. The developmental tasks for the young, middle, and older adult are included in the next chapter.

An American psychoanalyst, **Erik Erikson,** developed a theory of human development that linked psychological development with interactions with other people. Erikson understood life as divided into eight stages. Each stage has a psychosocial developmental task to be mastered, and an opposite negative trait that comes to the fore if the task is not mastered. Even if a developmental task is successfully mastered, a new situation may arise challenging the person to reaffirm his or her mastery. A brief listing of Erikson's developmental tasks through adolescence appears in Table 12–1. Throughout this chapter and the next, the ways that nutrition can influence psychosocial development are discussed.

Nutrition in Infancy

Infancy refers to the first year of life. To be more specific, for the first 28 days of life, the baby is a newborn or neonate. From day 29 to the first birthday the baby is an infant.

TABLE 12–1 Erikson's Theory of Psychosocial Development

Stage of Life	Developmental Task	Opposing Negative Trait
Infancy	Trust	Distrust
Toddler	Autonomy	Doubt
Preschooler	Initiative	Guilt
School-age child	Industry	Inferiority
Adolescent	Identity	Role confusion

Growth

During infancy, certain milestones are used to judge the adequacy of the baby's growth. The first year of life is critical for the growth of essential organs.

Expected Milestones

The only time human beings grow faster than in the first year after birth is the 9 months before birth. A baby's birth weight should double by age 4 to 6 months and triple by age 1. Thus an infant who weighs 7 pounds at birth should weigh 14 pounds at 6 months and 21 pounds at 1 year. From a birth length of about 20 inches, the baby grows to about 30 inches by age 1.

The rate of growth is more significant than absolute values. Is the infant progressing at a reasonable pace? A gain of 5 to 8 ounces per week is expected during the first 4 or 5 months. Thereafter, a gain of 4 or 5 ounces per week until the first birthday would be reasonable. Evidence suggests that breast-fed and formula-fed infants have different growth rates after 3 months of age. Formula-fed boys were significantly heavier than breast-fed boys at each month between ages 7 to 18 months. For girls the differences occurred between 6 and 18 months of age. The recommendation is for separate growth charts for breast-fed infants. (Dewey, et al, 1992).

During the first few days after birth, the baby loses weight as it adjusts to its new environment and food supply. The amount of weight lost should not exceed 10 percent of the birth weight. The newborn usually regains to its birth weight within 14 days.

Critical Tissue Growth

The period most critical to brain development extends from conception into the second year of life. Brain cells increase most rapidly before birth and during the first 5 or 6 months after birth. To reach the maximum brain growth, the baby needs optimal nutrition. Once this period of brain cell division and growth is completed, no further growth is possible. Improved nutrition after age 2 will not increase the number of brain cells. Conversely, severe protein-calorie malnutrition in the last trimester of pregnancy or the first 6 months of life may decrease brain cells by as much as 20 percent.

Development

Development refers to the process of changing to a mature individual involving psychosocial and physical changes, usually including an increase in size.

Psychosocial Development

The infant's developmental task is to learn to **trust.** The parent who responds promptly and lovingly to the infant's cries is teaching the baby to trust. If the caregiver handles the infant gently one time and roughly the next, the baby learns to mistrust. In situations where physical care is provided, but no tender relationships, infants may actually suffer stunted physical growth. This occurs often enough so that **failure to thrive** (FTT) has become a medical diagnosis for severely underweight infants. The developmental task of trust, if achieved, lays the foundation for future human relationships. If not accomplished, it lays a foundation also, but for mistrust and suspiciousness.

An infant can explore the world through feeding and foods. New foods encourage experimentation. Babies like to poke their fingers in the food. They attempt to feed themselves but turn the spoon upside down on the way to their mouths. Consistent acceptance from the parent will teach the infant to trust his or her world. The same behavior should not receive a laugh one time and a scolding the next.

Physical Development

Development proceeds at a different pace in various tissues and organs. Proper feeding practices are based on the maturation rate of body organs.

GASTROINTESTINAL SYSTEM   Infants do not develop a sense of taste until they are 3 to 4 months old. Because salivary and pancreatic amylases are inadequate for several months, complex carbohydrates are indigestible at birth.

Infants have to be fed often. A newborn's stomach holds about an ounce. By 1 year of age, the stomach will hold about 8 ounces. An adult's stomach, on the other hand, can hold about 2 quarts.

An infant's intestinal tract is also immature. It resembles a chain-link fence rather than a sieve. It allows whole proteins to be absorbed into the bloodstream. The more mature intestine permits absorption of amino acids but not whole proteins. This has major ramifications for the introduction of semisolid foods.

NERVOUS SYSTEM   Nervous tissue, bile, and hormones all require fat and cholesterol for their growth and development. Because of the rapid growth of the brain and the nervous system, the infant requires adequate fat and even cholesterol in its diet.

The **term infant** does have some well-developed reflexes. One of these is the **rooting reflex.** When the infant's cheek is stroked, the head turns toward that side to nurse.

For the first 3 or 4 months, the infant suckles by using an up-and-down motion of the tongue. If semisolid food is offered at this time, the natural motion of the tongue tends to spit it out. This, too, affects wise choices of food for infants.

After 4 months, the infant can suck using orofacial muscles. The tongue moves back and forth instead of up and down. At this point, semisolid food is more likely to be swallowed than spit out.

By 6 months of age, the infant has enough hand-to-eye coordination to put food and other objects into its mouth. A 7-month-old infant can chew appropriate foods.

URINARY SYSTEM   An infant's kidneys are immature. They have limited capacity to filter solutes. Not until the end of the second month can the infant's kidneys excrete the waste of semisolid foods. As is discussed later, however, feeding of semisolids often is delayed another 2 months. By the infant's first birthday, the kidneys have reached full functional capacity.

Nutritional Needs of the Term Infant

A normal pregnancy is 38 to 42 weeks. See Clinical Application 12–4 (page 218) for definitions of prematurity. Because breast milk is naturally suitable for human infants, its characteristics are the standard for infant formulas, which copy many of the qualities of breast milk.

Protein

Because of the extensive tissue building that occurs, an infant needs 2.5 to 3.5 grams of protein per kilogram of body weight. The 1-year-old infant requires only 2 grams of protein per kilogram of body weight. Compare this with the recommended amount of protein for an adult, 0.8 grams per kilogram of body weight. Proportionally, the infant needs 250 percent of the adult requirement.

The protein in breast milk is easy for the infant to digest. Sixty percent of the protein in breast milk is lactalbumin, with an amino acid pattern much like that of the body tissues. The infant's body can absorb it easily and, without much processing, can use it for building tissue.

Energy

Infants have high metabolic rates. Normal pulse rate is 120 to 150 per minute; normal respiratory

---

CLINICAL APPLICATION 12–1

Honey Is a Danger to Infants

No honey should be given to an infant until after the first birthday because it frequently contains organisms that an infant cannot fight off.

Bees may contaminate honey with botulism spores acquired from plants or the soil. These spores are not destroyed by processing. If ingested by the infant, the spores become active in its intestinal tract and produce a toxin. This is a potentially serious, even a fatal situation because the toxin affects the nervous system.

Botulism spores hide in many places. Honey is not the only source. Other foods and even dust contain botulism spores. In fact, in only 20 percent of the reported cases of infant botulism had the infant been fed honey. However, keeping honey out of the infant's diet lessens the risk considerably. The child's intestinal tract is better able to expel the botulism **spores** once the child reaches the age of 1 year.

---

source of carbohydrate the infant should not have is honey (see Clinical Application 12–1).

FAT An infant needs 30 to 55 percent of kilocalories from fat as a concentrated source of energy, thus compensating for his or her small stomach capacity. The developing nervous system also requires fat because approximately 60 percent of the structural material of the brain consists of lipids, mainly arachidonic and docosahexaeneic fatty acids (Phylactos, 1994). Since breast milk contains the necessary lipase to begin digestion for the infant, about 95 to 98 percent of the fat in human milk is absorbed. Box 12–1 identifies research linking cognitive development to breast-feeding. Because of their need for fat, 1- to 2-year-old children should drink whole milk.

EVALUATION The best indicator of adequate kilocaloric intake is a normal growth rate according to standard growth charts. These measurements should be made every 3 months. They can be graphed on growth charts such as those that appear in Appendix D.

rate is 30 to 50 per minute. Because of the large proportion of skin surface to body size, temperature regulation takes significant energy. Crying may double the metabolic rate.

A newborn requires 100 to 120 kilocalories per kilogram of body weight per day. If our 154-pound (70-kilogram) man consumed at the rate of a newborn, he would take in 7000 to 8400 kilocalories per day. By the end of the first year of life, the infant requires only 80 to 100 kilocalories per kilogram of body weight.

CARBOHYDRATE As is the case with protein, the carbohydrate in breast milk is easily digested by the infant. The lactose in breast milk is a source of galactose, which is necessary for brain cell formation. One

Vitamins

In the RDA table, vitamins are specified for infants aged 0 to 6 months and 6 to 12 months (see Appendix F). Infants need all the vitamins that other humans need, but in different amounts. Severe vitamin B_{12} deficiencies with grave neurological deterioration have been described in 4- to 8-month-old infants. Half the breast-feeding mothers were vegetarians, half were not (Graham, Arvela, and Wise, 1992). Human breast milk contains more vitamin C, but less vitamin D, than cow's milk. The cholesterol in breast milk functions as a precursor of vitamin D that is produced in the skin. For infants who receive some exposure to sunlight, this is a benefit. Because of other hazards of exposure to sun, however, a vita-

---

BOX 12–1 RESEARCH LINKS COGNITIVE ABILITIES TO BREAST-FEEDING

Preterm breast-fed infants showed significantly higher IQ scores at age 8 than formula fed infants even after controlling for social class and education (Lucas, et al, 1992). One possible explanation is that until recently infant formula did not contain arachidonic and docosahexaenoic fatty acids, the main components of brain tissue (Phylactos, et al, 1994). Long-term follow-up also showed the importance of breast-feeding to cognitive development. Adolescents who as full-term infants were breast-fed longer than 12 weeks tested significantly better in verbal and reasoning IQ than those breast-fed less than 12 weeks (Greene, et al, 1995).

min D supplement may be a wiser choice. Parents should consult their primary health care provider in this regard.

Special situations that demand vitamin supplementation are discussed later in this chapter.

Minerals

Infants need the same minerals as other human beings. Breast milk contains only one-third the sodium, potassium, and chloride and one-eighth the phosphorus of cow's milk. This dilution accommodates the limited function of the infant's kidneys. Breast milk also contains less iron than cow's milk, but the infant absorbs 49 percent of it compared with 10 percent from cow's milk. Likewise, 50 to 60 percent of the calcium in breast milk is absorbed by the infant, compared with 25 to 30 percent of the calcium in cow's milk. The zinc in breast milk is absorbed better than that in cow's milk as well.

These differences in mineral content affect the osmolality of the milk. See Clinical Application 12–2 for additional information on the extra minerals' effect on the workload of the kidneys. The data will show why unmodified cow's milk is inappropriate for young infants.

Water

The infant's body is about 75 percent water. By the age of 1, the body has converted to the adult proportion of about 60 percent water. The daily turnover of water in the infant is approximately 15 percent of body weight. Breast milk contains more water than cow's milk. Even in desert climates, an infant can be adequately hydrated on breast milk alone. An infant will regulate its intake of formula to obtain sufficient energy. If the formula is dilute, the baby will take more of it; if concentrated, less. This self-regulating mechanism is not perfect, however, since the infant may consume excess formula to quench its thirst.

The Breast-Fed Infant

Breast-feeding in the United States declined between 1984 and 1989 from 60 to 52 percent of newborns breast-fed and from 24 to 18 percent breast-fed at six months of age (Freed, 1993). Subsequently a national goal was established to increase the percentage of infants breast-fed by the year 2000. The targets are: 75 percent of infants to be breast-fed in early infancy and 50 percent through 5 or 6 months of age (U.S. Department of Health and Human Services, 1990). By contrast, in Scandinavia, the belief that it is unethical to feed infants synthetic formulas necessitates a system of human milk banks (Sturman, and Chesney, 1995). The use of supplementary bottle feeding is a risk to successful breast-feeding. Nurses in Toronto and Kansas City have learned to cup feed infants who could not be put to breast. This is a procedure in common use in Africa (Milford, 1995).

Infancy is the only time in life when a single food is the entire diet. All breast milk is not alike but rather adjusts to the infant's needs. Breast milk varies from mother to mother and even in one mother with the time of day.

Composition of Breast Milk

Breast milk compensates for the shortcomings of the infant's digestive system. Its composition varies within a feeding and during the weeks an infant is nursing.

CLINICAL APPLICATION 12–2

Renal Solute Loads

When selecting a formula, it is important to distinguish two measures of osmotic pressure. One is the osmotic pressure the formula presents to the gut. The other measure examines what remains to be excreted by the kidney after digestion and absorption have taken place. These leftovers are excess electrolytes and by-products of protein metabolism. The osmotic pressure of these leftovers presented to the kidney for disposal is called the *renal solute load*. It varies considerably from one formula to another. When dealing with an infant's immature digestive and urinary systems, selecting an appropriate formula may be crucial to health. Below is a comparison of several infant feedings with the intestinal osmolality and the renal solute load listed. As always, the standard of comparison is human breast milk.

Milk/Formula	Intestinal Osmolality (mOsm/kg)	Renal Solute Load (mOsm/L)
Human breast milk	300	101
Similac 60/40	260	96
Similac	290	105
Isomil	250	122
SMA	300	128
3.3 percent cow's milk	275	275

COLOSTRUM The milk secreted for the first 2 to 4 days after the birth of the baby is *colostrum*. It is a thin, yellow, cloudy fluid. Colostrum is high in proteins such as immunoglobulins, in fat-soluble vitamins, in minerals, and is low in fat.

TRANSITIONAL MILK This milk follows colostrum production and lasts about through the second week after delivery. Transitional milk contains lactose, fat, and water-soluble vitamins at the level of mature milk. It is also produced in larger quantities than colostrum.

MATURE MILK As breast-feeding becomes established, the mother produces mature milk. It varies in composition. At 3 months, for instance, immunoglobulins comprise a smaller portion of the proteins than was true when the baby was younger.

During a feeding, the constituents of the milk change. The milk contains more fat at the end of a feeding than in the beginning. Mature breast milk generally is 2 percent fat at the beginning of a feeding and up to 7 percent at the end. Fat provides satiety, or a feeling of fullness or satisfaction. If the infant received high-fat milk at the beginning of a feeding, it might become contented and stop nursing. The variation in content also offers the infant a variety of taste experiences. Despite the fact that some of their milk contains 7 percent fat, breast-fed infants at 1 year have serum cholesterol levels equal to formula-fed infants.

Unique Advantages to Breast-Feeding

There are two advantages to breast-feeding that cannot be duplicated by formulas. The first is the protection against disease provided by a mother's milk. The second is the lessening of the possibility of allergies in the infant. Even a few weeks of breast-feeding would benefit the infant.

PROTECTION AGAINST DISEASE Research shows that breast-fed infants are sick less frequently than formula-fed babies. This is most important in developing countries where sanitation, hygiene, and immunization are major public health issues. Gastrointestinal infections are the leading cause of infant mortality worldwide. In fact, fluid and electrolyte imbalances caused by infection kill more children than any other disease or disaster.

Breast-feeding promotes a particular kind of bacteria, *Lactobacillus bifidus*, in the baby's intestine rather than *Escherichia coli*. Although the normal adult intestine harbors *E. coli*, it can cause diarrhea in children. The *L. bifidus* also suppresses the growth of other organisms, such as staphylococci, shigella, and protozoa, which can cause disease.

Among the infection-fighting agents in breast milk are white blood cells (WBCs). Each cubic millimeter contains 4000 WBCs. This concentration is nearly as great as occurs in the blood. Most of these WBCs are macrophages that kill microorganisms.

Breast milk also contains the protein immunoglobulin A (IgA), an antibody against viruses and bacteria. Many proteins, if taken orally, would be digested. IgA, however, is resistant to acidity and enzymes that break down protein, so it is effectively transferred to the infant in the mother's milk. Moreover, IgA is supplied in the greatest amount during the first 3 months of lactation when an infant's immune system is the weakest.

PREVENTION OF ALLERGIES The infant's gastrointestinal tract can permit the passage of whole proteins into the bloodstream. These proteins can stimulate an allergic response in susceptible infants. Contrary to earlier opinion, infants can be allergic to their own mother's milk. Breast-fed infants whose mothers avoided dairy products, eggs, fish, peanuts, and soybeans had fewer and milder cases of eczema than breast-fed infants of mothers consuming unrestricted diets (Chandra, Purl, and Hamed, 1989). The occurrence rate is less than that in infants who become allergic to cow's milk. Once an infant becomes allergic to cow's milk, the risk of other allergies developing increases. Fortunately, most infants outgrow food allergies by age 2. Breast-feeding for 6 months or longer is required to prevent eczema until age 3. Exclusive breast-feeding for more than 1 month seems beneficial in preventing food allergies with its peak prevalence at 3 years and respiratory allergies with a peak prevalence at 17 years (Saarinen, and Kajosaari, 1995).

Galactosemia Precludes Breast-Feeding

The infant's lack of an enzyme to metabolize galactose is an absolute contraindication to breast-feeding. This condition of **galactosemia** is inherited as an autosomal recessive trait and occurs once in every 40,000 to 50,000 live births. The infant is fed a substitute formula containing no lactose or galactose.

The Formula-Fed Infant

As good as it is, even breast-feeding has some disadvantages. Among them is the inability of others, including the father, to feed the infant. Infants can be well nourished with commercial formulas, which are modified cow's milk products made to nearly duplicate breast milk. Earlier, in the chapter we compared breast milk to unmodified cow's milk, not to commercial baby formulas.

Characteristics of Formulas

The processing of infant formulas in the United States has been regulated by law since 1980. These products have been so well received that 95 percent of formula-fed infants receive commercial products rather than a homemade formula. Commercial formulas for full-term infants must contain 20 kilocalories per ounce. The formula osmolality may be no more than 400 milliosmoles per kilogram. Commercial formulas are designed to imitate human breast milk but they differ from it in protein, fat, and mineral content.

Formulas contain more protein than breast milk. The cow's milk proteins do not contain the optimal amino acids for human infants, so enough protein is included in the formula to provide a sufficient distribution of amino acids.

The saturated fats of cow's milk are poorly digested by the infant. In infant formulas, the saturated fats are removed and replaced by vegetable oils.

Formulas are treated to lower the sodium content of the cow's milk, but most formulas still contain more sodium than breast milk. SMA is the lowest in sodium, with 6.5 milliequivalents per liter. This is a trifle lower than breast milk, with 7 milliequivalents per liter.

Formulas can be purchased with or without added iron. Formulas without iron contain less than 1 milligram per quart, and formulas with iron contain 12 milligrams per quart.

Formula Preparations

Commercial formulas come in three forms: powder (to mix with water), liquid concentrate, and ready-to-feed. Less waste occurs with the powdered formula. A smaller amount can be mixed for the young infant. Opened cans of liquid formula may be stored covered in the refrigerator but must be used within 48 hours. Prepared bottles of formula should be discarded once they have been out of the refrigerator for 1 hour or have been offered to the infant.

In Western countries with safe drinking water supplies, the use of clean rather than sterile technique often is sufficient. The parents will receive specific instructions from their health care workers. Nevertheless, separate utensils should be kept for formula preparation. Parents should be cautioned that equipment cannot be adequately sanitized in a microwave oven. Extreme caution is required if a microwave oven is used for infant foods. Heat may be unevenly distributed and continues to build up in the food even after it is removed from the oven.

Parents must be impressed with the need to feed the infant the correct strength formula. Either too concentrated or too diluted a formula can cause severe electrolyte imbalances, even death.

Feeding Techniques

Contrary to the rigid feeding practices of some years ago, the current practice is to feed the infant when it is hungry. Most of the time the infant evolves a schedule whereby it demands a feeding approximately every 4 hours. By the age of 2 to 3 months, the baby probably will have eliminated one feeding so the schedule is five times a day. By 6 months most infants are feeding four times a day.

The baby is positioned in the crook of the arm almost as if breast-feeding. The parent's or caregiver's touch is important to the infant's development. The nipple hole should be large enough for milk to drip out without shaking. The bottle should be tipped so that the nipple is kept full of milk at all times. This prevents the infant from swallowing air while feeding. "Propping" an infant with a bottle is never acceptable because (1) choking is a real hazard and (2) the infant needs to be held to develop a closeness with the parent or caregiver. Figure 12–1 shows the infant and caregiver concentrating on each other during the feeding.

The daily formula intake for an infant should be 1.5 to 2 ounces per pound of body weight. At this rate, a 7-pound baby would take 10.5 to 14 ounces a day. An infant of this size would be feeding six times a day, so it would take 1.75 to 2.3 ounces per feeding. A 14-pound baby would be taking 21 to 28 ounces in four feedings of 5.25 to 7 ounces. A single feeding should never exceed 8 ounces.

Special Formulas

Manufacturers have devised formulas for special needs. Infants who are allergic to cow's milk, those with galactosemia or lactose intolerance, and those with fat absorption problems all need special formulas. See Clinical Application 12–3 for a brief description of soy formulas. Unfortunately, soy proteins may also cause allergies in as many as 35 percent of infants allergic to cow's milk (Moon, and Kleinman, 1995). Soy milk formula did not protect high-risk infants from eczema (Chandra, Pari, and Hamed, 1989). Other special formulas can be prescribed for infants with multiple allergies.

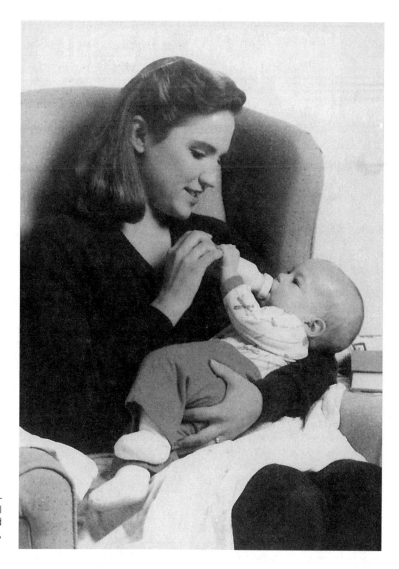

FIGURE 12–1 Babies are held close to the caregiver for bottle feeding so that their psychological as well as physical needs can be met. (Used and reprinted with permission of Ross Laboratories, Columbus, OH.)

The full-term infant's digestive, nervous, and urinary systems are immature. How, then, are the littlest humans, the premature infants fed? Clinical Application 12–4 summarizes some of the nutritional problems and appropriate interventions used for premature infants.

Hazards of Formula-Feeding

On a few occasions, improperly manufactured formulas have been responsible for vitamin and mineral deficiencies in infants. This is unacceptable, certainly, but rare. A more common hazard, and one an individual nurse can monitor, is the improper preparation and use of formulas by the parent. For-

---

CLINICAL APPLICATION 12–3

Soy Protein Formulas

Several formulas based on soy protein are available for infants with special needs. Most of them contain no lactose. Two commonly used soy products are ProSobee and Isomil SF. Many others are available. Temporary lactose intolerance sometimes follows diarrhea because of damage to the intestinal mucosa. In this situation, soy formulas may be useful temporarily until the infant's intestinal function returns to normal.

Premature Infants

Premature infants are born before 37 weeks gestation. A low-birth-weight (LBW) infant weighs less than 2500 g at birth. A very low-birth-weight (VLBW) infant weighs 1000 g (2.2 lb) or less. An infant can be both premature and LBW or VLBW. Not all premature infants weigh less than 2500 g. Nor are all LBW infants premature, but birth weight is the most potent single predictor of an infant's future health status. LBW infants are 20 times more likely to die as normal-weight infants. Although LBW infants make up just 7 percent of the births in the United States, they comprise almost 66 percent of deaths in the first year of life. There is a substantial association between intellectual function and LBW, even greater with VLBW.

Compared with full-term infants, premature infants have an even larger proportion of their bodies as water. They have less protein and fat. Their bones are poorly calcified and their muscles are poorly developed. There is almost no glycogen. The sucking reflex is not developed prior to the 32nd or 34th week of gestation. As a result, premature infants often require tube feeding through the gastrointestinal tract or intravenous feeding. Tube feeding will conserve energy even in an infant who is able to suck. Tube feedings at body temperature produced fewer gastric residuals than formula administered at room temperature or 50°F. No difference was noted between the last two (Gonzales, et al, 1995). Esophageal peristalsis is absent and the esophageal sphincter is weak, leading to increased danger of aspiration. The liver is immature in enzyme systems and in iron stores. Fat digestion is limited by decreased activity of pancreatic lipase. Fat absorption is limited by a deficiency of bile salts.

Protein digestion and absorption functions are relatively intact. Carbohydrate absorption also is intact, but digestion is limited by decreased pancreatic and salivary amylase activity and delayed development of lactase.

Special formulas for premature infants are designed to provide for the infant's growth needs despite the immature digestive system. Glucose polymers and medium-chain triglycerides are used to construct a formula that will take advantage of the infant's digestive capabilities. The premature infant has high energy needs. If given 120 kcal/kg of body weight enterally, the infant will grow at about the same rate as if still in the uterus. Special growth grids for premature infants are available. These are based on conceptual age or the expected due date.

Vitamin supplements are needed because the infant's intake is so small. Maximal transfer of vitamin E across the placenta occurs just before full-term delivery. Vitamin E stabilizes red blood cell membranes. If deficient, the infant suffers from hemolytic anemia. The other function of vitamin E is the possible contribution to preventing **retrolental fibroplasia** in infants receiving oxygen.

Premature infants may need to have their diet supplemented with the minerals calcium, phosphorus, and sodium. Rickets of prematurity can occur in the second postnatal month due not to the lack of vitamin D but to the lack of calcium and phosphorus. Prematurity is associated with increased dental caries, however fluoride intake recommendations are established for full-term infants only (Zlotkin, Atkinson, and Lockitch, 1995). Sodium needs will increase as the infant grows. Monitoring serum and urine sodium levels will alert the physician to the infant's changing needs.

Not all mothers of premature infants can establish lactation. The milk of those who do differs significantly from the milk of mothers who deliver at term: the breast milk of the mother of a premature baby has more protein and sodium but insufficient calcium, phosphorus, and magnesium. As is true with full-term infants, the mother's antibodies cannot be duplicated by formula.

---

mulas can be (1) the wrong dilution, (2) prepared with contaminated water, or (3) kept at feeding temperature too long. Body temperature is "just right" for bacteria to multiply, whether in the body or in a formula bottle.

Choice of Breast or Bottle

In this country, infants can be well nourished whether breast- or formula-fed. To raise a child successfully takes more than simply supplying the correct ratio of nutrients. No mother should be forced into breast-feeding because it meets the physician's or nurse's needs. Her informed decision should be supported enthusiastically.

Semisolid Foods

Contrary to folklore, no proof exists that the early feeding of solid food to infants promotes their sleeping through the night. At 3 months, 75 percent of infants sleep all night, regardless of diet.

When to Start

If solid foods are introduced too early, the infant may develop allergies because of the permeability of the intestine, which at this age permits whole proteins to be absorbed. Infants given 4 or more types of solid food before 4 months of age had 2.35 times the risk of childhood eczema as infants not so fed. The number of foods, not specific foods increased the risk (Fergusson, Horwood, and Shannon, 1990). Most physicians recommend starting semisolid foods at about 4 to 6 months of age. Figure 12–2 shows an infant trying cereal for the first time.

The infant should achieve voluntary control of swallowing at about 3 to 4 months. Before being offered solid food, the infant should be able to control his or her head and trunk. With this ability the baby can turn away when satisfied. By this time the infant has doubled its birth weight, is drinking 8 ounces of formula, and yet becomes hungry in less than 4 hours.

In introducing solid food it is important to follow the infant's lead. To avoid later feeding problems, solid foods should be started when the baby is interested. Babies this age are hungry and not fussy about tastes. They learn from adults, though, so the parent should avoid showing distaste for particular foods.

How to Feed

New foods should be introduced one at a time, so if a problem develops, it can be readily identified. A food should be tried for 3 to 5 days before the infant

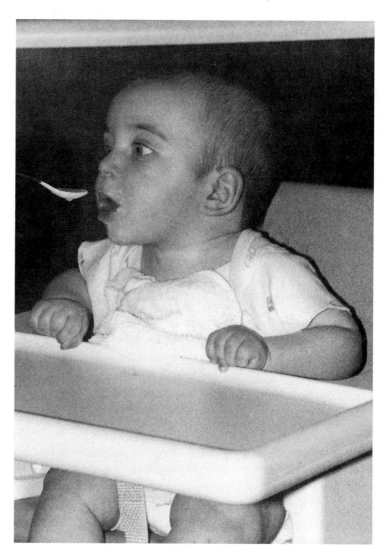

FIGURE 12–2 This 5-month-old baby is experiencing semisolid food for the first time. His readiness is clear. Notice how eager he is, how focused on the spoon.

TABLE 12–2   Suggested Schedule for Infant Foods

Age of Infant	Food	Rationale/Precautions
4 months	Infant cereal mixed with formula	Because of risk of allergies, rice offered first; wheat after age 12 months. Read labels: some mixed infant cereals contain wheat.
5 to 6 months	Strained vegetables	Less sweet than fruits; less likely to be rejected if offered first.
6 to 7 months	Strained fruits	Will be well accepted; humans have strong preference for sweets.
6 to 8 months	Finger foods (bananas, crackers)	Encourages self-feeding. Different textures may aid speech development.
7 to 8 months	Strained meats	Offer variety. See Clinical Application 12–5
10 months	Strained or mashed egg yolk	Start with 1/2 tsp. Due to possible allergy, delay egg white till 1 year old.
10 months	Bite-sized cooked foods	Select appropriate foods. See Clinical Application 12–5.
12 months	Foods from adult table	Select suitable foods, prepared according to baby's abilities.

is permitted to reject it. Only a taste or two is sufficient for the first try. Even if the baby takes the food eagerly, small amounts should be given to keep a sufficient appetite for milk.

The parent should heat a small amount to serve the infant. Food that has been heated and not consumed should be discarded to prevent possible contamination with salivary enzymes and bacteria. Food that has been opened but not heated can be stored in the covered jar in the refrigerator if it will be used in 2 to 3 days. A commonly used schedule for introducing new foods appears in Table 12–2. The baby's physician may modify this to meet individual needs.

This is a critical time in the infant's life. Eating adult foods is a skill that the baby must learn. However, the foods must be items the infant can chew and swallow safely. See Clinical Application 12–5 for tips on how to avoid choking accidents.

Weaning the Infant

Teaching the infant to use a cup is a gradual process. Often the baby will show an interest in the cup at 4 to 6 months. For these early experiments water can be offered.

Most mothers will begin serious weaning when the breast-fed infant is 7 to 8 months old. The best advice is to wean the child to formula and not to unmodified cow's milk.

The bottle-fed infant may not be ready to give up the bottle until 12 to 14 months of age. If bedtime bottles have not been used, weaning will proceed more rapidly.

It is best to change one feeding period at a time. Use the new schedule for 5 days or so, and then substitute the new method for a second feeding. Allowing the infant to set the pace will make the task easier.

CLINICAL APPLICATION 12–5

Avoiding Choking Accidents

Each year several hundred infants are asphyxiated by food. This is a hazard for older children as well. On average, one death every 5 days is reported in children from infancy to 9 years of age.

Hot dogs, or frankfurters, are involved most often. Hot dogs, apples, cookies, and biscuits cause choking most often in infants. Peanuts and grapes are the most dangerous for 2-year-old children, while 3-year-olds still face a risk from hot dogs.

Other foods that are often implicated in choking accidents are listed below. Because there are many other foods the child can eat safely, the prudent course is to avoid all of the foods listed. If a choking incident occurs, any caregiver needs to be able to administer cardiopulmonary resuscitation (CPR) should it become necessary. Training in CPR should be sought by all parents or parents-to-be. Small children should always be supervised while they are eating.

Hard shaped Foods	Stringy Foods	Sticky Foods	Plug Foods
Apples	Beans	Bread	Grapes
Carrots	Celery	Chewing gum	Hot dogs
Cookies		Peanut butter	
Corn			
Hard candy			
Nuts			
Peanuts			
Popcorn			
Raisins			
Raw vegetables			
Seedy items (e.g., watermelon)			

TABLE 12–3   Nutritional Problems in Infancy

Problem	Intervention	Comments
Regurgitation	Handle baby gently. Burp well; sit up after feeding.	Very common for first 6 months; not serious unless vomiting is projectile or bile-tinged.
Hiccoughs	Offer water to drink. Continue regular feedings.	May be caused by swallowed air.
Constipation	1/2 oz prune juice with 1/2 oz water; or 1/2 tsp dark corn syrup per feeding	Rare in breast-fed infants.
Burns to mouth	Shake formula after heating; test well.	Formula warmed in microwave oven continues to increase in temperature after removal.
Nursing-bottle syndrome	Do not use milk or juice as bedtime bottle. Do not put sweetener on pacifier.	See Clinical Application 3–1.

Special challenges are encountered by health care providers attempting to teach Western child care ways to immigrants. Learning the mothers' beliefs, carefully monitoring the infants' progress, and adapting advice to balance culturally mandated practices are appropriate strategies (Thomas, and de Santis, 1995).

Nutritional Problems in Infancy

Iron-deficiency anemia is the most prevalent nutritional deficiency in children in the United States. Other problems related to nutrition are allergies, cow's milk protein-induced intestinal injury, colic, and diarrhea. Additional problems of nutrition in infancy are summarized in Table 12–3. Some home remedies are included. If the infant does not improve rapidly, however, medical attention should be sought.

Iron-Deficiency Anemia

Sometimes a child drinks so much milk that he or she does not take in enough iron-rich foods. The result is iron-deficiency anemia.

OCCURRENCE   It is estimated that 24 percent of children between the ages of 6 months and 2 years have iron-deficiency anemia. This deficiency is ten times more prevalent in poor families than those with a higher socioeconomic status. In Great Britain, Asian children seem to have a higher prevalence than white children, possibly because the luxury status of milk in some tropical countries leads parents to overvalue its benefit to children (Duggan, 1993).

EARLY DIAGNOSIS   To be sure that iron deficiency is diagnosed promptly in infants and toddlers, routine monitoring of the hemoglobin level is necessary through the infant's second birthday. Normal hemoglobin levels are 14 to 24 grams per 100

milliliters in the newborn, 10 to 15 grams per 100 milliliters in the infant.

TREATMENT OF IRON-DEFICIENCY ANEMIA   Treatment may be medication, iron-fortified foods, and/or foods naturally high in iron. Treatment should produce a normal hemoglobin level in 1 to 2 months (Deglin, and Vallerand, 1995). Red meats, especially liver, are high in iron. The parent should offer the iron-rich foods at the beginning of the meal when the infant is hungry. After the baby has eaten the strained or pureed foods, breast milk or formula may be given.

To help prevent iron-deficiency anemia, tea should only be offered to a child after the first birthday, if at all. As little as 1 cup of tea per day decreases the absorption of iron from both plant sources and milk in 6- to 12-month-old infants. (Merhav, et al, 1985).

A number of special circumstances make vitamin and/or mineral supplementation desirable. Some of these situations appear in Table 12–4.

Allergies

Introducing certain foods too early increases the likelihood of allergies developing.

COMMON FOOD ALLERGENS IN INFANCY   An **allergen** is a substance that provokes an abnormal, individual hypersensitivity. One common allergen is cow's milk protein. Although it affects only 1 to 3 percent of children, an allergy to cow's milk can be a big problem for the affected families. Special formulas without cow's milk protein are available.

Allergen—A substance that provokes an abnormal, individual hypersensitivity.

TABLE 12–4 Vitamin-Mineral Supplementation for Infants

	Prescribed for	Situation
Vitamin		
D	Breast-fed infants	If sunlight exposure to head, arms, hands is less than 1 hour per week
E	Premature infants	See Clinical Application 12–4.
K	All infants	Given immediately before birth to mother or after birth to baby
C	2-week-old formula-fed infants, if vitamin is not in formula	Synthetic preferable to juices. Orange juice, especially, may be allergen.
Folic acid	Evaporated milk formula-fed infant	Sterilizing heat destroys folic acid.
B$_{12}$	Breast-fed if mother is strict vegetarian	
Minerals		
Calcium	Premature	See Clinical Application 12–4.
Phosphorus	Premature	See Clinical Application 12–4.
Iron	When birth weight has doubled	Iron-fortified formula is available.
Fluoride	All, shortly after birth, unless fluoride is in water used for formula or in supplemental fluid given breast-fed infant.	Fluoride is not secreted in breast milk.

The identification of allergies to orange juice has stimulated a major change in infant feeding. Formerly, infants were given orange juice as the first food to complement evaporated milk formulas. However, there is enough vitamin C in both breast milk and commercial formulas to prevent scurvy. Currently, if additional vitamin C is needed, a synthetic product is usually prescribed to avoid the allergens in orange juice.

Wheat protein and egg-white protein can also be allergens to infants. Other foods that have caused allergies in infants are peanut butter, other nuts, and chocolate. Peanuts and peanut products are probably the leading cause of fatal and near fatal **anaphylaxis** caused by food (Sampson, 1996). Of special concern are hidden ingredients in mixed products and contamination from a prior batch of food on the processing line.

SIGNS AND SYMPTOMS   Allergies to foods may produce signs and symptoms beyond the gastrointestinal tract. Food allergies can cause skin and respiratory problems. The infant may have **hives,** eczema, or other rashes; asthma, bronchitis, wheezing; or a runny nose, called allergic rhinitis.

The signs and symptoms of food allergies may appear as long as 5 days after exposure to the allergen. Thus, if 5 days are allowed to elapse between the introduction of each new food, chances are that the allergen will be identified more readily. In some cases involving older children or adults, the allergen may be inhaled from cooking vapors rather than in-

gested (Garcia-Ortiz, 1995). (See Box 12–2 for a discussion of cross-sensitivity to latex among persons allergic to various foods.)

TREATMENT OF ALLERGIES   It is easier to prevent allergies than to diagnose and treat them. If there is a family history of allergies, the best course may be for the mother to breast-feed and to avoid common allergens in her diet. Ironically, the soy formula used to treat children allergic to cow's milk protein also can cause allergies. A longer delay before introducing common allergy-provoking foods is wise for families with histories of allergies.

Many infants outgrow these food sensitivities by age 1 or 2. It is important not to permanently exclude foods from the diet based on the first year's experience. The physician should be reminded of the diet limitation so that an appropriate time can be chosen to reintroduce the offending foods. An exception is allergy to peanuts and other nuts, which is rarely outgrown (Sampson, 1996).

Cow's Milk Protein-Induced Intestinal Injury

Approximately 1 percent of infants incur intestinal injury from cow's milk protein. The signs include failure to thrive, fever, vomiting, diarrhea that may test positive for blood, and anemia resulting from the blood loss. Treatment consists of removing cow's milk protein from the diet, possibly until age 2. Gluten-containing foods should also be removed from the diet if the intestinal injury is severe. Other

---

BOX 12–2   LATEX ALLERGIES AND FOOD HYPERSENSITIVITY

Individuals allergic to latex have demonstrated hypersensitivity to foods botanically unrelated to latex. Among the fruits identified are: avacado, chestnut, banana, kiwi, papaya, and fig. Anaphylaxis occurred in many of those cases (Blanco, et al, 1994; Llatser, Zambrano, and Guillaumet, 1994). Latex allergy should be ruled out in individuals allergic to any of those goods before performing clinical procedures utilizing latex gloves (Rodriquez, et al, 1993).

---

foods often causing symptoms in these children, citrus fruits, chocolate, eggs, nuts, peas, and fish, are avoided until age 2 (Savilahti, 1981).

Colic

An estimated 10 to 20 percent of infants experience colic (Jacobson, and Melvin, 1995). Infantile colic frustrates parents but generally resolves by the time the baby is 3 months old. The infant with colic is unhappy and fussy. It may cry for hours, starting late in the afternoon, just when its caregivers are also tired and cranky.

POSSIBLE CAUSES   Any time multiple, diverse treatments are proposed, it is likely that the basic cause of a condition is unknown. This is the case with colic. Spasms of the muscles of the colon are blamed, hence the name colic. The baby's abdomen is tense and its legs are drawn up to the abdomen. Distention may result from swallowing air. The pain seems to be relieved by the passage of gas or flatus.

For the bottle-fed baby the nipple holes may be too big or too small, increasing the amount of air swallowed. If the infant is overfed, bacteria will ferment the excess milk in the intestine, forming gas.

The breast-fed infant might be swallowing air because of incorrect nursing position. Breast-fed infants seem to get gas from some of the same foods that give adults gas. Garlic, onion, broccoli, brussels sprouts, cabbage, and sauerkraut intake by the mother have all been suggested as contributing to infantile colic. Other foods that may cause problems, particularly if eaten in excess, are pickles, nuts, berries, citrus fruits, and chocolate. It is also possible that the baby may be allergic to antigens in the mother's milk. In one study, colic stopped when the breast-feeding mother stopped drinking cow's milk.

Other contributing factors may include fatigue or chilliness in the baby or tensions or emotional upsets in the mother. Compared to mothers of noncolicky infants, mothers of infants with colic were more bothered by the infants' temperament and were more likely to characterize the infants as difficult (Jacobson, and Melvin, 1995). Allergies or lactose intolerance should be ruled out first.

TREATMENT OF COLIC   Because of the lack of knowledge as to specific causes, many treatments have been devised. Holding the baby upright, burping, or giving it some warm water sometimes helps. Diluting the formula or offering cold formula has been successful with some babies. Other interventions reported to soothe colicky infants are swaddling, carrying the infant, using a pacifier, rocking, and soft repetitive sounds (Jacobson, and Melvin, 1995).

Even though their baby's condition is stressful for them, the parents should try not to be overly concerned. Most infants grow and gain weight despite the colic and colic usually disappears with or without treatment at about 3 months of age.

Diarrhea

Seventy-five percent of an infant's body weight is water, 54 percent of it extracellular. For this reason, an infant is at special risk of rapid dehydration from diarrhea.

CAUSES OF DIARRHEA   Infants are subject to osmotic diarrhea. Overfeeding and food intolerances are common causes of diarrhea. Apple juice may produce diarrhea in infants, owing to carbohydrate malabsorption. Zinc deficiency is being investigated as contributing to diarrhea in developing countries (Sazawal, et al, 1995).

PATHOPHYSIOLOGY   As a result of diarrhea, the wall of the intestine may become inflamed. This diminishes the amount of lactase produced, so the infant

---

Hives (urticaria)—Sudden swelling and itching of skin or mucous membranes, often caused by allergies; if the respiratory tract is involved, may be life-threatening.

exhibits a temporary lactose intolerance. Distension, cramps, and osmotic diarrhea ensue.

TREATMENT OF DIARRHEA Electrolyte solutions, discussed in Chapter 9, "Water and Body Fluids," are life-saving not only in developing countries but also in North America. New hypotonic oral rehydration solutions are being tested (Penny, and Lanata, 1995). An infant should take 120 milliliters of fluid per kilogram of body weight per day plus an amount equal to the liquid lost in the stools. Liquids at room temperature are often better tolerated than warm or cold beverages. This intake should maintain fluid balance unless the insensible water losses due to fever or environmental heat or humidity are excessive. Loss of 5 percent of body weight indicates dehydration and demands medical attention.

After 12 hours, if the diarrhea seems to be lessening, half-strength formula can be offered. If the diarrhea returns, the infant may have developed a temporary lactase insufficiency. Lactose-free formula may be needed.

WHEN TO CALL THE PHYSICIAN Although diarrhea is common in infants, it can be life-threatening. A parent should seek medical treatment immediately if the child has lost 5 percent of body weight, the diarrhea amounts to ten or more stools in 24 hours or is marked by a large volume of fluid loss. Other signs requiring immediate medical attention are a fever of 101°F or higher, vomiting, or a lack of improvement after 24 hours of home care.

Nutrition in Childhood

Childhood covers the growth periods of the toddler (1 to 3 years), the preschool child (3 to 6 years), and the school-age child (6 to 12 years). Fortunately, the child's nutritional needs become more like those of adults after the first birthday.

Nutrition of the Toddler

The toddler is 1 to 3 years old. During these years growth is slower and, although activity increases, the need for kilocalories decreases compared with infancy. So the child's appetite slackens.

Nevertheless, the child has to eat. How and what the family eats will influence the child's tastes for many years. How family members treat one another and the toddler at mealtimes and at other times is more important than the precise amount of food the toddler swallows at each meal.

Psychosocial Development

The psychosocial development task of the toddler is to build **autonomy,** or independence. The child still lives a sheltered life. Parents must take the toddler to playmates or bring playmates home.

Between 1 and 3 years come the "terrible twos." In Erikson's terms the child is learning to be autonomous. Every 2-year-old knows the word "No." One way parents can assist the toddler to achieve autonomy is to encourage choices from acceptable alternatives. See Figure 12–3. If the parent insists on the consumption of certain items, the child may learn to use food rejection as a means of gaining attention. Later, more serious eating problems may result from such interactions.

Physical Growth and Development

During toddler years, growth slows. The expected weight gain in the second year may be just 4 to 6 pounds. Height may increase by about 4 inches. By age 2, though, head circumference reaches two-thirds of its final size and the brain cells stop reproducing.

The toddler is aptly named. One of the skills being acquired during this time is walking upright. As this skill is being perfected, the child's muscles of the back, buttocks, and thighs are enlarging. The bones are becoming more mineralized and baby fat is disappearing.

Along with the gross motor skill of walking, the toddler's fine motor control improves. Eating utensils can be used with more finesse. The spoon is likely to reach the mouth still filled with food.

The toddler's mouth is more sensitive than an adult's mouth. Foods are eaten better at lukewarm temperatures rather than hot. Thus, dawdling at the table may have a physiological basis.

Nutrition Fundamentals

The toddler needs all the essential nutrients. The need for many nutrients increases proportionately with body size throughout the growth years. These needs, plus the poorer appetite and behavior patterns of toddlers, stretch the parents' ingenuity and patience.

FOOD LIKES Toddlers like finger foods. From a variety of finger foods, the child learns about texture. Toddlers prefer plain foods to most mixtures. Familiar combinations, though, may be relished. Some popular dishes are macaroni and cheese, spaghetti, and pizza.

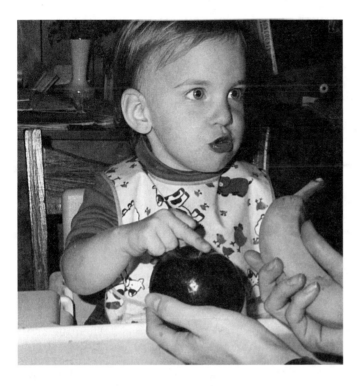

FIGURE 12–3 Autonomy is achieved in small steps. This 19-month-old girl is choosing her dessert.

MEALTIMES   Toddlers are learning social skills as well as good nutritional habits. Eating is a social experience for adults most of the time; toddlers appreciate company also. Visiting other homes might introduce food items and experiences not encountered at home.

Keeping to a regular schedule will help maintain the child's intake. A 1-year-old's stomach holds just 1 cup. Eating regular meals and nutritious snacks helps to avoid fatigue and controls the appetite. However, if high-sugar snacks are used to assuage hunger before a meal, the more nutritious foods at the meal may be taken poorly.

NEW FOODS   After the pureed foods of infancy, parents will be pleased to offer more attractive plates to the toddler. Brightly colored foods are appealing. Nevertheless, chewing may not be well developed. Tough meat is not for the toddler. Grinding the meat several times may make it safer and easier to eat.

All of the foods that were not recommended until after the first birthday can be gradually introduced. These include unmodified cow's milk, egg white, wheat, citrus fruits, seafood, chocolate, and nut butters. The careful parent will continue to introduce foods one at a time and watch for reactions.

Because of the toddler's small stomach capacity, small servings are all that can be tolerated. A serving is one fourth to one fifth the size of an adult serving. A good rule of thumb is to serve 1 tablespoonful for each year of age.

Daily intake should include one serving of a vitamin C-rich fruit or vegetable and one serving of a green leafy or yellow vegetable. Difficult as it may be, the parent should limit sugar and encourage consumption of fiber in cereals as well as in other foods. Iron-enriched cereals are the best choices.

Offering three meals and three nutritious snacks daily will increase the likelihood of the toddler obtaining sufficient nourishment. Because there are so many choices, the wise parent will avoid hazardous foods (review Clinical Application 12–5). Sometimes all that is necessary is chopping the food into very tiny pieces. Still, the toddler who is eating should not be left alone.

Because the kidneys become mature about age 1, the toddler can tolerate salt in moderation. The liking for salty foods is an acquired taste. Because of the association between salt and high blood pressure later in life, the prudent parent will discourage the consumption of heavily salted foods.

MILK AND FAT INTAKE   Because iron-deficiency anemia is common in toddlers, milk intake may have to be curtailed to no more than 1 quart per day to maintain the appetite for iron-enriched cereals, meats, and iron-rich fruits and vegetables. The term "milk anemia" refers to iron deficiency anemia caused by overconsumption of milk and underconsumption of iron-rich foods.

The American Academy of Pediatrics recommended the adult proportions of fat and cholesterol for children over 2 years of age. In contrast, the Canadian Pediatric Society recommended tapering fat intake from 50 percent of kilocalories at age 2 to 30 percent by the end of adolescence (Olson, 1995).

Nutrition of the Preschool Child

The preschool child requires all the nutrients necessary for other human beings. This is a delightful time of enthusiastic learning, much of which concerns food, since it is consumed every day.

Psychosocial Development

Erikson's theory postulates **initiative** as the psychosocial task to be mastered by the preschool child. Within their capabilities, children should be encouraged to set and achieve some goals of their own. Children can participate in planning and preparation of meals. They should be prompted to help in the kitchen, but not just with the cleanup. Preschool children love to make fancy cookies and showy relishes. Making even simple things like gelatin desserts gives the child a sense of accomplishment.

By making the meal a social time and eating slowly themselves, parents can encourage the same behavior in the child. Exemplifying good manners will be more productive than criticizing the child's manners. Having company their own age is helpful. Children have been observed to stay at the table longer and to eat more in the company of their peers. Exchanging visits with a friend's child will begin to broaden the child's horizons.

Physical Growth and Development

From the third to the sixth year, a child continues to gain 4 to 5 pounds per year. A gain in height of about 2 inches per year is average. Adequacy of growth should be assessed every 6 to 12 months. Growth charts remain the standard against which a given assessment is judged.

Nutrition Fundamentals

Preschool children are very active. A 3-year-old may need 1300 to 1500 kilocalories per day. But the child may have little appetite.

An adaptation of the Food Pyramid for preschoolers appears in Table 12–5. A serving of meat, fruit, or vegetable is 1 tablespoonful per year of age. A serving of breads and cereals is a half to one slice of bread or 1/2 cup of cereal or pasta. A serving of milk is still 1 cup.

DEVELOPING GOOD HABITS   The preschool child responds best to regular mealtimes. When the adult meal will be served late, the parents have to decide if it would be better to allow the child to socialize with adults at a late meal or to feed the child early.

But these children, like the toddlers, cannot eat enough in only three meals to meet their needs. By age 3, a child is able to verbalize hunger. A good supply of wholesome snacks will serve the conscientious parent well. Such items as cottage cheese, low-fat yogurt, fresh fruit, raw vegetables, milk, fruit juices, graham crackers, or fig bars all are nutrient dense and low in fat. So long as the parent still has control over the child's world, concentrated sweets such as candy and soda pop should be strictly limited.

Tableware appropriate for the preschool child will ease tensions during mealtimes. Unbreakable dishes

TABLE 12–5   Food Pyramid for the Preschool Child

Food Group	Number of Servings	Serving Suggestions
Bread/Cereal	Six or more	Select whole-grain breads and iron-fortified cereals.
Fruit	Two or more	Include 4 oz of orange juice or other food high in vitamin C.
Vegetable	Three or more	Include one vegetable high in vitamin A. Crisp-cooked, warm rather than hot vegetables preferred.
Meat	Two servings	Child-size servings of red meat is essential for RBC synthesis.
Milk	Three servings	Not to be overdone at expense of blood-forming nutrients. Low-fat milks are now permissible.

that are designed for stability, with deep sides to permit scooping the food onto a spoon or fork, are a practical choice. Small glasses and cups, also unbreakable, with a squat design and low center of gravity, will serve the child's and the parents' needs well.

It is not too early to emphasize the importance of cleanliness. Regularly washing hands before meals and brushing teeth after meals will cultivate good health habits.

NEW FOODS As with younger children, new foods should be offered one at a time in small amounts. Trying something new is most acceptable at the beginning of the meal when the child is hungriest. A taste or two is sufficient if new foods are offered at regular intervals.

Parents have the advantage over their children of being able to select the food. Items the parents dislike will not regularly grace the family table. Children, too, should be permitted their preferences. This advice is not permissive, just practical. If an argument over food develops into a power struggle, as sometimes happens, the child will never admit to liking it, even when it turns out to be quite tasty.

Nutritional Problems

Iron-deficiency anemia continues to be a significant problem for children of this age. The other concern is that of dental caries.

IRON-DEFICIENCY ANEMIA Children in low-income families are particularly subject to iron-deficiency anemia. Black and Hispanic children in the United States have been found to be low in iron, vitamin C, and vitamin A. Fortunately, the situation is improving. In 1985, 3 percent of the 6-month to 6-year-old children in low-income households were anemic compared with 8 percent in 1975. This change is attributed to the Women, Infants, and Children's Program (WIC). The WIC program provides specific goods and nutritional services to low-income pregnant women and young children.

DENTAL CARIES The destruction of tooth enamel by dental caries, discussed in Chapter 3, "Carbohydrates," is a problem for all economic groups. The "baby" teeth, as well as the permanent teeth, deserve care and professional attention. Brushing the teeth correctly may mean that the parent has to do it. Regular dental checkups should be a part of the preschool child's routine. Adequate dentition supports good nutrition.

SPECIAL ASSESSMENT TECHNIQUES Box 12–3 shows a nutrition screening tool for use with children up to 6 years old. The questionnaire is filled out by the primary caregiver to help identify probable nutrition problems.

Nutrition of the School-Age Child

By this time, few modifications in foodstuffs are necessary to accommodate the child. A balanced diet suitable for adults, emphasizing protein, vitamins, and minerals will also be good for a school-age child.

Psychosocial Development

The developmental task of the school-age child is to develop **industry.** These are the years to build competence in many different skills. School work, sports, hobbies, and chores at home permit the child to recognize the worth of work. Making and keeping commitments is part of this learning process.

The school-age child can participate in planning menus, shopping for food, preparing the meals, and cleaning up afterwards. See Figure 12–4. As with younger children, limiting the child to a scullery role will be more likely to foster a sense of inferiority than habits of industry.

Basic dietary habits are formed by the time a child enters school. Peer-group acceptance and approval is very important. Interactions with other children and school experiences expose a child to different foods and different cultures.

Growth and Health

By age 6, the child should weigh twice as much as at age 1. Suppose that our 7-pound infant who weighed 21 pounds at 1 year gained 5 pounds in the second year and 4 pounds per year through age 6. At age 6, the child would weigh 42 pounds, an amount that is twice the 1-year weight.

By school age, the effects of good or poor nutrition will begin to be apparent. The well-nourished child will display most of the qualities listed in Table 12–6. The poorly nourished child will be lacking in a significant number of these qualities.

Nutrition Fundamentals

School-age children, especially those 8 to 10 years old, generally have good appetites and they like almost all foods. However, vegetables are the least liked of the food groups. A new recommendation for fiber intake during childhood and adolescence is age plus 5 grams per day. Sixty-five percent of 6- to

BOX 12–3   A NUTRITION SCREENING TOOL FOR YOUNG CHILDREN

The PEACH Survey consists of 17 "yes" or "no" questions carrying weights from 1 to 4. It is designed to be self-administered by a child's primary caregiver. The tool was validated on children from birth to age 5 against a pediatric dietitian's assessment. A score of 4 or more indicates a probable nutrition problem.

PEACH* Survey

Agency: _____   Date: _____

Child's Name: _____   Date of Birth: _____

Address: _____   Phone #: _____

_____

Please circle YES or NO for each question as it applies to your child.

Does your child have a health problem (do **not** include colds or flu)? If yes, what is it?	YES NO	1
Is your child: Small for age: _____ Too thin? _____ Too heavy? _____ (If you check any of the above, please circle YES)	YES NO	3
Does your child have feeding problems? If yes, what are they?	YES NO	3
Is your child's appetite a problem? If yes, describe:	YES NO	1
Is your child on a special diet? If yes, what type of diet?	YES NO	2
Does your child take medicine for a health problem (Do **not** include vitamins, iron, or fluoride)? Name of medicine(s):	YES NO	1
Does your child have food allergies? If yes, to what foods?	YES NO	1
Does your child use a feeding tube or other special feeding method? If yes, explain:	YES NO	4
Circle YES if your child does **not** eat any of these foods: Milk __ Meats __ Vegetables __ Fruits __ (Check all that apply)	YES NO	1
Circle YES if your child has problems with: Sucking __ Swallowing __ Chewing __ Gagging __ (Check all that apply)	YES NO	3
Circle YES if your child has problems with: Loose stools __ Hard stools __ Throwing Up __ Spitting Up __ (Check all that apply)	YES NO	3
Does your child eat clay, paint chips, dirt, or any other things that are not food? If yes, what?	YES NO	2
Does your child refuse to eat, throw food, or do other things that upset you at mealtime? If yes, explain:	YES NO	2
For infants **under 12 months** who are bottle fed. Does your child drink less than 3 (8-ounce) bottles of milk per day:	YES NO	1
For children **over 12 months**: (Check if applies and cirlce the YES) Is your child **not** using a cup? __ Is your child **not** finger feeding? __	YES NO	1
For children **over 18 months**: Does your child still take most liquids from a bottle?	YES NO	2
Circle YES if your child is **not** using a spoon?	YES NO	2

Total = ☐

The Parent Eating and Nutrition Assessment for Children with Special Health Needs (PEACH) survey

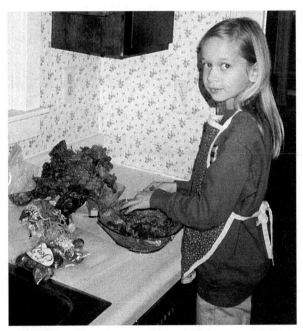

FIGURE 12–4 After-school chores could include making the salad for dinner.

11-year-old children consume less than this amount (Williams, 1995).

Breakfast is very important. The child needs energy and other nutrients to last until lunch. Breakfast should contain one-fourth to one-third of the day's nutrients. Research has demonstrated a positive effect of breakfast on thinking especially in children at nutritional risk (Pollitt, 1995).

The school-age child needs adequate protein intake for developing muscle and laying down bone matrix. Calcium is necessary to build dense bones. The body anticipates the adolescent growth spurt. The greatest retention of calcium and phosphorus precedes the rapid growth of adolescence by 2 years or more. Therefore, a liberal intake of milk and milk products before the age of 10 gives a child a great advantage. Calcium supplementation increased bone density 3 to 5 percent over 3 years in prepubertal twins compared to their identical twins receiving placebos (Johnston, et al, 1992).

Exercise

Exercise can help the school-age child achieve growth and development in several areas. Weight-bearing exercise stimulates the osteoblasts, the bone-building cells. Exercise balances intake and activity for weight control. Conversely, lack of exercise and excessive time spent watching television have been correlated with fatness. If long hours spent with television are accompanied by consumption of multiple snacks, the risk for obesity rises greatly. Exercise, especially team sports, fosters interactions with peers. Activities that are likely to become lifetime interests should be especially encouraged. Not many adults play football. A skill at tennis, though, may provide an outlet for many years.

Problem Areas

School-age children are generally so active that they may have trouble sitting still. Requiring 15 to 20 minutes at the table for meals will increase the likelihood of a complete meal being eaten. One study found 10 percent of school-age children skipped breakfast.

One study reported 6- to 10-year-old children received at least the RDA for all nutrients surveyed and consumed more than 200 percent of the RDAs for protein, vitamin C, folate, and vitamin B_{12} (Devaney, Gordon, and Burghardt, 1995).

Some children are bothered by caffeine. Eight ounces of hot chocolate or 12 ounces of cola contain 50 milligrams of caffeine. Two such beverages in a

TABLE 12–6 Indications of Good Nutrition in the School-Age Child

General appearance	Alert, energetic
	Normal height and weight
Skin and mucous membranes	Skin smooth, slightly moist; mucous membranes pink, no bleeding
Hair	Shiny, evenly distributed
Scalp	No sores
Eyes	Bright, clear, no fatigue circles
Teeth	Straight, clean, no discoloration or caries
Tongue	Pink, papillae present, no sores
Gastrointestinal system	Good appetite, regular elimination
Musculoskeletal system	Well-developed, firm muscles; erect posture, bones straight without deformities
Neurological system	Good attention span for age; not restless, irritable, or weepy

60-pound child are the equivalent of 8 cups of coffee in a 175-pound man. If the child has difficulty sleeping or has an irregular pulse, the first factor to investigate is caffeine intake.

In contrast, little scientific evidence exists to link sugar consumption to hyperactivity (Kinsbourne, 1994; Wolraich, et al, 1994; Wolraich, Wilson, and White, 1995). Some few children might be adversely affected, but widespread occurrence has been disproved.

Nutrition in Adolescence

Adolescence is the period that extends from the onset of **puberty** until full growth is reached. For most individuals, adolescence occurs between the ages of 12 and 20. Adolescence is second only to infancy in the nutritional requirements necessary for normal growth and development.

Psychosocial Development

The developmental task of adolescents is to achieve their own **identity,** including accepting their capabilities. In this process, teenagers "try on" various identities. Peers exert a major influence on a teenager's decisions. Adolescents pick up fads instantly and drop them just as suddenly. Food fads are part of the same pattern.

Physical Growth and Development

The term *growth spurt* is accurate. A teenager who may seem not to grow as much as others the same age will suddenly sprout like a weed, seemingly overnight. Boys and girls differ in the timing and completion of the growth spurt. Table 12–7 summarizes adolescent growth spurts. Growth is not completed at ages 15 to 19, only the growth spurt.

Zinc is essential for male sexual maturation. Before a person eliminates red meat from the diet he or she should consider the best sources of zinc—shellfish and red meat.

TABLE 12–7 Adolescent Growth Spurts

	Age in Years	
Status	Boys	Girls
Begins	12 to 13	10 to 11
Peaks	14	12
Completed	19	15

Nutrient Needs of the Adolescent

Because of their growing and developing bodies, adolescents need more energy, vitamins, and protein than the school-age child or the adult.

Energy

The adolescent may require 60 to 80 kilocalories per kilogram of body weight per day. This amounts to 2700 to 3600 kilocalories for a 100-pound teenager. Boys need more kilocalories than girls. A 15-year-old girl requires 2100 kilocalories compared to a 15-year-old boy's requirement of 3000 kcalories. The boy may be in a growth spurt, whereas the girl has probably completed hers.

Vitamins and Minerals

Emotional or physical stress can increase the utilization of vitamin C by three or four times.

The adolescent athlete may need up to 6000 kilocalories per day. Thiamin and niacin are related to energy expenditure and riboflavin is needed for protein utilization. Therefore, the need for these B-vitamins is increased in the athlete. A training table laden with extra whole-grain or enriched bread and milk, should meet these vitamin needs. High-school athletes seem more likely to use vitamin and mineral supplements than other teenagers (Sobal, and Marquart, 1994). Teaching or counseling may be indicated to increase the likelihood of informed decision making.

Fiber

Adolescents 12 to 18 years old are the least likely age group to meet the "age plus 5" level of fiber intake. Seventy-seven percent of boys and 89 percent of girls consumed less than this amount (Williams, 1995).

Food Pyramid Modification

The adolescent diet should consist of the adult distribution of foods except that three servings of milk or milk products should be ingested. Since one fourth the adolescent's kilocalories come from snacks, these "between-meal meals" should be nutritionally dense and chosen to balance the diet.

Problem Areas

Both adolescent boys and adolescent girls surveyed exceeded 200 percent of the RDAs for vitamins C and B_{12}. Boys also exceeded 200 percent of the

RDAs for protein and sodium. Girls reported less than the RDA for calcium, 87 percent for 11 to 14 year olds, and 80 percent for 15 to 18 year olds (Devaney, Gordon, and Burgherdt, 1995). The RDAs are appropriate standards for population groups, but not individuals. Two common nutritional problems of teenagers are overenthusiastic weight control and poor choices of foods.

Reduction Diets

Adolescents with BMIs greater than 30 should be referred for medical diagnosis and follow-up (Himes, and Dietz, 1994). However, many dieting teens are not overweight. Self-prescribed reduction diets are common among American women and girls. Unfortunately, Americans are lured by the "quick fix," promising instant results. Most often the diet consultants who promise quick results do so with an unbalanced diet. The weight control chapter addresses principles of safe weight reduction as well as bulimia and anorexia nervosa.

Poor Choices of Foods

Fast-food restaurant chains have made remarkable changes in their selections. They are now offering items such as salads, lower fat salad dressings, and low-fat milks. There are some healthy choices possible. However, the old standbys on the fast-food menus are generally higher in kilocalories, fat, sugar, and sodium than are similar items prepared at home.

As undesirable as a steady diet of fast food might be, it cannot be blamed for causing acne. About 80 percent of adolescents suffer from acne, starting about age 12 to 13 in girls and 14 to 15 in boys. Acne is caused by sex hormones stimulating the sebaceous glands. The skin becomes oilier and the ducts to the glands sometimes plug up, permitting the accumulation of harmful bacteria. There is as yet no convincing evidence that dietary indiscretions cause acne.

Summary

During periods of rapid growth the need for nutrients is critical. The lack of nutrients or the excessive intake of certain substances during such periods may cause serious, permanent damage in the individual.

While infants require the same nutrients as adults, they need them in different amounts. Breast milk is especially suited to the human infant because the protein, fat, and carbohydrate in breast milk are tailored to the infant's digestive capabilities. After the age of 4 months, semisolid and then solid foods are added to the diet gradually. Nutritional problems in infancy include iron-deficiency anemia, allergies, colic, and diarrhea.

Childhood includes the growth periods of the toddler, the preschool child, and the school-age child. Growth and development during childhood are not as rapid as during infancy. However, total amounts of nutrients recommended continue to increase with age so that the body's needs are met. Toddlers and preschoolers often develop iron-deficiency anemia.

During adolescence, the final growth spurt of childhood occurs. Physical growth and development are rapid and sexual maturity is attained. Energy, protein, vitamins, and minerals are needed in increasing amounts. Adolescent girls often lack enough calcium in their diets. Major problems in adolescents are self-prescribed reduction diets and poor choices of food.

> **Puberty**—Period of life at which the physical ability to reproduce is attained.

Case Study 12–1

Baby L, a 9-month-old girl, is being evaluated in a well-baby clinic. Her birth weight was 8 lb 4 oz. Her present weight is 20 lb 8 oz.

Mrs. L states that the baby is taking 10 oz of formula four times a day. The baby sleeps a lot between feedings. Mrs. L gives the baby cereal or fruit after the formula three times a day. She has not offered the baby vegetables or meats. The formula she is using contains 1 mg of iron per quart.

The nurse notes that Baby L is pale. Her mucous membranes, including the conjunctiva on the lower eyelid, are very light pink. Blood test results show that Baby L's hemoglobin is 8 g per 100 ml.

The physician may prescribe medical interventions. In addition, the nurse begins to implement the following nursing care plan.

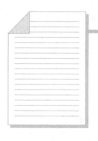

NURSING CARE PLAN FOR BABY L

Assessment

Subjective Data	Inactive for age
	Taking 40 oz of formula per day
	Few solids taken after formula
Objective Data	Pale skin, mucous membranes
	Hemoglobin 8 g per 100 ml

Nursing Diagnosis

Nutrition, altered: less than body requirements
Related to limited access to iron-rich foods as evidenced by pale skin and mucous membranes, hemoglobin 8 g/100 mL

Desired Outcome/ Evaluation Criteria	Nursing Actions	Rationale
Will take one serving of meat per day and one serving of vegetable per day in 3 weeks	Teach Mrs. L to offer semisolid food to Baby L before offering formula.	Offering the semisolid food when the baby is hungry increases the amount consumed.
Will increase hemoglobin to 9 g/100 mL in 3 weeks	Teach Mrs. L to limit Baby L to 32 oz of formula per day.	Limiting the amount of milk the infant takes will increase its appetite for iron-rich foods.
	Instruct Mrs. L to change to the iron-fortified preparation of the baby's formula.	Changing preparations will increase the available iron from 1 mg per quart to 12 mg per quart. The RDA for a 6- to 12-month-old infant is 10 mg.
	Instruct Mrs. L to introduce one iron-rich vegetable or meat to Baby L every 5 days.	Adding iron-rich foods will increase the iron available for absorption. The baby should be taking vegetables and meats, but the 5-day trial period should be maintained to monitor for allergies.

Study Aids

Chapter Review

1. A nurse in a clinic would identify which of the following infants as needing additional assessment of growth?
   a. Baby girl A, 4 months old, birth weight 7 pounds 6 ounces, present weight 14 pounds 14 ounces
   b. Baby boy B, 2 weeks old, birth weight 6 pounds 10 ounces, present weight 6 pounds 11 ounces
   c. Baby boy C, 6 months old, birth weight 8 pounds 8 ounces, present weight 14 pounds 8 ounces
   d. Baby girl D, 2 months old, birth weight 7 pounds 2 ounces, present weight 9 pounds 10 ounces

2. Which of the following are advantages of breast milk that formula does not provide?
   a. Less fat and cholesterol
   b. More antibodies and less risk of allergy
   c. More fluoride and iron
   d. More vitamin C and vitamin D

3. Which of the following combinations of foods are appropriate for a 6-month-old infant?
    a. Cocoa-flavored wheat cereal, orange juice, and strained chicken
    b. Graham crackers, strained prunes, and stewed tomatoes
    c. Infant cereal, mashed banana, and strained squash
    d. Mashed potatoes, strained beets, and chopped hard-cooked egg

4. If a family is following the dietary guidelines of the National Research Council, which of the following is it important not to eliminate from the school-age child's diet?
    a. Caffeine
    b. Fat
    c. Salt
    d. Sugar

5. Which of the following individuals is at greatest nutritional risk?
    a. 3-month-old infant being fed commercial formula
    b. 3-year-old child who drinks 3 cups of milk a day
    c. 8-year-old child who eats four chocolate chip cookies and drinks 2 glasses of milk after school
    d. 16-year-old girl who is pregnant and attempting weight loss

Clinical Analysis

1. Mrs. T is having her 2-month-old son checked in the well-baby clinic. She tells the nurse that the baby is not sleeping through the night yet. Mrs. T's mother advised her to start the infant on cereal to "fill him up" at bedtime. Despite the nurse's instructions, Mrs. T says she is going to try her mother's idea. Which of the following would be most important if Mrs. T chooses to start the cereal?
    a. Following the cereal with a bedtime bottle to wash it down
    b. Making cream of wheat very thin and feeding the baby with an eyedropper
    c. Putting infant cereal into a bottle and enlarging the nipple hole
    d. Using infant rice cereal mixed with formula

2. Ms. C has given a 24-hour dietary recall for her 18-month-old son. The nurse is alert to identify common causes of choking. To avoid choking accidents, which of the following groups of foods would be considered safest for a toddler?

    a. Apple quarters, green beans, and chicken noodle casserole
    b. Grapes, carrot strips, and macaroni and cheese
    c. Diced peaches, mashed potatoes, and spaghetti
    d. Watermelon chunks, cheese-stuffed celery, and sliced frankfurters

3. Ms. K has delivered a 3-pound 8-ounce premature infant. She had planned to breast-feed. Upon which of the following statements should the nurse base her teaching?
    a. Premature infants can sometimes be successfully breast-fed.
    b. Because of their larger proportion of body weight as water, prematures need supplemental water after every feeding.
    c. Formula feeding is advisable because room temperature feedings are better absorbed than those at body temperature.
    d. Breast feeding a premature offers no advantage to the infant and is difficult for the mother because of the necessary supplements.

Bibliography

Beckholt, AP: Breast milk for infants who cannot breastfeed. JOGNN 19:216, 1990.
Blanco, C, et al: Latex allergy: Clinical features and cross-reactivity with fruits. Ann Allergy 73:309, 1994.
Borowitz, D: Pediatric nutrition. In Feldman, EB: Essentials of Clinical Nutrition. FA Davis Company, Philadelphia, 1988.
Campbell, MK, and Kelsey, KS: The PEACH survey: A nutrition screening tool for use in early intervention programs. J Am Diet Assoc 94:1156, 1994.
Chandra, RK, Puri, S, and Hamed, A: Influence of maternal diet during lactation and use of formula feeds on development of atopic eczema in high risk infants. Br Med J 299:228, 1989.
Deglin, JH, and Vallerand, AH: Davis's Drug Guide for Nurses, ed 4. FA Davis Company, Philadelphia, 1995.
Devaney, BL, Gordon, AR, and Burghardt, JA: Dietary intakes of students. Am J Clin Nutr (suppl) 61:205S, 1995.
Dewey, KG, et al: Growth of breast-fed and formula-fed infants from 0 to 18 months: The DARLING study. Pediatrics 89:1035, 1992.
Duggan, MB: Cause and cure for iron deficiency in toddlers. Health Visitor 66:250, 1993.
Ewan, PW: Clinical study of peanut and nut allergy in 62 consecutive patients: new features and associations. Br Med J 312:1074, 1996.
Fergusson, DM, Horwood, LJ, and Shannon, FT: Early solid feeding and recurrent childhood eczema: A 10-year longitudinal study. Pediatrics 86:541, 1990.
Forgac, MT: Timely statement for the American Dietetic Association: Guidelines for healthy children. J Am Diet Assoc 95:370, 1995.
Freed, GL. Breast-feeding, time to teach what we preach. JAMA 269:243, 1993.

Garcia-Ortiz, JC, et al: Bronchial asthma induced by hypersensitivity to legumes. Allergol Immunopathol Madr 23:38, 1995.

Glenn, FB, Glenn, WD, and Duncan, RC: Fluoride tablet supplementation during pregnancy for caries immunity: A study of the offspring produced. Obstet Gynecol 143:560, 1982.

Gonzales, I, et al: Effect of enteral feeding temperature on feeding tolerance of premature infants. Neonatal Network 14:39, 1995.

Graham, MV, and Uphold, CR: Health perceptions and behaviors of school-age boys and girls. Journal of Community Health Nursing 9:77, 1992.

Graham, SM, Arvela, OM, and Wise, GA: Long-term neurologic consequences of nutritional vitamin B_{12} deficiency in infants. J Pediatr 121:710, 1992.

Greene, LC, et al: Relationship between early diet and subsequent cognitive performance during adolescence. Biochemical Society Transactions 23:376S, 1995.

Himes, JH and Dietz, WH: Guidelines for overweight in adolescent services: Recommendations from an expert committee. Am J Clin Nutr 59:307, 1994.

Jacobson, D, and Melvin, N: A comparison of temperament and maternal bother in infants with and without colic. Pediatr Nurs 10:181, 1995.

Jacobsson, I, and Lindberg, T: Cow's milk proteins cause infantile colic in breast-fed infants: A double-blind crossover study. Pediatrics 71:268, 1983.

Johnston, CC, et al: Calcium supplementation and increases in bone mineral density in children. N Engl J Med 327:82, 1992.

Kemp, SF, and Lockey, RF: Peanut anaphylaxis from good cross-contamination [letter]. JAMA 275:1636, 1996.

Kinsbourne, M: Sugar and the hyperactive child. N Engl J Med 330:355, 1994.

Latser, R, Zambrano, C, and Guillaumet, B: Anaphylaxis to natural rubber latex in a girl with food allergy: Pediatrics 94:736, 1994.

Lucas, A, et al: Breast milk and subsequent intelligence quotient in children born preterm. Lancet 339:261, 1992.

Lust, KD, Brown, JE, and Thomas, W: Maternal intake of cruciferous vegetables and other foods and colic symptoms in exclusively breast-fed infants. J Am Diet Assoc 96:46, 1996.

Merhav, H, et al: Tea drinking and microcytic anemia in infants. Am J Clin Nutr 41:1210, 1985.

Moon, A, and Kleinman, RE: Allergic gastroenteropathy in children. Annals of Allergy, Asthma, and Immunology 74:5, 1995.

Morse, JM, et al: The effect of maternal fluid intake on breast milk supply: A pilot study. Can J Public Health 83:213, 1992.

Muecke, L, et al: Is childhood obesity associated with high-fat foods and low physical activity? J Sch Health 62:19, 1992.

Mulford, C: Swimming upstream: Breastfeeding care in a non-breastfeeding culture. JOGNN 24:464, 1995.

Nicklas, TA: Dietary studies of children: The Bogalusa Heart Study experience. J Am Diet Assoc 95:1127, 1995.

Olson, RE: The dietary recommendations of the American Academy of Pediatrics. Am J Clin Nutr 61:271, 1995.

Penny, ME, and Lanata, CF: Zinc in the management of diarrhea in young children. N Engl J Med 333:873, 1995.

Phylactos, AC, et al: Polyunsaturated fatty acids and antioxidants in early development. Possible prevention of oxygen-induced disorders. Eur J Clin Nutr (suppl 2) 48:S17, 1994.

Pollitt, E: Does breakfast make a difference in school? J Am Diet Assoc 95:1134, 1995.

Rodriquez, M, et al: Hypersensitivity to latex, chestnut and banana. Ann Allergy 70:31, 1993.

Saarinen, UM, and Kajosaari, M: Breastfeeding as prophylaxis against atopic disease: Prospective follow-up study until 17 years old. Lancet 346:1065, 1995.

Sampson, HA: Managing peanut allergy. Br Med J 312:1050, 1996.

Savilahti, E: Cow's milk allergy. Allergy 36:73, 1981.

Sobal, J, and Marquart, LF: Vitamin/mineral supplement use among high school athletes. Adolescence 29:835, 1994.

Sturman, JA, and Chesney, RW: Taurine in pediatric nutrition. Pediatr Clin North Am 42:879, 1995.

Thomas, JT, and de Santis, L: Feeding and weaning practices of Cuban and Haitian immigrant mothers. J Transcult Nurs 6:34, 1995.

Thorp, FK, Pierce, P, and Deedwania, C: Nutrition in the infant and young child. In Halpern, SL (ed): Quick Reference to Clinical Nutrition, ed 2. JB Lippincott Company, Philadelphia, 1987.

Tuttle, CR, and Dewey, KG: Impact of a breastfeeding promotion program for Hmong women at selected WIC sites in Northern California. J Nutr Educ 27:69, 1995.

US Department of Health and Human Services: Healthy People 2000. US Department of Health and Human Services, Washington, DC, 1990.

Wharton, BA, Balmer, SE, and Scott, PH: Faecal flora in the newborn. Adv Exp Med Biol 357:91, 1994.

Williams, CL: Importance of dietary fiber in childhood. J Am Diet Assoc 95:1140, 1149, 1995.

Williams, CL, Bollela, M, and Wynder, EL: A new recommendation for dietary fiber in childhood. Pediatrics 96:985, 1995.

Wolraich, ML, et al: Effects of diets high in sucrose or aspartame on the behavior and cognitive performance of children. N Engl J Med 330:301, 1994.

Wolraich, ML, Wilson, DB, and White, JW: The effect of sugar on behavior or cognition in children. JAMA 274:1617, 1995.

Zlotkin, SH, Atkinson, S, and Lockitch, G: Trace elements in nutrition for premature infants. Clin Perinatol 22:223, 1995.

CHAPTER 13

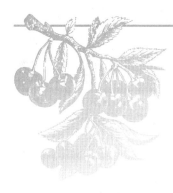

Life Cycle Nutrition:
The Mature Adult

LEARNING OBJECTIVES

After completing this chapter, the student should be able to:

1   Identify the food groups most likely to be lacking in the diets of adults and foods which are often eaten in excess.
2   Describe the changes in the older adult's body that impact nutritional status.
3   Explain how a nutritional assessment of an older adult would differ from that of a younger one.
4   Illustrate ways in which food could be used to aid psychosocial development.
5   List several suggestions to improve food intake for older persons in a variety of living situations.

The life cycle of human growth and development continues throughout the adult years. Both psychosocial and physical development proceeds as a person matures. This chapter discusses the impact on nutrition of the physiological and psychosocial changes that occur during young, middle, and older adult years. Because much of the material in this book is based on the nutritional needs of the average adult, the main focus of this chapter is the older adult. Overall food consumption of Americans poorly matches the Food Pyramid recommendations as Figure 13–1 illustrates. On average, Americans consume about 67 grams of fat (13 1/2 teaspoons) per day, which amounts to 37 percent of their kilocalories (National Live Stock and Meat Board, 1994). All adults averaged more than 34 percent of their kilocalories as fat, between 41 and 49 percent of kilocalories as carbohydrate, and less than 18 percent of kilocalories as protein. Vitamin C intake averaged more than 100 milligrams for all groups (Block, and Subar, 1992). Whites of high socioeconomic status reduced their consumption of high-fat foods (1989–1991 compared to 1965) and followed other dietary guidelines to a greater extent than did either whites or blacks of middle or low socioeconomic status (Popkin, Siega-Riz, and Haines, 1996).

Young Adulthood

We define young adulthood as ages 18 through 39. Not all 18-year-olds are adults, developmentally. Nor are all 40-year-olds middle-aged in thought or behavior. Chronological age is a convenient means of sorting people but has limited applicability to an individual.

Developmental Task of Young Adulthood

When identifying the patient's stage of psychosocial development, chronological age is not as important as a person's life situation. During the early years of young adulthood, the individual may be completing the adolescent task of identity. In many cases, our educational system demands dependency past the age of 18. According to Erikson, the developmental task of young adulthood is **intimacy.** For example, couples who delay commitment to a life partner until their thirties and forties will probably be working at achieving intimacy, whereas other 40-year-old persons may be tackling the task of generativity.

To achieve intimacy, the individual strives to build reciprocal, caring relationships. Intimacy suggests sexuality, but these relationships are not necessarily sexual. Solid friendships are based on intimacy, the revealing of oneself to another. The negative side of intimacy is isolation. Here, perhaps more than with the other developmental tasks it is apparent that a person chooses what he or she is to become.

Nutrition in the Young Adult

Throughout this book, the RDAs for individual nutrients, as well as dietary guidelines, have been specified. The age categories cited in the literature differ from our division into young, middle, and older adulthood. Across all the age groupings, however, most adults do not consume recommended intakes.

Minerals

All the 18- to 34-year-old men averaged at least 14 milligrams of iron daily (RDA is 10). The same age women, however, averaged 9 and 11 milligrams (RDA is 15) with white women the lowest (Block, and Subar, 1992).

Black men and women aged 18 to 34 years old had the lowest calcium intake, averaging less than 800 milligrams daily. It is not discernable from these data if any of these individuals aged 19 to 24 averaged 1200 milligrams of calcium intake, their recommended RDA (Block, and Suba, 1992).

Fat and Fiber

Because fiber is valuable in assisting the excretion of cholesterol, a high-fiber intake would be desirable if cholesterol intake is high. Of 18 to 34 year olds, only white women averaged less than 300 milligrams of cholesterol per day. Only black and Latino men averaged even half the recommended 25 grams of fiber daily (Block, and Subar, 1992).

Fruits and Vegetables

Fruits and vegetables are good sources of fiber as well as vitamins and minerals. Survey data indicates only 6 percent of adults aged 19 to 29 consumed at least two servings of fruit and three servings of vegetables on the day recorded (Patterson, et al, 1990).

Consumption of recommended levels of either fruits or vegetables was slightly better: 25 percent of adults aged 19 to 29 consumed three servings of vegetables, and 22 percent had two servings of fruit. This compares with 27 percent of those aged 30 to 54 for vegetables and 26 percent of the same group for fruits (Patterson, et al, 1990).

Actual Consumption Pyramid
U.S. Total

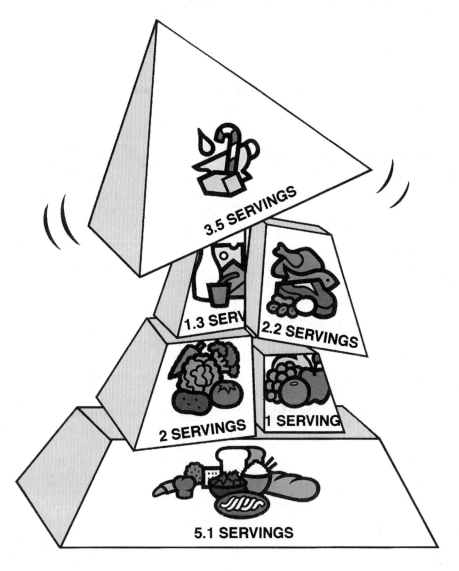

Eating in America Today, Edition II
A Dietary Pattern and Intake Report
commissioned by the
National Live Stock and Meat Board

FIGURE 13–1 The tumbling pyramid. Actual consumption of foods in the United States shows the meat group as the only food group for which intake corresponds with recommendations. (From Eating in America, ed 2, National Live Stock and Meat Board, courtesy of National Cattlemen's Beef Association, with permission.)

Although 24-hour recall data is insufficient to evaluate an individual's nutritional status, data from large groups can serve to identify problem areas. The conclusion here is that the average young adult does not eat well. If these adults feed their children the same limited fare, the next generation will learn no better.

Middle Adulthood

The middle adult years are those between ages 40 and 65. Mandatory retirement rules in the past - designated age 65 as the beginning of old age. Now the entry and exit points for middle age are more flexible.

Developmental Task of Middle Adulthood

To achieve **generativity** the person guides the next generation to adopt similar values and follow a path parallel to the mentor's. In this way, a middle-aged adult can attain a measure of immortality. This can be accomplished through influencing not only one's own children, but also one's students or one's protégé at work.

Nutrition in Middle Adulthood

As is true of the young adult, only a small minority of middle-aged adults report meeting or exceeding their RDAs or dietary guidelines on a given day.

Minerals

All the averages of men aged 35 to 49 exceeded the RDA for iron. Women aged 35 to 49 consumed even less iron than younger women, averaging 8 to 10 milligrams daily (RDA is 15). Again, white women consumed the least iron and Latino women consumed the most iron. After age 51, the RDA for women drops to 10 milligrams. Even so, only Latino women aged 50 to 64 averaged this much iron intake (Block, and Subar, 1992).

Of 35 to 49 year olds, only white and Latino men's average calcium intake exceeded the RDA. After age 51, the RDA for women is 1200 milligrams. Of 50- to 64-year-old women, blacks reported the least calcium intake, averaging 544 milligrams, and Latinos the most calcium intake at 691 milligrams (Block, and Subar, 1992).

Fat and Fiber

Of the 35 to 64 year olds, white, black, and younger Latino women averaged less than 300 milligrams of cholesterol daily. Only Latino men averaged even half of the recommended fiber intake (Block, and Subar, 1992).

Fruits and Vegetables

Middle-aged adults consumed a slightly better diet in regard to fruits and vegetables than did young adults.

Eight percent of adults aged 30 to 54 met the Food Pyramid standard by eating at least two servings of fruit and three servings of vegetables on the day recorded. Another 27 percent of adults aged 30 to 54 consumed three servings of vegetables but less than two servings of fruit. Almost as many, 26 percent, achieved the fruit standard but not the vegetable (Patterson, et al, 1990).

Older Adulthood

Older adults traditionally have been defined as those over the age of 65. For years, that was the typical retirement age.

Changes in the Elderly Population

Our older population is changing demographically. In 1900, the **life expectancy** was 45 years. Currently, the life expectancy for women is 78 years and for men it is 71 years. In 1900, 4 percent of the population was over age 65; now the percentage is at 12 percent and growing. Barring major calamities, by early in the next century 20 percent of the population will be over 65 years of age; 11 percent will be over 75 years of age. The fastest growing segment of the population is people older than 85.

This transformation is attributed to improved sanitation, increased concern about safety, and control of communicable diseases. In 1900, 1 in 10 infants died; now the figure is 1 in 100, despite the fact that smaller infants are surviving. In the days of the "Wild West," a woman usually died before her youngest child left home, and a man could have one horse his entire adult life. The average life span of horses is 25 years. The work world was harsh. Children worked in heavy industry. The death of one miner a week in a relatively small mining operation was commonplace.

Today the major causes of death in adults are heart

TABLE 13–1   Erikson's Theory of Psychosocial Development in Maturity

Stage of Life	Developmental Task	Opposing Negative Trait	Use of Food to Achieve Task
Young adult	Intimacy	Isolation	Arranging candlelight dinner
Middle adult	Generativity	Stagnation	Teaching someone to prepare family favorite or ethnic dishes
Older adult	Integrity	Despair	Using food fragrances or memories of food to reminisce

disease, cancer, and stroke. All of them are linked to lifestyle, including a nutritional component.

Distinctions Among Older Adults

As a group, older adults display a wide range of interests and abilities. Some will be content to stay at home and work in the garden. Others will travel extensively. Only 10 percent are confined in any serious way. A roomful of 3-year-old children will be more like one another than a roomful of 70-year-old adults. In old age, people become more like themselves, accentuating traits they have had all along. Many older persons have difficulty changing their behavior patterns, including those related to food.

Illness and nutrition are interrelated. Of recently hospitalized elderly persons, 31 percent were classified as undernourished compared to 7 percent of those living at home. Only 43 percent of the hospitalized groups showed no sign of undernutrition compared to 86 percent of the at-home group (Mowé, Bøhmer, and Kindt, 1994).

The stereotype of the old folks in a nursing home is just that, a stereotype. Only 5 percent of older adults live in nursing homes. However, that 5 percent represents more than 1 million clients. This subgroup of the older population has special nutrient needs. Up to 50 percent cannot feed themselves. Often they have very low calcium intakes and low intakes of vitamin A, vitamin C, thiamin, riboflavin, and iron. If they do not get sufficient sun exposure or do not consume fortified dairy products, they are at increased risk for vitamin D deficiency.

Psychosocial Development

The developmental task for older adults to achieve is **integrity.** Those who accomplish this task will look back on their lives as worthwhile. Although they may have suffered some failures and have some regrets, they are able to see their lives in perspective. They can forgive themselves for their faults because they know they did the best they could with what they had. A technique to help the older person achieve integrity is reminiscence. See Table 13–1 for an application of Erikson's theory to maturity.

Socially, the older adult faces tremendous adjustments when a spouse of many years dies. The accompanying depression and new responsibility for tasks the spouse performed may significantly affect food intake. Analysis of home health care clients found social or friendship networks did not predict dietary intake (Payette, et al, 1995).

The Aging Body

Just as adolescents face a changing body image, so do older adults. Even without frank disease, the physical abilities of the older adult diminish. Middle-age spread gives way to dwindling bulk and waning strength. Living with their bodies challenges the old to adjust. Among the body systems significantly changed in the aging process are the integumentary, sensory, gastrointestinal, urinary, musculoskeletal, nervous, endocrine, and cardiovascular systems.

Integumentary System

Many changes take place in the skin as a person ages. As subcutaneous fat is lost, the skin becomes dry and wrinkled. Less elasticity is present to spring back after a pinch, so using this method to test for dehydration is unreliable. The older adult also loses some of the ability to synthesize vitamin D from sunshine. An 80-year-old person requires almost twice as much time in the sun to produce a given amount of vitamin D as a 20-year-old (Ryan, Eleazer, and Egbert, 1995).

Life expectancy—The probable number of years that persons of a given age may be expected to live.

Sensory System

Four senses become markedly less acute as a person ages: vision, hearing, taste, and smell. Because the sense receptors do not deteriorate equally, some of the sense loss is attributed to changes in the central nervous system. Again, extensive variations exist among individuals.

Eyes

Vision is reduced. The person sees reds, oranges, and yellows better than blues and violets. Clouding of the lens of the eye, a **cataract,** decreases overall vision. The fine print labeling food items may be illegible to the elderly. Older eyes do not adjust well to glare. These changes in vision may make grocery shopping burdensome. Food preparation may become not only difficult but also hazardous if the person cannot see adequately. Poor vision was associated with lower protein and energy intakes in home health care clients independent of other medical conditions (Payette, et al, 1995).

Ears

The sound receptors in the inner ear deteriorate. First to be lost is the ability to perceive high tones. The older person with poor hearing usually will hear men's voices better than women's. Hearing aids do not fully compensate for the hearing loss. In fact, they often magnify sideline noise to the point of distraction. The result may be social isolation when it becomes too laborious to interact with others. Socializing at meals may become embarrassing or frustrating, and thus avoided.

Nose and Tongue

For the sense of taste to function well, the sense of smell must also be intact. Food tastes bland when a person has a head cold. Older adults have dulled senses of smell and taste. The peak acuity of the sense of smell is between 20 and 40 years of age. In the tongue, receptors for sweet and salty taste deteriorate before those for bitter and sour. For this reason, older persons may lavish sugar and salt on their food.

Gastrointestinal System

Particularly crucial to nutriture is the gastrointestinal system. Hundreds of processes are required for the proper digestion, absorption, and metabolism of foods. Many functions of the gastrointestinal system decline significantly in older people.

By the age of 65, 41 percent of Americans are **edentulous** or toothless. This proportion is declining due to more frequent efforts at restoration (Miller, 1995). The major cause of tooth loss in the older adult is not dental caries but **periodontal disease,** which affects the gums. Dentures, like hearing aids, only partially substitute for the real thing. Furthermore, a denture cannot be effective if the underlying tissue is in poor condition.

The production of saliva decreases sharply in the older adult. This results in **xerostomia.** Chewing and swallowing become more difficult and food intake may be affected. Also with age, less mucus and smaller quantities of enzymes are secreted. Decreased amounts of gastric acid are secreted after the age of 50. An extreme case, **achlorhydria,** the absence of hydrochloric acid in the stomach, may interfere with protein digestion and with vitamin and mineral absorption. Vitamin B_{12} and iron are of special concern.

Intestinal **motility** decreases because of lessened muscle tone. Medications may interfere with electrolyte balance, also diminishing muscle tone. By the age of 70, the liver loses 18 percent of its weight and has reduced capabilities.

Urinary System

The kidneys lose about 10 percent of their weight by the time an adult reaches the age of 70. At age 80, the blood flow to the kidneys is one-half of what it was at age 35. This compromised kidney function makes reliance on urine samples for nutrient analyses less reliable in the elderly. Renal function can be measured by a **blood urea nitrogen** (BUN) test. An increase in the BUN level usually indicates a decrease in function. Patients with even slightly elevated BUNs may not be able to excrete the waste products from protein metabolism. Thus care must be taken when giving high-protein nutritional supplements to older persons with elevated BUNs.

Musculoskeletal System

The major loss of body mass in the older adult is loss of muscle mass. By age 70, skeletal muscle diminishes by 40 percent. Because muscle is a more active tissue than fat, energy needs decline with the diminished muscle mass.

Perhaps more noticeable than the overall loss of muscle is the loss of height in older people. The average lifetime loss of height amounts to 2.9 centimeters (1.16 inches) in men and 4.9 centimeters (1.96 inches) in women. A major cause of this loss of height is osteoporosis. The bone loss amounts to about 8 percent per decade after age 35, so that by the age of 70, 25 percent of the bone structure is gone.

Joint surfaces are roughened by **arthritis.** By the age of 50, one-half of all adults have this degenerative joint disease. Arthritis impairs the use of the hands for opening jars, chopping raw foods, and cutting cooked foods at the table. Arthritis also impairs the operation of the mandibular joint of the jaw for chewing.

Nervous System

By the time a person reaches old age, the brain has endured a lifetime of stressors. Brain cells are not replaced as they are destroyed. Consequently, the number of brain cells is decreased. Blood flow to the brain decreases due to narrowing of the arteries. Thirst sensation becomes less operative, increasing the risk of uncompensated dehydration. Adaptation to stress is less effective as people age. For instance, **mortality** from heat stroke rises sharply after age 60. The brain requires glucose for fuel. Performance by elderly individuals on memory tests was better following glucose ingestion rather than saccharin (Gold, 1995).

Endocrine System

The older person is slowing down. Resting energy expenditure (REE) decreases, especially in the brain, skeletal muscle, and the heart. The older adult's REE may be 10 to 12 percent less than a younger person's. Lost muscle mass is replaced, if at all, by adipose tissue that is less active metabolically than muscle.

Cardiovascular System

As the older adult continues to age, there is (1) a decrease in cardiac output and (2) a slower heart rate. In response to exercise, the heart rate does not increase as effectively as in youth, nor does it return to normal as rapidly. Because of these diminishments, the elderly are at risk for diseases of the heart. Dietary modifications for heart disease are discussed in Chapter 19, "Diet in Cardiovascular Disease."

Nutrition in the Older Adult

Older adults reported more healthy eating habits than the young and middle-aged adults. Thirteen percent of adults aged 55 to 74 achieved the Food Pyramid standard for fruits and vegetables. Three servings of vegetables but less than two servings of fruit were consumed by 28 percent. Another 40 percent met the fruit standard but not the vegetable one (Patterson, et al, 1990).

Available evidence suggests that older persons need almost the same intake from all nutrients as do other adults, with the exception of kilocalories. Energy needs decrease with age. Thus, there is less leeway for indiscretions and empty kilocalories in the diet.

Energy Nutrients

Estimates of the decrease in energy needed by older adults average about 5 percent per decade after the age of 40. As with younger people, the simplest criterion for the suitability of intake is the maintenance of a healthy body weight.

The current recommendation is that older adults should have at least 30 minutes a day total of moderate activity. It can be 30 minutes at one time or two 15-minute sessions or three 10-minute sessions. An exercise routine should be introduced gradually (Foreyt, 1995). On average, physically active people live longer than inactive people, even if exercise is

---

Cataract—Clouding of the lens of the eye.

Edentulous—The state of having no teeth.

Periodontal disease—Any disorder of the supporting structures of the teeth.

Xerostomia—Dry mouth caused by decreased salivary secretions.

Achlorhydria—Absence of free hydrochloric acid in stomach.

Motility—Ability to move spontaneously.

Blood urea nitrogen (BUN)—The amount of nitrogen present in the blood as urea, often elevated in renal disorders.

Arthritis—Inflammatory condition of the joints, usually accompanied by pain and swelling.

Mortality—The death rate; number of deaths per unit of population.

started late in life. Exercise reduces risk of chronic diseases and makes individuals feel healthier and look younger.

Distribution of Energy Nutrients

The proportion of energy to be obtained from each of the energy nutrients is changed slightly for older adults. They should derive 50 to 60 percent of their kilocalories from carbohydrates. Fats should contribute 20 to 30 percent of the kilocalories. Limiting fats should also increase comfort, mainly because fat absorption is delayed in older persons, causing early satiety.

Latino women came closest to meeting these guidelines, averaging 49 percent of kilocalories from carbohydrates and 34 percent from fats. All the women averaged less than 300 milligrams of cholesterol. Only Latino men averaged even half the recommended daily amount of fiber (Block, and Subar, 1992).

An intake of protein at the level of 0.8 gram per kilogram of healthy body weight still should amount to 12 percent of total kilocalories. Some authorities suggest increasing the protein allotment for the elderly. No consistent relationship between protein intake and serum albumin level has been found in elderly people, however (Freedman and Ahronheim, 1986). One reason for this may be related to liver function. A normally functioning liver is necessary to construct albumin molecules from the ingested protein and resulting amino acids. If liver function is impaired, no amount of intake will produce normal blood albumin levels. Mortality rates from all causes were highest in persons over 71 years of age with the lowest serum albumin levels and decreased with increasing albumin levels. It is uncertain if serum albumin reflects nutritional status or disease presence and severity (Corti, et al, 1994). For a given individual, serum albumin levels can indicate nutritional status, pathology, or both. An additional reason for moderate protein intake concerns calcium use. A high protein intake also increases calcium loss in the urine.

Vitamins

Vitamin intake and usage are potential problems for the elderly. Deficiencies of vitamins A, D, C, and niacin, and B_{12} are most frequently of concern. Excesses are possible, also, especially in persons who self-medicate on megadoses of vitamins.

Fat-Soluble Vitamins

Because fat-soluble vitamins are stored in the body, it may take a long time for a deficiency to present clinical signs. Assessment of the individual is the only means to pinpoint a person's practices and risks.

Vitamin A plays a role in bone metabolism. In the elderly, excessive levels of vitamin A are associated with increased bone loss.

Most of a person's vitamin D is synthesized in the skin. This process is substantially reduced in the older adult. Milk is an excellent source of vitamin D because of fortification. The elderly person who is likely to be deficient in vitamin D, then, is the one who stays indoors and does not consume enough milk or milk products.

Water-Soluble Vitamins

The RDA for older adults is the same amount of vitamin C, 60 milligrams, as for younger adults. Older adults living at home generally have a better vitamin C status than those living in institutions. The independent elderly may spend more on fruits and vegetables than institutions do, or the vitamin C in foods may be destroyed by poor cooking and serving practices in institutions.

Eating patterns affect the intake of B vitamins. Older adults who eat little meat and consume little milk or milk products containing tryptophan are at risk for niacin deficiency.

Older adults have decreased gastric juice, which contains intrinsic factor. Because of this, senior adults may develop a vitamin B_{12} deficiency, especially those with limited meat consumption. The meat group supplies 66 percent of the total dietary vitamin B_{12} (National Live Stock and Meat Board, 1994).

Minerals

Minerals of particular concern in the elderly are iron and calcium. None of the individuals over 65 years averaged the RDA for calcium. Men averaged over 700 milligrams (RDA, 800), black women averaged 536 milligrams (RDA, 1200), and white and Latino women averaged 623 and 646 milligrams, respectively (Block, and Subar, 1992). See Table 8–1 for alternate recommendations for calcium intake and Clinical Application 8–3 to review research on osteoporosis.

Iron absorption is impaired by decreased gastric acidity, whether due to aging or to antacid use. All

TABLE 13–2 Signs of Dehydration in the Elderly

Body System	Sign
Skin and mucous membranes	Skin warm and dry
	Decreased turgor; pinch test may be inaccurate due to loss of elasticity
	Furrowed tongue
	Elevated temperature
Cardiovascular	Elevated pulse
Urinary	Increased specific gravity
	Increased urinary sodium
Musculoskeletal	Weakness
Neurological	Confusion

the men over 65 years of age, but none of the women, averaged at least 10 milligrams of iron daily (Block, and Subar, 1992). Anemia is not always the result of aging or nutritional deficits. Hidden blood losses should be suspected and their sources sought in the anemic elderly person, just as in younger clients.

Water

Many older persons have problems maintaining fluid balance. Sometimes the difficulty is self-inflicted. Loss of sphincter muscle tone in women and difficulty urinating in men may prompt older people to limit fluids. Older adults need 6 to 8 glasses of water per day, enough to produce about 1.5 liters of urine.

Dehydration in the elderly can result in abnormal functioning. One of the signs of dehydration in the elderly is confusion. If no one is alert to these mental changes, the person may compound his or her difficulties by forgetting to take medications or eat meals. Table 13–2 lists the signs of dehydration in the elderly.

Patients who are immobilized may need as many as 12 to 14 glasses of water per day. Immobility increases the calcium loss from bones. The high serum calcium level is controlled by the kidney. A large fluid intake keeps the urine dilute so that the calcium does not form stones.

Common Problems Related to Nutrition

Although constipation, obesity, and low protein intake are common problems that are not unique to the elderly, they do represent special **geriatric** concerns.

Constipation

A person may complain of acute **constipation,** which is the lack of stools, or chronic constipation, which is general difficulty passing bowel movements. Recommended methods to achieve bowel regularity include increasing fluid intake, consuming high-fiber foods, taking time for elimination, and exercising.

Doubling the person's water intake, medical conditions permitting, is the first step. Loading the diet with fresh fruits and vegetables is the second. Time should be set aside every day to have a bowel movement, preferably in the morning after drinking a warm beverage. Lastly, exercise promotes regular bowel movements.

Older adults sometimes adopt the routine use of laxatives to correct bowel habits. For such persons, the program mentioned above will not provide instant resolution. If the regimen is adhered to, however, it is possible to overcome even long-standing constipation.

Obesity

Since weight control is discussed in a later chapter, only brief mention of obesity in the elderly appears here. For a person to have lived more than 65 years, some correct lifestyle choices must have been made. Weight reduction should be pursued if it is needed to treat current problems, such as diabetes mellitus, but not to prevent new ones (Feldman, 1988). Only modest changes should be suggested and these should be introduced gradually. Concentrating on changing one behavior at a time may help avert further weight gain. For example, a client who is gaining weight could substitute skim milk for whole or 2 percent milk.

Low Protein Intake

The main reason older adults do not eat enough protein is the lack of money. To rectify the situation, the federal government, with an amendment to the Older Americans Act, established meal programs for senior citizens. Low-cost meals are offered at central gathering places and/or delivered to the homebound. Figure 13–2 illustrates a group of senior citizens participating in one such meal program.

> **Geriatrics**—The branch of medicine involved in the study and treatment of diseases in the elderly.

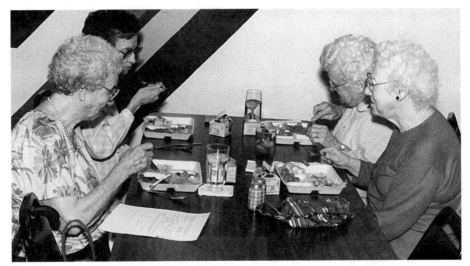

FIGURE 13–2   This group of senior citizens is participating in a federal meal program. The program provides not only food but also a social activity and a regular schedule.

A serum albumin level of less than 3.5 grams per deciliter is a criterion for visceral protein depletion and is used to justify a diagnosis of malnutrition for Medicare and Medicaid. It was also the most frequently found indicator for pressure ulcers in nursing home residents (Gilmore, et al, 1995).

Again, individual assessment is the key to planning nutritional care. For example, milk-based supplements that are both nutrient-dense and easy to consume might be a dietary recommendation for the person who cannot chew. To accommodate dentures, the person may reduce his or her intake of meats, fresh fruits, and vegetables, and may need assistance selecting appropriate substitute items. Dietary intake in home health care clients was not related to masticatory ability, however (Payette, et al, 1995). A recommended procedure for learning to eat and drink with dentures is discussed in Clinical Application 13–1.

The Nursing Process and the Elderly

Although elderly persons are not all alike, they do share some common problems that occur frequently enough to bear special mention. These are listed as topics to be assessed in the elderly in Table 13–3.

Suggestions to increase the nourishment of elderly clients appear in Table 13–4. Keep in mind that there is no single answer suitable for every problem. The nurse's role in nourishing the hospitalized elderly client is discussed in Clinical Applica-

tion 13–2. Obtaining adequate food for a client undergoing many diagnostic procedures may tax the nurse's ingenuity.

Nutrition Education for Adults

Because none of the age groups of adults are remarkable in complying with the recommended food intake, some general suggestions for improvement are pertinent to the majority of adults. As always, for individual counseling an individual assessment is needed.

Fat consumption is excessive, especially in the poor. Modifications in food preparation techniques could decrease these fat kilocalories. For example, an estimated 71 percent of the time, poultry is eaten

---

CLINICAL APPLICATION 13–1
Learning to Eat with Dentures

Persons need to learn to use dentures one step at a time. The steps are in exactly the same order as those used by infants learning to eat. The person should first practice swallowing liquids with the dentures in place. After this is mastered, soft foods can be chewed. Lastly, the person should learn to bite regular foods with the dentures. Splitting up the learning process into manageable units helps to make this process less frustrating for the new denture wearer.

TABLE 13–3 Topics to be Assessed in the Elderly*

Oral Cavity Function
- Difficulty tasting, changes in taste perception
- Bleeding gums, dry mouth
- Difficulty chewing, toothaches, poorly fitting dentures
- Foods client is unable to eat

Meal Management
- Who shops? Where? Ease of making food decisions?
- Transportation problems?
- Budgeting a concern? Knowledge to make informed choices?
- Who cooks? Knowledge and skill level?
- Refrigeration, storage, and cooking facilities?
- Ability to manage containers: jars, cans, bottles

Psychosocial Factors
- Where are most meals eaten?
- Mealtime companions?
- Recent change in living conditions?
- Satisfaction with situation?

* In addition to the normal assessment, that is, appetite or weight changes, bowel habits.

TABLE 13–4 Increasing Food Intake in the Elderly

Get the Person Ready for Meals
- Provide oral hygiene before meals to freshen and moisten mouth.
- Suggest smokers refrain for 1 hour before meal to increase appetite.
- Allow 4 to 5 hours between meals and supplements to permit hunger to develop.

Promote Social Interaction
- Encourage potluck meals with friends for those who live alone.
- Combine meal at senior center with an activity of interest.
- Encourage alert nursing home residents to choose compatible mealtime companions.
- Control the noise in the dining room to avoid overstimulating those with hearing aids.

Serve Food Attractively
- Vary textures, colors, flavors.
- To increase vegetable intake, offer raw, crisp-cooked, or marinated vegetables as appetizers.
- Use "good" dishes and flatware, centerpieces, tablecloths, or place mats.
- Provide enough nonglaring light to see food clearly.

Obtain Outside Help
- Home health aide to shop, do basic fix-ahead preparations
- Meals on Wheels for homebound
- Food stamps, surplus commodity programs for those eligible
- Instructional materials on food purchasing, storage, cooking from county extension service

CLINICAL APPLICATION 13–2

Hospitalization of the Elderly

With the exception of obstetrics and pediatrics, elderly clients dominate as consumers of health care. Eighty percent of the elderly, compared with 40 percent of people less than 65 years old, have one or more chronic diseases.

Older persons are unable to tolerate starvation for more than 5 days because they lack nutritional reserves (Feldman, 1988). Serving no food to a client because of diagnostic tests is starvation. The conscientious nurse obtains meals or feedings for the client who was NPO (i.e., who was allowed "nothing by mouth") for breakfast and lunch. There is nothing magical about the times of 8 AM–12 NOON–6 PM for meals. The committed nurse will arrange for adequate nourishment for clients, despite scheduling difficulties. Dietary staff have no idea when an individual client is finished with tests for the day until notified by the nurse.

without efforts to minimize its fat content. For pork the estimate is 68 percent of the time (Thompson, et al, 1992).

Fruit and vegetable consumption is very low. Neither fruits nor vegetables were consumed by 11 percent of adults surveyed. Almost half of the adults, 45 percent, reported having no servings of fruit or juice, and 22 percent had no servings of vegetables. Even when two servings of vegetables were reported, 21 percent of the adults consumed two servings of the same vegetable (Patterson, et al, 1990).

Most adults could benefit from instruction in the key concepts of nutrition: balance, variety, and moderation. The alert nurse has an important contribution to make in identifying knowledge deficits and impaired health practices related to nutrition. This responsibility applies to all clients receiving nursing care, not only those with obvious nutrition-related medical diagnoses.

Summary

Surveys have indicated that a majority of adults do not follow the Food Pyramid guidelines or the RDAs for some nutrients. Of special concern is excessive fat intake. Low fiber intake is another problem. Adequacy of vitamin and mineral intake is in question because 91 percent of persons did not consume the recommended two servings of fruits and three servings of vegetables in the period surveyed. These data suggest the need for nutrition education among adults.

Changing social, economic, and physical circumstances affect the nutritional status of the elderly client. When a spouse dies, grief, depression, and poor appetite often overcome the widow or widower.

Learning to live on Social Security benefits, pensions, and savings may place a strain on some elderly persons.

With age, secretions decrease along the entire gastrointestinal tract. Nutrients that require an acid medium for maximum utilization, including vitamins C and B_{12}, will be affected. Lack of outdoor activity, dislike for milk, and decreasing effectiveness of the skin's synthesis of vitamin D all place the older person at risk for vitamin D deficiency. The senses of taste and smell become less keen. Having to wear dentures may compound the problem of inadequate intake. Decreased mobility and declining vision can cause food procurement and preparation to become even more difficult.

However, all elderly persons are not affected equally by the aging process, nor are they equally adept at adapting to its effects. This makes an individual assessment crucial to providing adequate nutritional care.

| Case Study 13–1 | Mr. E is a 75-year-old widower. He recently had surgery for cataracts and subsequently gave up driving his car. His home is two blocks off the bus route and eight blocks from the nearest supermarket. Mr. E has moderately painful knees from arthritis. He has been taking the bus to the supermarket every other day so that he could manage one package on the way home. He has confided to the nurse in his doctor's office that he is ready to "just give up. It's too much trouble to eat anymore." Mr. E's weight today is 160 lb, 5 lb less than last month. |

NURSING CARE PLAN

Assessment

Subjective Data   Restricted vision led to inability to drive a car safely

Dependent on public transportation

Painful knees

Verbalized discouragement with procuring food

Objective Data   Weight loss of 5 lb in past month

Nursing Diagnosis	Health maintenance, altered: related to impaired mobility outside of home, as evidenced by verbalization to nurse and weight loss of 5 lb in past month.	
Desired Outcome/ Evaluation Criteria	**Nursing Actions**	**Rationale**
Mr. E will acknowledge need for assistance with meals to stop losing weight by end of visit today.	Discuss Mr. F.'s weight change with him. Determine what kind of assistance he would accept.	Clients are likely to change behaviors only if the new behavior is acceptable to them.
Given several options of community support, Mr. E will select one and begin to implement the change within 3 days.	Describe Senior Citizen Nutrition Program, Meals on Wheels, home health aide shopping service, and door-to-door Care-a-Van service. Explore social support available from family and less restricted friends.	Clients may know about these programs but prefer to remain independent. Allowing the client some time to choose makes the choice more his own.
	Nurse to follow-up with telephone call in 3 days.	Following up with a telephone call shows the nurse is committed to working through this problem with Mr. E.

Study Aids

Chapter Review

1. The actual consumption of food in the US is closest to the recommended Food Pyramid in which area?
   a. Fats, oils, and sweets
   b. Milk, yogurt, and cheese
   c. Meat, poultry, fish, dry beans, eggs, and nuts
   d. Vegetables
   e. Fruits
   f. Bread, cereal, rice, and pasta

2. The sense of taste diminishes with age. Which of the following sensations usually are missed first?
   a. Bitter and sour
   b. Salty and sour
   c. Salty and sweet
   d. Sour and sweet

3. A nurse making a home visit routinely screens for dehydration in elderly clients. Which of the following would the nurse assess?
   a. Body temperature and urine specific gravity
   b. Tongue condition, pulse rate, and muscle strength
   c. Skin turgor and heart and lung sounds
   d. Client's Intake and Output records

4. Which of the following conditions is likely to contribute to vitamin D deficiency in older adults?
   a. Atrophied skin, dislike for milk, and indoor life
   b. Lack of exercise, failing hearing and vision
   c. Slowed peristalsis, diminished secretion of intrinsic factor
   d. Achlorhydria and inability to chew meats

5. Ms. P is a 58-year-old retired cook who tells the clinic nurse she regrets not having had children and grandchildren. Which of the following activities might assist Ms. P to attain generativity?
   a. Editing a cookbook for her church group.
   b. Taking a class in ethnic cooking in preparation for her next trip.
   c. Serving on the Meals-on-Wheels Advisory Board.
   d. Volunteering to teach a special recipe at a local school.

Clinical Analysis

Ms. O is a 66-year-old retired schoolteacher who suffered a stroke 8 months ago. For the past 7 months she has resided in a nursing home. Ms. O has residual weakness on the right side. She has not mastered the use of tableware with her left hand. Her nurse is concerned because Ms. O weighs 125 pounds, compared with 135 pounds upon admission to the nursing home. The nursing assistants report that Ms. O takes a little of most foods but refuses to eat more than half of any of the foods.

1. The nurse discovers that a contributing factor in Ms. O's refusal to eat is embarrassment over her inability to control her lips. Which of the following outcomes would be appropriate in this case?
   a. Client will gain 5 pounds in the next 2 weeks.
   b. Client will consume 3/4 of the food served within 1 week.
   c. Client will feed herself with her left hand within the next 3 weeks.
   d. Client will consent to tube feeding

2. Which of the following nursing actions is appropriate initially to minimize Ms. O's embarrassment?
   a. Allowing her to eat her meals alone in her room
   b. Ordering finger foods that she can eat with her left hand
   c. Assigning her to a table with other stroke patients who feed themselves
   d. Instructing the nursing assistants to feed Ms. O privately

3. Which of the following activities could reasonably be expected to increase Ms. O's appetite?
   a. Participating in a craft session before lunch
   b. Taking a nap before dinner
   c. Practicing walking before lunch or dinner
   d. Watching television with her roommate after breakfast

Bibliography

Block, G, and Subar, AF: Estimates of nutrient intake from a good frequency questionnaire: The 1987 National Health Interview Survey. J Am Diet Assoc 92:969, 1992.

Coodley, G, et al: Malnutrition in the elderly. Geriatric Medicine Today 10:45, 1991.

Corti, M-C, et al: Serum albumin level and physical disability as predictors of mortality in older persons. JAMA 272:1036, 1994.

Feldman, EB: Essentials of Clinical Nutrition. FA Davis Company, Philadelphia, 1988.

Fiatrone, MA, et al: High intensity strength training in nonagenarians. JAMA 263:3029, 1990.

Foreyt, J: The 2nd Building Alliances to Communicate Food, Nutrition and Fitness. A Summary of Presentations, March 23–24, 1995. Food Marketing Institute, The American Dietetic Association, The President's Council on Physical Fitness.

Forgac, MT: Timely statement for the American Dietetic Association: Dietary guidance for healthy children. J Am Diet Assoc 95:370, 1995.

Freedman, ML, and Ahronheim, JC: Nutritional needs of the elderly: Debate and recommendations. Geriatrics 40:45, 1986.

Gilmore, SA, et al: Clinical indicators associated with unintentional weight loss and pressure ulcers in elderly residents of nursing facilities. J Am Diet Assoc 95:984, 1995.

Gold, PE: Role of glucose in regulating the brain and cognition. Am J Clin Nutr 61(suppl):9875, 1995.

Kerstetter, JE, Holthausen, BA, and Fitz, PA: Malnutrition in the institutionalized older adult. J Am Diet Assoc 92:1109, 1992.

Koehler, KM, Hunt, WC, and Garry, PT: Meat, poultry, and fish consumption and nutrient intake in the healthy elderly. J Am Diet Assoc 92:325, 1992.

MacLean, TB: Influence of psychosocial development and life events on the health practices of adults. Issues in Mental Health Nursing 13:403, 1992.

Miller, CA: Nursing Care of Older Adults, ed 2. JB Lippincott, Philadelphia, 1995.

Mowé, M, Bøhmer, T, and Kindt, E: Reduced nutritional status in an elderly population (>70 y) is probable before disease and possibly contributes to the development of disease. Am J Clin Nutr 59:317, 1994.

National Live Stock and Meat Board: Eating in America Today, ed 2. Chicago, 1995.

Patterson, BH, et al: Fruit and vegetables in the American diet: Data from the NHANES II survey. Am J Public Health 80:1443, 1990.

Payette, H, et al: Predictors of dietary intake in a functionally dependent elderly population in the community. Am J Public Health 85:677, 1995.

Popkin, BM, Siega-Riz, AM, and Haines, PS: A comparison of dietary trends among racial and socioeconomic groups in the United States. N Engl J Med 335:716, 1996.

Ryan, C, Eleazer, P, and Egbert, J: Vitamin D in the elderly. Nutr Today 30:228, 1995.

Small, SP, Best, DG, and Hustins, KA: Energy and nutrient intakes of independently-living, elderly women. Can J Nurs Res 26:71, 1994.

Thompson, FE, et al: Sources of fiber and fat in diets of US women aged 19 to 50: Implications for nutrition education and policy. Am J Public Health 82:695, 1992.

CHAPTER 14

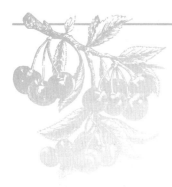

Food Management

LEARNING OBJECTIVES

After completing this chapter, the student should be able to:

1 Describe the conditions under which microbiologic food illnesses can occur.

2 Discuss the information on food labels.

3 Identify foods that are likely to harbor disease-producing microbiologic organisms.

4 Describe one systematic approach to identify nutritional hazards in a person's diet.

5 Teach clients how to prevent foodborne illnesses.

Competent meal management requires some knowledge of food safety. Each American eats more than 1000 pounds of food each year. Considering the number of people involved in the growth, distribution, preparation, and service of food, our food safety record is excellent. The US food supply is as safe, wholesome, and nutritious as any in the world.

The Food and Drug Administration (FDA) has set up a list of food safety problems. Problems are ranked in descending order of importance, considering the number of people affected by a problem and the severity of the problem. The FDA's list of food safety priorities is:

1. Microbiologic hazards
2. Nutritional hazards
3. Environmental pollutants
4. Natural food intoxicants
5. Food additives

In this chapter, each of these food safety concerns are discussed.

Microbiologic Hazards

Microbiologic hazards include single-cell and multiple-cell organisms such as bacteria, viruses, molds, and parasites that can invade the food supply through direct, indirect, or intermediary means. These microorganisms may be carried from one host to another by animals, including humans, inanimate objects including food, and environmental factors, such as air, water, and soil. Many microorganisms cause disease. Under certain conditions, food can turn into a vehicle for disease transmission.

Most foodborne diseases infect the tissues of the digestive tract, resulting in gastric distress. Symptoms of gastric distress include abdominal pain, nausea, vomiting, diarrhea, and cramps. If prolonged, the resultant diarrhea can lead to dehydration or other complications, some of which can be fatal. More severe symptoms include fever and neurological disorders. Foodborne disease can last for a few hours or for several days.

Bacterial Foodborne Disease

Bacteria are everywhere. Doorknobs, countertops, hands, eyelashes, mouths, some water supplies, and food are a few of the many places where bacteria can be found. The type of food, the presence or absence of oxygen, the moisture content of the food, and the acidity or alkalinity of the food's environment determine bacterial growth rates. The length of time food is held at a given temperature also affects bacterial growth rates. Given sufficient time, bacteria can frequently adapt to all types of foods and to all conditions of moisture, acidity, oxygen, and temperature. Most bacteria adjust to a new environment in about 4 hours. For this reason, vulnerable foods should not be eaten if held at room temperature for more than 4 hours.

Bacterial growth refers to an increase in the numbers of organisms. Under ideal conditions, cell numbers can double every half hour: one becomes two, two become four, and four become eight. A single bacterial cell can multiply to 33 million after 12 hours.

The following conditions are necessary for microbiologic food illness to occur:

Source of bacteria—The bacteria must come in contact with the food.
Food—The food must permit the bacteria to grow and either increase in number or produce a poisonous toxin.
Temperature—The temperature must be favorable for the growth of bacteria. 45°F to 140°F is the temperature range in which most bacteria multiply rapidly. (Note: room and body temperature are in this range.) (See Figure 14–1).
Time—Enough time must elapse for bacteria to grow and/or produce a toxin.
Ingestion—An unsuspecting person must eat the food that contains the toxin or bacteria.

Bacteria are frequently odorless, tasteless, and colorless. Without laboratory analysis there is no way to tell whether a food will cause illness. For this reason, proper food handling to prevent the growth of bacteria is the best insurance against food poisoning. Bacterial foodborne diseases are usually subdivided into two groups, food infections and food intoxications.

Food Infections

A **food infection** is an illness caused by eating food containing a large number of disease-producing bacteria. Symptoms of food infections occur 12 to 36 hours after consumption of the offending food.

SALMONELLA Probably the best known genus of bacteria responsible for foodborne illness is **Salmonella.** The infection, called **salmonellosis,** is transmitted by the consumption of contaminated foods or contact with an infected person. Some foods support the growth of *Salmonella* better than others. Clinical Application 14–1 lists guidelines for the safe handling of eggs, a common **vehicle** for salmonella transmission.

Elderly persons, infants, pregnant women, and people with illnesses that impair their ability to fight infections are at highest risk. In these persons, a relatively small number of bacteria could cause severe illness. Please refer to Clinical Application 14–2 for a discussion of clients with suppressed immune systems. A healthy person would require a much larger number of bacteria to cause illness. Most of the recent deaths caused by *Salmonella* have occurred

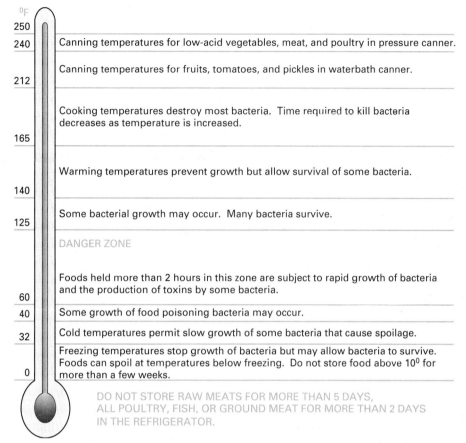

°F

250
240 — Canning temperatures for low-acid vegetables, meat, and poultry in pressure canner.

— Canning temperatures for fruits, tomatoes, and pickles in waterbath canner.
212

— Cooking temperatures destroy most bacteria. Time required to kill bacteria decreases as temperature is increased.
165

— Warming temperatures prevent growth but allow survival of some bacteria.
140

— Some bacterial growth may occur. Many bacteria survive.
125

DANGER ZONE

— Foods held more than 2 hours in this zone are subject to rapid growth of bacteria and the production of toxins by some bacteria.
60
40 — Some growth of food poisoning bacteria may occur.

32 — Cold temperatures permit slow growth of some bacteria that cause spoilage.

— Freezing temperatures stop growth of bacteria but may allow bacteria to survive. Foods can spoil at temperatures below freezing. Do not store food above 10⁰ for
0 more than a few weeks.

DO NOT STORE RAW MEATS FOR MORE THAN 5 DAYS, ALL POULTRY, FISH, OR GROUND MEAT FOR MORE THAN 2 DAYS IN THE REFRIGERATOR.

FIGURE 14–1   A temperature guide to food safety. (From the US Department of Agriculture.)

among the elderly in nursing homes (Department of Health and Human Services, 1990).

Typhoid fever is caused by one type of *Salmonella* bacteria. This illness is spread by food and water contaminated by feces and urine of clients and carriers.

Other types of bacteria cause food infections. *Shigella* and *Campylobacter* are other examples of disease-producing bacteria.

Food Intoxication

Food intoxication is an illness caused by the consumption of a food in which bacteria have produced a poisonous toxin. The onset of symptoms is very rapid (1 to 8 hours) since the bacteria have already produced the offending toxin before food consumption. There often is no fever because a toxin causes the illness rather than an infection. Symptoms of this disorder last for a day or two but are usually so severe that exhaustion and dehydration can produce serious aftereffects. Three bacteria are respon-

sible for the majority of reported cases of food intoxication: *Staphylococcus*, *Clostridium perfringens*, and *Clostridium botulinum*. The extent to which a person may suffer the effects of a toxin depends on (1) how much is ingested and (2) the person's susceptibility.

Food Infection—An illness acquired through contact with food or water contaminated with disease-producing microorganisms.

Salmonellosis—A bacterial infection manifested by the sudden onset of headache, abdominal pain, diarrhea, nausea, and vomiting. Fever is almost always present.

Vehicle—Contaminated inanimate objects that transmit disease; examples are water, food, utensils.

Food Intoxication—An illness caused by the consumption of a food in which bacteria have produced a poisonous toxin.

STAPHYLOCOCCAL POISONING One of the most common species of bacteria that produce a poisonous toxin is **Staphylococcus aureus,** often referred to as staph. Staph have been reported to be in the nasal passages of 30 to 50 percent of healthy people and on the hands of 20 percent of all healthy people. Infected cuts, boils, and burns also harbor this organism.

Good personal hygiene prevents the contamination of food. Heat destroys the bacteria but not the toxin the bacteria already have produced. Because heat does not destroy the toxin, control of temperature alone will not provide protection. Prevention of staph poisoning must include good personal hygiene *and* temperature control. Signs and symptoms of staphylococcal poisoning appear suddenly after 2 to 6 hours and generally subside within 24 hours. These include abdominal cramps, nausea, vomiting, diarrhea, fever, headache, and sweating.

CLOSTRIDIUM PERFRINGENS **Clostridium perfringens** produces a toxin that causes lower gastrointestinal distress. The symptoms include a sudden onset of colic followed by diarrhea and nausea. Vomiting and fever are usually absent. Careful control of a food's temperature and good personal hygiene can protect a person from this food infection.

BOTULISM **Clostridium botulinum** is another bacterium that produces a toxin. The resulting disease is **botulism.** The organism is found in soils throughout the world and can be found in the intestinal tracts of domestic animals. Vegetables grown in contaminated soil harbor this organism.

Botulin, the toxin produced by *C. botulinum* is so poisonous that a single ounce is enough to kill the world's population. Symptoms usually begin 12 to 36 hours but can occur as early as 3 hours after the consumption of the contaminated food. The toxin affects the nervous system, leading to dizziness, headache, double vision, and paralysis. The paralysis leads to respiratory and heart failure.

The spores of *C. botulinum* grow under anaerobic (without air) conditions. Canned foods are processed to be anaerobic, thus they provide an ideal medium for the growth of this bacterium. Home-canned, nonacid fruits and vegetables, faulty pro-

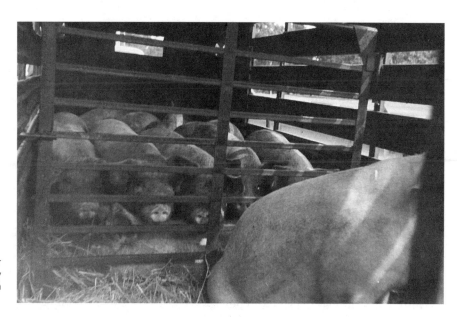

FIGURE 14–2 Swine may harbor *Trichinella spiralis,* which can easily be destroyed by cooking pork to an internal temperature of 160°F.

cessed commercially canned tuna, and improperly packaged smoked fish all have transmitted botulism.

Botulism can be avoided by properly processing and preparing susceptible foods. A reliable home-canning food guide should be consulted regarding proper time, pressure, and temperature required to kill spores for each specific food. As an additional precaution, all home-canned foods should be boiled for at least 10 minutes to destroy botulinal toxins.

In summary, bacteria need food, moisture, warmth, and time to grow. Usually we cannot control the food source (the food is the source) or moisture content of food to decrease bacterial growth. We can control how long and at what temperature food is held and handled. The longer food is held at room temperature and the more food is handled, especially between 45°F and 140°F, the more likely it is to house harmful bacteria.

Parasitic Infections

A **parasite** is an organism that lives within, upon, or at the expense of a living host without providing any benefit to the host. There are several parasites that can live in animals used for food by human beings. When a person eats an animal infected with a parasite, he or she also consumes the parasite. This can result in illness. The parasites discussed in this text are *Trichinella spiralis* and tapeworms.

Trichinella spiralis

Trichinella spiralis is a worm that becomes embedded in the muscle tissue of pork Fig. 14–2. A pig may eat meat from an animal that harbors the worm in its muscle. The worm produces a larva that is protected from animal (including human) digestion. The larvae mature in the animal's stomach in 5 to 7 days. The adult worms then invade the lining of the small intestine, where they reproduce. The original worm's larvae enter the bloodstream of the animal and are carried to all parts of the body. They then penetrate the muscles, form cysts, and remain alive and infective for months. The cycle is completed when another animal eats the muscle containing the live *Trichinella spiralis* larvae.

When a human being eats the larvae, usually in undercooked pork, he or she develops **trichinosis.** The symptoms of trichinosis usually appear 9 days after eating the infected meat, but this time can vary from 2 to 28 days. This period of time is called the **incubation period.** The incubation period is the

---

Botulism—An often fatal form of food intoxication caused by the ingestion of food containing poisonous toxins produced by *Clostridium botulinum.*

Parasite—An organism that lives within, upon, or at the expense of a living host.

Trichinosis—The infestation of *Trichinella spiralis,* a parasitic roundworm, transmitted by eating raw or insufficiently cooked pork.

Incubation period—The time it takes to show disease symptoms after exposure to the offending organism.

length of time it takes to show disease symptoms after exposure to the offending organism. The first symptoms, which mimic food poisoning, are nausea, vomiting, and diarrhea. When the larvae migrate into the muscles, systemic symptoms develop. These include fever, swelling of the eyelids, sweating, weakness, and muscular pain. Death due to heart failure may result.

Tapeworms

Tapeworms are acquired by humans through the ingestion of raw seafood or undercooked beef and pork. Hogs and steers become intermediate hosts when they graze on sewage-polluted pastures. Tapeworm infestation can occur when human wastes contaminate freshwater streams and lakes, animal pastures, or feed. Symptoms of a tapeworm infection may be trivial or absent. Some people in whom the worms are attached to the jejunum develop vitamin B_{12} deficiency, anemia, and massive infections with diarrhea. Obstruction of the bile duct or intestine can also be a complication.

Viral Infections

A **virus** is a microscopic parasite that is entirely dependent on the nutrients inside host cells for its metabolic and reproductive needs. Viruses may invade the cells of people, animals, plants, and bacteria to survive and thereby cause disease. Food frequently serves as a vehicle for some viruses, including those that cause influenza and infectious hepatitis. Food can become contaminated in its growing environment or during processing, storage, distribution, or preparation. Some viruses are found in the intestinal tract of infected humans. If an infected person neglects to wash his or her hands after defecation and then handles food, the virus can contaminate the food and passed on to unsuspecting consumers.

Hepatitis A virus

The hepatitis A virus causes infectious hepatitis, a liver disease. This virus can be found in water that has been contaminated with raw sewage and in shellfish harvested from fecally contaminated water. During food processing, hepatitis A can be transmitted when polluted water is used or by fecal contamination by insects or rodents. Infected workers can transmit the virus through sandwiches, baked goods, or any other food that is handled. Thus there are three ways the virus can be spread:

polluted water, insects and rodents, and infected food handlers.

The onset of viral hepatitis A is abrupt with fever, malaise, anorexia, nausea, and abdominal discomfort. A few days later the client may develop jaundice. Table 14–1 summarizes food handling tips related to microbioligic hazards.

Substances Made Poisonous by Other Organisms

The consumption of toxic fish and plants can cause illness. Molds can also produce disease. Some molds, however, are beneficial.

Toxic Seafood

The tissue of fish and shellfish can be naturally toxic to humans even when the fish is fresh. The fish may not show any outward signs of illness and there is usually no way to tell whether the fish is toxic or not. Because most fish toxins are stable to heat, they are not destroyed by cooking. **Paralytic shellfish poisoning** outbreaks have been reported after the consumption of poisonous clams, oysters, mussels, and scallops. *Ciguatera* is the name of a toxin produced by an organism that frequently infects larger fish such as snapper, grouper, and barracuda. From time to time the concentration of this toxin occurs in large amounts and causes the ocean to appear red. Coastal waters are routinely monitored for the presence of the organism that produces ciguatera. If excessive numbers of the organism are found, a "red tide" alert is made. The best prevention is to avoid eating fish caught during a red tide.

Scromboid fish poisoning is caused by the presence of undesirable bacteria. This poisoning occurs in fish such as tuna, mackerel, bonito, and skipjack. The bacteria produce a toxin on fish flesh after they have been caught. Scromboid fish poisoning can be prevented by the adequate refrigeration of freshly caught fish.

Molds

Molds are the most widely encountered microorganism. Molds are spread by air currents, insects, and rodents. Some molds are beneficial. For example, molds are used to manufacture several types of cheese and soy sauce.

Like bacteria, molds are often involved in food spoilage and are a nuisance in the food industry. A number of molds grow well in cold storage but are easily destroyed by a mild heating process where temperatures of 140°F or higher are reached. Molds

TABLE 14–1   Food Handling Tips Related to Specific Agents and Susceptible Foods

Infective Agent and Susceptible Foods	Food-Handling Tips
Salmonella species Meat, eggs, poultry, milk, and products made with these foods	Wash hands especially after defecation and after preparing uncooked meat, poultry, and eggs. Wash all surfaces and utensils that come in contact with meat, eggs, and poultry thoroughly. Refrigerate prepared food in small containers. Thoroughly cook all foodstuffs from animal sources. Avoid recontamination within the kitchen after cooking. (For example, do not allow food that has been cooked to come into contact with utensils used in the preparation of raw meats.) Never serve raw eggs, fish, and undercooked meats (see Clinical Application 14–2). Do not allow infected people to handle food. Instruct children to wash their hands after handling pet turtles, ducklings, or chicks.
Typhoid fever Any food or water	Wash hands after urination and/or defecation. Avoid contaminated water and ice.
Staphylococcus aureus Bruised poultry, processed meats, cheeses, ice cream, mixed dishes such as potato salad and spaghetti	Personal hygiene: hand washing, avoid handling food when you have infected cuts, boils, and burns (see Figure 14–1). Temperature control: store food between 40°F and 140°F (see Figure 14–2); do not eat food held at room temperature for longer than 4 hours.
Clostridium perfringens Meats, stews, gravies, large masses of food	Cool food rapidly in shallow containers that are no more than 4 in deep. Heat all leftovers to at least 165°F. Hold all hot food above 140°F.
Clostridium botulinum Canned foods Large masses of food with an air-free center	Never taste food from a bulging container. Do not serve home-canned food to institutionalized clients. Follow manufacturer's directions when home canning and use only equipment that has been carefully cleaned. Avoid home-smoked fish. Do not store home-smoked fish in plastic bags.

Table continued on following page

grow on bread, cheese, fruits, vegetables, starchy foods, preserves, grains, and a wide variety of other products. **Aspergillus** molds produce a series of **mycotoxins** called **aflatoxins** that may be present in peanuts or peanut products. Many experts believe aflatoxins to be the most potent liver toxin and cancer-producing agent known.

The best advice is to discard moldy bread as the mold may have penetrated the rest of the item and not be visible to the naked eye. Mold on natural cheese can be safely removed and the remainder of the cheese eaten because the mold is not as likely to have penetrated the rest of the cheese.

Nutritional Hazards

Nutritional hazards are the number two safety risk according to the FDA. Although problems associated with an unbalanced diet occur frequently, clinical symptoms of illness are not as acute and severe as those arising from microbiologic hazards. Illness

Virus—Very small noncellular parasite that is entirely dependent on the nutrients inside host cells for its metabolic and reproductive needs.

TABLE 14–1   Food Handling Tips Related to Specific Agents and Susceptible Foods (Continued)

Infective Agent and Susceptible Foods	Food-Handling Tips
Trichinella spiralis Pork and pork products	Feed swine only cooked garbage. Use pest control measures. Cook all pork to an internal temperature of 160°F (US Dept. of Agriculture, 1990). Exposure of pork cuts or carcasses to low-level gamma irradiation effectively sterilizes and, at higher doses, kills trichina-encysted larvae. Adapt and enforce regulations that allow only certified trichinae-free pork to be used in raw pork products (Benenson, 1995).
Tapeworms Raw seafood and undercooked beef and pork	Do not eat raw seafood (sashimi) and meat. Educate the public to prevent fecal contamination of soil, water, and human and animal food.
Hepatitis A virus Water and any food	Good personal hygiene including hand washing. Infected people should not handle food. Avoid contaminated water and shellfish harvested from fecally contaminated water. Use pest control measures. A vaccine is now available and should be considered for those at risk of infections, i.e., international travelers.

from a food infection or food intoxication poses an immediate danger.

Two different topics are covered in the following sections of this text: food labeling laws and a method the health care worker can utilize to assist in the evaluation of a client's dietary status. Knowledge of these topics can help avoid nutritional hazards associated with consumption of an unbalanced diet.

The Food Label

"The Food Label," was developed by the federal government to provide up-to-date, easier-to-use nutrition information (see figures). Features include:

1. *Standardized Format:* Every label has the same layout and design and is entitled "Nutrition Facts." Some very small packages may use a simplified format.
2. *Serving Sizes:* All serving sizes listed on similar products are stated in identical household and metric measures to allow comparison shopping.
3. *Daily Values:* The bottom half of the "Nutrition Facts" panel shows either the minimum or maximum levels of nutrients that should be consumed each day for a healthful diet. For example, the value listed for carbohydrates refers

to the minimum level while the value for fat refers to the maximum level.

4. *Percent Daily Values:* The percent daily values are based on a 2000 kilocalorie diet and make judging the nutritional quality of a food easier.
5. *Health Claims:* The Food and Drug Administration allows only seven specific claims about the relationships between:

- *Fat and cancer risk*
- *Saturated fat and cholesterol and heart disease risk*
- *Calcium and osteoporosis risk*
- *Sodium and hypertension risk*
- *Fruits, vegetables, and grains that contain soluble fiber and heart disease risk*
- *Fruits and vegetables and cancer risk*

6. *Descriptors:* terms like "low," "high," and "free" must meet legal definitions. Following is a list of key words and what they mean:

   Free: less than 0.5 grams of fat per serving and tiny or insignificant amounts of cholesterol, sodium, and sugar

   Low: 3 grams of fat (or less) per serving; also low in saturated fat, cholesterol, and/or kilocalories

   Lean: less than 10 grams of fat, 4 grams of saturated fat, and 95 milligrams of cholesterol per serving. ("Lean" is not as lean as "Low.")

Extra Lean: 5 grams of fat, 2 grams of saturated fat, and 95 milligrams of cholesterol per serving. (Leaner than "Lean," "Extra Lean" is still not as lean as "Low.")

Light (Lite): 1/3 fewer kilocalories or 1/2 the fat of the original; no more than 1/2 the sodium of the higher-sodium version.

Cholesterol Free: less than 2 milligrams of cholesterol and 2 grams (or less) of saturated fat per serving.

High: a food "High" in a particular nutrient must contain 20 percent or more of the Daily Value for that nutrient.

Good Source Of: one serving contains 10 to 19 percent of the Daily Value for a particular vitamin, mineral, or fiber.

7. Ingredients are listed in descending order by weight. The list is required on almost all foods, even standardized ones like mayonnaise and bread. (See Figures 14–3 and 14–4.)

Examples of Questions Used to Evaluate Dietary Status

Reviewing a client's reported intake or actual food consumption and comparing this to the Food Pyramid guide can assist in the identification of some nutrients that may be lacking in a person's diet. Table 14–2 lists the recommended number of servings needed each day according to sex, age, and physiological state (breast-feeding or pregnant). The following method of comparing a client's daily intake to the Food Pyramid is suggested:

1. Did the client consume at least the recommended servings of grains for his or her sex, age, and physiological state? Nutrients supplied by this group include carbohydrate, thiamin, iron, and niacin. A person who does not eat enough grains may be deficient in these nutrients. In addition, this group supplies fiber.
2. Did the client consume recommended servings

The Food Label at a Glance

Descriptors
The FDA has set specific definitions for:
- free
- light
- more
- good source
- high
- low
- reduced
- less

For fish, meat, and poultry:
- lean
- extra lean

Ingredients
are listed in descending order by weight, and the list is required on almost all foods, even standardized ones like mayonnaise and bread.

Health claim
message referred to on the front panel is shown here.

FROZEN MIXED VEGETABLES
IN SAUCE

- Low Fat
- Cholesterol Free
- Good Source of Fiber
See back panel for nutrition information

(See back panel for message on saturated fat and cholesterol and heart disease.)

NET WT. 8.9 oz. (252 g)

Ingredients: Broccoli, carrots, green beans, water chestnuts, soybean oil, milk solids, modified cornstarch, salt, spices.

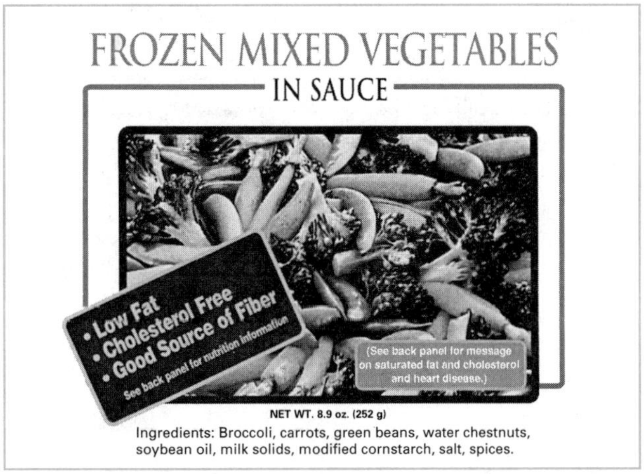

"While many factors affect heart disease, diets low in saturated fat and cholesterol may reduce the risk of this disease."

Source: Food and Drug Administration 1993

Health Claims
can carry information about the link between certain nutrients and specific diseases. For such a "health claim" to be made on a package, FDA must first determine that the diet-disease link is supported by scientific evidence. At this time, FDA is allowing seven specific claims about the relationships between:

- fat and cancer risk
- saturated fat and cholesterol and heart disease risk
- calcium and osteoporosis risk
- sodium and hypertension risk
- fruits, vegetables, and grains that contain soluble fiber and heart disease risk
- fiber-containing grain products, fruits, and vegetables and cancer risk
- fruits and vegetables and cancer risk.

FIGURE 14–3 The food label at a glance. The food label must include descriptors, ingredients, and only certain allowed health claims in a standardized format. (From the Food and Drug Administration, 1993.)

The Food Label at a Glance

Serving sizes are stated in both household and metric measures and reflect the amounts people actually eat.

Nutrition Facts

Serving Size 1/2 cup (114g)
Servings Per Container 4

Amount Per Serving

Calories 90   Calories from Fat 30

	% Daily Value *
Total Fat 3g	**5%**
Saturated Fat 0g	**0%**
Cholesterol 0mg	**0%**
Sodium 300mg	**13%**
Total Carbohydrate 13g	**4%**
Dietary Fiber 3g	**12%**
Sugars 3g	
Protein 3g	

Vitamin A	80%	●	Vitamin C	60%
Calcium	4%	●	Iron	4%

* Percent Daily Values are based on a 2,000 calorie diet. Your daily values may be higher or lower depending on your calorie needs:

	Calories	2,000	2,500
Total Fat	Less than	65g	80g
Sat Fat	Less than	20g	25g
Cholesterol	Less than	300mg	300mg
Sodium	Less than	2,400mg	2,400mg
Total Carbohydrate		300g	375g
Fiber		25g	30g

Calories per gram:
Fat 9   ●   Carbohydrate 4   ●   Protein 4

* This label is only a sample. Exact specifications are in the final rules.
Source: Food and Drug Administration 1993

Calories from fat are shown on the label to help consumers meet dietary guidelines that recommend people get no more than 30 percent of their calories from fat.

% Daily Value shows how a food fits into the overall daily diet.

The **list of nutrients** covers those most important to the health of today's consumers, most of whom need to worry about getting too much of certain items (fat, for example), rather than too few vitamins or minerals, as in the past.

The label of larger packages must tell the number of calories per gram of fat, carbohydrate, and protein.

Daily Values are maximums, as with fat (65 grams or less); others are minimums, as with carbohydrate (300 grams or more). The daily values for a 2,000- and 2,500-calorie diet must be listed on the label of larger packages. Individuals should adjust the values to fit their own calorie intake.

FIGURE 14–4 The food label at a glance. This figure illustrates and describes information that can be found on a food label. The standardized format facilitates comparison shopping.

TABLE 14–2 How Many Servings Do You Need Each Day?

	Women and Some Older Adults	Children, Teen Girls, Active Women, Most Men	Teen Boys and Active Men
Calorie level*	about 1600	about 2200	about 2800
Bread group	6	9	11
Vegetable group	3	4	5
Fruit group	2	3	4
Milk group	**2–3	**2–3	**2–3
Meat group	2, for a total of 5 oz	2, for a total of 6 oz	3 for a total of 7 oz

* These are the calorie levels if you choose low-fat, lean foods from the five major food groups and use foods from the fats, oils, and sweets group sparingly.
** Women who are pregnant or breast-feeding, teenagers, and young adults to age 24 need three servings.
SOURCE: USDA: Food Guide Pyramid—A Guide to Good Eating. Consumer Information Center, Pueblo, Colorado.

of fruits? After counting the number of servings of fruits eaten, check for a reliable source of vitamin C. It is difficult for a client to meet his or her vitamin C allowance without including fruits or some vegetables in the diet. Other nutrients in this group are fiber, iron, potassium, folic acid, carbohydrate, and other trace minerals. Remember, many fruits function as a scrub brush for the teeth and intestines. If an individual's diet is low in fruits ask about his or her dentation. The client may avoid this fruit (especially raw) because of chewing problems. The client may also have a problem with elimination.

3. Did the client consume the recommended number of servings of vegetables? After counting the servings of vegetables, check for a reliable source of vitamin A. It is difficult for an individual to meet his or her vitamin A allowance without including some vegetables in the diet. Many of the comments listed under fruits also apply to the vegetable group such as: nutrients high in this group, fiber, potential dentation, and elimination problems if not part of the diet, etc.

4. Did the client consume the appropriate amount of milk for his or her age, sex, and physiological state? If not, the diet may be lacking in calcium, vitamin D, and riboflavin. Double check for other reliable sources of calcium such as cheese and foods made with milk.

5. Did the client consume the number of recommended servings from the meat group for his or her age and physiological state? If not, the diet may be lacking in protein, iron, and B-vitamins. Remember, the meat group also includes cheese, eggs, beans, and other protein-rich foods.

Environmental Pollutants

A great many people are concerned about environmental pollution. Although the problem is widespread, situations that pose a severe and immediate danger to health are uncommon. The US Environmental Protection Agency (EPA) regulates any pesticide that may be present in food and sets tolerance levels to provide a high margin of safety. See Box 14–1 for a discussion of issues in food preparation and processing.

Chemical Poisoning

Chemical poisoning is caused when people eat toxic substances that may be intentionally or accidently added to foods during growing, harvesting, processing, transporting, storing, or preparing foods. Two general types of chemical poisoning can occur. They are heavy-metal and chemical-product contamination pesticides.

Heavy Metals

Several metals can be toxic. Sources of metals in the soil include parts of rocks and minerals that have weathered to produce soil; water erosion of soil particles; metals as added ingredients or impurities in fertilizers; pesticides containing metals; metals in manure and sludge; and metals in airborne dust. The origin of airborne dust is industrial and mining waste, fossil fuel combustion products, radioactive fallout, pollen, sea spray, and meteoric and volcanic material. Airborne dust eventually settles to the ground and becomes part of the soil. Plants may grow normally but contain levels of selenium, cadmium, molybdenum, or lead that are toxic to humans.

BOX 14–1 ISSUES IN FOOD PROCESSING AND PREPARATION

Outbreaks of serious disease have been linked to changes in food preparation and processing. In botulism, the anaerobic organism secretes a toxin in airtight food packages. Years ago in Alaska, botulism was traced to the substitution of plastic bags for clay pots in the preparation of a Native American dish. Similarly, smoked fish packaged in plastic bags rather than in waxed paper and wooden crates were identified as the source of the disease in Michigan.

Mad Cow Disease (bovine spongiform encephalopathy [BSE]) in Britain has a similar history. BSE is one of several subacute degenerative diseases of the brain with very long incubation periods and causing no demonstrable inflammatory or immune response. The causative agent is a prion, a proteinaceous infectious agent, that is extremely difficult to destroy. It is resistant to heat, pressure cooking, ultraviolet light, irradiation, bleach, formaldehyde, and weak acids. Even autoclaving at 135°C for 18 minutes does not eliminate infectivity.

A change in the British processing of animal carcasses for animal feed in 1982 began the transmission the infective agent to cattle. The practices of boiling under pressure to 160°C and using a solvent to extract fat from the central nervous system, fell by the wayside as a result of the deregulation of the industry. Four years after deregulation, in 1986, the first British case of BSE was confirmed. In 1988, protein from ruminants was banned as ruminant feed. Specific bovine organs were banned in human food in 1989, and in fertilizer in 1991. Various export bans were imposed from 1990 to 1994.

By March 1995, more than 146,000 confirmed cases of BSE were recorded in Britain. The incubation period is usually between 3 and 6 years, and since British beef cattle are usually slaughtered at about 2 years of age, it is certain that the BSE agent had entered the human food chain.

Whether humans can and will contract a spongiform encephalopathy, Creutzfeldt-Jakob disease, from the BSE agent is the focus of intense debate. Experts differ as to the effectiveness of the species barrier, the role of genetic susceptibility, the dose necessary to produce disease, and the efficiency of natural oral transmission as opposed to laboratory or surgical inoculation.

What is clear from both the botulism and the spongiform encephalopathy outbreaks is that drastically altering proven food-processing procedures without verifying equivalent safety can be dangerous. In the case of serious diseases, the hazard is substantial.

The toxic action of metals is believed to be important in enzyme poisoning. For example, mercury, lead, copper, beryllium, cadmium, and silver have been found to inhibit the enzyme **alkaline phosphatase.** One function of alkaline phosphatase is in the mineralization process of bone. Some disease states associated with the consumption of toxic minerals include rickets and bone tumors. Lead ingestion has been linked to mental retardation in children and spontaneous abortions in pregnant women. (See Clinical Application 8–5.)

Mercury is extremely toxic and is widely distributed over the surface of the earth. In the 1950s, a well-publicized incident occurred in Japan. A large chemical plant poured industrial waste containing mercury into a bay. Area residents who ate fish from the bay complained of numbness of the extremities, slurred speech, unsteady gait, deafness, and visual disturbances. Mental confusion and muscular incoordination were apparent in all the clients.

Chemical Products

Chemical foodborne illness is also associated with chemical products such as detergents, sanitizers, pesticides, and other chemicals that may enter the food supply. After consumption, the symptoms of chemical poisoning appear in a few minutes to a few hours, but usually apppear in less than 1 hour. Nausea, vomiting, abdominal pain, diarrhea, and a metallic taste are common complaints with chemical foodborne illnesses.

We all keep many chemicals in our homes. When compounds such as detergents and cleaners are used for the wrong purpose or in excessive amounts, they can cause illness and death. Chemical poisoning can be prevented by:

1. Using each product for its intended use and in the amounts recommended
2. Reading the label before use
3. Keeping chemicals in their original containers
4. Never storing or transporting chemicals in containers used to store food. They may be mistaken for food or beverages.

Pesticides are chemicals used to kill insects or rodents. Improperly used pesticides have caused poisonings when they were accidentally mixed with food. The use of pesticide-containing aerosols around foods and packaging materials and in food preparation areas can be dangerous.

According to a 1989 survey by the Food Marketing Institute, pesticide residues in food appear to be the number one concern to the public. **Residues** are trace amounts of any substance remaining in a product at the time of sale. Three governmental agencies are involved in the regulation of products that enter the US food supply:

• The Environmental Protection Agency (EPA)
• The Food and Drug Administration (FDA)
• The United States Department of Agriculture (USDA) Food Safety and Inspection Service (FSIS)

The EPA regulates the use of potentially harmful pesticides that are used in food production. Included among its duties is that of establishing tolerance levels for pesticides.

The FDA, in addition to its other functions, regulates animal drugs, including food additives, and environmental contaminants. This includes setting tolerance levels for these residues in edible foods. In setting a tolerance level, the FDA determines the highest dose at which a residue causes no ill effects in laboratory animals. This is called the **tolerance level.** The tolerance level is then divided by a factor ranging from 100 to 1000 to account for possible differences between animals and humans. This assumes that humans are 10 times more sensitive than the most sensitive animal species tested. In addition, a further assumption is made that children and the elderly are 10 times as sensitive as others. This is the 100-fold safety factor, which is derived by multiplying 10 times 10. A large margin of safety is built into residue limits established for compounds involved in the production of human food.

The Food Safety and Inspection Service (FSIS) enforces the residue limits in meat and poultry. The FDA is responsible for foods other than meat and poultry. When an illegal residue is found, the FDA can conduct an investigation and the FSIS can detain future shipments from the violating producer.

Natural Food Intoxicants

Many foods (unprocessed or uncooked) contain natural components that can harm health. All foods are made up of chemicals, some of which can alter the way the body uses nutrients. For example, some foods contain chemicals that inactivate vitamins. Healthy people who eat well-balanced diets should not worry about natural food intoxicants. Illness from naturally occurring toxic compounds in foods is not common in this country. However, if an individual eats large amounts of a single food at one time, he or she may experience the effects of natural food intoxicants. The best protection against the effects of natural food intoxicants is to eat a wide variety of foods. This will limit exposure to any one toxic compound.

Food Additives

Additives may be introduced into food deliberately or accidentally.

Intentional Use of Additives

Additives are intentionally added directly to food during processing for several reasons. Steroids and antibiotics are intentionally used in animal production for various reasons.

Reasons for the Use of Additives

There are four reasons additives are intentionally used:

1. To maintain or enhance a food's nutritional value: frequently vitamins, minerals, and different forms of fiber are added to food.

> **Tolerance level**—The highest dose at which a residue causes no ill effects in laboratory animals.
>
> **Additive**—A substance added to food to increase its flavor, shelf life, characteristics such as texture, color, aroma, and/or other qualities.

2. To maintain a food's quality: many additives are used to prevent the growth of microorganisms and extend a product's shelf life. Some additives, called antioxidants, are used to prevent fats in food from deteriorating. Antioxidants are substances that prevent chemical breakdown by preventing or inhibiting the uptake of oxygen. Many researchers believe antioxidants protect an individual from cancer.

3. To assist in processing, transporting, or holding a food: one additive that helps facilitate the processing of food is an **emulsifier.** An emulsifier helps to evenly distribute the molecules of two liquids that normally do not mix. Mayonnaise is an example of an emulsified product. Baking soda and baking powder are other commonly used additives. These substances cause such products as cakes to rise and improve their texture and volume as well.

4. To improve the way a food tastes, looks, or smells: artificial colors, flavors, and sweeteners all fall into this category.

Table 14–3 lists the types of common food additives.

Use of Steroids in Animal Production

Hormones or steroids have been approved by the FDA for use in beef cattle and sheep. Currently, the only FDA-approved hormones for animal use are the anabolic (growth-promoting) steroid implants. Steroids are given to the animal in the form of implants, which are deposited underneath the skin on the back side of the animal's ear. Implants improve feed efficiency (the animal's ability to grow on a given amount of food), reduce the cost of meat production, and result in the production of carcasses with more lean meat and less fat. The implants are composed of natural or synthetic steroid sex hormones: estrogens, androgens, progestins, and combinations thereof (Ritchie, 1990).

Many consumers are concerned about the health hazards of eating beef and sheep with steroid residues. Implantation results in some increase in the hormone content of beef tissue. Beef muscle from an implanted steer contains 0.022 nanograms per gram of steroids compared to 0.015 nanograms per gram in the muscle of nonimplanted steer. (A nanogram equals one billionth of a gram.) These

TABLE 14–3   Common Food Additives

Type of Additive	Reasons Used	Examples
Acidity control agents	Influence flavor, texture, and shelf life	Sodium bicarbonate Citric acid Hydrogen chloride Sodium hydroxide Acetic acid Phosphoric acid Calcium oxide
Antioxidants	Prevent discolorization Protects fats from rancidity	Vitamin C Vitamin E BHT and BHA
Flavors	Food enhancers	Hydrolyzed vegetable protein Black pepper Mustard Monosodium glutamate
Leavening agents	Used to make dough rise	Sodium acid phosphate Sodium aluminum phosphate Monocalcium phosphate Yeast
Preservatives	To extend shelf life	Sulfur oxide Benzoic acid Propionic acid EDTA
Stabilizers and thickeners	To enhance texture	Sodium caseinate Gum arabic Modified starch Pectin

numbers really do not mean much unless you compare them with the amount of the same steroid produced daily in the human body. Before puberty, a boy produces 41,000 nanograms of estrogen and progesterone daily. A pregnant woman produces 20 million nanograms. These steroids are also present naturally in our food supply. A 3-ounce serving of potatoes contains 225 nanograms and a 3-ounce serving of cabbage contains about 2000 nanograms of these steroids. The fact is that the hormone content of beef, whether implanted or not, contains very low levels of steroids as compared with levels naturally produced by the human body or naturally present in foods.

Use of Antibiotics in Animals

Many consumers are also concerned that using antibiotics in animal production poses a human health risk. These compounds are used in animal production in two basic ways: (1) to treat specific diseases, and (2) to maintain health and well-being, thus promoting growth and feed efficiency. The antibiotics penicillin and tetracycline have received the most attention. The two issues raising the most controversy are (Ritchie, 1990):

1. Do antibiotic residues in meat consumed by humans cause development of resistant bacteria in the human body?

   Most experts think not, because the residues of antibiotics in meat are very low.

2. Does the feeding of antibiotics to animals increase levels of disease-resistant bacteria, which may be transferred to humans via bacteria-contaminated meat?

   The use of antibiotics does appear to increase the proportion of resistant bacteria in the animal's body. However, the transfer of resistant bacteria from animals to humans, resulting in illness, has not been adequately studied.

In summary, the controversy on the use of antibiotics in meat remains unresolved.

Accidental Use of Additives

Some additives have entered the food supply accidentally. For example, chemicals may be added to food through contact with surfaces that have been cleaned with solutions that contained the chemical.

Food Selection, Storage, and Handling Guidelines

Even experts have difficulty monitoring all the toxic substances in the food supply. Thus, it is impossible for the average consumer to be aware of all the poisonous substances found in foods. This section of the chapter offers some guidelines that, if followed, will help decrease the risks of food-borne disease. Table 14–1 discusses food handling tips related to specific infective agents.

Food Selection

The greater the variety of foods consumed, the less likelihood of exposure to contaminants of any single food item. Remember that contaminants of natural origin are present in foods.

Food Storage

Proper storage of food helps ensure that there will be minimal contamination of the food from any source. The following guidelines should be followed when storing food:

- Containers used to store food should be covered to provide physical protection for the food.
- Food should be stored in locations that provide minimal risk of contamination from other foods.
- Stored food should be properly labeled to prevent confusion due to similar appearances.
- Proper temperature control of stored food is important to control the growth of disease-producing organisms. The use of thermometers in refrigerators and freezers is recommended.
- Food storage immediately following food preparation is important. Hot food items should be stored in such as manner that they can cool quickly. Allowing hot food to cool to room temperature prior to placing it in the refrigerator is an unsafe practice.

Sanitation and Personal Hygiene

The cleanliness of people involved in food handling and a clean working environment are essential to the prevention of foodborne disease. An unclean person cannot handle food in a sanitary fashion. Smoking and eating while preparing food may result in food contamination. Personal practices such as scratching the head, placing fingers in or about the mouth or nose, and sneezing may contaminate food. Work surfaces in the food preparation area should be clean. Food handlers should always wash their hands after touching themselves. The wearing of soiled clothing while preparing food increases the risk of foodborne disease. Frequent hand washing with soap is the best insurance against food contamination. In fact, the most common way sources of disease are transmitted from a food handler to food is by the hands. Needless to say, it is essential to always wash your hands after using the toilet.

Preventing Cross-Contamination

Cross-contamination refers to the spreading of a disease-producing organism from one food to another. This may happen when a food preparer handles raw meat, eggs, or milk and then handles fruit, lettuce, or bread products that will be served uncooked. The cook transfers the offending substance or organism to the uncooked food item. Organisms can also be transferred to nonfood items such as a cooking utensil and then passed on to the food or a person.

Cooked meat should not be allowed to come in contact with raw meat. This includes the drippings of raw meat. For example, storing raw meat above cooked meat in the refrigerator is inviting trouble. As raw meat drips, the drippings could fall on the cooked meat, thus contaminating it. Nor should consumers use the same utensils for raw meat and foods intended to be served uncooked. Never use the same platter to carry raw meat to the grill and then to carry cooked meat to the table. Instead, the platter should be washed in hot, soapy water between uses.

Safe Food Preparation

Food is the least protected during actual food preparation because of necessary handling, possible contamination from the environment, and the room's temperature. Food should always be prepared with the least amount of hand contact. All work surfaces that come in contact with raw meats should be thoroughly cleaned using soap and hot water. Cooking utensils should be used whenever possible. Raw fruits and vegetables should be thoroughly washed. Potentially hazardous foods requiring cooking should be cooked to heat all parts to at least 140°F. In addition, poultry, poultry stuffings, stuffed meats, and stuffings containing meat should be cooked to at least 165°F. Fresh pork needs to be cooked until at least 160°F.

Safe Cooling and Reheating

Food should be thawed properly. This can be done in refrigerated units at a temperature that should not exceed 45°F. This can also be accomplished under running water at a temperature of 70°F or below. Using the microwave oven to thaw food is a safe method as long as the thawing is part of a continuous cooking process. After thawing the food should be cooked immediately. All foods that have been cooked and then refrigerated should be reheated to a safe temperature of 165°F.

Frozen food items will soon bear a new kind of label that is designed to turn a special color if the food item undergoes an undesirable increase in temperature during transit. The label will thereby warn both food retailers and consumers that the food may be unsafe to eat.

Summary

Thousands of substances besides nutrients are present in foods. Most of these substances are harmless in the amounts typically eaten if the food item is selected, stored, and prepared under recommended conditions. Many foods contain toxic substances naturally. Only in recent years have we been able to detect and measure these toxic substances. It stands to reason that a particular food is safe if our ancestors have eaten it for countless generations with no resulting disease. The human body appears able to safely handle small amounts of toxic substances without injury.

The FDA ranks pathogenic (disease-causing) microorganisms as the most dangerous food-related public health threat. An individual is more likely to suffer from a foodborne illness due to microbiologic contamination than from any other source. Most microbiologic hazards can be controlled by following good principles of food handling. Selecting a wide variety of foods, storing the foods appropriately, and preparing foods correctly all help prevent illness. Health care workers should teach the use of food labels and the risks of microbiologic and residual chemical hazards of foods to their clients.

Cross-contamination—The spreading of a disease-producing organism from one food, person, or object to another food, person, or object.

Case Study 14–1   Ms. N is a 95-year-old woman who is 5 ft tall and weighs 122 lb (dressed without shoes). She has just been admitted to the nursing home. During the routine nursing admission process, Ms. N requested an eggnog every night at 8:00 PM. She stated she dislikes package mixes and would prefer her eggnog made with whole milk, ice cream, and a raw egg. Ms. N's physician has ordered an eggnog at HS (Latin for hour of sleep, or just before bedtime) q.d. (every day). Ms. N stated she has always drunk a homemade eggnog every night for the past 50 years. The client's daughter has stated she makes her mother an eggnog each day from raw eggs.

NURSING CARE PLAN FOR MS. N

Assessment

Subjective Data   Client stated she drinks an eggnog made with a raw egg each day. Client's daughter stated she makes her mother such a beverage.

Objective Data   Height: 5 ft, 0 in Weight: adm 122 lb 100 percent RBW Age 95

Nursing Diagnosis   Infection, potential for: unsafe food behavior related to knowledge deficit as evidenced by client's statement, "I eat one raw egg each day," and the client's age.

Desired Outcome/ Evaluation Criteria	Nursing Actions	Rationale
The client will state that raw eggs can make one ill.	Provide verbal and written information to the client and the client's daughter on the relationship between food illness and *Salmonella* infection.	Elderly clients are particularly at risk from salmonellosis.
	Have the client and the client's daughter state that raw eggs are hazardous.	Verbal recognition of a hazard is the first step in behavioral change.
The client will accept an eggnog made from pasteurized egg product.	Request the dietitian send an eggnog made with pasteurized egg product to client at bedtime each day.	The risk of salmonellosis from pasteurized eggs is lower than from raw eggs.
	Chart acceptance or rejection of the beverage.	Acceptance of the modified eggnog will increase long-term compliance.

Study Aids

Chapter Review

1. Trichinosis is most frequently transmitted by:
   a. Raw milk
   b. Infected pork
   c. Raw vegetables
   d. Wild mushrooms

2. The term "lean" on a food label means the product contains:
   a. Less than 0.5 grams of fat per serving
   b. 3 grams of fat (or less) per serving
   c. Less than 10 grams of fat, 4 grams of saturated fat, and 95 milligrams of cholesterol per serving

3. Foods commonly contaminated with Salmonella are:

a. Eggs
b. Raw vegetables
c. Canned foods
d. Whole grains

4. The best method to control the spread of food-borne illness is by:
a. Wearing gloves when handling food
b. Proper hand washing
c. Taking food supplements
d. Avoiding certain foods

5. A person who excludes all breads, grains, and cereals from the diet is likely to lack adequate:
a. Calcium, vitamin D, and riboflavin
b. Carbohydrate, thiamine, iron, and niacin
c. Vitamin A, calcium, and carbohydrate
d. Carbohydrate, zinc, and vitamin C

Clinical Analysis

1. Ms. P has brought her 80-year-old mother, Mrs. Q, to the Ambulatory Care Clinic for treatment for severe diarrhea of 24 hours duration. In addition to performing any diagnostic tests and instructing the client and daughter about prescriptions, the nurse should:
a. Document all food consumed during the past seven days
b. Inquire about food practices in the home
c. Inspect Mrs. Q's passport for foreign travel in the past month
d. Document the client's immunization status

2. If a jar or can of food shows signs of spoilage, the person should:
a. Boil the food before eating
b. Discard the food item
c. Skim off the top of food in the can, discard, and bring the remainder to a boil before using.
d. Taste the food

3. A nurse is making a home visit to follow up a toddler's progress after an ear infection. She notices the mother's cleaning caddie contains an open soda bottle. The nurse should:
a. Ignore the cleaning caddie because that is not the purpose of the visit
b. Inquire about gastrointestinal upsets in the child
c. Instruct the mother on the safe storage of cleaning agents
d. Assess the amount of sugar sweetened soda the family consumes

Bibliography

Almond, JW: Will bovine spongiform encephalopathy transmit to humans? Br Med J 311:1415, 1995.

American Institute for Cancer Research. Newsletter 48, Summer, 1995. US Department of Agriculture. A Quick Consumer Guide to Safe Food Handling. Home and Garden Bulletin No. 248, September, 1990.

Benenson, AS (ed): American Public Health Department: Control of Communicable Disease Manual ed 16. American Public Health Association, Washington, DC, 1995.

Collee, JG: A dreadful challenge. Lancet 347:917, 1996.

Collinge, J, and Rossor, M: A new variant of prion disease. Lancet 347:916, 1996.

Day, M: Maddening inaction. Nursing Times 91:14, 1995.

Dealler, SF: UK adults' risk from eating beef. Lancet 347:195, 1996.

Department of Health and Human Services: unpublished memorandum. Public Health Services: Center for Disease Control. Questions and Answers about Salmonella. Atlanta, June 8, 1990.

Diringer, H: Proposed link between transmissible spongiform encephalopathies of man and animals. Lancet 346:1208, 1995.

Gore, SM: More than happenstance: Creutzfeldt-Jakob disease in farmers and young adults. Br Med J 311:1416, 1995.

Food Marketing Institute. Trends. Consumer Attitudes and the Supermarket. Food Marketing Institute, Washington, DC, 1990.

Graven, R: Meals, Microbes, and You: A Sanitation Program for Food Service Personnel. Cornell University, Ithaca, NY.

Kimberlin, RH: Creutzfeldt-Jakob disease [Letter]. Lancet 347:65, 1996.

Lefferts, LY, and Schmidt, S: Mold: The fungus among us. Nutrition Action. Center for Science in the Public Interest, Washington DC, 1991.

Morris, GK: Salmonella Enteritidis: Assessment and Risk. Nutrition Close-Up. Egg Nutrition Center, Washington, DC, September 1990.

Owen, AL: The impact of future foods on nutrition and health. J Am Diet Assoc 90:1217, 1990.

Patterson, WJ, and Dealler, S: Bovine spongiform encephalopathy and the public health. Journal of Public Health Medicine 17:261, 1995.

Penner, KP: Contaminated raw seafood. Nutrition and the MD 16(6), 1990.

Ridley, RM, and Baker, HF: The myth of maternal transmission of spongiform encephalopathy. Br Med J 311:1071, 1995.

Ritchie, HD: Agriculture on the stand: Are modern practices safe? Michigan State University, 1990 (unpublished paper).

Roberts, GW: Furrowed brow over mad cow. Br Med J 311:1419, 1995.

Steelman, VM: Creutzfeldt-Jakob disease: Recommendations for infection control. Am J Infect Control 22:312, 1994.

Tabizi, SJ, et al: Creutzfeldt-Jakob disease in a young woman. Lancet 347:945, 1996.

Tyler, KL: Risk of human exposure to bovine spongiform encephalopathy. Br Med J 311:1420, 1995.

Watson, L: Safety and Regulation of Plant Biotechnology. Plant Biotechnology, Monsanto St. Louis, Missouri, 1995.

Will, RG, et al: A new variant of Creutzfeldt-Jakob disease in the UK. Lancet 347:921, 1996.

CHAPTER 15

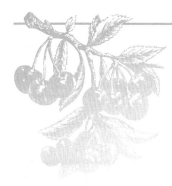

Nutrient Delivery

LEARNING OBJECTIVES

After completing this chapter, the student should be able to:

1 Identify three routes used to deliver nutrients to clients and potential complications with two of these routes.
2 Discuss the kinds of commercial formulas available for oral and tube feedings.
3 Discuss why it is important to carefully control the concentration, rate, and volume of a formula delivered to a client.
4 List at least five reasons for the high incidence of malnutrition in institutionalized clients and the interventions nurses can use to combat malnutrition.
5 Describe suggested procedures for administering medications through feeding tubes.

Food services in health care facilities have two major functions: the preparation and physical delivery of meals to clients, and the nutritional care of clients. The nutritional care of clients includes three areas:

1. Assessing the client's need for nutrients
2. Monitoring the client's nutrient intake
3. Counseling the client about nutritional needs

Quality nutritional care saves both the client and society health care dollars and preventable hardship.

Food Service in Institutions

All nurses need to become familiar with some aspects of the food service in the organizations where they are employed. Specific duties of nurses are often related to meal service patterns.

Meal Service Patterns

Most institutions serve not only three meals to clients each day but also several between-meal feedings. Feedings between meals are available for clients in need of extra nutrients, those who desire extra food, or those unable to consume sufficient kilocalories at the regular mealtimes. It is important for nurses to become familiar with the times meals are served to clients.

The dietary and nursing departments need to coordinate their respective schedules so clients receive their food while it is hot and attractive. The administration of medications sometimes must also be coordinated with meal delivery schedules. Scheduling the client for diagnostic tests, blood work, and educational sessions should be coordinated with the meal service schedule.

Nutritional Care Services

Institutions vary in the types of nutritional services available to clients. A larger teaching hospital or medical center frequently has nutrition professionals who specialize in the treatment of a particular type of client. For example, a critical care dietitian has special training to assess, plan, implement, and counsel clients in high-risk stages of trauma, disease, and processes involving nutritional support. In this situation other health care workers can rely on the critical care dietitian to provide technical support. At the other end of the spectrum, in a small community hospital or a long-term care facility, a dieti-

tian may be present only on a part-time basis or as a consultant. Thus, other health care workers must plan to make the best use of the dietitian's services when he or she is available. In this situation the nursing staff needs to assume more responsibility for the nutritional care of clients.

Assessment, Monitoring, and Counseling

Nutritional care is a joint responsibility of the dietary and nursing departments. Assessing, monitoring, and counseling activities are usually done in collaboration.

Assessment

Some dietary departments screen clients for nutritional problems during admission. Those clients who are found to be at a nutritional risk have a complete nutritional assessment, which usually includes the following:

1. Height, weight, and weight history
2. Laboratory test values
3. Food intake information
4. Potential food-drug interactions
5. Mastication and swallowing ability
6. Client's ability to feed himself or herself
7. Bowel and bladder function
8. Presence of *pressure ulcers*
9. Food allergies and intolerances
10. Any other factors affecting nutritional status, such as food preferences, cultural and religious beliefs about food
11. Determination of body composition
12. Severe burns, trauma, infection, or other physiological stress that increases nutrient needs and is likely to prolong hospital stay

In some health care facilities, nurses are responsible for screening clients for nutritional problems. If the nurse finds a client at a nutritional risk, she or he should make a referral to the dietitian.

All residents in long-term care facilities are required to have a nutritional assessment performed by a registered dietitian. The assessment identifies clients at a nutritional risk. The care plan should reflect nutritional problems identified during the assessment.

Monitoring

All clients should be reassessed or monitored at appropriate intervals. Some clients in hospital intensive care units require continuous monitoring. Other clients require reassessment daily.

The client care conference is a productive method to monitor clients. It is most effective if all health care workers come prepared. Prior to the conference, information on the nutritional care of the client should be gathered including:

1. The client's initial nutritional assessment
2. The client's present body weight and weight history
3. A record of the client's recent food acceptances
4. Any changes in the client's medical condition
5. The client's diet order

With the above information, most changes in the client's nutritional status can be easily identified. Weight loss is easily determined. A review of the client's food acceptance record, if available, can verify whether such a weight loss is likely a result of poor food intake.

Those clients determined to be at a nutritional risk because of poor food intake should be treated. Treatment may include a nutritional supplement, between-meal feedings, a change in diet, or a change in feeding status. For example, perhaps a client's condition has deteriorated to the point where he or she has a self-care deficit in feeding. In this case, the client's feeding status would need to be changed from self-feed to feed. Monitoring the client's weight, laboratory values, and food intake is an important part of delivering quality nutritional care.

Counseling

All clients should be evaluated for nutritional counseling. The assumption that a client is not expected to be discharged and therefore is not entitled to education is unjustified. Educating the client about nutritional concerns helps the client assume responsibility for his or her own care, thus promoting self-esteem and a sense of worth.

Diet Manuals

Current accreditation standards require all institutions to have a diet manual available to all health care workers. The diet manual defines all diets used in the facility and includes information about the particular food service operation. A soft diet may vary slightly from one institution to another. For example, one soft diet may allow lettuce, whereas another does not. This is because a diet manual is approved and developed jointly by all health care

professionals in a facility. Regional food preferences and the unique training of the facility's medical staff and other professionals influence the choice of food items allowed and avoided on special diets.

Usually, the administrative dietitian is responsible for initiating the selection of a diet manual or for writing the manual. Most aspects of the nutritional care given to clients are covered in such a manual, including nutritional supplements stocked by the pharmacy, purchasing, and/or dietary departments; dietary preparation for diagnostic procedures; kilocalorie count procedures; meal service delivery schedules; client educational services; a listing of foods allowed, restricted, and avoided on the various diets; and nursing procedures to follow when transmitting a diet order. When preparing the manual, the dietitian usually consults with other department heads and members of the medical staff. After the manual is written, it must be approved by the facility administrator and the medical staff. Physicians are usually requested to follow the manual when prescribing diets for clients. The medical staff, nursing department, and other professionals in the hospital can and do influence the nutritional care given to clients by participating in the diet manual approval process.

Diet Orders

The physician is responsible for ordering a diet for the client. Just as you cannot administer a medication to a client without a medication order, you cannot legally choose a diet for a client without a physician's order. One of the functions of the diet manual is to define a diet. The diet manual is the first place to look when clients request food items that are not being served to them. As defined in the diet manual, perhaps the food item is restricted or not allowed on the client's prescribed diet.

SPECIAL DIETS   The purpose of a special or modified diet is to restore or maintain a client's nutritional status. This can be accomplished by modifying one or more of the following aspects of the diet:

1. Basic nutrients such as calcium, iron, sodium, potassium, and so forth may be increased, decreased, or eliminated.
2. Kilocalories may be either restricted or increased.
3. Texture or consistency of foods may be altered, for example, only clear liquids may be served.
4. Seasonings such as pepper may be restricted or eliminated.

All modified diets are variations of the general diet, since the client still needs all the essential nutrients. For this reason, each modified diet must be carefully planned to provide each of the essential nutrients or a documented reason why one or more essential nutrients are not provided.

Much confusion results when the terminology in the diet order is not the same as the terminology in the diet manual. For example, a low-salt diet may not be the same as a low-sodium diet as defined in the diet manual. Physicians may persist in ordering a low-salt or low-sodium diet even though the diet manual requests that all sodium-restricted diets be ordered in units of sodium such as 2-gram sodium or 4-gram sodium. Many facilities have eliminated this confusion by defining a low-sodium and low-salt diet in the diet manual. The definitions for both low-salt and low-sodium diets differ markedly from one facility to another. Other vague diet orders are *salt-free*, *diabetic*, *regular diabetic*, *low-fat*, *fat-free*, and *as tolerated*. The nursing or dietetic staff should clarify all vague diet orders with the physician before the client is served. All health care workers should become familiar with the terminology in the facility's diet manual.

Diet manuals are not usually designed to be used directly for client instruction. Much of the information in the diet manual is directed to physicians and other health care workers to assist in the implementation of special diets. For example, many diet manuals describe indications and contraindications for use of a particular diet. An **indication** is the circumstance that indicates when the diet should be used. A **contraindication** describes circumstances when the diet should not be used. The diet manual also lists nutrients deficient in a particular diet. This type of information may alarm and confuse some clients.

COMMON DIET ORDERS Some of the common diet orders are *clear liquid*, *full liquid*, *soft*, and *general* or *regular*. A clear liquid diet is any transparent liquid that can be poured at room temperature. Gelatin, some

juices, broth, tea, and coffee are clear liquids. A clear liquid diet is nutritionally inadequate. However, clear liquid complete nutritional supplements are available. A full liquid diet is any liquid that can be poured at room temperature. Milk, custard, thinned hot cereals, all fruit juices, ice cream, and all items allowed on the clear liquid diet are allowed on most full liquid diets. The major difference between a clear liquid and a full liquid diet is that the latter contains milk and milk products (Table 15–1).

Soft diets vary greatly from one facility to another. For example, a mechanical soft diet is ordered when the client has only a few or no teeth (edentulous). A soft diet is ordered following surgery when easily digested foods are required. A facility that specializes in treating clients with eye, ear, nose, and throat disorders may have many types of soft diets. A pureed diet consists of foods soft enough to be mashed easily in the mouth and safely swallowed. Table 15–2 lists recommended foods on a pureed, mechanical soft, and soft diet. A general or regular diet means that the client is on an unrestricted diet. Frequently, an "as tolerated" or "progressive" diet may be prescribed. This means a clear liquid diet is to be served initially and the diet advanced (full liquid to soft to general) as the client tolerates. The nurse is usually responsible for determining the client's tolerance for food just prior to tray delivery.

Diets for Diagnostic Procedures

Many diagnostic procedures that require dietary preparation are performed in hospitals. There are dozens of diagnostic procedures, and of course not every procedure will be discussed in this text. Instead we will concentrate on why it is important to follow the facility's diet manual when preparing a client for a procedure.

POOR CLIENT PREPARATION A poor dietary preparation can force a client to have an expensive procedure repeated or postponed. For example, Figure

TABLE 15–1 Composition of Liquid Diets

Diet	Protein (g)	Fat (g)	Carbohydrate (g)	Sodium (mEq)	Potassium (mEq)	Kilocalories
Clear liquid	5	trace	70–95	65	20	375
Clear liquid with three 6 oz servings of Citrotein	30	1	140–165	80	30	750
Full liquid	50	55	205	110	65	1500

SOURCE: Adapted from Pemberton, CM, et al: Mayo Clinic Diet Manual: A Handbook of Dietary Practice, ed 6. BC Decker, Philadelphia, 1988, p 47.

TABLE 15–2   Consistency Modifications—Recommended Foods

Food Group	Pureed Diet	Mechanical Soft Diet	Soft Diet
Soups	Broth; bouillon; strained or blenderized cream soup	Broth; bouillon; strained or blenderized cream soup	Broth; bouillon; cream soup
Beverages	All	All	All
Meat	Strained or pureed meat or poultry; cheese used in cooking	Ground, moist meats, or poultry; flaked fish; eggs; cottage cheese; cheese; creamy peanut butter; soft casseroles	Moist, tender meat, fish, or poultry; eggs, cottage cheese; mild flavored cheese; creamy peanut butter; soft casseroles
Fat	Butter; margarine; cream; oil; gravy	Butter; margarine; cream; oil; gravy; salad dressing	Butter; margarine; cream; oil; gravy; crisp bacon; avocado; salad dressing
Milk	Milk; milk beverages; yogurt without fruit, nuts, or seeds; cocoa	Milk, milk beverages; yogurt without seeds or nuts; cocoa	Milk, milk beverages; yogurt without seeds or nuts; cocoa
Starch	Cooked, refined cereal; mashed potatoes	Cooked or refined ready-to-eat cereal; potatoes; rice; pasta; white, refined wheat, light rye bread or rolls; graham crackers as tolerated	Cooked or ready-to-eat cereal; potatoes; rice; pasta; white, refined wheat, light rye or graham bread, rolls, or crackers
Vegetables	Strained or pureed; juice	Soft, cooked, without hulls or tough skin as in peas and corn; juice	Soft, cooked, vegetables; limit strongly flavored vegetables and whole-kernel corn, lettuce and tomatoes
Fruit	Strained or pureed; juice	Cooked or canned fruit without seeds or skins; banana; juice	Cooked or canned fruit; banana; citrus fruit without membrane; melon; juice
Desserts	Gelatin; sherbet; ice cream without nuts or fruit; custard; pudding; fruit ice; Popsicle	Gelatin; sherbet; ice cream without nuts or fruit; custard; pudding; fruit ice; Popsicle	Gelatin; sherbet; ice cream without nuts; custard; pudding; cake; cookies without nuts or coconut; fruit ice; Popsicle
Sweets	Sugar; honey; jelly; candy; flavorings	Sugar; honey; jelly; candy; flavorings	Sugar; honey; jelly; candy; flavorings
Miscellaneous	Seasonings; condiments	Seasonings; condiments	Seasonings; condiments

SOURCE: From Pemberton, CM, et al: Mayo Clinic Diet Manual: A Handbook of Dietary Practice, ed 6. BC Decker, Philadelphia, 1988, p 49, with permission.

15–1 shows two colon roentgenograms, or x-ray studies. Figure 15–1 (A) is a roentgenogram from a poorly prepared client. Feces in the colon block the view of structures within the colon. Figure 15–1 (B) shows the colon of a well-prepared client. There is an absence of fecal material and the entire length of the colon can be visualized.

Some roentgenograms are not only expensive but also uncomfortable. The client must have the procedure repeated if necessary bodily structures cannot be visualized. Although the specific dietary prepara-

tion for x-ray studies of the colon may vary from one facility to another, dietary preparations usually include some similarities. The client should be instructed not to eat or drink anything after midnight

Indication—A circumstance that indicates when a treatment should or can be used.

Contraindication—Any circumstance indicating that a treatment should not be given.

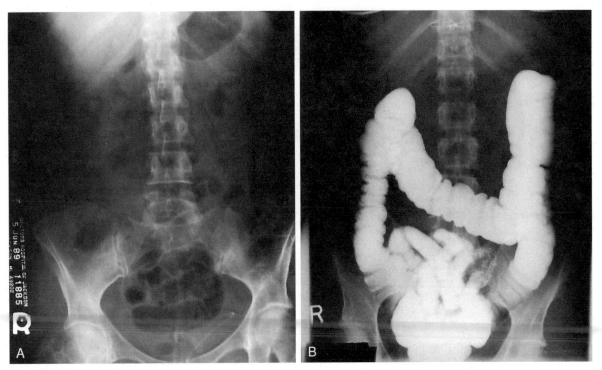

FIGURE 15–1 (*A*) Image of a client who was poorly prepared for a barium enema. (*B*) Image of a client who was adequately prepared for a barium enema. (Courtesy of Dr. Russell Tobe.)

on the day of the imaging study. In addition, the client may need to follow a clear liquid diet for 12 to 48 hours prior to the procedure.

Many clients have x-rays studies performed as outpatients. The nurse working in a physician's office is usually responsible for dietary instruction prior to these procedures. A reliable diet manual should be consulted before the scheduling of clients for such studies.

MISDIAGNOSIS A poor dietary preparation can lead to a misdiagnosis. For example, a blood sample for a fasting blood glucose (FBS) test should be drawn on a fasting individual. **Fasting** means that the client has not had any food or fluid by mouth for at least 8 hours prior to the test. If the client eats before the procedure, his or her glucose level may be elevated. This may cause a misdiagnosis of diabetes. A misdiagnosis may cause a client unnecessary anxiety and expense.

Importance of Nutritional Care

Malnutrition associated with both acute and chronic disease is common in hospital settings. **Acute** means

that the illness is characterized by a rapid onset, severe symptoms, and a short course. **Chronic** means that the illness is characterized by a long duration. The presence and importance of malnutrition has been increasingly recognized over the past 15 to 20 years.

Malnutrition is one of the most common diseases affecting the care of hospitalized patients. According to one study, on admission, 200 of the 500 clients studied were malnourished (McWhirtner, 1994). Many clients become increasingly more malnourished while in the hospital. Measurements of food intake in at-risk groups leave no doubt as to the main cause of hospital-induced malnutrition: many clients do not consume enough food (Dickerson, 1995).

Malnutrition is associated with a 25 percent morbidity and a 5 percent mortality. **Morbidity** is defined as the state of being diseased. Mortality is defined as the death rate. A malnourished client is thus more likely to be sicker and run a higher risk of death than a well-nourished client with the same diagnosis. Because malnutrition affects morbidity and mortality, it is also associated with a prolonged hospital stay.

Iatrogenic Malnutrition

The term **iatrogenic malnutrition** was first used in 1974 (Butterworth and Blackburn, 1975). Iatrogenic malnutrition is a less offensive phrase than induced malnutrition by a physician or an institution. Routine hospital practices such as extended periods of food or nutrient deprivation due to treatments or diagnostic tests that interfere with the client's meal schedule or cause a lack of appetite are related to the high prevalence of malnutrition. Drug therapy may also affect a client's appetite. Some drugs cause drowsiness, lethargy, nausea, and anorexia. Problems related directly to an illness, such as pain, unconsciousness, paralysis, vomiting, and diarrhea can also interfere with eating.

Today many institutions have written policies and procedures for both nurses and dietitians to follow to minimize the likelihood of iatrogenic malnutrition. Clinical Application 15–1 discusses several undesirable practices of health care workers and the duties that dietitians and nurses should perform to combat institutional malnutrition.

Methods of Nutrient Delivery

Nutrients can be delivered to the client orally in foods or supplements, by a tube feeding, or parenterally through veins. An **enteral tube feeding** means the feeding of an appropriate formula or liquid via a tube to a client's gastrointestinal tract. A **parenteral feeding** designates any route other than the gastrointestinal tract, such as intravenous.

Oral Delivery

Most institutionalized clients are fed orally. All of the factors mentioned throughout this text influence whether or not the food items served are actually consumed by the client. Whenever possible, the client should be encouraged to eat foods, not only as an optimal way to obtain nutrients but also because it is beneficial for the client to continue to experience the normal psychologic and physical pleasure associated with eating.

The Menu

An institution's menu can be selective or nonselective. A selective menu is similar to a restaurant menu in that clients can choose the specific menu items that appeal to them. Everyone has food likes and dislikes. What appeals to one client may not appeal to another. Clients eat best when they fill out their menu, or a close significant other does so for them. Marking the menu is one way in which a client can participate daily in care planning.

Some institutions do not have a selective menu. Only one menu is prepared and served to all clients. A nonselective menu is less expensive than a selective menu.

Eating Environment

Health care workers need to create as pleasant an environment as possible immediately before and during mealtime. The room should be checked for objectionable odors, sounds, and sights. Obviously, a full bedside commode or an emesis basin discourages eating. The client should be prepared to eat when the tray arrives. Cleaning the client's hands and face facilitates enthusiasm about eating. The client's bedside table should be cleared of all miscellaneous items so that the table can be used for the client's tray. Because all food loses temperature quickly, unnecessary delays in serving the tray should be avoided. The client should be properly positioned to eat. This includes elevating the head of the bed (if condition permits) and positioning the bedside table to the correct height.

Some clients may find the odor of food offensive. For these clients it is best for the nurse not to uncover the food items directly in front of them, so as to minimize the risk of nausea.

Feeders versus Self-Feeders

Some clients must be fed. Food should be offered in bite-size portions and in the order that the client prefers. The temperature of all hot liquids should be checked against the inside of the nurse's wrist before these items are offered to the client. Clients should not be rushed during feeding. Talking with the client while feeding makes mealtime more pleasant and signals to the client that he or she is not rushed. Sitting while feeding the client also indicates a willingness to spend time with the client and encourages relaxation.

Fasting—The state of having had no food or fluid by mouth for eight hours.

Enteral tube feeding—The feeding of a formula by tube into the gastrointestinal tract.

Parenteral feeding—Feeding administered by any route other than the gastrointestinal tract.

Undesirable Practices Affecting Hospitalized Clients and Methods to Combat Iatrogenic Malnutrition

Some practices performed by health care professionals are undesirable. Many of these practices can affect the nutritional health of hospitalized clients. The result may be iatrogenic malnutrition. However, undesirable practices can be avoided and methods have been established for dietitians and nurses to combat institutionally induced malnutrition.

Undesirable Practices Performed by Health Care Professionals

1. Failure to record actual height and weight of clients
2. Diffusion of the responsibility for client care, that is, among nurses, physicians, dietitians, and other health care workers
3. Prolonged intravenous feedings of only glucose in water or saline
4. Failure to observe and document clients' food intake
5. Withholding meals because of diagnostic tests
6. Administering tube feedings in inadequate amounts, of uncertain composition, and under unsanitary conditions
7. Ignorance of the composition of vitamin mixtures and other nutritional products by all health care team members
8. Failure to recognize increased nutritional needs due to injury or illness
9. Failure to ascertain whether the client is optimally nourished before surgery and failure to provide adequate nutritional support after surgery
10. Failure to appreciate the role of nutrition in the prevention of and recovery from infection, with an unwarranted reliance on antibiotics
11. Lack of communication among physicians, nurses, and dietitians

12. Delay of nutritional support until a client is in an advanced state of depletion, which is irreversible

Methods for Dietitians and Nurses to Combat Iatrogenic Malnutrition

Duties to be completed by the dietitian:

- Description of recent food consumption patterns, eating habits, and meal composition (diet history)
- Circumstances of food purchase, storage, and preparation in the home (diet history)
- Estimate of daily average kilocaloric consumption (assessment)
- Estimate of energy expenditure—for example, low, average, or high level of physical activity (assessment)
- Estimate of possible nutrient deficiencies, based on suspected imbalances (assessment)
- Food tray viewed (monitoring)

Duties to be completed by the nursing staff:

- While hospitalized, documentation of actual food consumption, including any provided by nonhospital sources (monitoring)
- Estimate of fluid intake (monitoring)
- Estimate of stool frequency, urinary losses, losses by suction tube, drainage, and so forth (monitoring)
- Behavior patterns, vomiting, unusual comments clients make about food (assessment and monitoring)
- Careful recording of weight at regular intervals (monitoring)

Adapted from Butterworth and Blackburn, 1975, p 8.

In a long-term care facility, it is important that a client's ability to feed himself or herself be reevaluated at regular intervals. Any client's condition can change, and health care workers need to constantly be aware of any changes in the client's condition.

Assisting the Handicapped Client

A client with a handicap may require either total or partial assistance with eating. Partial assistance may include opening milk cartons and plastic bags containing condiments and eating utensils, buttering the bread, and cutting the meat. Blind clients may be able to feed themselves once they are told where the food is placed on the plate. Food placement described as hours on a clock is the usual technique.

Some clients can feed themselves but they may be very slow, clumsy, and messy. A towel under the chin may assist in cleanup. Offering hot beverages in small amounts may minimize the likelihood of an accident.

Sometimes the type of food offered to clients may influence whether or not they can feed themselves. The consistency of food offered to the client is one example. A thin liquid may cause some clients to choke. A thicker substance such as yogurt may be better tolerated. Finger foods such as French fries or hard-cooked eggs are better accepted by some handicapped people. The handicapped client's food tolerances and preferences are best learned by observation and simply by asking the client what he or she can tolerate.

Health care workers should encourage clients to remain as independent as possible in all the activities of daily living, including eating. If a client cannot feed himself or herself, an evaluation should be made. Some clients' inability to feed themselves may be related to neuromuscular disabilities. Many special eating devices have been developed to assist these clients. The occupational therapist has had special training in the selection and fitting of such eating devices.

Supplemental Feedings

Many clients are unable to consume sufficient kilocalories and/or nutrients because of anorexia or an increased need. The first step with this type of client is to offer additional foods at or between meals. Any between-meal feedings must adhere to the client's diet order. A kilocalorie count should be started for poor eaters; kilocalorie counts are one method to monitor the effectiveness of nutritional care. If the client will not accept the supplemental feedings, another treatment approach may need to be implemented.

Liquid supplementation is often useful because liquids are better accepted than solids by many clients. Many debilitated clients seem to feel less full after drinking a beverage than after eating a comparable number of kilocalories and nutrients in foods. Liquid supplements can include milk, milk shakes, and instant breakfast drinks. Many different commercially prepared liquid formulas are available. Four different types of supplements are used as oral feedings: modular supplements, intact or "polymeric" formulas, elemental or "predigested" formulas, and disease-specific formulas.

MODULAR SUPPLEMENTS   A **modular supplement** contains only one nutrient. These are designed for clients who require the addition of only one nutrient. Moducal, Nutrisource CHO, Polycose, and Sumacal are supplements produced by different manufacturers that contain only carbohydrate. Medium-chain triglycerides supply only one form of lipid. Microlipid is another example of a of lipid supplement. Modular supplements for protein in-

clude Pro Mod, Propac, Pro-Mix, and Casec. Modular supplements are available in a liquid or powder form. Modular supplements may be added to foods, other types of oral supplements, or tube feedings.

INTACT OR "POLYMERIC" FORMULAS   An **intact** or **"polymeric" formula** is used when the GI tract is functional and the client needs all of the essential nutrients in a specified volume. There are dozens of these products on the market. A complete supplement should always be used when the formula is the sole source of nutrition is the formula. Ensure, Sustacal, Resource, and Meritene are examples of complete nutritional supplements. Some complete nutritional supplements are also designed as tube feedings. The consistency and flavor of a feeding designed to be tube-fed will probably not be acceptable to the client when fed orally.

Intact formulas differ from one another. Some contain lactose and some do not. Some provide fiber. The product may be a powder for reconstitution, a liquid, or a pudding. It may be flavored or unflavored. The percent of kilocalories derived from carbohydrates, fats, and proteins may be different. The carbohydrate, fat, and protein may be derived from various sources. For example, the protein source in Meritene is concentrated skim milk, while the protein source in Ensure is sodium and calcium caseinates and a soy-protein isolate. For many reasons the source of any of the three energy nutrients may be important. For example, Meritene is not a good supplement to use for a client with a lactose intolerance. Citrotein is a clear liquid polymeric formula.

Commercial supplements should be used only after the client's requirements for nutrients have been assessed. Some health care workers still think that if some is good, more is better and therefore encourage the client to consume greater amounts of oral supplement. Excess nutrients, however, are rarely beneficial. Not only do clients become frustrated because they cannot consume all of the supplement served to them, but to do so may be medically harmful. Many organs in the human body are in a stress

---

Modular supplement—A nutritional supplement that contains a limited number of nutrients, usually only one.

Intact or "polymeric" formula—An oral or enteral feeding that contains all the essential nutrients in a specified volume.

situation in the poorly nourished client. Why subject the client's kidneys or liver to unnecessary work if the nutrients cannot be used efficiently? Clinical Calculation 15–1 demonstrates a suggested procedure to follow when determining the volume of an oral supplement to serve to a client.

ELEMEMTAL OR "PREDIGESTED" FORMULAS Another group of oral supplements includes **elemental or "predigested" formulas.** Examples of elemental or predigested formulas include Flexical, Vital, and Vivonex. The nutrients in these formulas are easier to digest or partially digested. For example, mal-

---

CLINICAL CALCULATION 15–1

How Much Oral Supplement Is Indicated?

1. Place client on a kilocalorie count.
2. Calculate client's kilocalorie allowance.
3. Select an appropriate oral supplement for the client. Some hospitals allow clients to taste several supplements and choose the one most palatable to them.
4. Determine the difference between the client's recorded food intake and kilocalorie allowance.
5. Determine the kilocaloric concentration of the formula. This can be done by referring to either the appropriate table in the diet manual or the supplement's label. Usually formulas are between 1.0 to 2.0 kcal/mL.
6. Determine how many milliliters of formula are needed to meet the client's kilocalorie allowance.
7. Divide the total milliliters needed by the number of feedings to be offered.
8. Calculate the client's protein allowance (0.8 g/kg).
9. Check to make sure that the client's protein allowance will be met by the combination of recorded protein intake and volume to be provided in the supplement. Also check to make sure that the client will not be receiving more than twice the RDA for protein.

Example:

1. Assume that the client ate 550 kcal.
2. Assume that the client is a woman who weighs 60 kg, is 55 years of age, and is 5 ft, 6 in tall. (Review Chapter 6, "Energy Balance" if necessary to calculate kilocalorie allowance; the 30 kcal per kilograms was taken from the table in that chapter.)

   Client needs approximately 30

   kcal/kg = 30 kcal/kg × 60 kg

   kcal allowance = 1800 kcal

3. Assume that the client has tasted several supplements and prefers Sustacal Liquid.
4. The client's kilocalorie allowance is 1800 kcal.

   The client ate   550 kcal

   The difference is 1250 kcal

5. Sustacal Liquid contains 1.0 kcal/mL (information obtained from the product's label).
6. The client needs 1250 mL of Sustacal Liquid.

$$\frac{1250 \text{ kcal}}{1 \text{ kcal/mL per milliliter}} = 1250 \text{ mL}$$

7. The client stated she would prefer to drink this feeding six times per day—some on each tray and at three between-meal feedings.

$$\frac{1250 \text{ mL}}{6 \text{ feedings}} = 210 \text{ mL per feeding*}$$

8. Assume from the client's recorded food intake that she is eating about 10 g of protein per day. A woman weighing 60 kg has a protein allowance of 0.8 g/kg.

   60 kg × 0.8 g/kg = 48 g of protein

   Subtract the 10 g eaten from trays −10

   The supplement should provide at least 38 g of protein and no more than 86 g (48 × 2-10) of protein.†

9. Sustacal Liquid contains 61 g of protein per 1000 mL or 0.061 g/mL.

   1250 mL × 0.061 g/mL = 76.25 g of protein

   The client's protein allowance will more than be met by 1250 mL of Sustacal Liquid and food, but will not exceed the 200% guideline.

---

*This product is available in both quarts and 240-mL units. Some institutions stock only 240-mL units and may prefer to dispense this feeding in 240-mL units. In this situation, divide 240 mL into 1250 mL. The client would need only 5.2 feedings per day. This would be offered to the client in four feedings of 240 mL for a total of 960 mL and one feeding of 290 mL to equal the 1250 mL.

† It is important that the feeding and food not provide more than twice the client's protein allowance. In this case, 48 × 2 = 96 g. As the client is eating about 10 g of protein per day and will consume about 76 g more in the supplement, her total protein intake would be approximately 86 g/day. This amount does not exceed twice her RDA for protein and is therefore acceptable.

trodextrins, corn syrup solids, oligosaccharides, and glucose polymers are rapidly hydrolyzed by maltase and oligosaccharidases, which are apt to be present in higher concentrations than lactase.

Protein is either partially or totally predigested. Partially predigested protein (small peptides) offer an advantage over totally predigested protein (single amino acids). Peptides and free amino acids do not inhibit each other's transport, so that absorption of nitrogen is actually improved by the inclusion of small peptides. Easier-to-digest fats include medium-chain triglycerides. Partially digested fats include mono- and diglycerides.

Predigested formulas contain little lactose and residue and may be given orally or through a tube. These formulas are very expensive and are designed only for use with clients with limited gastrointestinal function and/or metabolic disorders. They are less palatable than intact feedings, so client acceptance is sometimes a problem when they are administered orally.

DISEASE-SPECIFIC FORMULAS   The last group of oral supplements includes those designed for clients with specific metabolic problems. For example, special formulas are available for clients with liver (*Hepatic-Aid,* Travasob Hepatic) and kidney disorders (*Suplena, Amin-Aid,* Travasob Renal). These special formulas are discussed in subsequent chapters.

Oral supplements are also used extensively to wean clients from both tube and parenteral feedings. Once a client ceases to consume foods orally, a transition period is always necessary to wean the client back to oral feedings.

Enteral Tube Feeding

Tube feedings are the second way nutrients can be delivered to clients. Some medical conditions may render oral feeding impossible, insufficient, or impractical. Table 15–3 lists several common conditions in which a tube feeding is indicated.

Tube feedings, like oral supplements, can be made from table foods or purchased commercially prepared. If money is tight and the client has no impairment of digestion and absorption, he or she can be taught to prepare a tube feeding from table foods prior to discharge. Home-prepared tube feedings are less expensive than commercially prepared feedings but more prone to contamination. Many of the commercial products described under the previous section can be used in the tube-fed client.

TABLE 15–3   Conditions Indicating a Tube Feeding*

Condition	Examples
Client has mechanical difficulties that make chewing and/or swallowing impossible or difficult	Obstruction of the esophagus, weakness or nausea, mouth sores, throat inflammation
Client has an intestinal disease and cannot digest or absorb food adequately	Malabsorption syndromes
Client refuses to eat or cannot eat	Anorexia nervosa, senile dementia
Client is unable to consume a sufficient amount of food because of clinical condition	Coma, serious infections, trauma victims, clients with large kilocalorie requirements

* Other conditions will be discussed in subsequent chapters.

Use the Gut and Make It Work

The gut should always be used to the extent possible. Oral supplements should be considered before tube feeding; tube feeding should always be considered before intravenous feeding. Tube feeding is safer, cheaper, and more physiological than an intravenous feeding, in other words, it mimics normal feeding conditions. Nutrients should be supplied intact as opposed to predigested if the client has normal digestion. **Intact nutrients** are nutrients that are not predigested. With intact nutrients the body must keep producing all the secretions and enzymes necessary for digestion. This forces the gut to function.

Tube Placement

Tubes can enter the body either through the nose or by a surgically made opening. The most common tube insertion method is through the nose. If the client is fully alert during the procedure, he or she

Elemental or "predigested" formula—Formula that contains either partially or totally predigested nutrients.

Intact nutrients—Nutrients that have not been predigested.

can assist in passing the tube by swallowing. A **nasogastric (NG) tube** runs from the nose to the stomach. A **nasoduodenal (ND) tube** runs from the nose to the duodenum. A **nasojejunal (NJ) tube** runs from the nose to the jejunum. These types of tubes are designed for short-term use only because of client discomfort and tissue irritation.

A critical responsibility of nurses is assessment of feeding tube placement. The most reliable method of determining nasoenteral tube placement upon insertion is radiography (Fater, 1995). Unfortunately, feeding tubes migrate (after x ray) and move out of the stomach. This places the client at risk for aspiration because the tube has inadvertently entered the trachea. The ideal method for determining feeding tube placement has yet to be determined (Fater, 1995). Nurses must remain alert to new research findings in this area of current research.

When a tube is needed long-term or cannot be inserted through the nose, an **ostomy,** or surgically formed opening, is created. An **esophagostomy** is a surgical opening into the esophagus through which a feeding tube is passed. A **gastrostomy** is a surgical opening in the stomach through which a feeding tube is passed. A **jejunostomy** is a surgical opening in the jejunum through which a tube is passed.

Each tube location has advantages and disadvantages. One advantage of a feeding ostomy located in the intestines is that the client is the least likely to regurgitate the feeding. **Regurgitate** means to cause to flow backward. Regurgitation is more likely when a feeding is administered to clients through a nasogastric tube, esophagostomy, or gastrostomy. During regurgitation the feeding backs up. If the feeding backs up into the client's lungs, a lung infection can develop. When a client has inhaled fluids regurgitated from the stomach, he or she may develop aspiration pneumonia. **Aspiration** is the state whereby a substance has been drawn into the nose, throat, or lungs. Most studies show an aspiration rate of 30 to 40 percent with tube feedings (Galindo-Ciocon, 1993). Aspiration pneumonia can be a fatal complication of a tube feeding (or improper oral feeding). Another advantage of a jejunostomy is that it bypasses esophageal or gastric outlet obstructions.

Contamination

Unfortunately, tube feedings provide an excellent environment for the growth of microorganisms. When a tube feeding becomes contaminated with bacteria, the client receiving the feeding may become ill and may suffer from gastrointestinal problems such as nausea, vomiting, or diarrhea. For this reason, many hospitals and nursing homes use only commercially prepared tube feedings (as opposed to those prepared in-house from table foods). Commercial feedings are packaged under sterile conditions. Most hospitals do not have a sterile area in their dietary departments. Even commercially prepared formulas can become contaminated if they are not handled safely after opening.

To eliminate contamination, first check the can for the correct product, flavor, expiration date, and signs of contamination such as swelling. If the can is swollen, notify your supervisor. Do not administer a feeding from a damaged can. Other cans in the same shipment should be checked for contamination.

Good personal hygiene is important. The following recommendations will reduce the possibility of contamination:

- Always wash your hands before opening the can.
- Wash the top of the can carefully before opening.
- Shake the can well before opening.
- If a can opener is needed, be sure it is clean.
- Transfer the formula into a clean container.
- Use sterile, bottled, or boiled water to dilute formula (if indicated).
- Label any remaining formula carefully with the client's name, room number, the date the formula was opened, amount in the container, name of the product, and other pertinent information. Other information may include whether the formula is diluted or contains medications, vitamins, or other additives.
- Store the formula in the refrigerator in a covered container. When a new supply of formula is received, place it in the rear of the storage area so that the older formula is used first.
- Once opened, most formulas should be discarded after 24 hours.

Administration

Tube feedings can be administered either continuously, intermittently, or by bolus. Clogging of the tube occurs significantly more often with continuous rather than intermittent feedings (Galindo-Ciocon, 1993).

CONTINUOUS FEEDING Many professionals feel that a **continuous feeding** is preferable. A continuous feeding is always recommended for formulas delivered directly into the small intestine. One recommended rate is 30 to 50 milliliters per hour, in-

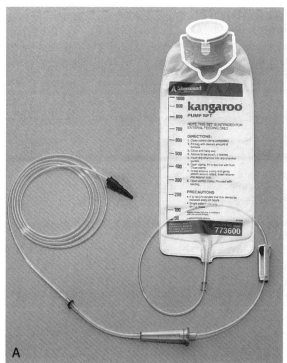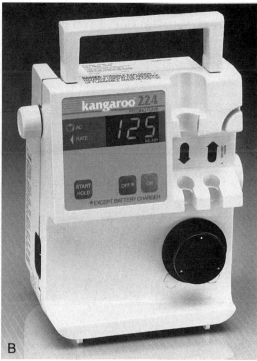

FIGURE 15–2 Equipment used to deliver a specific volume and rate of a formula to a client. (*A*) This is a pump set. The nurse would pour the formula into the top of the bag. (*B*) This is a feeding or infusion pump (necessary for a continuous feeding). The flow rate of the formula is maintained with this device. (Photographs were provided courtesy of Sherwood Medical, St. Louis, MO. Kangaroo is a registered trademark.)

creasing daily by 25 milliliters per hour to the rate necessary to provide energy needs. This gradual increase in the formula's volume gives the client's gastrointestinal tract a chance to adjust to the formula. This will assist in the prevention of many complications seen in tube-fed clients. Safety precautions for continuous feedings include (1) flushing the tube with water every 4 to 6 hours; and (2) allowing no more than a 4-hour hang time for each bag of formula unless the formula is packaged in a sterilized delivery system. This will assist in preventing contamination and bacterial growth.

Figure 15–2 illustrates some of the equipment used to deliver a specific volume and rate of a formula to a client. An infusion pump is necessary for precise control of a continuous feeding.

INTERMITTENT FEEDING An **intermittent feeding** means giving a 4- to 6-hour volume of feeding solution over 20 to 30 minutes. Clients tolerate intermittent feedings much better than bolus feedings because these feedings more closely approximate normal eating behavior. The tube needs to be flushed after each feeding to minimize bacterial growth and prevent contamination.

BOLUS FEEDING A **bolus feeding** means giving a 4- to 6-hour volume of feeding solution within a few minutes. A client is thus fed only four to six times per day. Feedings given by this method are frequently poorly tolerated, with clients complaining of abdominal discomfort, nausea, fullness, and cramping. Some clients, however, can tolerate bolus feedings after they have had a period of adjustment to the tube feeding. Bolus feedings are usually poorly tolerated for feedings that enter the intestines. The adjustment period should follow the procedure described above, that is, the volume of feeding is slowly increased. Clients on bolus feedings should be in-

Ostomy—A surgically formed opening.

Continuous feeding—Delivery of a tube feeding on an ongoing basis.

Intermittent feeding—Giving a 4- to 6-hour volume of a tube feeding over 20 to 30 minutes.

Bolus feeding—Giving a 4- to 6-hour volume of a tube feeding within a few minutes.

TABLE 15–4   Common Mechanical, Gastrointestinal, and Metabolic Complications of Tube-Fed Clients and Prevention Strategies

Complication	Prevention Strategy
Mechanical	
Tube irritation	Consider using a smaller or softer tube
	Lubricate the tube before insertion
Tube obstruction	Flush tube after use
	Do not mix medications with the formula
	Use liquid medications if available
	Crush other medications thoroughly
	Use an infusion pump to maintain a constant flow (Fig. 15–2)
	Feeding should not be started until tube placement is radiographically confirmed
Aspiration and regurgitation	Elevate head of client's bed greater than or equal to 30 degrees at all times
	Discontinue feedings at least 30 to 60 minutes before treatments where head must be lowered (e.g., chest percussion)
	If the client has an endotracheal tube in place, keep the cuff inflated during feedings
	Test pH of aspirate with pH paper or meter
	a. pH of tracheobronchial secretions is alkaline, >7.4
	b. pH of gastric secretions is acidic <5.0
	c. As the tube moves from the acid stomach to the alkaline duodenum, pH will change from acid to alkaline
	Place a black mark at the point where the tube, once properly placed, exits the nostril
Tube displacement	Replace tube and obtain physician's order to confirm with x-ray imaging
Gastrointestinal	
Cramping, distention, bloating, gas pains, nausea, vomiting, diarrhea*	Initiate and increase amount of formula gradually
	Bring formula to room temperature before feeding
	Change to a lactose-free formula
	Decrease fat context of formula
	Administer drug therapy as ordered, e.g., Lactinex, kaolin-pectin, Lomotil
	Change to formula with a lower osmolality
	Change to formula with a different fiber content
	Practice good personal hygiene when handling any feeding product
	Evaluate diarrhea-causing medications the client may be receiving (e.g., antibiotics, digitalis)
Metabolic	
Dehydration	Assess client's fluid requirements before treatment
	Monitor hydration status
Overhydration	Assess client's fluid requirements before treatment
	Monitor hydration status
Hyperglycemia	Initiate feedings at a low rate
	Monitor blood glucose
	Use hyperglycemic medication if necessary
	Select low-carbohydrate formula
Hypernatremia	Assess client's fluid and electrolyte status before treatment
	Provide adequate fluids
Hyponatremia	Assess client's fluid and electrolyte status before treatment
	Restrict fluids
	Supplement feeding with rehydration solution and saline
	Diuretic therapy may be beneficial
Hypophosphatemia	Monitor serum levels
	Replenish phosphorus levels before refeeding
Hypercapnia	Select low-carbohydrate, high-fat formula
Hypokalemia	Monitor serum levels
	Supplement feeding with potassium if necessary
Hyperkalemia	Reduce potassium intake
	Monitor potassium levels

* The most commonly cited complication of tube feeding is diarrhea.

structed not to recline for at least 2 hours following the feeding. Tubes should be irrigated (flushed) after each bolus feeding to prevent contamination. **Irrigation** means flushing water through the tube or cavity.

Potential Complications

Complications fall into three categories: mechanical, gastrointestinal, and metabolic. Table 15–4 reviews the mechanical gastrointestinal, and metabolic complications of tube-fed clients and lists system-specific prevention strategies. Metabolic complications will be discussed later chapters.

Osmolality

The osmolality of a solution is based on the number of dissolved particles in the solution. The greater the number of particles, the higher the osmolality.

At a given concentration, the smaller the particle size, the greater the number of particles present. Oral supplements and tube feedings with a high osmolality draw body fluid into the bowel, resulting in a fluid imbalance. The symptoms are diarrhea, nausea, and flushing. The osmolality of normal body fluids is approximately 300 milliosmoles per kilogram. Predigested nutrients have a higher osmolality than intact nutrients. An **isotonic** feeding has an osmolality of 300 milliosmoles, the same osmotic pressure as body fluids. Table 15–5 lists the osmolality of selected formulas.

There is a great variation from one individual to another in sensitivity to the osmolality of oral supplements and tube feedings. All clients need a period of adjustment to a formula with a high osmolality. The majority of clients are able to develop a tolerance to a high-osmolality formula. Some clients, however, are more likely to develop symptoms of an intolerance. These include debilitated clients, clients with gastrointestinal disorders, preoperative and postoperative clients, gastrostomy

and jejunostomy clients, and clients whose gastrointestinal tract has not been challenged by food for a significant period of time.

Administration of Medications to a Tube-Fed Client

All health care workers should be aware of potential drug-food interactions so that proper steps can be taken to minimize or avoid complications (see Chapter 16, "Food, Nutrient, and Drug Interactions). Clinical Application 15–2 discusses suggested procedures for administering medications through feeding tubes. Medications can be physically incompatible with the tube feeding. This may be related to changes in the feeding's viscosity (thickness), or flow characteristics. Some medications may also cause the feeding to separate, granulate, or coagulate.

Monitoring the Tube-Fed Client

The tube-fed client requires special monitoring. The purpose of the monitoring is to check for tolerance to the feeding and to determine if the nutritional status of the client is declining, stable, or improving (Quality Assurance Committee of the American Dietetic Association, 1984). The categories of factors that should be monitored include physical factors, intake factors, and laboratory data. Clinical Application 15–3 discusses factors that should be routinely monitored in each of these categories.

Metabolic, fluid, and electrolyte complications can occur during enteral nutritional support. Adequate monitoring of the client on an enteral feeding is not merely cost-effective but critical to ensure successful therapy.

Home Enteral Nutrition

Many clients on tube feedings are being discharged from hospitals and nursing homes. Most hospitals and nursing homes that discharge clients on home enteral nutrition (HEN) have a **nutrition support service.** The delivery of effective nutritional support requires a team effort. Team members usually include the physician, pharmacist, nurse clinician, dietitian, and social worker. Team functions vary from one facility to another. Members of nutrition sup-

TABLE 15–5   Osmolality of Selected Formulas

Formula	Milliosmoles*/hg	Description
Stresstein	910	Elemental formula
Vivonex HN	810	Elemental formula
Ensure	450	Intact or polymeric
Isocal	300	Intact or polymeric

* Please note the wide range in osmolality of the various formulas.

Nutrition support service—A team service that assesses, monitors, and counsels clients on enteral and parenteral feedings.

Procedures for Administering Medications through Feeding Tubes

Procedures for the administration of medications through feeding tubes may vary slightly from one institution or facility to another. The following suggested procedures, however, are common in most facilities:

1. If possible, administer drugs in liquid form.
2. If the drug is not available in liquid form, consult with the pharmacist; he or she may be able to procure a liquid form or similar drug provided by the American Society of Hospital Pharmacists in Pediatric Extemporaneous Formulation List of the manufacturer's suggestions.
3. Exercise caution when calculating equivalent liquid doses. Many liquid dosage forms are intended for pediatric use and the dose of the drug must be adjusted appropriately for adults.
4. Administer crushed tablets only when no other alternatives are available.
5. If crushed tablets are administered, crush the tablet to a fine powder and mix with water. Do not crush any tablet on the list of oral drugs that should not be crushed. Do not crush drugs with a sustained-release action or an enteric coating. If in doubt, consult with the pharmacist.
6. Administer each drug separately. Do not mix all the medications for one dosing time. Flush with at least 5 mL (1 tsp) of water between each medication.
7. Flush the tube with at least 30 mL of water before giving the medication and before restarting the tube feeding.
8. To avoid causing gastric irritation and diarrhea, drugs that are hypertonic or irritating to the cells that line the gastrointestinal tract, such as potassium chloride, should be diluted in at least 30 mL of water prior to administration.
9. If the medication is ordered to be added to the feeding, observe the feeding after the addition for any reaction or precipitation. Shake the solution thoroughly. Label the feeding with at least the name and amount of the drug added, the time, date, and your initials.
10. Drugs usually administered with meals to avoid gastric irritation, such as indomethacin, should also be diluted with water prior to administration.
11. Sustained- or slow-release formulations of drugs that are used for once-daily dosing may need to have divided dosing schedules when administered in liquid form.

Adapted from Wright, 1986, p. 33.

Physical and Intake Factors and Laboratory Data to Monitor in the Client Receiving Nutritional Support

Clients who are receiving nutritional support such as tube feeding require special monitoring. This is done (1) to check for tolerance to the feeding and (2) to determine the effect of the feeding. Many physical factors and intake factors are routinely monitored; certain laboratory data are monitored as well. Physical factors to routinely monitor include:

- A change in gastrointestinal tract function
- Abdominal discomfort or gas
- Stool consistency, frequency, odor, and color (when the onset of diarrhea occurs without a formula change, consider medication rather than feeding as probable cause; potential formula factors include rapid administration, cold feedings, fat malabsorption, lactase deficiency, protein malnutrition, bacterial contamination, or high osmolality). Constipation may be caused by dehydration, impaction, and/or obstruction (Feldman, 1988).
- Gastric retention, that is, formula remains in the stomach (formula has too high an osmolality) (Feldman, 1988).
- Weight changes (should not exceed 1/4 to 1/2 lb per day)
- Intake and output
- Temperature
- Client's physical condition
- Psychological impact of the feeding

Intake factors to routinely monitor include:

- Volume ordered
- Volume actually administered
- Adequacy of intake compared to needs (kilocalorie/protein count)

Laboratory data to monitor include:

- Urinary glucose/serum glucose
- Serum electrolytes
- Calcium-to-phosphorus ratio
- CBC with differential
- Liver function tests
- Urinary urea nitrogen (if available)
- Transferrin (if available)
- Retinol-binding protein
- Skin testing (to assess immunocompetence)
- BUN/creatinine
- Serum albumin
- Cholesterol/triglycerides (should be tested at least 6 hours after lipid infusion has stopped)

Adapted from the Quality Assurance Committee of the American Dietetic Association, 1984, p. 89 with permission.

BOX 15–1   INDICATION FOR PPN AND TPN

PPN (PERIPHERAL PARENTERAL NUTRITION)

PPN is indicated when the energy needs of the client do not exceed 2000 kcal per day and the client is not expected to require nutritional support for longer than 10 days.

TPN (TOTAL PARENTERAL NUTRITION)

Potential candidates for TPN include those clients who are anticipated to require nutritional support for longer than 10 days and have an increased requirement for energy. Examples of such situations follow:

1. Preoperative preparation of severely malnourished clients: Cancer of the esophagus and stomach, severe peptic ulcer disease, dysphagia, amyotrophic lateral sclerosis (ALS) (Lou Gehrig's disease), and congenital abnormalities.
2. Postoperative surgical complications: Prolonged ileus, obstruction, peritonitis, short-bowel syndrome, etc.
3. Inflammatory bowel disease: Regional enteritis, Crohn's disease, ulcerative colitis, etc.
4. Inadequate oral intake or malabsorption: Metastatic carcinoma on chemotherapy or radiation therapy, acute pancreatitis, coma, massive burns, chronic malnutrition, anorexia, major trauma, hepatic insufficiency, hypermetabolic states, etc.

---

port teams assess, monitor, and educate clients. Some nutrition support service team members also arrange for client follow-up in outpatient clinics or in the home.

Parenteral Nutrition

Parenteral nutrition is the third way nutrients can be delivered to the client. Nutrients are delivered to the client through the veins (intravenously) in parenteral nutrition. **Peripheral parenteral nutrition** (PPN) means to feed the client via a vein away from the center of the body. In **total parenteral nutrition** (TPN) the client is fed via a central vein. TPN and PPN can be used to provide partial or total daily nutritional requirements. Clients who cannot or should not be fed through the gastrointestinal tract are some of the candidates for TPN and PPN. Box 15–1 describes both indications for PPN and TPN.

Peripheral Parenteral Nutrition (PPN)

Intravenous (IV) feedings are routine in most health care institutions. IV solutions usually contain water, dextrose, electrolytes, and occasionally other nutrients. IV solutions are used to maintain fluid, electrolyte, and acid-base balance. Intravenous solutions do contain kilocalories. Clinical Calculation 15–2

describes how to calculate the kilocalorie content of an intravenous solution.

Amino acids and fat can be supplied peripherally. To prevent ketosis, intravenous lipid emulsions should contribute no more than 60 percent of the total kilocalories provided. Dextrose concentrations are limited to approximately 10 percent since peripheral veins are unable to withstand concentrations greater than 900 milliosmoles per kilogram (Moore, 1993). Thus, PPN has often failed to provide adequate kilocalories and other nutrients for repair and replacement of losses. PPN has been used to supplement a partially successful enteral nutrition program.

A new system for PPN (called all-in-one or three-in-one) has been developed that allows a higher osmotic load (1200 to 1350 milliosmoles per liter) to

---

Peripheral parenteral nutrition (PPN)—An intravenous feeding via a vein away from the center of the body.

Total parenteral nutrition (TPN)—An intravenous feeding via a central vein that provides total nutrition.

CLINICAL CALCULATION 15–2

Calculation of Kilocalories in IV Solutions

D_5W means 5 percent dextrose in water. The subscript following the D tells you the percent of dextrose in the solution. Other common concentrations of sugar and water are $D_{10}W$ and $D_{50}W$.

A 5 percent concentration of dextrose means 100 mL of water contains 5 g of dextrose. A 10 percent concentration of dextrose means 100 mL of water contains 10 g of dextrose. A 50 percent concentration of dextrose means 100 mL of water contains 50 g of dextrose. A simple proportion should be used to calculate the amount of kilocalories in any given volume of a solution.

The formula is:

$$\frac{\text{percent of concentration}}{100 \text{ mL}} \quad \text{as} \quad \frac{x \text{ grams of dextrose}}{\text{volume of solution client received}}$$

For example, a client has received 2000 mL of D_5W

$$\frac{5 \text{ g of dextrose}}{100 \text{ mL}} \quad \text{as} \quad \frac{x \text{ grams of dextrose}}{2000 \text{ mL}}$$

Proportions are solved by cross-multiplication and division: (5 g × 2000 mL) divided by 100 mL = 100 g of dextrose. One gram of carbohydrate given intravenously provides 3.4 kcal; thus 100 g × 3.4 kcal/g = 340 kcal.

---

be delivered peripherally. Lipids, amino acids, and dextrose are all incorporated in one container. Tolerance of this higher osmotic admixture in peripheral veins might be attributed to the buffering and dilution effects of intravenous fats in combination with the higher pH of the amino acid solutions and the addition of heparin to the admixture (Hoheim, 1990).

The ratio of nonprotein to protein kilocalories is important in peripheral feedings. This is discussed in the chapter on stress.

Total Parenteral Nutrition (TPN)

When nutrients are infused into a central vein, parenteral nutrition is often referred to as TPN or **hyperalimentation.** Hyperalimentation is actually a misnomer because it implies that the solution exceeds nutritional requirements. The **superior vena cava** is one of the largest diameter veins in the human body and is often used for TPN. Total parenteral nutrition can deliver greater nutrient loads because the blood flow in the superior vena cava

rapidly dilutes these solutions 1000-fold (Feldman, 1988). Concentrations for both dextrose and amino acids are determined by the client's needs. Clinical Calculation 15–3 explains and demonstrates the calculation of a sample TPN solution.

INSERTION AND CARE OF TPN LINE   The physician inserts the TPN line usually through the subclavian vein and into the superior vena cava (Fig. 15–3). It can be inserted at the client's bedside using strict aseptic technique. The TPN solution is a sterile mixture of glucose, amino acids, vitamins, and minerals. The pharmacist usually prepares the TPN solution. Lipids are usually administered to the client in a separate solution. Vitamins B_{12}, K, and folic acid are given to the client separately.

Total parenteral nutrition has both advantages and disadvantages. Central TPN should not be carried out without experienced personnel and proper facilities. One disadvantage of TPN is that it takes a highly trained staff to provide safe administration and close monitoring. This makes the therapy expensive. The nurse is responsible for assessing, monitoring, and educating the client destined for home TPN. The clinical dietitian on the TPN team usually has an advanced degree and special training. The dietitian is responsible for constant nutrition assessment, monitoring, interpretation of data, and calculating formula needs with the physician.

MONITORING   Careful administration of the TPN solution is important. Most reputable institutions have a strict protocol that must be followed by all health care professionals. A **protocol** is a description of steps to be followed when performing a procedure. Protocols vary widely from one institution to another. Most TPN protocols include the following: a slow start, a strict schedule, close monitoring, instructions for increasing the volume, maintenance of a constant rate, and instructions on a slow withdrawal. The solution may require adjustment. This can be done by increasing or decreasing any or all of the nutrients. Both careful monitoring of the client's response to TPN and taking corrective measures when needed are essential for safe administration of these solutions.

Many metabolic complications are possible with TPN. Rapid shifts of potassium, phosphorus, and magnesium intracellularly result in a lowering of their concentrations in the serum. The TPN solution may need to be altered if there is a drop in the serum values of these electrolytes. Providing glucose in excess of kilocaloric needs can result in several problems, including carbon dioxide retention with respiratory difficulty. High glucose content of TPN

Calculation of a Sample TPN Solution
TPN Energy Nutrient Content

TPN solutions are usually packed in 500 cc bags. Pharmacists prefer to use dextrose and amino acids in 500 cc bags and vary the concentration of the nutrients to achieve the appropriate nutritional parameters. For example, a 500 cc bag of dextrose mixed with a 500 cc bag of amino acids equals 1000 cc. Lipids are usually provided as 250 cc of 20 percent lipid (1/2 bag) or 500 cc (one bag) of 10 percent lipid. The client's needs for kilocalories, protein, and fat can be accommodated by individualizing the concentration of each energy nutrient. For example, dextrose can be ordered from 5 to 70 percent, noted as "D_5, D_{40}, D_{50}," etc. Commonly used concentrations of amino acids are 5 percent, 8.5 percent, and 10 percent.

NUTRITIONAL VALUES USED IN COMPUTATIONS OF TPN SOLUTIONS

Dextrose	= 3.4 kcal/g
20 percent lipid	= 2.0 kcal/cc
10 percent lipid	= 1.1 kcal/cc
Protein	= 4.0 kcal/g
1 g of nitrogen	= 6.25 g protein

Calculate the total kilocalories, nonprotein kilocalories, grams of nitrogen, calorie/nitrogen ratio, and percent kilocalories from fat in 500 cc D_{50}, 500 cc 10 percent amino acids, and 250 cc 10 percent lipid.

Dextrose	Percent concentration × volume = grams of dextrose	0.50 × 500 = 250 g dextrose
	Grams of dextrose × 3.4 kcal/g = kcal of solution	250 g dextrose × 3.4 kcal/g = 850 kcal
Amino acids	Percent concentration × volume = grams of protein	0.10 × 500 cc = 50 g protein
	Grams of protein × kcal/g = protein kcal	50 g protein × 4 kcal/g = 200 kcal
Lipids	Kcal/cc × volume in cc = fat kcal	1.1 × 250 cc = 275 kcal
Total kilocalories	Add kcal from dextrose, protein, and lipid	850 + 200 + 275 = 1325 kcal
Percent kilocalories from fat	Kcal from fat divided by total kcal = percent fat kcal	275 ÷ 1325 = 21 percent fat

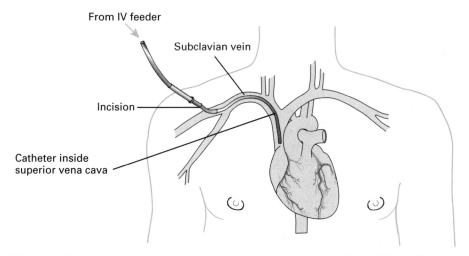

FIGURE 15–3   TPN line placement via subclavian vein to superior vena cava. (From Williams, SR: Essentials of Nutrition and Diet Therapy, ed 6. Times Mirror/Mosby College Publishing, St. Louis, 1990, with permission.)

solutions also leads to hyperglycemia. Therefore, glucose levels should be assessed regularly. Liver function test results will become abnormal after an excess glucose load. Excess glucose may lead to hyperlipidemia and fatty deposits in the liver. The avoidance of metabolic complications directly related to a glucose overload is one reason TPN clients need to be monitored closely. These complications can be avoided by providing only an appropriate and not an excessive amount of kilocalories. In addition, an initial slow infusion at low concentrations prevents complications.

TRANSITION AND COMBINATION FEEDINGS   Clients need a transition period from TPN to oral feedings. Some physicians prefer to wean clients from TPN by using tube feeding. Other physicians prefer to avoid the tube and wean clients orally. In the latter case, as the client's oral intake increases, the TPN solution is gradually withdrawn. Expect the client who has been on TPN for a significant period of time to experience some difficulty with oral feedings. One of the problems with TPN is that the gut does not have to work during its administration. Consequently the gut will have undergone some atrophy. Oral foods should be offered slowly during the weaning process. Some physicians avoid this problem by allowing some clients to consume a clear liquid or light diet while on TPN, if their condition permits.

HOME PARENTERAL NUTRITION   Increasingly, clients are being discharged on TPN. Clients need adequate follow-up by either the hospital or a community home agency.

Summary

The nutritional care of clients is a joint responsibility of the dietary and nursing departments. All nurses who work in institutions need to know not only how meals are distributed to clients but also current meal service schedules. This will have an impact on the administration of medications and the scheduling of clients for procedures. Nutritional care includes three areas: assessing the client's need for nutrients, monitoring nutrient intake, and counseling clients about nutritional needs.

Nutrients can be delivered to clients orally, via tube feeding, and/or parenterally. One principle is followed when selecting a feeding route: if the gut works, use it to maximum capability. Every means should be attempted to assist clients to eat orally and independently. Oral feedings should be considered before tube feeding. Tube feeding should be considered before intravenous feeding. Intravenous feeding can be delivered peripherally or centrally. Clients on either tube feedings or intravenous feedings need to be closely monitored.

A case study and a sample plan of care follow. Both are designed to show you how the information you have studied in this chapter can be used in nursing practice.

Case Study 15–1   P was brought in to the emergency room by ambulance with his mother. The mother stated her son was hit by a car while riding his bike. P is 11 years old, 4 ft, 11 in tall, and weighs 89 lb. The client's mother stated her son was well prior to the accident. In the emergency room it was observed that both his eyes were surrounded by contusions, his throat and the left side of his face were swollen. Communication with the client was at first minimal because it was painful for him to speak. An intravenous solution of D_5W was started in the emergency room. He was also shown to have a fractured femur. Surgery was required to reset the bone. The physician determined that traction would be necessary. P is expected to require traction, and thus hospitalization, for 3 to 5 weeks.

Five days later, P is still having problems swallowing. He has not progressed beyond sips of clear liquids. The kilocaloric count showed an average daily intake of 395 kcal, with only 8 g of protein for the past 3 days. P appears to be in pain when he swallows and has choked twice on larger sips of the clear liquids. The client speaks only in single words or short sentences. It is still painful for him to talk. The swelling in his esophagus has decreased enough to allow the insertion of a small silicone feeding

tube. The physician has ordered a nasogastric feeding tube with Enrich. The order reads:

Day 1 Continuous drip 50 mL/h 1/2 strength
Day 2 Continuous drip 50 mL/h 3/4 strength
Day 3 Continuous drip 50 mL/h full strength
Day 4 Continuous drip 84 mL/h full strength

Enrich contains 1.1 kcal/mL and 39.7 g of protein per 1000 mL. P may have ice chips and small amounts of clear liquids in addition to the tube feeding as desired. The physician stated, "The client will remain on a tube feeding until he can consume his kilocalorie requirement orally. This client requires adequate nutrition to enable the femur to heal properly." P is not expected to be discharged on a home enteral tube feeding. His prognosis is good and he is expected to make a full recovery.

The physician inserted the nasogastric tube himself because of the swelling in the esophagus and the danger of a perforation. The nurse assisted at the client's bedside. The client held the nurse's hand tightly as the tube was inserted. He had a worried look on his face, increased facial perspiration, and increased pulse/respirations during the procedure.

NURSING CARE PLAN FOR P

Assessment

Subjective Data   Client held hand tightly during nasogastric tube insertion and appeared worried, apprehensive, and jittery.

Objective Data   Client is a trauma victim who showed increased perspiration and increased pulse/respirations during the tube insertion procedure.

Nursing Diagnosis   Fear: Client fear related to enteral nutrition therapy and situational crisis as evidenced by facial tension during tube insertion and increased pulse/respirations and perspiration.

Desired Outcome/ Evaluation Criteria	Nursing Actions	Rationale
The client will state he needs the food in the tube feeding to heal his leg until he is eating better.	Explain enteral nutrition therapy procedures as performed.	A tube feeding is unfamiliar to most clients. Knowledge about the procedure may relax the client.
	As the client's condition permits, be available for listening and talking. Encourage the client to acknowledge and express feelings.	The client needs to vent his feelings about both the tube feeding and the situational crisis (the accident).

Study Aids

Chapter Review

1. Modular formula feedings:
   a. Always have a low osmolality
   b. Are designed for clients with malabsorption
   c. Contain a limited number of nutrients
   d. Are always predigested

2. A(n) _____ provides all of the essential nutrients in a specified volume.
   a. Intact or polymeric formula
   b. Modular feeding
   c. Intravenous feeding
   d. Elemental or predigested formula

3. Careful administration of total parenteral nutrition does *not* include:
   a. A slow start
   b. Close monitoring
   c. Abrupt withdrawal
   d. A strict schedule

4. Diarrhea in the tube-fed client is most likely to be caused by the following:
   a. A continuous infusion feeding
   b. A bolus feeding
   c. A fluid deficit
   d. Insufficient kilocalories

5. Which of the following is *not* a recommended procedure for administering medications through a tube feeding?
   a. Mix all the medications together, crush thoroughly, mix with water, and add to the formula.
   b. If at all possible, use medications in the liquid form.
   c. Flush the tube with at least 30 milliliters of water prior to giving the medication and before resuming the tube-feeding formula.
   d. If a medication is ordered to be added to the formula, observe the feeding after the addition for any reaction or precipitation.

Clinical Analysis

1. Mr. J, 58 years old, visits his physician with a complaint of abdominal pain. He is scheduled for a diagnostic work-up, which will include a **barium enema** (x-ray study of his colon). Prior to this procedure, the nurse should instruct the client to:
   a. Eat a large breakfast on the day of the examination, such as orange juice, cereal, toast, scrambled eggs, and milk.
   b. Drink ample fluids on the morning of the examination, including at least 12 ounces of juice, 1 cup of gelatin, and broth.
   c. Take nothing orally after midnight on the day of the examination and consume only gelatin, clear broth, tea, coffee, and grape, apple, or cranberry juice on the day before the examination.
   d. Drink milk, juices, and coffee and eat only strained cream soups, ice cream, and gelatin on the day before the examination and take nothing orally after midnight.

2. Ms. L has a jejunostomy. She was discharged from the hospital last week after receiving instructions on home care from the nutrition support service. The local pharmacy is out of the Vivonex formula she has been instructed to use. As the nurse, you recommend that:
   a. She substitute Ensure
   b. She substitute Polycose
   c. She contact the Nutrition Support Service for instructions
   d. She substitute an intact or polymeric formula

3. Mr. W has been receiving a tube feeding of Ensure via nasogastric tube for 3 weeks via a bolus infusion. He has just started to have loose stools (300 milliliters each × 6 today). You should first suspect the following to be responsible for the diarrhea:
   a. A new medication added to his treatment plan
   b. Bacterial contamination
   c. Intolerance to the bolus delivery method
   d. Lactose intolerance

Bibliography

Butterworth, CE: The skeleton in the hospital closet. Nutrition Today 9:8, 1975.

Butterworth, CE, and Blackburn, GL: Hospital malnutrition and how to assess the nutritional status of a patient. Nutrition Today 10:8, 1975.

Davis, AE, et al: Preventing feeding-associated aspiration. MEDSURG Nurs. 4:111, 1995.

Dickerson, J: The problem of hospital-induced malnutrition. Nurs Times 91:44, 1995.

Fater, KH: Determining nasogastric feeding tube placement. MEDSURG Nurs 4:27, 57, 1995.

Galindo-Ciocon, DJ: Tube feeding: Complications among the elderly. Journal of Gerontological Nursing 19:17, 1993.

Hoheim, TA, et al: Clinical experience with three-in-one admixtures administered peripherally. Nutrition in Clinical Practice 5:118, 1990.

Hui, YH: Human Nutrition and Diet Therapy. Wadsworth Health Sciences, Monterey, CA, 1983.

McWhirtner, JP: Incidence and recognition of malnutrition in hospital. Br Med J 308:946, 1994.

Moore, MC: Pocket Guide to Nutrition and Diet Therapy. CV Mosby, St Louis, 1993.

Pagana, KD, and Pagana, TJ: Diagnostic Testing and Nursing Implications. CV Mosby, St Louis, 1992.

The Quality Assurance Committee of the American Dietetic Association: Suggested Guidelines for Nutrition Management of the Critically Ill Patient. American Dietetic Association, Chicago, 1984.

Wright, B: Enteral feeding tubes as drug delivery systems. Nutr Supp Serv 6:33, 1986.

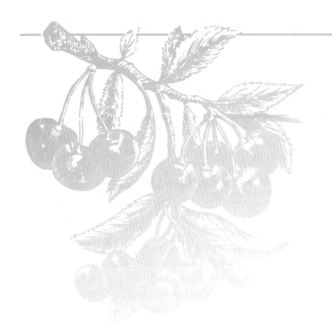

UNIT THREE

Clinical Nutrition

CHAPTER 16

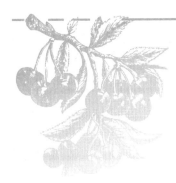

Food, Nutrient, and Drug Interactions

LEARNING OBJECTIVES

After completing this chapter, the student should be able to:

1 Explain the importance of proper scheduling of medications in relation to food intake.

2 Identify two groups of clients likely to experience food-drug interactions.

3 Recognize certain food and drug interactions discussed in the text.

4 Describe four ways in which nutrients and drugs can interact and give an example of each.

5 Discuss one food-drug interaction that is potentially life-threatening and design nursing interventions to avoid this possibility.

6 Relate sodium-water balance to the effects of lithium.

This chapter explains and gives examples of the different ways in which drugs interact with foods (including beverages), nutrients (including nutrient formulas and supplements), and the nonnutrient components of foods. In no sense is the discussion exhaustive. Pharmaceutical references should be used when administering medications.

A drug is a substance other than food intended to affect the structure or function of the body. As used in the text, the term "drug" includes alcohol and both prescription and over-the-counter drugs. As is the practice in most hospitals, we use the **generic name** of the drug.

The Effects of Drugs on Nutritional Status

Any person taking a drug risks potentially harmful effects from food and drug interactions. Nutritional status can be affected because these interactions can alter (1) food intake, (2) the absorption of nutrients or drugs, (3) the metabolism of nutrients or drugs, and (4) the excretion of nutrients or drugs. Some known interactions are considered clinically desirable and result in the control of a disease process. For example, by restricting a client's dietary vitamin K, the effect of warfarin (an anticoagulant) is prolonged. However, many effects resulting from food and drug interactions are undesirable. These include nutritional deficiencies, growth retardation in children, loss of disease control, and acute toxic reactions. Some persons, especially the elderly, are at higher risk than others for suffering unwanted effects.

Identifying Clients at High Risk

Persons at highest risk for food and drug interactions are those who (1) take many drugs, including alcohol, (2) require long-term drug therapy, or (3) have poor or marginal nutrition. These and other risk-increasing factors are listed in Clinical Application 16–1. The elderly are particularly vulnerable because they are more likely to have several of the risk factors mentioned.

Over one-third of 311 retirement community residents reported using alcohol with a high-risk medication. Half the residents who reported some alcohol intake also took antihypertensive drugs, perhaps without knowing that alcohol alone exacerbates hypertension. Over one-quarter of the residents took aspirin and one-fifth took other nonsteroidal anti-inflammatory drugs that with alcohol can cause in-

creased bleeding time and gastric inflammation and bleeding (Adams, 1995). Individuals receiving these medications are likely to be on long-term regimens, increasing the risk of adverse effects. See Fig. 16–1.

The elderly are also more prone to food-drug interactions as a result of self-medication, noncompliance, and changes in their nutritional-status needs associated with aging. Clinical Application 16–2 lists factors that should trigger investigation of the client's risk of drug-nutrient interactions.

Minimizing Food and Drug Interactions

Known adverse outcomes of food and drug interactions can be offset by changes in drug dosage, diet, or both. Because drugs often increase or decrease the absorption of nutrients, it may be necessary to change (1) the route of administration, (2) the dose of a drug, (3) the time interval between doses, and/or (4) whether or not the drug is administered with food. For example, therapeutic drug levels may not be achieved or may take longer to build if less drug is absorbed due to an interaction with food. This could prolong a disease or prevent its cure. Dosage adjustments often will minimize such effects.

Certain foods or nutrients (including supplements) may be (1) added to the diet, (2) deleted from the diet, or (3) required in increased or reduced amounts to counterbalance adverse nutrient-drug interactions. For example, protein inhibits the absorption of phenytoin, an anticonvulsant drug, whereas carbohydrate increases its absorption.

CLINICAL APPLICATION 16–1

Factors Increasing the Risk of Drug-Nutrient Interactions

The risk of a drug-nutrient interaction is increased if a client:

- *Is malnourished*
- *Consumes alcohol*
- *Takes a high-potency vitamin or mineral supplement*
- *Is receiving many drugs*

or if the client's drugs:

- *Are given with meals*
- *Are instilled into a feeding tube*
- *Are prescribed long-term to control chronic disease*
- *Are known to cause malabsorption or have antinutrient effects*

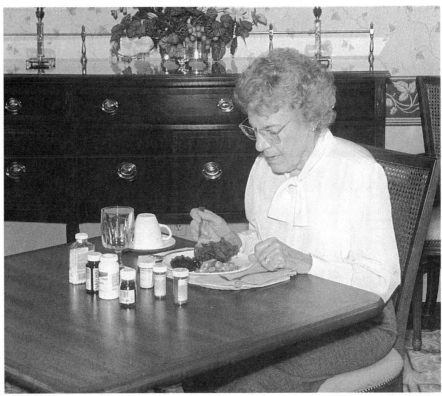

FIGURE 16–1 This woman displays several risk factors for drug-nutrient interactions. She is elderly, is on a multiple drug regimen, and takes some of her medications with a meal.

Depending on the desired therapeutic effect, dietary intake of protein and/or carbohydrate may be modified.

Food and drug interactions can be complex, especially if the client is on a multiple-drug regimen or is at high risk for other reasons. Having a sound knowledge of potential food and drug interactions is an important function of health care professionals. Physicians, dietitians, pharmacists, and nurses have a joint responsibility in being aware of and controlling such interactions (Lasswell, et al, 1995). The clinical pharmacist can be a valuable ally of the nurse when scheduling medications for optimal effect. Likewise, the clinical dietitian may be asked to assess a client's risk for food-drug interactions. A good reference library on the clinical unit is also helpful in providing information.

CLINICAL APPLICATION 16–2

Screening Clients at Risk of Drug-Nutrient Interactions

Further nutritional assessment may be in order if the client:

1. Reports a recent weight change
2. Abuses alcohol
3. Consumes a modified diet, including one characterized by significant changes in protein content
4. Takes medication with meals
5. Has a worsening of signs and symptoms of the disease
6. Displays laboratory values indicating nutrient depletion
7. Receives medications known to interfere with nutrition

Generic name—The name given to the drug by the original developer; usually the same as the official name given to it by the Food and Drug Administration.

The Effects of Drugs on Foods and Nutrients

A number of drugs have a variety of effects on foods and nutrients: (1) drugs can affect food intake; (2) drugs can alter the absorption of nutrients through both luminal and mucosal effects; (3) the metabolism of nutrients can be affected by drugs; and (4) drugs can increase or decrease the excretion of certain nutrients.

The Effects of Drugs on Food Intake

Even before food is ingested, drugs can affect food intake. Several drugs increase or decrease appetite, interfere with the senses of taste and smell, and cause gastric irritation. Food is sometimes used to temper these and other side effects of drugs.

Decreased Appetite

CNS stimulants, including dextroamphetamine and methylphenidate, both used in the treatment of narcolepsy or the management of attention deficit disorder (ADD), have the effect of depressing the desire for food. One of the side effects of these stimulants in children is slowed growth. Dextroamphetamine is more likely to interfere with growth than methylphenidate.

Antineoplastics, drugs or agents that prevent the development, growth, or proliferation of malignant cells, are notorious for causing a loss of appetite (anorexia). Other side effects including severe nausea, vomiting, and **stomatitis** exacerbate the anorexia. Examples of such antineoplastic drugs are bleomycin, plicamycin, and vincristine.

Poor appetite can also result from drugs that cause a dry mouth. Many antihistamines, including brompheniramine and diphenhydramine, decrease saliva output, thereby causing anorexia.

When assessing a client with a weight-loss history or a client taking drugs known to cause food and drug interactions, nurses should review the client's drug regimen. Both physician-prescribed and self-prescribed drugs and nutritional supplements are pertinent to include in a nutritional assessment.

Increased Appetite

Some antidepressants, such as doxepin, may promote appetite and lead to marked weight gain. Another such drug, bupropion, can either increase or decrease appetite.

Medroxyprogesterone, a female hormone used as an oral contraceptive and in cyclic hormone therapy after menopause, also increases appetite. This hormone occurs naturally in the second half of the menstrual cycle and in pregnancy (to support the growth requirements of the mother and fetus). To minimize its effects, several nursing interventions might be appropriate: increasing the fiber content of the client's diet and encouraging the client to drink 6 to 8 glasses of water daily, to eat slowly, and to chew food thoroughly.

Changes in Taste or Smell

The senses of taste and smell influence the response to foods. Some drugs alter the perception of these senses making foods and beverages taste bitter, metallic, or unpleasant. Although this usually leads to a decreased appetite, some individuals will try to rid themselves of the sensation by eating constantly.

Acetylsalicylic acid (ASA), more commonly known as aspirin, is a drug used to control pain or to reduce fever. It also is taken in small daily doses to decrease the risk of heart attacks. One gram of ASA, about three adult-dose tablets, increases the taste perception of bitterness.

An anti-infective reserved for tuberculosis and other serious infections, streptomycin, is excreted in the saliva. One result is a metallic or bitter taste even when the drug is administered by intramuscular injection.

Lithium carbonate, an antimanic drug, causes a strange, unpleasant taste sensation. Other common side effects of this drug related to nutritional intake are dry mouth, anorexia, nausea, vomiting, and diarrhea. Lithium carbonate also has serious interactions with a person's fluid and electrolyte balance (discussed later in the chapter).

Penicillamine, a drug given for heavy metal poisoning or for **Wilson's disease,** in which a genetic defect prevents excretion of copper, causes a loss of taste and smell. This side effect is caused by zinc deficiency because zinc also binds with penicillamine.

Nursing interventions that may help a client with taste changes include providing good oral hygiene before meals and avoiding bitter foods in favor of the other taste sensations—sweet, sour, or salty.

Gastric Irritation

Drugs that cause gastric irritation are often taken with food to reduce this side effect. Chronic use of aspirin can lead to gastric bleeding and anemia. Taking aspirin with food, milk, crackers, or a full glass of water reduces the likelihood of stomach irritation. Other nonsteroidal anti-inflammatory drugs (NSAIDs) and potassium chloride are also associated with gastric irritation.

The Effects of Drugs on Nutrient Absorption

Drugs can affect the absorption of nutrients in several ways. Drug-induced alterations in absorption are categorized according to two general mechanisms of action: the luminal effect or the mucosal effect.

Luminal Effects

The **luminal effect** refers to drug-induced changes within the intestine that affect the absorption of nutrients or drugs without altering the intestine itself. These drug-induced changes may affect peristalsis, pH, or the formation of complexes.

PERISTALSIS   Laxatives may interfere with the absorption of nutrients and other drugs because they stimulate peristalsis and thus cause a rapid transit time of intestinal contents. Long-term use may result in physical dependence and electrolyte imbalances. Two laxatives, bisacodyl and phenolphthalein (common ingredients in over-the-counter preparations), interfere with the uptake of glucose, water, calcium, sodium, and potassium.

A relatively short period of malabsorption with diarrhea may interfere with the absorption of vitamin K. This in turn enhances the activity of warfarin, especially if intake of green vegetables has been sparse. One physician advises halving the dose of warfarin during an attack of diarrhea (Black, 1994). However, clients should consult their own physicians.

Other drugs may slow peristalsis and thus cause a slow transit time. The long-term use of either docusate sodium, a stool softener, or chlorpromazine, an antipsychotic drug, results in the increased absorption of cholesterol, an undesirable side effect in most clients.

CHANGES IN PH   The absorption of weakly acidic drugs takes place in the stomach whereas the absorption of neutral and alkaline drugs takes place in the small intestine. Drug-induced changes in the pH of these sites influence the absorption of both nutrients and drugs. For example, an acid pH is necessary for folic acid absorption. It is also required for intrinsic factor to combine with vitamin B_{12} (extrinsic factor) for the absorption of vitamin B_{12}. Because long-term antacid or potassium chloride therapy neutralizes gastric acidity, the result is a decrease in the absorption of both folic acid and vitamin B_{12}. Antacids and potassium also decrease the absorption of iron because an acid medium is necessary to convert ferric iron (Fe^{3+}) to ferrous iron (2^{+}), the more absorbable form.

FORMATION OF COMPLEXES   Sometimes, foods or nutrients bind with or form complexes with drugs. This combining can increase, decrease, or prevent the absorption of one or the other.

Cholestyramine, a lipid-lowering agent, binds with bile salts, which increases the excretion of cholesterol. Unfortunately, it may also bind with the fat-soluble vitamins A, D, E, and K. These vitamins are then excreted along with the cholesterol. Because vitamin K is not stored in the body in significant amounts, cholestyramine therapy can lead to a deficiency of prothrombin and hemorrhage. However, water-soluble forms of these vitamins are available for patients who need them. Cholestyramine also interferes with the absorption of folic acid, vitamin B_{12}, calcium, and iron, necessitating vigilant monitoring of nutritional status.

Mineral oil, a lubricant, is sometimes used as a laxative. The fat-soluble vitamins dissolve in the indigestible oil and are excreted; calcium and phosphorus are excreted too. Therefore, taking mineral oil long-term on a daily basis is undesirable. Children and elderly adults with relaxed cardiac sphincters are at risk for aspiration pneumonia if the mineral oil is regurgitated. Alternate medications are preferable for these clients.

Mucosal Effects

The luminal effects do not affect the tissues or organs. In contrast, **mucosal effects** are drug-induced changes that affect the absorption of nutrients or

---

Antineoplastic—A drug or other agent that prevents the development, growth, or proliferation of malignant cells.

Stomatitis—An inflammation of the mouth.

Luminal effect—Drug-induced changes within the intestine that affect the absorption of nutrients or drugs without altering the intestine itself.

Mucosal effect—Drug-induced changes within the intestine that affect the absorption of drugs or nutrients by damaging or altering the tissues.

drugs by damaging or altering tissue structures. Mucosal effects include decreased digestive enzymes, damaged intestinal mucosa, and inhibited transport mechanisms.

DECREASED DIGESTIVE ENZYMES   Hundreds of enzymes are involved in digestion. Many drugs, including alcohol, can destroy the structural integrity of digestive organs by damaging tissues. This usually causes decreased enzyme production, resulting in poor nutrient absorption.

Long-term alcohol consumption damages the pancreas, decreasing enzyme production. Thus the breakdown of amino acids and fats, chiefly governed by the action of pancreatic enzymes, is slowed or insufficiently completed. The result is reduced or poor absorption of amino acids and fats.

DAMAGED INTESTINAL MUCOSA   A number of drugs contribute to the malabsorption of drugs by their damaging effect on the intestinal mucosa. Some drugs produce general malabsorption; other drugs are more specific and decrease the absorption of only certain nutrients.

Alcohol abuse causes several changes in the intestinal mucosa that lead to the malabsorption of many nutrients. Most commonly affected are thiamin and magnesium, but folic acid, niacin, and pyridoxine also may be malabsorbed.

Because neomycin, an anti-infective, inhibits protein synthesis in bacteria, it is sometimes used to reduce the bacterial count in the bowel before intestinal surgery. Changes produced in the intestinal mucosa by neomycin lead to the decreased absorption of fat; vitamins A, D, and K; folic acid; and vitamin B_{12}. This malabsorption is not likely to cause problems when the drug use is short-term.

Gastrointestinal tract cells, because of their short service life and rapid turnover, are killed by many antineoplastic drugs, such as methotrexate. Consequently methotrexate administration results in the malabsorption of vitamin B_{12}, folic acid, and calcium.

Colchicine, an antigout drug, also inhibits the absorption of vitamin B_{12}, folic acid, and calcium. In addition, colchicine reduces the absorption of fat, lactose, and carotene.

INHIBITED TRANSPORT MECHANISMS   Several nutrients have to be helped across the intestinal membrane to the bloodstream. A number of drugs impair the absorption of nutrients through their effects on the transport mechanism. For example, the sedative/hypnotic drug glutethimide impairs the transport of calcium.

Para-aminosalicylate, an antitubercular drug, is administered for a prolonged period (1 to 2 years) to be effective. This drug interferes with the uptake and transport of vitamin B_{12} across the mucosal wall. When taking a client history, then, the nurse should gather any pertinent data, not just data concerning *recent* changes in a client's life or health.

Phenytoin, a drug used to control epileptic seizures or heart rhythm irregularities, is structurally similar to folic acid. They compete for the same receptors in the small bowel (Berg, et al, 1995). Reduced folic acid absorption also occurs with sulfasalazine, an anti-inflammatory agent used to treat ulcerative colitis. The decrease in absorption is due to the inhibited transport of folic acid.

The Effects of Drugs on Nutrient Metabolism

Many drugs alter the metabolism of nutrients. Two commonly prescribed classes of drugs, corticosteroids and beta-adrenergic blocking agents, change the way the body uses energy nutrients. Drugs also disrupt vitamin metabolism by a variety of mechanisms.

Alteration of Energy Nutrient Metabolism

Beta-adrenergic blocking agents, such as atenolol and metoprolol, are given for hypertension and angina. These drugs decrease lipolysis and muscle glycogenolysis, thus decreasing the amount of fat and glucose available for energy. The mechanism by which protein is altered is unclear, but the end result of long-term treatment with beta-blockers may be increased body fat, decreased fat free mass, and a resting energy expenditure reduction of 8 to 17 percent (Lamont, 1995).

Corticosteroids are hormones produced by the adrenal gland. Pharmaceutical doses of these drugs are given for their anti-inflammatory effects. The side effects of the drug are signs and symptoms like those of the disease called Cushing's syndrome, which results from oversecretion of corticosteroids. The metabolism of all the energy nutrients is affected. Corticosteroids stimulate the conversion of fat and protein to glucose. Hyperglycemia results, or preexisting diabetes is worsened. Corticosteroids increase the catabolism of the matrix of the bone, inhibit the osteoblasts from building new bone, and prevent the liver from processing vitamin D. When this lack of vitamin D results in insufficient calcium being absorbed by the intestine, parathyroid hormone causes withdrawal of calcium from the bones, and osteoporosis is the consequence. Similar protein wasting affects the skin and skeletal muscle, producing easy bruising and weakness. Corticosteroids also cause a redistribution of fat deposits to the trunk, the back of the neck, and the face so that the person eventually develops a "moon face" and "buffalo hump."

Interference with Vitamin Metabolism

Although vitamins have specific and singular functions in the body, several mechanisms can interfere with their proper metabolism. The same vitamin may be affected by different drugs at various phases of its metabolism.

Anti-infectives destroy intestinal bacteria, which synthesize vitamin K (Conly, and Stein, 1994). Sometimes buttermilk or yogurt is effective in replacing the intestinal bacteria.

The molecular structure of warfarin, an anticoagulant drug, resembles that of vitamin K. Warfarin achieves its therapeutic effect by "fooling" the liver into using it in place of vitamin K to manufacture prothrombin. Warfarin also interferes with the synthesis of clotting factors VII, IX, and X. Eating large amounts of food high in vitamin K during anticoagulant therapy with warfarin decreases or may even negate the desired effect of the drug. Clients should not stop eating foods containing vitamin K, but they should avoid wide swings in the amounts eaten. A problem might arise if they eat a lot of green leafy vegetables one day and none for several days.

Methotrexate, an antineoplastic agent, is an antagonist of folic acid. It successfully destroys cancer cells because they, too, require folic acid for DNA replication. In the process, normal body cells' efforts to divide are thwarted.

Both the antitubercular drug isoniazid and the antiparkinson agent levodopa form a complex with pyridoxine. The kidney then excretes this complex in the urine rather than returning it to the bloodstream. The interaction can also move in the opposite direction. The amount of pyridoxine in a normal diet creates no problem. Supplemental pyridoxine may be added to a levodopa regimen to correct a deficiency. However, this will decrease the effectiveness of levodopa.

An anticonvulsant, phenytoin, interferes with the liver's processing of vitamin D. Clients receiving long-term therapy need an estimated 15 to 25 micrograms of vitamin D daily to prevent rickets or osteomalacia.

The Effects of Drugs on Nutrient Excretion

Drugs usually cause excessive excretion, rather than retention, of nutrients. Drugs can act on the excretion of nutrients in four ways: they can (1) compete with nutrients for binding sites, (2) form chemical bonds with the nutrient, (3) deplete the nutrient supply in the body's tissues, and (4) interfere with the kidneys' reabsorption of the nutrient back into the bloodstream.

Competition for Binding Sites

Many drugs circulate in the bloodstream attached to plasma proteins. These plasma proteins serve a similar function in relation to some nutrients. The plasma protein and its hitchhiker drug or nutrient form a large particle. Sometimes there are too few binding sites for all the drug or nutrient. When that happens, excess drug or nutrient accumulates as free, small particles in the bloodstream. The kidney is likely to excrete these small particles rather than to restore them to the bloodstream. One common drug that interferes in this manner with a nutrient is acetylsalicylic acid, or aspirin. It displaces folic acid from its plasma protein. The kidney then excretes the folic acid in the urine.

Formation of Chemical Bonds

To combat heavy metal poisoning, an antidote drug that combines chemically with the metal is administered. The drug plus the metal then is excreted harmlessly. As with many treatments, the drug is not specific and will combine with nutrients as well as the noxious heavy metal. An example of this type of interaction involves penicillamine. It forms a stable bond with zinc, copper, and other metals, causing excessive excretion, thus possibly leading to deficiencies.

Depletion of Nutrients in Tissues

As part of its overall catabolic effect, the anti-inflammatory glucocorticoid prednisone depletes tissues of ascorbic acid. The ascorbic acid accumulates in the blood and is excreted. Because ascorbic acid is necessary for the healing of wounds, one side effect of prednisone and other corticosteroids is poor wound healing.

When alcohol is present, folic acid leaks from the liver into the bloodstream. Its fate from there is excessive excretion in the urine, leading to folic acid deficiency.

Interference with Reabsorption by Kidney

Many diuretic agents prevent normal reabsorption of sodium into the bloodstream within the kidney. This increases the amount of sodium excreted by the kidney into the urine. Along with the sodium, water is also excreted. Often the drug is not specific enough to dispose of sodium alone. Many diuretics also cause loss of potassium. Sometimes the client must take pharmacologic doses of potassium chloride to prevent hypokalemia. One diuretic, furosemide, produces calcium loss in addition to potassium loss by the same mechanism. In contrast, other diuretics are potassium-sparing, eliminating the need for supplementation. In a study of drug-nutrient interactions, between 11 and 36 percent of long-term care facility clients were shown to be at risk for hyper- or **hypokalemia,** serum potassium outside the normal range (Lewis, Frongillo, and Roe, 1995).

Table 16–1 summarizes the effects of drugs on foods and nutrients.

The Effects of Foods and Nutrients on Drugs

Foods and nutrients can decrease, delay, or increase the absorption of drugs. They can also cause alterations in drug metabolism.

The Effects of Foods on Drug Absorption

In some cases the interaction of food with a drug can be used to therapeutic advantage. In other situations, knowledge of interactions will aid the health care team to schedule meals and medication doses to the best advantage of the client.

Decreased or Delayed Absorption

Food, nonnutrient components of foods, or nutrients in food may decrease or delay the absorption of drugs. Drug bioavailability may vary as much as 50 percent, depending on the drug–meal relationship (Lewis, Frongillo, and Roe, 1995). Food delays the absorption of cortisone, a glucocorticoid used as an anti-inflammatory drug. Taking cortisone with food produces a more consistent blood level of the drug. Other factors, such as a drug's susceptibility to acid degradation or its ability to form insoluble complexes, also influence whether a drug is administered with food or between meals.

Food in the stomach, acidic fruit or vegetable juices, and carbonated beverages increase gastric acidity. Anti-infectives particularly susceptible to acid degradation are penicillin G, cloxacillin, and ampicillin. An acid medium breaks down these drugs, producing a less effective blood level. To diminish such acid degradation, these anti-infectives are administered between meals.

Drugs formulated to dissolve in the intestine rather than in the stomach are **enteric-coated;** an acid-resistant shell covers the active ingredient (see Fig. 16–2). The stomach normally is acid and the duodenum alkaline. Milk raises the pH of the stomach, making it more alkaline. Taking enteric-coated drugs with milk, then, will allow the coating to dissolve early and therefore will decrease the action of the drug. One of these drugs is erythromycin, an anti-infective. It should not be taken with milk. Alcohol and hot beverages can also cause premature erosion of the enteric-coating on drugs.

Tetracycline, an anti-infective, combines with the salts of iron, magnesium, aluminum, and calcium to form insoluble compounds. This decreases the absorption of the drug. For this reason, tetracycline should not be administered within 1 to 3 hours of iron supplements or iron-containing foods (red meat, egg yolks), milk or other dairy products, or antacids containing magnesium, aluminum, and/or calcium.

Amino acids compete for absorption with levodopa, a drug used in the management of Parkinson's disease. Separating the dose from high-protein intake by 3 hours improves absorption. Protein also delays the action of phenytoin (an anticonvulsant) and inhibits the absorption of theophylline, a bronchodilator used to treat asthma.

A high-fiber meal decreases the absorption of digoxin, a drug used to treat congestive heart failure by slowing and strengthening cardiac contractions. The pectin in apples and jelly reduces the absorption of acetaminophen, an analgesic. Absorption of isoniazid is lowest with a high carbohydrate meal. It should be given with the client fasting.

Increased Absorption

Foods and nutrients may also increase or facilitate the absorption of drugs. Some drugs are affected in one or more ways by one or more nutrients. Levodopa, the drug used in the management of Parkinson's disease, has a second interaction with food. Whereas protein delays the absorption of levodopa, carbohydrate facilitates it. Giving levodopa with carbohydrate-rich snacks improves the absorption of the drug. Similarly, protein delays the anticonvul-

TABLE 16–1   The Effects of Drugs on Nutrients

Drug Group	Drug	Effects/Action on Nutrient	Mechanism of Action
ALTERATION IN FOOD INTAKE			
Analgesic	Acetylsalicylic acid	Decreases appetite	Altered taste; gastric irritation
Antineoplastic	Bleomycin, plicamycin, vincristine	Decreases appetite	Side effects: anorexia, nausea, vomiting, and stomatitis
Antihistamine	Brompheneramine, diphenhydramine	Decreases appetite	Side effect: dry mouth
Antidepressant	Bupropion	Increases/decreases appetite	Side effects
CNS stimulant	Dextroamphetamine, methylphenidate	Decreases appetite	Depressed desire for food
Antidepressant	Doxepin	Increases appetite	Side effect
Antimanic	Lithium carbonate	Decreases appetite	Altered taste; side effects: dry mouth, anorexia, nausea, and vomiting
Hormone	Medroxyprogesterone	Increases appetite	Effect of hormone
Chelating agent	Penicillamine	Decreases appetite/overeating	Altered taste and smell
Anti-infective	Streptomycin	Decreases appetite/overeating	Altered taste
ALTERATION IN NUTRIENT ABSORPTION			
Alcohol	Alcohol (ethanol)	Decreases absorption of amino acids, fat, thiamin, folic acid, niacin, magnesium, and pyridoxine	Decreased enzyme production, damaged intestinal mucosa
Antacid; Electrolyte therapy	Antacids; Potassium	Decreases absorption of folic acid, vitamin B_{12}, and iron	Changes in pH
Laxative	Bisacodyl, phenolphthalein	Interferes with uptake of glucose, potassium, calcium, sodium, and water	Altered peristalsis
Lipid-lowering agent	Cholestyramine	Interferes with absorption of vitamins A, D, K, B_{12}, folic acid, and calcium	Formation of complexes
Antigout agent	Colchicine	Malabsorption of vitamin B_{12}, folic acid, calcium; reduces absorption of fat, lactose, and carotene	Damaged intestinal mucosa
Stool softener	Docusate sodium	Increases absorption of cholesterol	Altered peristalsis
Sedative/hypnotic	Glutethamide	Leads to calcium deficiency	Impaired transport mechanism
Antineoplastic	Methotrexate	Decreases absorption of vitamin B_{12}, folic acid, and calcium	Damaged intestinal mucosa

Table continued on following page

sant action of phenytoin, but the presence of carbohydrate increases the absorption. Protein inhibits the absorption of theophylline (a bronchodilator), but fat or carbohydrate accelerates its absorption. A high-carbohydrate, low-protein diet decreased the number of wheezing spells suffered by asthmatic children receiving theophylline (Feldman, 1980).

Hypokalemia—Potassium depletion in the circulating blood; less than 3.5 mEq/L in adults.

Enteric-coated—Type of drug preparation designed to dissolve in the intestine rather than in the stomach.

TABLE 16–1   The Effects of Drugs on Nutrients (Continued)

Drug Group	Drug	Effects/Action on Nutrient	Mechanism of Action
ALTERATION IN NUTRIENT ABSORPTION			
Laxative—lubricant	Mineral oil	Decreases absorption of vitamins A, D, E, and K, calcium, and phosphorus	Formation of complexes
Anti-infective	Neomycin	Decreases absorption of fat, fat-soluble vitamins, vitamin B_{12}, lactose, iron, sucrose, sodium, potassium, calcium	Damaged intestinal mucosa
Antitubercular	Para-aminosalicylate	Reduces absorption of vitamin B_{12}	Inhibited transport mechanism
Anticonvulsant	Phenytoin	Reduces absorption of folic acid	Inhibited intestinal enzymes
Anti-inflammatory	Sulfasalazine	Reduces absorption of folic acid, iron	Inhibited transport mechanism
ALTERATION IN NUTRIENT METABOLISM			
Alcohol	Alcohol (ethanol)	Amino acids poorly utilized	Damaged intestinal mucosa
Anticonvulsant	Anticonvulsants	Folic acid and vitamin D deficiency	Impeded conversion of vitamin D to intermediate form
Anti-infective	Broad spectrum antibiotics	Decreased vitamin K synthesis	Destruction of intestinal bacteria
Corticosteroid	Corticosteroids	Decreases glucose tolerance; produces tissue wasting, "moon face," and "buffalo hump"	Glyconeogenesis; protein catabolism; mobilization of fats
Hormones in oral contraceptives	Estrogen/progesteron	Folic acid, vitamin B_6, and vitamin B_{12} deficiencies; increased serum lipid levels	Multiple mechanisms
Antitubercular	Isoniazid	Pyridoxine deficiency	Increased urinary excretion
Antiparkinson	Levodopa	Pyridoxine deficiency	Increased urinary excretion
Antineoplastic	Methotrexate	Folic acid deficiency	Destruction of GI tract cells
Anticoagulant	Warfarin	Depletes vitamin K	Interference with synthesis of clotting factors
ALTERATION IN NUTRIENT EXCRETION			
Analgesic	Acetylsalicylic acid	Increases excretion of folic acid	Competition for binding sites
Alcohol	Alcohol (ethanol)	Increases excretion of folic acid	Nutrient not retained in liver
Diuretic	Furosemide	Increases excretion of sodium, potassium, and calcium	Interference with reabsorption by kidneys
Chelating agent	Penicillimine	Increases excretion of metals, esp. zinc and copper	Formation of chemical bonds
Glucocorticoid	Prednisone	Increases excretion of vitamin C	Catabolism of tissues

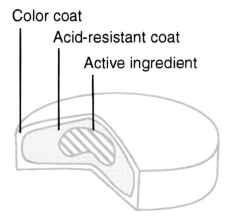

FIGURE 16–2 Diagram of an enteric-coated tablet. Substances that penetrate the acid-resistant coating defeat the purpose of this type of tablet. (From Clayton, BD, and Stock, YN, p 56, with permission.)

Fatty foods enhance the absorption of griseofulvin, an antifungal drug. For a person on a low-fat diet, the drug can be administered either in a **micronized** form or in a low-fat suspension. The pharmacist can suspend the drug in a small amount of corn oil.

The Effects of Foods on Drug Metabolism

Foods can alter the metabolism of drugs. One metabolic food-drug interaction can be life-threatening.

Monoamine Oxidase Inhibitors

The usual abbreviation for this group of drugs is **MAO inhibitor.** Several antidepressants are MAO inhibitors and some other drugs produce similar reactions. See Table 16–2.

MECHANISM OF DRUG ACTION   These drugs prevent the breakdown of tyramine and dopamine, chemicals necessary for proper functioning of the nervous system. The drugs' therapeutic effect is to increase the concentration of epinephrine, norepinephrine, serotonin, and dopamine in the central nervous system, thus counteracting depression.

In the peripheral nervous system the MAO inhibitors also prevent the release of norepinephrine that builds up in the nerves. The stores of norepinephrine become especially high in the nerves that regulate the size of blood vessels. The result is a decreased ability to constrict peripheral blood vessels. The vasodilation thus produced leads to hy-

potension. To compound the situation, the drugs also inhibit the body's normal response to a low blood pressure, an increased heart rate. Thus the individual displays the unusual combination of hypotension and bradycardia.

EFFECT OF FOODS ON MAO INHIBITORS   Some foods contain **tyramine,** a metabolic intermediate product in the conversion of the amino acid tyrosine to epinephrine. Foods containing degraded protein, such as aged cheese, are high in tyramine. When a client on MAO inhibitors consumes foods or beverages high in tyramine, the drugs prevent the normal breakdown of tyramine. As a consequence, the tyramine oversupply leads to excessive epinephrine, producing hypertension. Sometimes the blood pressure is severely elevated, which can cause intracranial hemorrhage.

As in many situations, an individual's response to tyramine varies. Several factors interact to determine the severity of reaction: (1) the amount of tyramine ingested, (2) the dose of the MAO inhibitor, (3) client susceptibility, and (4) the time between the drug dose and tyramine-containing meal.

TYRAMINE-RICH FOODS   Many foods contain enough tyramine to create problems for the person receiving MAO inhibitors. These include foods and beverages such as cheese, beer, and chianti wine, in which aging is used to enhance flavor. The amount of tyramine varies even in different samples of a particular food. Table 16–2 describes the tyramine-restricted diet. Since this interaction can be life-threatening, the best advice to give a client is to avoid all foods capable of causing problems, even though a small amount of the food, or a given batch of a product, might be safe.

Effects of Other Nutrients

Certain nutrients increase the amount of a drug in the bloodstream, thus increasing or decreasing the risk of toxicity. For example, fat displaces the an-

---

Micronize—To pulverize a substance into very tiny particles.

Monoamine oxidase (MAO) **inhibitor**—A class of antidepressant drugs that may have critical interactions with foods.

Tyramine—A monoamine present in various foods that will provoke a hypertensive crisis in persons taking MAO inhibitors.

TABLE 16–2 Tyramine-Restricted Diet

Description	Indication	Adequacy
Restricts food with naturally high levels of tyramine.	Used when clients receive drugs classified as monoamine oxidase inhibitors (MAOs) and those with MAO activity. *Antidepressants:* Isocarboxazid; Phenelzine; Tranylcypromine *Anti-infectives:* Furazolidone; Isoniazid *Antineoplastics:* Procarbazine	Adequate in all nutrients according to the current Recommended Dietary Allowance if the individual makes appropriate food choices.

Foods	To Avoid	To Use Moderately
Breads and cereals	None	None
Fruit and vegetables	Avocados Bananas Figs Broad (fava) beans Chinese pea pods Eggplant Italian flat beans Mixed Chinese vegetables	None
Dairy	Aged cheese (brick, blue, brie, cheddar, Camembert, Swiss, Romano, Roquefort, mozzarella, Parmesan, provolone) Yogurt	Gouda cheese Processed American cheese
Meat and fish	Any canned meat Beef or chicken liver Sausage (bologna, salami, pepperoni, summer) Fish (caviar, dried fish, salt herring)	
Beverages	Ale, beer, sherry, red and white wines	Coffee, colas, hot chocolate (1–3 cups per day)
Other	Chocolate, bouillon and other protein extracts, meat tenderizer, soy sauce, yeast concentrates	

tianxiety drug diazepam from **protein binding sites,** thus increasing the amount of unbound drug circulating in the bloodstream. This increased serum concentration leads to increased activity of the drug.

Warfarin achieves anticoagulation by fooling the liver into accepting it as vitamin K. For maximum therapeutic effect, the amount of foods high in vitamin K consumed should be consistent, not excessive one day and scanty the next. Table 16–3 summarizes instructions for clients taking warfarin products.

Correct potassium and calcium levels are necessary for adequate muscle function, including that of the heart. Hypokalemia or hypercalcemia increases the risk of toxicity from digitalis. Clients receiving digitalis and loop diuretics, a common combination, require careful monitoring.

Premature infants have immature respiratory systems. Although they need oxygen to survive, it can become toxic to them. Vitamin E protects these infants from bronchopulmonary dysplasia due to oxy-

gen toxicity. Table 16–4 summarizes the effects of foods and nutrients on drugs.

Occasionally a nutrient acts inadvertently as a carrier for a drug. For example, a woman was seen in a dermatology clinic for a persistent rash, worsened by sunlight. She habitually drank 500 milliliters of tonic water daily as a beverage. Tonic water is a carbonated mixer containing lemon, lime, sweeteners, and quinine, a drug used to treat malaria and nocturnal leg cramps. The amount of quinine in the water, 40 milligrams in 500 milliliters, was much less than that given to pharmacologically to adults Among quinine's side effects, however, is a skin rash. Once the woman ceased drinking tonic water, her skin problem was cured (Wagner, Diffey, and Ive, 1994).

Effects of Non-nutrient Intakes

Although it is not a nutrient, caffeine is part of a person's oral intake and it should be included in a di-

TABLE 16–3   Dietary Restrictions for Oral Anticoagulant Therapy

Avoid	One Serving Per Day, 1 Cup Raw or 1/2 Cup Cooked	Check with Prescriber If Large Increases or Decreases
Kale (except garnish)	Broccoli	Green vegetables
Parsley (except garnish)	Brussels sprouts	Garbanzo beans
Natto (Japanese)	Spinach	Lentils
	Turnip or other greens	Soybeans or soybean oil
		Liver

etary assessment. Caffeine increases the effect of theophylline and stimulants. In some users, caffeine produces effects similar to other psychoactive substances of dependence: tolerance, withdrawal, persistent desire or unsuccessful efforts to control use, and continued use despite knowledge of persistent physical or psychological problems related to its use (Strain, et al, 1994).

Another non-nutrient, marketed as a food supplement is Mahuang. This is the main plant source of ephedrine, a drug with central nervous system stimulating effects, which is used in many over-the-counter decongestants and diet aids. In one case, a man took increasing amounts of a herbal diet supplement containing Mahuang over a 2-month period for weight control. He became uncharacteristically restless, sleepless, argumentative, aggressive, and so disorganized at work he was given a leave of absence. Discontinuation of the herbal supplement and a prescribed sedative returned him to normal in 3 days (Capwell, 1995).

The amount of Mahuang in the supplement was never ascertained. Since manufacturers of food supplements are not regulated by the FDA, the labels can omit quantities of active ingredients.

The Body's Homeostatic Mechanisms Affect Drug Excretion

In addition to nutritional status, the status of acid-base balance and fluid and electrolyte balance affect the excretion of drugs. To consider either acid-base balance or fluid and electrolyte balance in isolation risks oversimplifying the body's functions. The functions of these two regulatory systems are interwoven.

Acid-Base Balance

The kidney is the gatekeeper of the bloodstream. The contents of urine reflect the metabolic state of the body. The end products of the foods consumed and the drugs taken make the urine either more acid or more alkaline. Freshly voided urine usually has an acid pH, averaging about 6.0.

Alkaline Urine

Large amounts of citrus juices or a vegetarian diet cause the urine to become alkaline. When the body is producing alkaline urine, the kidney will take longer to excrete alkaline drugs. Higher levels of the drugs will remain in the bloodstream for a longer period. Examples of alkaline drugs are the cardiac antidysrhythmic quinidine; the tricyclic antidepressant imipramine; and the amphetamine stimulants. If the client's metabolism causes an alkaline urine, these drugs will give more pronounced and prolonged effects. Clients treated with these drugs should neither change the amounts of citrus juice they consume nor become vegetarians without consulting the physician.

The opposite effect occurs when a person's metabolism produces alkaline urine and the drugs are acidic. The kidney excretes acidic drugs faster than usual if the urine is alkaline. One acidic drug that should spring to mind immediately is acetylsalicylic acid. Another acidic drug is the barbiturate commonly used as an anticonvulsant, phenobarbital. The kidney will discard either of these drugs faster than normal if the patient is producing an alkaline urine.

Acid Urine

Large doses of ascorbic acid (vitamin C) make the urine more acidic. Vitamin C is sometimes given specifically for the purpose of acidifying the urine. For example, a urinary pH of 5.5 or less is necessary for the urinary anti-infective drug methenamine to be effective. In an acid urine, the

---

Protein binding sites—Various sites in the body tissues to which drugs may become attached, rendering the drug temporarily inactive.

TABLE 16–4   How Foods Affect Drugs

Effect	Type of Food/Nutrient	Action on Drug
Decrease in absorption	Amino acids in proteins	Inhibit absorption of levodopa, theophylline
		Delays action of phenytoin
	Calcium in dairy products	Combines with tetracycline to impair absorption
	High-fiber meal	Decreases absorption of digoxin
	Milk, alcohol, hot beverages	Cause premature erosion enteric-coatings
	Pectin in jelly, apples	Reduces absorption of acetaminophen
	Carbohydrate	Decreases absorption of isoniazid
Increase in absorption	Carbohydrate	Enhances absorption of levodopa, phenytoin, theophylline
	Fatty foods	Enhance absorption of griseofulvin
Altered metabolism	Caffeine	Enhances effect of theophylline
	Fat	Enhances activity of diazepam
	Tyramine-containing foods	May cause hypertensive crisis when combined with MAO inhibitors
	Vitamin E	Protects premature infants from oxygen toxicity

drug becomes ammonia and formaldehyde, both bactericidal chemicals.

Sulfonamides are another class of drugs given for urinary tract infections. One of the possible side effects of sulfonamides is **crystalluria,** crystallization of the drug in the urinary tract. Although some drugs crystallize more readily than others, this class of drugs is more likely to crystallize in concentrated or acid urine. For this reason, clients should be instructed to drink ample fluid. It may also be necessary to deliberately alkalinize the urine to prevent crystallization. Table 16–5 summarizes the effects of acid-base balance on the excretion of drugs.

Fluid and Electrolyte Balance

Fluid and electrolyte status also influences the effects of drugs. An increase or decrease in sodium, the mineral most closely associated with water balance, can affect the excretion of certain drugs. Imported licorice may cause serious imbalances in fluid and electrolyte status.

Sodium, Fluids, and Lithium Carbonate

Both sodium intake and increased fluid intake affect the antimanic drug lithium carbonate. This drug is absorbed, distributed, and excreted alongside of sodium. Therefore, decreased sodium intake with decreased fluid intake may lead to lithium retention. Conversely, increased sodium intake and increased fluid intake increase the excretion of lithium and decrease the antimanic effect, resulting in overmedication and worsening signs and symptoms of mania. Because of this important interaction, clients taking lithium

are taught to monitor the concentration or **specific gravity** of their urine.

Licorice

A flavoring agent, licorice, when taken to excess, can cause hypokalemia, sodium and water retention, hypertension, and alkalosis. This is an action of natural licorice only. It is imported into this country. The licorice commonly manufactured in the United States contains artificial flavoring and does not produce these ill effects. Imported licorice, however, may cause problems for clients on low-sodium diets or potassium-wasting diuretics.

Responsibilities of Health Care Professionals

The Joint Commission on the Accreditation of Healthcare Organizations mandates that clients be

TABLE 16–5   Effects of Urinary pH on Drugs

	Alkaline Urine	Acid Urine
Increased excretion	Acetylsalicylic acid	Amphetamines
		Imipramine
	Phenobarbital	Quinidine
Decreased excretion	Amphetamines	Acetylsalicylic acid
	Imipramine	
	Quinidine	Phenobarbital
Necessary for adequate effect	Sulfonamides	Methenamine

given information on the medications they receive including potential dietary interactions. Although the dietitian is charged with this responsibility, the successful completion of the task requires cooperation from the health care team. Charting Tips 16–1 pertains to client teaching.

Institutionalized clients do not necessarily receive maximum therapeutic effects from their medications. Researchers found only 50 percent of 424 doses of three cardiac medications (hydralazine, phenytoin, and propranolol) were administered correctly on a full stomach and 53 percent of 101 doses of captopril were correctly given on an empty stomach. In the 24 hours studied, only 15 percent of 153 clients received all their medication doses correctly timed with meals. This last group included the one client whose physician's order specified before meals in contrast to the 182 physicians' orders that did not include a reference to meals (Strong, et al, 1991).

Managing a medication regimen is a challenge worth accepting. The consequences of improper scheduling can be treatment failure, toxicity, and/or increased expense.

Summary

This chapter has only touched the surface of the subject of food and drug interactions. For every drug selected for discussion, many others were omitted. Commonly prescribed drugs and those with significant interactions with foods were included. In addition, we have discussed various modes of food and drug interactions.

Persons at highest risk for food-drug interactions are those who (1) take many drugs, including alcohol, (2) require long-term drug therapy, or (3) have poor or marginal nutrition. Food-drug interactions

CHARTING TIPS 16–1

✓ Record the client's knowledge at the start of your teaching.

✓ Identify information discussed.

✓ Indicate evidence, such as verbalization or recitation, that indicates client understood your teaching.

✓ Whenever possible, give the client a choice. If the client makes a choice, chart the decision as the client's.

✓ Document educational materials given to the client.

can affect (1) food intake, (2) absorption of nutrients or drugs, (3) metabolism of nutrients or drugs, and (4) excretion of nutrients or drugs.

Medications influence food intake. They can decrease or increase appetite, cause taste changes, or provoke gastric irritation.

Drugs affect nutrient absorption through luminal or mucosal effects. Food or nutrients can decrease, delay, or increase absorption of drugs.

In addition to interactions involving intake and absorption, foods and drugs can affect one another's metabolism. Two important nutrient-drug interactions are those of tyramine-containing foods with MAO inhibitors and of sodium and water with lithium carbonate.

Foods and drugs interact during excretion of waste products also. At special risk are clients in unstable acid-base or fluid and electrolyte balance or those with alterations in serum proteins.

Specific gravity—Weight of a liquid or solid substance compared with an equal volume of water taken as 1.000. Normal urine has a specific gravity from 1.010 to 1.025.

Case Study 16–1 Mrs. S, a 72-year-old client, is being seen by the home health nurse to reaffirm her suitability for independent living. She has a history of congestive heart failure for which she has been successfully treated with digoxin 0.125 mg daily for the past 6 months. Mrs. S takes the tablet with her usual breakfast of orange juice and tea.

Recently she has had difficulty with constipation. Obtaining information on bowel hygiene on her own, she decided to improve her nutritional intake by adding a high-fiber cereal to her breakfast.

After 1 week, her constipation has been relieved, but she now is becoming fatigued easily. When climbing a flight of stairs she finds it necessary to rest twice en route.

The nurse asked Mrs. S to weigh herself. Mrs. S reported she had gained 5 lb in 2 weeks. Based on the above data and her observations, the home health nurse prepared a nursing care plan. The portion of it pertinent to food and drug interactions appears below.

NURSING CARE PLAN FOR MRS. S

Assessment

Subjective Data	Easily fatigued
	Short of breath < 1 flight of stairs
	History of constipation, relieved by addition of high-fiber cereal to diet
	Medications—digoxin, 0.125 mg daily in morning with breakfast.
Objective Data	Alert, oriented, cooperative. Vital signs normal except pulse 90 beats per minute. Weight gain—5 lb over 2 weeks.

Nursing Diagnosis   Health maintenance, altered: related to food-drug interaction as evidenced by beginning signs of heart failure.

Desired Outcome/ Evaluation Criteria	Nursing Actions	Rationale
Client will revise medication or meal schedule immediately to maximize effectiveness of digoxin.	Teach client to separate digoxin dose from high-fiber foods.	High-fiber foods decrease the absorption of digitalis preparations.

Study Aids

Chapter Review

1. Which of the following clients would be at greatest risk for food-drug interaction?
   a. A 50-year-old man with no current disease
   b. A 75-year-old woman with several chronic diseases requiring medication
   c. A 12-year-old within normal limits on the height and weight chart
   d. A 25-year-old pregnant woman

2. Which of the following are ways in which food and drugs interact?
   a. Drugs may affect food intake.
   b. Either may affect the absorption of the other.
   c. Certain foods and drugs specifically interfere with the metabolism of the other.
   d. Nutrients and drugs can increase or decrease the rate of excretion of one another.
   e. All of the above are true.

3. It is recommended that levodopa be taken with carbohydrate-rich snacks but separated from any high-protein meal by 3 hours because:
   a. Glucose from the carbohydrate aids in the distribution of the drug.
   b. Carbohydrate causes the release of insulin, which is necessary for the absorption of levodopa.
   c. Amino acids compete with levodopa for absorption.
   d. Levodopa is likely to sensitize the person to various proteins.

4. A client taking lithium is most likely to display increased mania with:
   a. Decreased fluid intake and decreased sodium intake.
   b. Decreased fluid intake and increased potassium intake.
   c. Increased sodium intake and decreased potassium intake.
   d. Increased sodium intake and increased fluid intake.

5. Individuals taking the anticoagulant warfarin must be counseled to limit consumption to one serving per day of:
   a. Broccoli and spinach
   b. Vegetable oils
   c. Kale and parsley
   d. Dried apricots and dates

Clinical Analysis

Mr. AS is being admitted to a long-term care facility. He is a 45-year-old posttrauma client. The motor vehicle accident in which he became paralyzed below the waist also killed his wife and daughter. The accident occurred 6 months ago. In the meantime he has been treated at a rehabilitation center, but his depression interfered with his progress. After many trials of various antidepressants, he is now receiving phenelzine. The following questions relate to his care.

1. To ensure that everyone caring for Mr. AS is alerted to potential complications related to his drug therapy, the nurse begins a nursing care plan. The nursing diagnosis that best states this problem as described by the data is:
   a. Coping, ineffective individual: related to deaths of family members as evidenced by need for antidepressant therapy
   b. Risk for altered tissue perfusion, cerebral, related to inappropriate diet combined with phenelzine therapy
   c. Knowledge deficit related to potential food-drug interaction between tyramine-containing foods and monoamine oxidase inhibitor
   d. Bowel elimination, altered: related to paraplegia as evidenced by incontinence

2. Close attention to Mr. AS's diet is essential. Which of the following foods will he have to avoid completely?
   a. Baked beans, dates, and roast beef
   b. Sugar, molasses, and maple syrup
   c. Bologna, cheddar cheese, and wine
   d. Green beans, whole-wheat bread, and oranges

3. When teaching the nursing assistants about the dietary restrictions needed by Mr. AS, the nurse should be sure the nursing assistants understand that:
   a. The potential complication can be life-threatening.
   b. Mr. AS is to be kept unaware of the complication.
   c. As time goes on, the forbidden foods can be added to the diet slowly, one at a time.
   d. If Mr. AS does not cooperate in his dietary care, his paralysis is likely to worsen.

Bibliography

1994 Joint Commission Accreditation Manual for Hospitals. Volume 1: Standards. Joint Commission on Accreditation of Health Care Organizations, Oakbrook Terrace, IL, 1993.

Ackley, BJ, and Ladwig, GB: Nursing Diagnosis Handbook, ed 2. Mosby, St. Louis, 1995.

Adams, WL: Potential for adverse drug-alcohol interactions among retirement community residents. J Am Geriatr Soc 43:1021, 1995.

Berg, MJ: Folic acid improves phenytoin pharmacokinetics. J Am Diet Assoc 95:352, 1995.

Black, JA: Diarrhoea, vitamin K, and warfarin [Letter]. Lancet 344:1373, 1994.

Brensilver, JM, and Goldberger, E: A Primer of water, Electrolyte and Acid-Base Syndromes, ed 8. FA Davis Company, Philadelphia, 1996.

Capwell, RR: Ephedrine-induced mania from an herbal diet supplement [Letter]. Am J Psychiatry 152:647, 1995.

Clayton, BD, and Stock, YN: Basic Pharmacology for Nurses, ed 9. CV Mosby, St. Louis, 1989.

Conly, J, and Stein, K: Reduction of vitamin K_2 concentrations in human liver associated with the use of broad spectrum antimicrobials. Clin Invest Med 17:531, 1994.

Deglin, JH, and Vallerand, AH: Davis's Drug Guide for Nurses, ed 4. FA Davis Company, Philadelphia, 1995.

Feldman, CH: Effect of dietary protein and carbohydrate on theophylline metabolism in children. Pediatrics 66:956, 1980.

Harris, JE: Interaction of dietary factors with oral anticoagulants: Review and applications. J Am Diet Assoc 95:580, 1995.

Karch, AM: Lippincott's Nursing Drug Guide, JB Lippincott, Philadelphia, 1996.

Lamont, LS: Beta-blockers and their effects on protein metabolism and resting energy expenditure. J Cardiopulm Rehabil 15:183, 1995.

Lasswell, AB, et al: Family medicine residents' knowledge and attitudes about drug-nutrient interactions. J Am Coll Nutr 14:137, 1995.

Lewis, CW, Frongillo, EA, and Roe, DA: Drug-nutrient interactions in three long-term care facilities. J Am Diet Assoc 95:309, 1995.

Roe, DA: Handbook on Drug and Nutrient Interactions, ed 5. The American Dietetic Association, Chicago, 1994.

Strain, EC, et al: Caffeine dependence syndrome. JAMA 272:1043, 1994.

Strong, A, et al: Drug administration in relation to meals in the institutional setting. Heart Lung 20:39, 1991.

Wagner, GH, Diffey, BL, and Ive, FA: `I'll have mine with a twist of lemon' Quinine photosensitivity from excessive intake of tonic water [Letter]. Br J Dermatol 131:734, 1994.

Wilson, BA, Shannon, MT, and Stang, CL: Nurses Drug Guide, Appleton and Lange, Stamford, CT, 1996.

Woolf, G, et al: Acute hepatitis associated with the Chinese herbal product Jin Bu Huan. Ann Intern Med 121:729, 1994.

CHAPTER 17

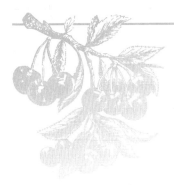

Weight Control

LEARNING OBJECTIVES

After completing this chapter, the student should be able to:
1 Discuss the effects of weight loss on the body.
2 Identify the medical, psychological, and social problems associated with too much and too little body fat.
3 Describe the healthy way to lose weight.
4 Discuss the dangers of inappropriate weight loss.
5 Describe the symptoms commonly exhibited by a client with anorexia nervosa and/or bulimia.

The diagnosis and consequences of obesity are far-reaching. Basic knowledge about theories of obesity and the principles basic to a weight loss formula are essential for researchers, practitioners, and clients. Principles of balances and imbalances in energy production and use are central to understanding the nature of and problems associated with obesity. As researchers discover new and more effective treatments for obesity, the effects of weight loss and the success rates for such treatments will be analyzed. Conclusions from longitudinal studies may then be used to further advance scientific knowledge about the causes, contributing factors, effective treatments, and psychological implications of obesity. As clients and health care personnel await the results of new studies, several options remain for managing obesity. Following a general discussion of obesity, these options will be discussed.

Energy Imbalance

Energy imbalance results when the number of kilocalories eaten does not equal the number used for energy. An individual can determine whether food intake is meeting energy needs by monitoring his or her weight. If more kilocalories are eaten than are used by the body, weight gain will occur. If fewer kilocalories are eaten than are used by the body (and protein intake is adequate), weight loss will occur. In cases where a single health care provider follows the progress of a client for an extended time, energy balance can be assessed by monitoring the client's weight history.

Basic Principles

There are two basic principles of energy imbalance. First, it takes a specific number of kilocalories to gain or lose a pound of body fat. Second, the body stores energy and uses stored energy in a highly specific manner.

The Five-Hundred Rule

To lose 1 pound of body fat per week, the individual must eat 500 kilocalories fewer per day than his or her body expends for 7 days. To gain 1 pound of body fat per week, the individual must eat 500 kilocalories more per day for 7 days than his or her body expends. The gain or loss of body fat need not occur during the course of a week; the kilocalorie surplus or deficit may occur over a month or year. The principle is the same. The total num-

ber of kilocalories required to gain or lose a pound of body fat is 3500.

Body Fat Stores

Excess kilocalories are stored as body fat in adipose tissue. The human body is able to store adipose fat tissue in unlimited amounts. This can lead to **obesity.** During a kilocalorie deficit, the body will first seek the energy necessary to sustain body functions in glycogen stores which are limited. When a kilocalorie deficit occurs for longer than about 1 day, the body will seek the energy necessary to sustain its functions in *both* body fat stores (adipose tissue) and body protein stores (organ and muscle mass).

The Client with Excessive Body Fat

Most health experts agree that there is a high prevalence of **overweight** and obese people in our society. There are many social, psychological, and health consequences for the overly fat client. At the same time, the entire scientific community struggles with how to define and diagnose overly fat clients. How a client is diagnosed often determines which treatment approach is indicated.

Diagnosing the Client with Excessive Body Fat

Diagnosing the client as underweight, normal weight, mildly obese, moderately obese, or severely obese is often necessary. How the client is classified often determines whether treatment is indicated and the kind of treatment that is appropriate. However, classifying the client with excessive body fat is often difficult for the health care professional. This is due in part to (1) the lack of universally accepted definitions and standards and (2) the widespread use of several different methods of diagnosis.

Energy imbalance—Situation in which kilocalories eaten do not equal the number used for energy.

Obesity—Excessive amount of fat on the body; obesity for women is a fat content greater than 33 percent; obesity for men is a fat content greater than 25 percent.

Overweight—10 to 20 percent above healthy body weight; 110 to 120 percent healthy body weight.

One major problem in diagnosing the overly fat client is that there is no universally accepted definition for the following words: overweight, mildly obese, moderately obese, and severely obese. This is why most authors define these terms at the beginning of each book or article on weight control that they publish. This text defines these terms and includes a discussion on three of the methods used to diagnose clients: percent healthy body weight, body mass index, and percent body fat. This section begins with a discussion of height and weight tables because these tables are used to calculate percent **healthy body weight** (HBW).

Height and Weight Tables

Height and weight tables have been used to diagnose the client with excessive body fat for years. Insurance companies developed the first height and weight table in 1908 based on insurable populations. Its original purpose was to determine insurance rates based on life expectancy studies. The medical community subsequently adopted this and similar tables for clinical use. In 1942 and 1943, the Metropolitan Life Insurance Company introduced the term **"ideal body weight"** and called its table "Ideal Weights for Men and Women." Nutrition researchers use the term "ideal" when reference is made to this height and weight table. The assumption of this table is that a stable body weight throughout the life cycle has a health benefit. The Desirable Weight for Height Table was introduced in 1959. The assumption of this table is that maintaining a lower-than-average weight has a health benefit. Nutrition researchers use the term "desirable" when reference is made to this height and weight table. The authors of this text have avoided the use of the terms "ideal" or "desirable" because these terms refer to specific height and weight tables (each of which are based on different assumptions of what constitutes a healthy body weight).

The height and weight table found in Table 2–6 is the 1983 Metropolitan Height and Weight Table, which was developed so as not to be labeled with any term denoting a value judgment. There is much controversy about this table now since it is skewed and does not reflect the entire population, only those individuals who applied for insurance. However, the 1983 Metropolitan Height and Weight Table is currently the most widely used table in most diet manuals and medical textbooks. The assumption of this table is that a modest increase in weight (2 to 13 pounds) throughout adulthood does not result in a decreased life expectancy. Thus, the weights in the 1983 table are about 2 to 13 pounds heavier than those in the 1959 table in each sex, frame size, and height category.

Much controversy exists concerning which height and weight table best meets the health needs of the population. In fact, many other organizations and researchers have developed their own height and weight tables because of a dissatisfaction with the Metropolitan Life Insurance Company's tables. It is important to realize that the height and weight tables of the Metropolitan Life Insurance Company are based on mortality or death rates. The weights presented are not necessarily the weights at which any individual is the healthiest, performs his or her job optimally, or even looks his or her best. Height and weight tables cannot replace a thorough physical assessment, an accurate diet history, information about exercise patterns, or measurement of a client's body fat content.

Body Mass Index

A client's body mass index (BMI) is his or her body weight in kilograms divided by height in meters squared. BMI can be determined without doing any calculations by using a chart called a **nomogram.** A nomogram is a chart that shows a relationship between numerical values. Figure 17–1 is a nomogram used to determine BMI. Note that the left side of the chart is labeled "weight" and the right side is labeled "height." To determine your BMI, place a ruler between your body weight (without clothes) on the left to your height (without shoes) on the right. Your body mass index is at the point where the line crosses the middle column.

A BMI of 20 to 25 kilograms per meters squared is normal. Overweight clients will have a BMI of 25 to 30. The obese client will have a BMI above 30 (National Research Council, 1989).

Percent Body Fat

Although a HBW expressed as a percent over 120 or a BMI in excess of 30 kilograms per meters squared may alert the health care worker that the client may fall outside acceptable guidelines, this is not always foolproof. Two examples are discussed to illustrate this concept.

First let us consider the 5 foot, 4 inch woman with shoes (1 inch heels) who has a medium frame size and was weighed wearing indoor clothing. According to the 1983 Metropolitan Height and Weight Table for Adults (see Table 2–6) she should weigh between 124 and 138 pounds. Let us review the calculation of HBW (Chapter 2): if we subtract 124

BOX 17–1   PERCENT HEALTHY BODY WEIGHT

Descriptive words such as underweight, normal weight, mildly obese, and so forth are often used in terms of percent body weight (HBW–Chapter 2). Healthy body weight can vary depending on which height and weight table is used. Classifications for body weight are commonly defined (Stunkard, 1984) as follows:

    Overweight: 10 to 20 percent HBW
    Obese: over 20 percent HBW
        Mildly obese: 20 to 40 percent overweight or 120 to 140 percent HBW
        Moderately obese: 41 to 100 percent overweight or 141 to 200 percent HBW
        Severely obese: greater than 100 percent overweight or more than 200 percent HBW.

pounds from 138 pounds, the difference would be 14 pounds; if we divide 14 pounds by 2 pounds, the answer would be 7 pounds; if we add 7 pounds to 124 pounds, the sum would be 131 pounds. Thus 131 pounds is this client's theoretical HBW. Suppose this client weighed 131 pounds. Her HBW would be 100 percent. Can we automatically conclude that this client is not obese? The answer is no.

The optimal body fat content for females is 18 to 22 percent. A more accurate definition of obesity for females is a body fat content of greater than 33 percent. A person at her HBW is metabolically obese if her body fat content exceeds 33 percent. The woman in the preceding example may have all of the health risks of obesity even at 100 percent HBW if her body fat content exceeds 33 percent.

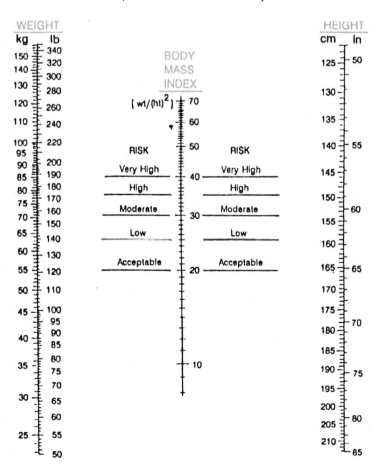

FIGURE 17–1 Nomogram for determining body mass index. (From the National Research Council: Diet and Health, 1989, with permission.)

Second, let us consider a 5 foot, 9 inch man with shoes (1-inch heels) who has a medium frame and was weighed wearing indoor clothing. According to the same table used above, this individual should weigh between 148 and 160 pounds. The same process can be used to derive his HBW. First, subtract 148 pounds from 160 pounds; the answer is 12 pounds. Next divide 12 pounds by 2 pounds; the answer is 6 pounds. When you add 6 pounds to 148 pounds, you have calculated his HBW, which is 154 pounds. Suppose this client weighed 205 pounds. Dividing 154 pounds into 205 pounds would equal 133 percent. Can we automatically classify this client as moderately obese? The answer is no. This client may have a body fat content of only 15 percent. Remember, the optimal fat content for men is 15 to 19 percent. The individual described above would most likely be a trained athlete and the excess weight would be the result of increased muscle mass. A fat content in excess of 25 percent is considered obese for males.

From these examples, we have demonstrated the importance of determining the percent of body fat for each client. At least half of the body fat is located just beneath the skin. Therefore, the measurement of skinfold thickness is the most commonly used technique to estimate a person's body fat content. In this chapter, the four-site measurement technique to determine percent body fat is discussed. This technique requires a minimum of calculations.

The worksheet in Clinical Calculation 17–1 can be used to assist in calculating a client's percent body fat using skin calipers. A total of 12 measurements should be taken at four different sites. The three numbers obtained at each site are averaged to give a value of one number per site. All of these numbers are added and compared with the number on a standard table to determine the client's percent body fat. This Body Fat and Skinfolds table is located in Appendix F. This procedure takes time and requires accurate measurements.

Other techniques to estimate body fat involve the use of tissue x-ray studies, ultrasound, electrical conductivity, bioelectrical impedance, computed tomographic scans, and magnetic resonance imaging scans. Many of these techniques to measure body fat are practiced only at major medical centers, because the technology to perform them is expensive.

Prevalence

Prevalence means the total number of cases of a specific disease in an existing population at a certain time. One in three Americans may be classified as ei-

---

CLINICAL CALCULATION 17–1

Calculating Body Fat Content Using the Four-Site Technique

Worksheet for Calculating Percent Body Fat Using Skin Calipers

Skinfold Measurements	1	2	3	=	Total ÷ 3 = Average
Biceps	__ +	__ +	__	= __	____
Triceps	__ +	__ +	__	= __	____
Subscapular	__ +	__ +	__	= __	____
Suprailiac	__ +	__ +	__	= __	____
Total value of the average of four sites: ____					

Procedure to Calculate Percent Body Fat Using Skin Calipers in Adults

1. Take skinfold measurements directly on the skin, not through clothing.
2. Pick up and hold the skinfold with one hand while measuring it with calipers held by the other hand.
3. Take three measurements at each of the four sites. Then average the three measurements of each skinfold to arrive at a final figure.

   - Biceps—measure the muscle belly of the biceps. This will generally be a point on the straightened arm just opposite the nipple.
   - Triceps
   - Subscapular—measure on the back just under the shoulder blade.
   - Suprailiac—measure approximately 1 in above the hip bone.

4. Add the averages of all skinfold sites to arrive at a total skinfold measurement.
5. To determe the percent body fat, compare the total measurement with the values in the appropriate Body Fat and Skinfolds table located in Appendix E.

(Adapted, courtesy of Jan Wohgulmuth, PT, Director of Physical Therapy at Doctor's Hospital of Jackson, Michigan)

---

ther overweight or obese. The prevalence of excess body weight is thus 33 percent (Table 17–1). Very few persons are classified as severely obese. Most of the people with excess body weight are mildly obese.

The development of excess body weight is strongly influenced by age and sex and economic, racial, and ethnic factors. The following are most likely to be overweight or obese: females, especially

TABLE 17–1 Classification and Percent Healthy Body Weight for a Reference Woman of 5 Feet, 4 Inches

Classification	Percent of Total 5 Foot, 4 Inch Obese Population	HBW	Reference 5 Foot, 4 Inch Woman (Medium Frame)*
Normal weight	None	95–105 percent	124–138 pounds
Mildly obese	90 percent	120–140 percent	157–196 pounds
Moderately obese	9 percent	140–200 percent	183–262 pounds
Severely obese	0.5 percent	200 percent	>262 pounds

* Weight in pounds with indoor clothing weighing 3 pounds; shoes with 1-inch heels.

black females; females below the poverty level; male Mexican Americans; and older persons.

Many experts are concerned about the prevalence of obesity in the nation's children. Estimates indicate that obesity is present in as many as 25 percent of children and adolescents and that obesity has increased up to 54 percent among children 6 to 11 years (Donnelly, 1995). Asian children have the lowest incidence of obesity. **Incidence** is defined as the frequency of occurrence of any event or condition over time and in relation to the population in which it occurs. Native Americans have the highest incidence of obesity. Clinical Application 17–1 discusses tips for weight control in young children.

Obesity prevalence in the United States has increased from 25 percent to 33 percent between 1976 to 1980 and 1988 to 1991 (Russell, 1995). Adult men and women are an average 7.9 pounds heavier in the latter period versus the former.

Consequences of Obesity

There are many adverse consequences to the problems of obesity. The distribution of body fat affects a person's susceptibility to medical problems, and the psychological ramifications of obesity are significant. Clients are often enmeshed in a tangle of cultural, religious, emotional, societal, and perceptual issues. Many clients find great difficulty in breaking the cycle of undesirable behaviors that contributes to obesity. This warrants an examination of each area to enhance understanding.

Social

The social consequences of obesity are connected to cultural expectations and the documented prejudice many obese people experience.

CULTURAL EXPECTATIONS Culture, in this context, refers to the convictions of a given people during a given period. Currently, many Americans are preoccupied with leanness. Leanness means being attractive and desirable. Fatness means being unattractive and undesirable. Yet, what is and has been considered attractive has changed over time. Leanness has not always been the preferred body build. During one period, the overly fat body was considered the most attractive. Carrying excess weight meant that the person was well-to-do; he or she could afford to overeat. Many experts feel that members of our society are slowly changing their perception of what is attractive. For example, the female with well-developed muscles is considered more attractive to many than her lean, not-as-muscular counterpart. The increased numbers of female body builders demonstrate this attitudinal change.

In the United States the obese client has been under intense pressure to lose weight. In an effort to be attractive, many obese clients try to lose weight. Over time, most people who lose weight regain the weight they have lost. When the reduced-weight obese person regains the weight lost, he or she often gains an additional few pounds over and above the original weight. Thus, a self-defeating cycle begins, which is described later in this chapter.

PREJUDICE DOCUMENTED Several classic studies show that obese persons are the objects of prejudice and unfair discrimination. In a 7-year follow-up study of women aged 16 to 24 years, obese women were less likely to have been married and had less schooling, lower incomes, and higher rates of household poverty than those with other chronic medical conditions (Gortmaker, et al, 1993). Health care workers should try to understand their own feelings about fatness, obesity, and obese persons. All too often, health care workers insult obese clients without even being aware of it. Clients benefit when health care workers are sensitive to their psychological needs. Above all else, the nurse should treat the obese client with respect, kindness, and patience.

Tips for Weight Control in Young Children

Obesity in young children is frequently genetic but it can be minimized by sound health habits. Following is a list of health habits that should be encouraged in young overweight children:

1. The more hours spent watching television, the heavier the child. For this reason, viewing time should be restricted to no more than 2 hours per day.
2. The more physical activity, the leaner the child. Thus the child should be encouraged to engage in all forms of physical activity. Examples of appropriate activity for very young children include ballet lessons, tricycle or bicycle riding, walking daily with another family member, swimming lessons, and sledding. Try to cultivate the enjoyment of year-round athletic activities in the child (Fig. 17–2).
3. The length of time the child spends chewing food may decrease the number of kilocalories the child spontaneously eats. Always serve fresh fruits and vegetables with every meal, including breakfast. Examples of low-kilocalorie snacks that require chewing include cut-up apples, peaches, pears, carrots, cucumbers, and green peppers.
4. Fat is the most concentrated source of calories. Try to limit the child's fat intake. Foods that contain fat include all meat, fish, and poultry. It is best to restrict the amount and the kind of meat, fish, and poultry eaten by the overweight child. The amount of meat a child should eat is frequently calculated by the dietitian. Some dairy products also are high in fat. The child should be encouraged to consume nonfat dairy products such as skim milk, partly skimmed cheeses, diet cheeses, and nonfat yogurt. Other sources of fat include salad dressings, margarine, nuts, seeds, oil, bacon, avocado, cream cheese, and sour cream.
5. Teach the child to be aware of what he or she eats and to recite after each meal what he or she has eaten.
6. Encourage the child to eat slowly. For example, serve a hot soup at the beginning of a meal. The child will have to wait for the soup to cool before it can be consumed.
7. Try not to make the child feel guilty about his or her weight problem. Again, recent research has shown that massive obesity in children is partly genetic. The child is *not* totally responsible for his or her present body weight. Try to be kind, patient, and considerate but firm.
8. Small daily decreases in energy expenditure may be significant over the course of a year. Lifestyle behaviors such as the use of television remote controls, telephone extensions, and garage door openers all decrease energy expenditure.

Psychological

Obesity can be associated with a range of psychological problems. In this section we discuss one aspect of the psychological consequences of obesity—body image disturbances.

BODY IMAGE DISTURBANCES **Body image** is defined as the mental picture a person has of himself or herself. A disturbed body image can manifest itself in two ways. First, people with distorted body images are dissatisfied with their bodies. Chronic complaints, demands for extra attention, and frequent negative statements made by clients about the way they look may be signs of an underlying body image disturbance. Second, persons with distorted body images frequently do not view their bodies realistically. For example, obese persons may view themselves as having certain body parts larger than they actually are. Later in this chapter the client with anorexia nervosa is discussed. People with anorexia nervosa, a mental health disorder, frequently have body image disturbances: very thin clients who have this condition frequently view themselves as overweight despite valid evidence contradicting this view.

Body image disturbance is not found in emotionally healthy obese individuals (Stunkard, and Mendelson, 1967). Body image disturbance is most common in young women of the middle and upper-middle classes who have been obese since childhood, many of whom have a generalized neurotic disturbance, and whose parents and peers criticized them for their obesity (Stunkard, and Burt, 1967; Stunkard, and Mendelson, 1961).

Medical

Obesity is considered a major health problem in the United States. Excessive body weight has been associated with both a decreased life expectancy and nonfatal disease risks.

LIFE EXPECTANCY The relationship between life expectancy and severe obesity is clear: the severely obese client has a shorter life expectancy than his or her lean counterpart. Less clear is the relationship of overweight, mild obesity, and moderate obesity to life expectancy. Some researchers are questioning whether these clients do have a shorter life expectancy. This is one reason for the current controversy over whether the medical community should be encouraging all overweight clients to lose weight.

DISEASE RISK Obesity is connected to many chronic diseases. Obesity is strongly linked to heart disease

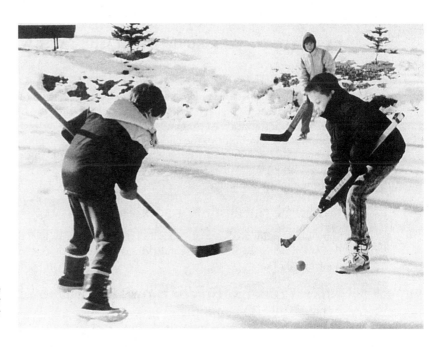

FIGURE 17–2 Youngsters who engage in year-round sports activities are better able to maintain their weights than other youths.

as well as high blood pressure, high cholesterol levels, and noninsulin-dependent diabetes (National Institute of Health Consensus Development Panel on the Health Implications of Obesity, 1985). Obesity is also associated with gallbladder disease, fatty liver, lung function impairment, endocrine abnormalities, childbearing and childbirth complications, trauma to the weight-bearing joints, excessive protein in the urine, and increased hemoglobin concentration. Overweight men have higher rates for colorectal and prostate cancer; overweight women have higher rates for cancer of the ovary and of the breast. There are many nonfatal risks associated with obesity. A nonfatal risk is a hazard that does not decrease life expectancy but does decrease the quality of life for an individual. Back and joint pain is one example of a nonfatal health risk.

The distribution of body fat affects risks. Abdominal obesity is more dangerous than gluteal-femoral obesity (Bjorntorp, 1986). **Abdominal obesity** means that the excess weight is between the client's chest and pelvis. The client with abdominal obesity is said to be shaped like an apple. Clients with abdominal obesity are especially vulnerable to the nonfatal risks associated with excessive body weight. **Gluteal-femoral obesity** means that the excess weight is around the client's buttocks, hips, and thighs. The client with gluteal-femoral obesity is said to be shaped like a pear. Clients with gluteal-femoral obesity are not as susceptible to the nonfatal risks associated with excessive body fat.

The treatment of obesity is an important means of controlling major chronic and degenerative diseases. For example, in some noninsulin-dependent diabetics, weight loss will lower blood glucose levels. Weight reduction therapy is also used to treat hypertension.

Theories about Obesity

Theories about obesity are plentiful (Box 17–2). The truth may be that any one of these theories may be accurate for a specific client but that none is true for everyone. For example, recent research has shown that obese mice have a deficiency of the hormone leptin. Some researchers have referred to the obesity gene (ob gene). The ob gene produces leptin, a hormone that, if all is working correctly, helps to prevent obesity. Leptin is produced by the adipocytes and travels through the blood presumably to the hypothalamus. Many experts think leptin acts as an afferent satiety signal. There is a strong correlation between serum leptin concentrations, percentage body fat, and the body-mass index.

Abdominal obesity—Excess body fat located between an individual's chest and pelvis.

Gluteal-femoral obesity—Excess body fat centered around an individual's buttocks, hips, and thighs.

BOX 17–2 FREQUENTLY ASKED QUESTIONS ABOUT THEORIES OF OBESITY

CAN A MALFUNCTIONING HYPOTHALAMUS CAUSE WEIGHT GAIN?

Appetite and satiety are regulated by a part of the brain called the hypothalamus. Satiety is the feeling of satisfaction after eating. Appetite refers to the pleasant sensation based on previous experience that causes a person to seek food for the purpose of eating. **Hunger** is the physical sensation caused by a lack of food, characterized by a dull or acute pain at or around the lower part of the chest. A malfunctioning hypothalamus could cause an individual to receive incorrect hunger signals, thus stimulating continued eating and signaling weight gain. Appetite, satiety, and hunger may be incorrectly processed by a malfunctioning hypothalamus.

IS OBESITY THE RESULT OF POOR METABOLISM?

Some obese individuals actually require fewer kilocalories for normal body functions than do lean individuals. Some obese individuals use kilocalories very efficiently and may have poor metabolism.

WHAT IS THE FUNCTION OF BROWN FAT, AND HOW DOES IT AFFECT OBESITY?

Brown fat, a special type of fat cell, accounts for less than 1 percent of total body weight. The function of brown fat is to burn kilocalories and release the energy as heat. Energy released as heat is not stored as body fat. Some obese people may have defective brown fat or less brown fat than lean people.

WHAT IS THE SET POINT THEORY?

The set point theory argues that each individual has a unique, relatively stable, adult body weight that is the result of several biologic factors. The obese person may have a higher set point than his or her lean counterpart.

WHY SHOULD THE NUMBER OF FAT CELLS IN THE BODY INFLUENCE WEIGHT?

Obese individuals have many more fat cells than do their lean counterparts. A kilocalorie deficit can reduce the fat in each cell but cannot break down the entire cell. Once manufactured, a fat cell exists until death. Empty fat cells pressure the reduced obese person to fill the depleted cells. The reduced obese person must learn to constantly ignore internal hunger signals. Although obese individuals are able to do this for a short period, long-term adaptation to hunger pains is difficult.

ARE THERE ANY ENZYMES IN THE METABOLIC CHAIN THAT CONTRIBUTE TOWARD OBESITY?

Lipoprotein lipase is an enzyme that is involved in the uptake of fatty acids for the manufacture of fat in individual fat cells. Research has shown that the activity of this enzyme increases during weight reduction. This action makes the fat cell even more efficient in synthesizing fats.

REFERENCES

Lindpaintner, K: Finding an obesity gene—A rate of mice and men. N Engl J Med 332:679, 1995.
Rohner-Jeanrenaud, F. and Jeanrenaud, B: Obesity, leptin, and the brain. N Engl J Med 334:324, 1996.

However, some obese mice have elevated levels of leptin in their serum. For this group of mice, the pathology is not a deficiency of leptin but perhaps a receptor or a postreceptor defect in the hypothalamus. Leptin studies have been done mostly in mice, not humans.

Identical twins raised in different environments (adopted and nonadopted) have been studied extensively. From these studies, many experts believe obesity is about 33 percent genetic and 66 percent environmental (food and exercise behaviors) (Romsos, 1996). Keep the theories in Box 17–2 in mind when counseling the client who is overweight, obese, or underweight. There is more than one cause for the development and maintenance of obesity.

Effects of Weight Loss on the Body

Weight loss affects body composition. The health benefits of weight loss are all related to a loss of body fat, not a loss of lean body mass.

Loss of Fat versus Loss of Water and Protein

Most people, especially the mildly and moderately obese, can lose only about 2 pounds of body fat a week by eating less. Any weight loss beyond that is probably due to loss of water and/or lean muscle tissue. There is always some loss of body protein along with body fat during weight loss. The loss of body protein from reduced food intake alone is greater than the loss of body protein from a combination of reduced food intake and regular exercise. Also, the greater the rate of weight loss, the more organ and muscle mass is lost. For example, Table 17–2 considers the client who loses 13 pounds of body weight over a 2-week period by diet alone.

Variation with the Severity of Obesity

The amount of lean body mass an individual loses during weight reduction also depends on the degree of severity of his or her obesity (Van Itallie, 1988). Severely obese clients can tolerate very low-calorie diets better than the moderately obese client. By tolerate, we mean that they conserve body protein during weight loss. This means mildly and moderately obese individuals are at a higher risk of becoming protein-depleted during rapid weight loss. Rapid weight loss (0.5 to 1.0 pounds per day), if sustained for many weeks, is associated with an excessive loss of lean body mass and protein depletion of the heart (Van Itallie, 1988). Malnutrition of the heart muscle can lead to sudden death. As individuals lose more and more fat during weight loss, their ability to conserve lean body mass decreases. Thus, the length of time an individual diets as well as his or her beginning total body fat content has an impact on the amount of lean body mass lost.

Success Rates for Weight Loss

Weight cycling and the type of diet eaten by the individual attempting weight loss can influence the success rate. Starvation and self-imposed dieting appear to result in eating binges once food is available and in psychological manifestations such as preoccupation with food and eating, increased emotional responsiveness and dysphoria (excessive anguish and depression), and distractibility (Polivy, 1996).

Weight Cycling

The individual who loses weight rapidly has a difficult time keeping the lost weight off. This is partly

TABLE 17–2   Example of the Yo-Yo Effect—Weight Loss and Regain

Patient Information	Weight		
	Before Dieting	After Dieting for 2 Weeks	After Regain
Body weight (pounds)	217	204	217
Body fat (pounds)	70	66	79
Percent body fat	32.2 percent	32.3 percent	36 percent
Lean body mass lost		2.5 lb muscle and organ mass	
		6.5 lb water	
		4 lb fat	
		13 total lb*	

* Does not take into account that most people regain more weight than they orginally lost.

Fat and lean body mass are inversely proportional. As one goes up, the other goes down. Water composition is directly proportional to lean body mass. About 72–73 percent of lean body mass is water. Over a 12-week period on the diet, about 15 lb of muscle and organ mass (not including water) may be lost.

because original weight loss is a combination of fat and lean body mass. Because it takes fewer kilocalories to support fat than protein tissue, weight regain occurs. Any weight regained is usually all body fat. When a client gains and loses weight repeatedly, the net result is called the **yo-yo effect,** also known as **weight cycling.**

Self-Prescribed Fad Diets

Many kinds of fad diets have come and gone. Typically, such diets limit the person to a few specific foods or food combinations.

For example, one common fad diet recommends the consumption of a high-fat diet. Carbohydrates are restricted. This diet does not meet the recommendations of The American Heart Association, the American Cancer Society, and the American Dietetic Association and may be harmful. High fat intake has been associated with many chronic and degenerative diseases. Another example of a fad diet is the grapefruit diet, on which the individual is allowed only grapefruit. Such a diet is not nutritionally balanced and cannot possibly lead to a healthy lifelong change in eating behaviors. See Box 17–3.

Treatment of the Client with Excessive Body Fat

The fact that an individual is obese by any standard does not automatically make him or her a suitable candidate for any available treatment plan. The following sections describe processes used to screen clients for weight reduction and for the various treatments available.

Screening

How do health professionals decide which obese clients would benefit from treatment and which would not? Not all clients should be encouraged to lose weight because repeated weight cycling is harmful. Inappropriate weight-loss methods, including repeated crash diets, can have damaging effects on physical health and psychological well-being (Foster, 1988; Van Itallie, 1984; Wadden and Stunkard, 1985).

Client screening is part of responsible weight-loss programs. Such screening usually focuses on gathering the following data (Petermarck, 1989):

1. Is weight loss indicated for this client? Is the client internally motivated to lose weight? The basic motivation to undergo treatment must originate from the client.
2. What level of health supervision is necessary? Are clients screened for psychosocial conditions that would make weight loss inappropriate? Are clients at medical risk, requiring a physician's care?
3. What factors in the client's history and lifestyle are relevant to the weight-loss program? For

---

BOX 17–3 PSYCHOLOGICAL CONSEQUENCES OF FOOD RESTRICTION

Food restriction either voluntary or involuntary has consequences. Xenophon in ancient Greece described a "ravenous hunger" in soldiers who had been deprived of food during a military campaign (Stunkard, 1993). During World War II Keyes, et al studied the effects of semistarvation on subjects (Keyes, et al 1948). Cocina and Dixon studied the effects of food deprivation on rats (Coscina and Dixon, 1983). In all of these studies, the subjects responded to food deprivation with extraordinarily similar behaviors. First, restrained eaters did not necessarily have much, if any, long-term weight loss. Second, restraining one's eating makes one highly susceptible to bouts of excessive eating even after restrictions are lifted. Third, study subjects exhibited cognitive and emotional changes when food was restricted including: heightened emotional responsiveness; cognitive disruptions, including distractibility; and a focus on food and eating (Polivy, 1996).

Health care providers need to caution clients about the consequences of restrained eating. Overweight clients need to be helped to give up their weight reduction diets and to be advised to eat balanced healthful diets. Obese clients need to be taught to incorporate their favorite foods into more moderate levels of intake and to increase their physical activity. A reduction in counterproductive "restraint" seems likely to produce both physical and psychological well-being (Polivy, 1996).

example, a weight-loss program that is costly may not be affordable for the low-income client.

The best candidates for weight reduction are those who express the desire to change their total lifestyle. The client must be motivated enough to agree to participate in a routine exercise program, follow a low-kilocalorie diet, and change lifelong food behaviors. A significant time investment on the client's part is also necessary. The capacity to succeed is best demonstrated by deeds rather than words (Van Itallie, 1988). For example, will the client attend all program sessions and self-monitor his or her food intake? In addition, the best candidates for weight reduction have implemented lifestyle modifications to limit and control stress. While all individuals experience some stress daily, highly stressful life events such as a recent divorce, the death of a significant other, or a change in a living situation or job status significantly decrease the chance of success.

MOTIVATION   Most individuals associate weight loss with being more attractive. The association between weight loss and wellness is a secondary consideration. The health benefits of weight loss are related to a loss of body fat, however, and not to a loss of lean body mass. The individual who loses a large amount of lean body mass as opposed to body fat derives minimal health benefits from weight loss.

Setting Realistic Goals

Nurses can assist clients in setting realistic goals for weight reduction. Many times the client has an unrealistic weight-loss goal. For example, the weight-reduction diet may be planned to allow for a loss of 1 pound per week, but the client may expect to lose 5 pounds per week. The female client may expect to lose enough weight to be able eventually to wear a size 5 dress, even though this is not a realistic expectation for a client who has a large frame.

VALUE OF WEIGHT MAINTENANCE   All overweight clients should be educated to stop gaining weight. A valuable service is provided by health care workers when they counsel clients on weight maintenance. Clinical Application 17–2 may be of assistance when counseling the client on weight maintenance.

The Triangle: Diet, Behavior Modification, and Exercise

Sound weight-control programs include nutrition education, instruction on behavior modification,

---

CLINICAL APPLICATION 17–2

Prevention and Control of Excess Body Fat

Weight maintenance is the key to weight control. How can we as health care workers help out clients to achieve and maintain a healthy body weight?

We know it takes more kilocalories to support body protein content than body fat content. Health care workers should first encourage patients to exercise more to increase their body protein content. Many experts believe that our society's increasingly sedentary lifestyle may be responsible for the increasing prevalence of obesity.

Second, eating fat is fattening. Here are some reasons to avoid dietary fat:

1. The client gets more usable kilocalories from fat (Pawlak, 1989). Teaspoon for teaspoon, fat contains more kilocalories than either carbohydrate or protein.
2. When eaten in excess, fat kilocalories are rapidly and effortlessly stored in fat cells (Pawlak, 1989). There is very little energy cost to convert fat in food to body fat. Carbohydrates in food must be converted to fat before carbohydrate can be stored in fat cells. This conversion requires an expenditure of kilocalories. Kilocalories used to convert carbohydrate in food to body fat are not stored as body fat.
3. The fat cell strongly resists release of its stored fat (Pawlak, 1989). Once a fat cell has been manufactured, there is no evidence that it can ever be broken down; it exists until death. When dieting, a person can reduce the amount of fat in each fat cell but not break down the cell completely. Some researchers believe that an empty fat cell sends a message to the reduced-obese person's brain to eat. The reduced-obese/overweight person must learn to cope with a message constantly coming from the brain to eat. This is another reason why it is very difficult for a client to keep weight off permanently. Prevention of weight gain is the easiest way to maintain a reasonable body weight.

Third, a low-fiber intake may predispose a client to obesity. Fiber has a high satiety value. Obesity is uncommon among the populations of countries where a high proportion of dietary kilocalories is consumed as starchy vegetables. Educating clients to eat the recommended six servings of starch and five to nine servings of fruits and vegetables may help clients achieve satiety. Many starches, fruits, and vegetables contain appreciable amounts of fiber.

Adherence to a low-fat and low-fiber diet will not always result in a permanent weight loss. An individual can still gain weight on a low-fat diet if he or she overeats foods high in carbohydrates. Portion control is important. For some people, the most valuable information on the food label is the serving size.

To summarize, the health care worker can educate clients to (1) exercise more, (2) eat less fat, (3) eat more fiber, and (4) use portion control.

and an exercise program. The best programs offer a lifelong support component. Recognition by the nutrition counselor and the client that it is far easier for the client to lose excess body fat than to keep the lost fat off is important for a good long-term client outcome.

Dietary Treatment

Weight-reduction diets can be divided into two types: the so-called very low-calorie diets and the low-kilocalorie diets. Clinical Application 17–3 lists three guidelines that clients and nurses can use to evaluate a low-kilocalorie, weight-reduction diet.

VERY LOW-CALORIE DIETS **Very low-calorie diets** (VLCD) contain approximately 400 to 800 kilocalories per day. A VLCD diet may include only very lean meat and vitamin and mineral supplements. A beverage form of the diet is also widely used. Weight loss on these diets is dramatic. The typical man loses about 6.6 pounds per week. The typical woman loses about 4.4 pounds per week.

This is not exclusively fat loss. Significant amounts of water and lean body mass are also lost. This is the key reason why mild and moderately obese clients should avoid VLCD. Grossly obese individuals not only have increased body fat but also increased lean body tissue compared with smaller individuals. Thus they can afford to lose more lean body mass than their less obese counterparts. **Cardiac arrhythmia,** or irregular heart action (heartbeat), has occurred suddenly and without warning in mildly and moderately obese individuals who have followed drastic weight-reduction regimens. Therefore, these diets should be undertaken under the direct supervision and instruction of the client's physician.

An important feature of VLCDs is that in addition to the diet, clients should receive a program of physical exercise and behavior modification in order to develop long-lasting lifestyle changes that could ensure maintenance of the weight loss achieved.

Low-Kilocalorie Diets

The most common tool used for teaching clients how to eat in order to lose weight is the American Diabetic and Dietetic Association's Exchange Lists. The ADA Exchange lists are located in Appendix A.

Nutritional counselors should encourage clients to make major behavioral changes in their eating habits slowly. The goal in weight-reduction counseling is to help the client make permanent lifestyle changes. The current recommendation is that clients should be encouraged to change only one to two negative food behaviors at a time. For example, if the nutrition counselor recommends that the client substitute skim milk for whole milk, it is not wise to simultaneously discourage the use of sweets. The goal is to encourage *permanent* changes in eating behavior, so the client needs time to make the necessary adjustments. With this in mind, perhaps it is best to review one exchange list at a time with some clients. Priority should be given to eliminating foods in the fat, milk, and meat lists that are high in fat and in which the client overindulges. The average woman will lose weight on a 1200-kilocalorie diet. Larger women and most men will lose weight on a 1500-kilocalorie diet.

Exercise

Exercise plays a critical role in the loss and maintenance of body weight. Exercise is important for increased energy expenditure, maintenance of lean body mass, and as part of a total change in lifestyle. For the greatest benefit, the exercise chosen should involve movement that increases the heart rate and is acceptable to the client. Walking, running, swimming, and bicycling are all good forms of exercise. The recommended exercise should be done on most or, preferably, all days of the week for a total of 30 minutes or more of moderate intense physical activity. This physical activity can include 2 miles of walking briskly, cycling, swimming, pulling a golf cart, leisurely canoeing, general household cleaning, mowing the lawn, or painting the house. Clients should be cautioned to gradually increase the intensity and the duration of the activity. Overdoing physical activity at the onset is one of the major reasons why people stop exercising.

CLINICAL APPLICATION 17–3

Guidelines for a Healthy Weight-Reduction Diet for the Overly Fat Client

Any healthy weight-reduction diet should meet the following guidelines:

1. It should contain at least 1200 kcal.
2. It should not exclude any of the five major food groups.
3. The rate of weight loss should be between 1 and 2 lb per week.

To identify those individuals at a major heart disease risk, all clients should be screened by a physician before exercise recommendations are made. Clients with known heart, lung, or metabolic disease should have a physician-supervised stress test before beginning an exercise program.

When following an exercise program, fluid intake should be adequate. Individuals should drink water before, during, and after exercise. Close attention to

TABLE 17–3 Weight Control: Behavior Modification Techniques

Self-Monitoring
- Keep a food diary and record all food intake.
- Keep a weekly graph of weight change.
- Keep an exercise diary.

Stimulus Control
- At home, limit all food intake to one specific place.
- Plan food intake for each day.
- Rearrange your schedule to avoid inappropriate eating.
- Sit down at a table while eating.
- At a party, sit a distance from snack foods, eat before you go, and substitute lower kilocalorie drinks for alcohol.
- Decide beforehand what you will order at a restaurant.
- Save or reschedule everyday activities for times when you are hungry.
- Avoid boredom; keep a list of activities on the refrigerator.

Slowed-Down Eating
- Drink a glass of water before each meal. Drink sips of water between bites of food.
- Swallow food before putting more food on the utensil.
- Try to be the last one to finish eating.
- Pause for a minute during your meal and attempt to increase the number of pauses.

Reward Yourself
- Chart your progress.
- Make an agreement with yourself or a significant other for a meaningful reward.
- Do not reward yourself with food.

Cognitive Strategies
- View exercise as a means of controlling hunger.
- Practice relaxation techniques.
- Imagine yourself ordering a side salad, diet dressing, low-fat milk, and a small hamburger at a fast-food restaurant.
- Visualize yourself enjoying a fresh apple in preference to apple pie.

thirst should be given to prevent dehydration. The thirst mechanism may not be adequate to prevent dehydration in many elderly persons and in individuals involved in heavy exercise during hot weather (Petersmarck, 1989). Such persons need to be taught to drink water even if they are not thirsty.

Behavior Modification

Permanent weight loss can only result from a permanent change in eating and exercise behaviors. The behavioral strategies most commonly applied in weight-reduction programs include self-monitoring, stimulus control, slowed-down eating, a reward system, and cognitive behavior modification. Table 17–3 lists specific techniques used to help clients modify their behaviors.

SELF-MONITORING   Clients keep their own food records, track their body weights, and record exercise completed during self-monitoring. Many clients come to regard self-monitoring of their food intake as the single most helpful strategy in a weight-reduction program (Foreyt, 1990, unpublished lecture). Recording of food intake seems to work best when clients know they must turn in the records to their nutritional counselor.

Requiring clients to monitor their weight is also a helpful behavioral strategy. When clients are gaining weight they tend to avoid scales and mirrors. Requiring clients to weigh themselves helps to keep them on their eating plan. Clients should also be asked to record what exercise is completed in a notebook. Again, the notebook should be reviewed regularly in the training program (Foreyt, 1990, unpublished lecture).

STIMULUS CONTROL   **Stimulus-control** strategies are designed to help clients rearrange their lifestyle to reduce the chances of inappropriate eating habits (Foreyt, 1990, unpublished lecture). Clients are taught to examine their behaviors to determine which ones may trigger them to eat inappropriately. For example, a truck driver may eat two doughnuts every morning for breakfast because he or she drives past the bakery on the way to work. The nutritional counselor may recommend that this client take a different route to work to reduce the probability of his or her buying doughnuts.

Very low-calorie diet (VLCD)—Diet that contains less than 800 kilocalories per day.

SLOWED-DOWN EATING   Some obese people eat very rapidly. It takes approximately 20 minutes from the time food has been eaten for the brain to receive the message that food has been consumed. An individual can consume many extra kilocalories in 20 minutes. Obese clients are frequently taught a number of behavioral techniques to slow down their eating.

REWARD SYSTEM   Many clients respond better to any type of suggested behavioral change when they are working for specific rewards. In one program, for example, whenever a client performs a desirable behavior he or she earns tokens. The tokens are redeemable at the hospital's gift shop for merchandise.

COGNITIVE STRATEGIES   Many weight-reduction programs include cognitive strategies. The goal of cognitive strategies is to increase the client's knowledge of his or her eating behaviors so that he or she can develop skills to cope with negative behaviors. Teaching the client to relax is one type of cognitive strategy. The use of imagery is another form of cognitive strategy, for example, asking clients to imagine themselves coping successfully with anxiety-arousing events.

Social Support Systems

Obesity is a chronic ailment. Since there are no known cures that significantly reduce obesity for most clients, a program should always include long-term continuing evaluation.

Psychotherapy

Obesity can be associated with a range of psychological problems. Some individuals have unresolved psychological problems that present insurmountable barriers to success in weight loss. In such cases, where the full benefit of the nutrition and exercise components of weight loss cannot be realized, mental health treatment should occur before or concurrently with weight-loss treatment (Petersmarck, 1989).

All clients enrolled in a weight-loss program should be helped to understand biologic and genetic factors that contribute to obesity. Such an understanding not only minimizes guilt and depression but also allows him or her to learn to accept responsibility for variables over which control can be achieved (such as food types, meal size, activity level). Nurses should try to help clients appreciate the limitations of weight loss.

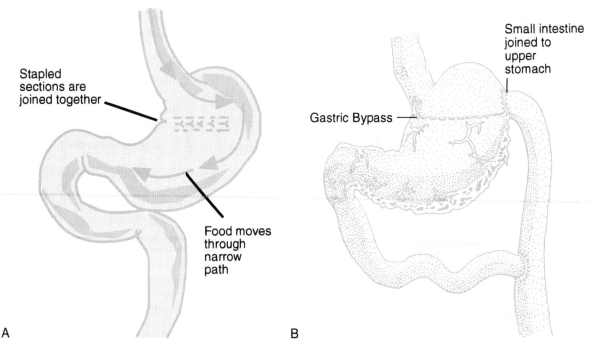

FIGURE 17–3   Illustrations of two common surgical procedures used to treat obesity: (*A*) gastric stapling and (*B*) gastric bypass.

Dieting can lead to depression in susceptible persons. In fact, kilocalorie restriction has been known to bring on suicidal behavior (Petersmark, 1989). The stress of kilocaloric restriction can also interfere with treatment of a chronic psychological disorder. Conversely, a number of psychological conditions can affect eating. For all of these reasons, a mental health professional should be part of any weight-reduction program.

Comparison of Weight-Loss Programs

Clearly, no one type of program is appropriate for all overweight or obese individuals. The expected rate of weight loss, unpleasant side effects, and program costs should all be considered objectively by nurses before referring any client to a program.

Other Treatment Approaches

Many drastic methods to lose weight have been and continue to be tried. Various types of surgical procedures, jaw wiring, acupuncture, and medications have all been used to promote weight loss.

SURGERY Many different surgical procedures have been and are being used to treat obesity. The removal of fat tissue through a vacuum hose is called **lipectomy.** This procedure is done more for cosmetic reasons than for weight control. A **jejunoileal bypass** involves the removal of a part of the small intestine. Clients lose weight after this procedure because they cannot absorb all the food they eat. This places these clients at a nutritional risk. All gastric (stomach) procedures either route food around (bypass) or through only part of the stomach (reduction). Diagrams of **gastric stapling** and **gastric bypass,** two common procedures, are shown in Figure 17–3. When the stomach is smaller or reduced, only a limited amount of food can be consumed at one feeding. This induces weight loss from reduced kilocalorie intake (Sims, May, 1985). Clinical Application 17–4 discusses problems clients often encounter after gastric surgery for weight reduction. Clinical Application 17–5 suggests general guidelines for these clients to follow.

The results that can be expected from gastric surgery procedures should always be spelled out to clients. No permanent effects can be promised, and having the surgery does not mean that afterward the client can overeat indefinitely without weight gain. Ninety percent of weight loss occurs in the first year,

---

CLINICAL APPLICATION 17–4

Complications of Gastroplasty and Gastric Bypass

There are many potential acute complications of gastric surgery for weight reduction. These include:

1. *Nausea, vomiting, bloating, and/or heartburn:* These signs and symptoms can be caused by overeating, not chewing food well, eating too quickly, drinking cold or carbonated beverages, using drinking straws, or eating gassy foods.
2. *Staple disruption (for gastric stapling procedures):* The result of loosened staples is that a larger intake of food is necessary before satiety can be achieved. Excessive food intake or vomiting can cause the staples to become disrupted.
3. *Obstruction:* An obstruction is the blockage of a structure. In this case, a blockage can occur close to the area stapled. A frequent cause of obstruction is poorly chewed food. The result is stomach pain, nausea, and vomiting.
4. *Dumping syndrome:* Intake of concentrated sweets and large quantities of fluids cause quick dumping of food into the small intestine. Abdominal fullness, nausea, diarrhea 15 minutes after eating, warmth, weakness, fainting, racing pulse, and cold sweats are symptoms of this syndrome.
5. Among the long-term risks is osteoporosis, due to decreased calcium absorption

---

and clients often begin to gain again in the second and third years. Only a minority achieve a weight as low as 125 percent of HBW. The procedure should be viewed as a tool to be used in conjunction with behavioral training—the small pouch helps clients learn to reduce the amount consumed and slows down intake. After the first year, due to stretching of the pouch or intestinal adaptation, much of the effect of the surgery can be overridden.

Gastric stapling—A surgical procedure on the stomach to induce weight loss by reducing the size of the stomach; also known as gastroplasty.

Gastric bypass—A surgical procedure that routes food around the stomach.

CLINICAL APPLICATION 17–5

Guidelines for the Client Following Gastric Surgery for Weight Reduction

The client who has had gastric surgery for weight reduction may find the following general guidelines helpful:

1. Eat three to six small meals per day.
2. Eat slowly.
3. Chew food thoroughly.
4. Eat very small quantities.
5. Stop eating when full.
6. Drink most fluids between meals.
7. Select a balanced diet.
8. Take a multivitamin-multimineral supplement.
9. Exercise regularly.

Jaw wiring, acupuncture, and medications have also been used to promote weight loss. Jaw wiring prohibits the consumption of food. This procedure had a poor long-term outcome because once the wires are removed, clients return to their former eating behaviors and the lost weight is regained.

MEDICATIONS AS SURGERY   Because most obese people cannot achieve prolonged weight loss with dietary restriction alone, the treatment of obesity with anorexigenic medications is now being considered by many physicians. The Food and Drug Administration has recently approved the use of dexfenfluramine and fenfluramine-phentermine for appetite control. These medications work by altering the metabolism of **serotonin,** a brain chemical. Serotonin helps send messages from brain cell to brain cell and is involved in neural mechanisms important in sleep and sensory perception. Emotions such as stress, fatigue, anxiety, irritability, and depression have all been linked to serotonin brain levels. The FDA said these medications could be used safely by individuals with a body mass index greater than 30 or by the slightly less obese patient with significant weight-related health problems such as elevated blood pressure, elevated cholesterol, or diabetes. Anorexigenic medications by themselves are not effective for long-term weight loss. Unfortunately, after the first 6 months of drug treatment, weight gain occurs in many patients despite continuation of drug therapy (Russell, 1995). Exercise and the consumption of a balanced and healthful diet are still the cornerstones of any weight reduction program.

The Client with Reduced Body Mass

The client with a reduced body mass is as difficult, if not more difficult, to treat than the overly fat client. Body fat has some important roles in insulation and protection of body organs. A client with a low body fat content usually has a loss of lean body mass as well, and loss of this functioning tissue gives clinicians concern. Women cease to ovulate and menstruate when the percent of body fat falls below a certain level.

Classification

Methods similar to those used to diagnose the overly fat client can be used to diagnose the client with reduced body mass. A person whose weight is more than 15 percent below HBW may be classified as underweight. A man with a body fat content of less than 15 percent and a woman with a body fat content of less than 18 percent may be classified as having a reduced body mass. A BMI less than 20 may indicate that the client has a reduced body mass.

Consequences

Long-term follow-up of studies indicates that extreme leanness is associated with increased mortality and decreased life expectancy. However, the causes of mortality are different from those associated with excess weight (National Research Council, 1989). The excessively lean person is almost twice as likely to succumb to respiratory diseases such as tuberculosis. In addition, these clients have a greater difficulty maintaining body temperature during cold weather. Infections and disturbances of the gastrointestinal tract are more likely in the underweight person as is fragile bone structure and osteoporotic changes.

Causes

A person may be underweight by virtue of genetics or because of a long-term or recent weight loss. As part of the nutrition screening process, a health care worker should ask the client about any change in body weight. A good question is, "Have you experienced any unintentional weight loss?" If the client responds yes, it is important to determine the time frame of the weight loss. However, a response such as "I have always been lean" indicates a lifetime pattern and may indicate that the client's leanness is genetic.

Rapid Loss Increases Risk

The greater the rate of weight loss, the more the client is at a nutritional risk. **Rate** means loss per unit of time. For example, a 20-pound weight loss in 2 weeks is a large rate of loss. Such a client has lost a large amount of lean body mass. However, a 20-pound weight loss during a 20-week period could be attributed mostly to a loss of body fat with a minimal loss of lean body mass. If the client began with surplus body fat stores, a loss of 20 pounds may not place this client at a high nutritional risk. If the client had a reduced body mass, even a slow weight loss may place him or her at a nutritional risk.

Not all changes in body weight are caused by insufficient kilocalorie intake. For example, a client may lose several pounds of body weight over the course of 1 day as a result of diuretic therapy. The weight loss in this situation would be due to water loss, not body fat or protein loss.

One method to determine whether a client is eating enough food is to monitor his or her food intake. Kilocalorie intake is monitored by visually recording actual food consumption and calculating the kilocalories eaten.

Eating Disorders

Eating disorders may be caused by psychological factors, resulting in nutritional problems. Many experts are concerned about the prevalence of anorexia nervosa and bulimia.

Anorexia Nervosa

Anorexia nervosa is a medical condition resulting from self-imposed starvation. Symptoms include:

1. Loss of 20 to 40 percent of usual body weight (UBW); refer to Clinical Calculation 17–2 to calculate UBW
2. Decreased resting energy expenditure (REE)
3. **Amenorrhea,** or the cessation of menstruation
4. Constipation
5. Hair loss
6. Abnormal sleeping patterns
7. Preoccupation with food
8. Body image disturbance
9. Denial of problem
10. Intake of only 500 to 800 kilocalories per day
11. Slow eating
12. Increased physical activity
13. Social isolation
14. Intense fear of becoming obese

CLINICAL CALCULATION 17–2

Percent Usual Body Weight

The health care worker can calculate the client's percent usual body weight (UBW). The formula is:

$$\frac{\text{Present weight}}{\text{Usual weight}} \times 100$$

A 5 percent weight loss in 1 month may not be significant. However, a 5 percent weight loss over a week may be significant. The kcal deficit may be related to a recent change in medication, an underlying but as yet undiagnosed condition, a recent change in living situation, or not taking the time to eat.

This disorder may be life-threatening. Although found primarily in adolescent girls and young women, approximately 4 to 6 percent of the cases occur in men (National Research Council, 1989). The client may resort to a variety of devices to lose weight, including starvation, vomiting, and laxative use.

Bulimia

Bulimia is much more common than anorexia nervosa, especially during adolescence and young adulthood (Halmi, et al, 1981). The prevalence of bulimia has been found to be as high as 13 percent in a college population. Bulimics binge and purge. **Binging** involves the consumption of as much as 5000 to 20,000 kilocalories per day. **Purging** is the intentional clearing of food out of the system by vomiting and/or using enemas, laxatives, and diuretics.

Anorexia nervosa—A mental disorder characterized by a 25 percent or greater loss of usual body weight, an intense fear of becoming obese, and self-starvation.

Amenorrhea—Cessation of menstruation.

Bulimia—Excessive food intake followed by extreme methods, such as self-induced vomiting and the use of laxatives, to rid the body of the foods eaten.

Treatment

There are many approaches to treatment of eating disorders, including behavioral therapy, family therapy, and group therapy. It is important to help the client discover the reason he or she chooses to eat, not eat, binge, or purge. Some of these clients are admitted to the hospital for treatment. Careful recording of kilocalories consumed is indicated. Sometimes nurses are asked to sit with these clients and watch them eat. These clients may attempt to hide food in their clothes, mouth, bedding, or anywhere else. It is sometimes necessary for the nurse to accompany these clients to the bathroom. Clients with eating disorders have been known to flush their food down the toilet. For these reasons, daily weights are often ordered by physicians for such clients.

Summary

Energy imbalance results from a malfunction of homeostatic mechanisms. The reason an individual eats more or fewer kilocalories than needed to maintain a stable body weight is not known. The overweight or obese individual has eaten more kilocalo-ries than he or she has used. The individual with a reduced body mass has eaten fewer kilocalories than he or she has used. One quarter of the US population is overly fat. The prevalence of individuals with excess body fat is increasing. Many experts attribute this to our increasingly sedentary society. At the same time, the prevalence of eating disorders such as anorexia nervosa and bulimia is also high. Many Americans are more concerned with their appearance than with their health. The nurse needs to help the client focus on the health benefits of weight control.

Americans are willing to spend substantial amounts of money in the hopes of improving their appearance. Over the long term, however, the pursuit of the perfect body frequently has a negative impact on one's health. Repeatedly following crash diets can have serious psychological and medical consequences.

Permanent weight loss can occur only when the individual makes a commitment to change his or her total lifestyle. Exercise; a well-balanced, low-kilocalorie diet; and behavior modification are all necessary parts of a sound weight-reduction program. Surgical interventions, acupuncture, and medications are also used to promote weight loss.

Case Study 17–1

R, admitted to the hospital for an evaluation of her weight loss, is 18 years old, is 5 ft, 2 in tall, weighs 80 lb, and has a medium frame. She is 64 percent of her healthy body weight. R's mother stated "My daughter is melting away to nothing. R runs every morning before school. She takes a 4-hour nap after school and is awake most of the night. She rarely eats with the family and will not go out to eat with us, although she talks about food constantly. Her beautiful hair looks terrible. She has not had a period in 6 months. I can hear her vomiting in the bathroom during the night." The client's only complaint is constipation. She denies she has any other problems. According to the client's medical history, her weight 1 year ago was 115 lb (HBW = 98 percent) and her assessment revealed a small frame.

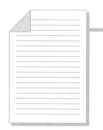

NURSING CARE PLAN FOR R

Assessment

Subjective Data Client stated during admission that "I need to lose weight." Per client's mother, client has been vomiting.

Objective Data Weight 1 year ago 115 lb and HBW 98 percent. Adm. weight 80 lb and HBW 64 percent. Cessation of menstruation.

Nursing Diagnosis Nutrition, altered: related to self-starvation as evidenced by client's admitted desire to lose weight and a HBW of 68 percent.

Desired Outcome/ Evaluation Criteria	Nursing Actions	Rationale
Client will state "I need to gain weight."	Educate client on the dangers of continued weight loss.	The client must be made to realize that continued weight loss is life-threatening.
Client will cease losing weight for 2 weeks.	Weigh client daily (in her underwear).	Body weight for this client would be a reliable indicator of energy balance, as the client is not edematous.
Client will gain 1 lb per week after weight loss has ceased until she attains her usual body weight.	Record food intake.	In tallying the client's daily kilocalorie count, the dietitian will need to include the kilocalories obtained from the food the nurse gives the client.
	Offer small quantities of food every 2 hours.	Anorexia nervosa clients frequently have diminished appetite, and small feedings are usually better tolerated.
	Reinforce the nutritional care plan prescribed by the physician and planned by the dietitian. This may require the support of Psychological Services.	Given the complexity of the problem, a team approach is indicated for clients with eating disorders.
	Refer client to Psychological Services.	Psychological services may be indicated because clients of this type are often resistant to increased food intake.

Study Aids

Chapter Review

1. To lose 2 pounds of body fat per week, an individual must eat _____ fewer kilocalories than used each day for 7 days.
   a. 1000
   b. 1500
   c. 2000
   d. 2500

2. A very rapid rate of weight loss (1 pound per day) in the mildly obese (Select the best response):
   a. Usually encourages permanent changes in behavior
   b. May lead to sudden death in some patients
   c. Will preserve lean body mass
   d. Fosters long-term weight maintenance

3. Which of the following statements is true?
   a. A client at 100 percent HBW is never overly fat.
   b. A normal BMI is 20 to 25.
   c. The obese female has a body fat content in excess of 22 percent.
   d. The healthiest range of body fat for males is 25 to 30 percent.

4. A client with reduced body mass _____.
   a. has an increased resting energy expenditure
   b. frequently complains of constipation
   c. is not likely to have a body image disturbance
   d. typically seeks the company of others

5. Any healthy weight-reduction diet should meet all of the following guidelines except one. Please select the *exception*.
   a. It should contain at least 1200 kilocalories.
   b. It should exclude all fats.
   c. It should include all of the major food groups.
   d. The rate of weight loss should be between 1 and 2 pounds per week.

Clinical Analysis

1. Mrs. R is a 40-year-old mother of three. She has arthritis in both knees. She weighs 165 pounds, has a medium frame, and is 5 feet, 3 inches tall. Her HBW is thus 128 percent. Her body fat content is 34 percent. Her physician has told her to lose weight, as this would help reduce her knee pain. According to Mrs. R she never thought she was overweight until she was 24 years old. At this time, her weight started increasing. When she weighed 140 pounds, she started to diet. One time she lost a total of 25 pounds, which she promptly regained plus an additional 5 pounds. The client described four additional weight cycles. Mrs. R claims she cannot exercise because "it is too painful on my knees." She has tried every conceivable type of diet, including a comprehensive medically supervised weight control program. Mrs. R states that for the past year, no matter how little she eats, she cannot lose weight even on a 1200-kilocalorie diet.

1. Mrs R:
   a. Apparently knows a great deal about low-kilocalorie foods, because she has successfully lost weight before
   b. Knows very little about foods, because she always regained the weight she lost
   c. Lacks motivation, because she has an inability to follow through with the appropriate behavior
   d. Should be discouraged from further attempts to control her weight

2. M had a slow weight gain for about 10 years. She asks for advice concerning how to best manage her weight. M leads a sedentary lifestyle, eats three well-balanced meals each day, and enjoys going out to dinner with her husband one night each week. M would most likely benefit from:
   a. Decreasing her meal frequency
   b. Increasing her physical activity
   c. Taking an anorexigenic medication
   d. Not going out to dinner with her husband each week

3. Mr. P wants to lose weight and weighs 115 percent of his healthy body weight. Initially, the nurse should advise Mr. P to:
   a. Follow a 1200 calorie diet
   b. Ask his doctor for a medication to assist in weight reduction
   c. Self-monitor and write down his food intake and physical activity
   d. Refer client to a surgeon for an evaluation

Bibliography

A losing formula: The liquid diet craze. Newsweek, April 30, 1990.

Allen, JD: A biomedical and feminist perspective on women's experiences with weight management. Western J Nurs Res 1615:524, 1994.

Bennett, W, and Gurin, J: The Dieter's Dilemma. Basic Books, New York, 1982.

Bjorntorp, P: Fat cells and obesity. In Brownell, KD and Foreyt, JP (eds): Handbook of Eating Disorders: Physiology, Psychology, and Treatment of Obesity, Anorexia, and Bulimia. Basic Books, New York, 1986.

Bray, GA: Brown tissue and metabolic obesity. Nutrition Today 17:23, 1982.

Bray, GA: Complications of obesity. Ann Int Med 103:1052, 1985.

Canning, H, and Mayer, J: Obesity: Its possible effect on college acceptance. N Engl J Med 275:1172, 1966.

Coscina, DV, and Dixon, LM: Body weight regulation in anorexia nervosa: Insights from an animal model. In Darby, PL, Garfield, PE, Garner, DM, et al (eds): Anorexia Nervosa: Recent Developments. Allan R. Liss, New York, 1983.

Crisp, AH: Treatment and outcome in anorexia nervosa. In Goodstein, RK (ed): Eating and Weight Disorders: Advances in Treatment and Research. Springer, New York 1983.

Donnelly, JE, et al: Preventing childhood obesity. Food and Nutrition News. National Live Stock and Meat Board. 67:1, 1995.

Environmental Nutrition: Winning at the Weight Loss Game: Choosing the Right Program. Environmental Nutrition Newsletter, December 1990.

Foreyt, JP: Unpublished lecture, Spring Michigan Dietetic Association Conference, Michigan State University, East Lansing, 1990.

Foster, G, et al: Resting energy expenditure, body composition, and excess weight in the obese. Metabolism 37:467, 1988.

Ginsburg-Feller, F: Growth of adipose tissue in infants, children, and adolescents: Variations in growth disorders. Int J Obes 5:1981.

Gortmaker SL, et al: Social and economic consequences of overweight in adolescence and young adulthood. N Engl J Med 329:1008, 1993.

Grubbs, L: The critical role of exercise in weight control. Nurse Practitioner 18:4, 1993

Guthrie, H: Introductory Nutrition, ed 6. CV Mosby, St Louis, 1986.

Halmi, KA, Falk, JR, and Schwartz, E: Binge-eating and vomiting: A survey of a college population. Psychol Med 11:697, 1981.

Harrison, JE: Metabolic bone disease. In Jeejeebhoy, KN (ed): Current Therapy in Nutrition. Decker, Toronto, Canada, 1988.

Keyes, A, Brozek, J, Mickelson, O, et al. The Biology of Human Starvation. 2 vols. University of Minnesota Press, Minneapolis, 1950.

Larkin, JC, and Pines, HA: No fat persons need apply: Experimental studies of the overweight stereotype and hiring preference. Sociology of Work and Occupations 6:312, 1979.

Lindpaintner, K: Finding an obesity gene—A tale of mice and men. N Engl J Med V 332:679, 1995.

Mayer, J: Overweight: Causes, Cost and Control. Prentice-Hall, Englewood Cliffs, NJ, 1968.

National Dairy Council: Weight Management: A Summary of Current Theory and Practice. National Dairy Council, Rosemont, Illinois, 1985.

National Institute of Health Consensus Development Panel: Health Implications of Obesity. Ann Intern Med, 103:1073, 1985.

National Research Council: Diet and Health Implications for Reducing Chronic Disease Risk. Report of the Committee and Diet and Health, Food and Nutrition Board, Commission on Life Sciences. National Academy Press, Washington, DC, 1989.

Pate, RR: Physical activity and public health: A recommendation from the Centers of Disease Control and Prevention and the American College of Sports Medicine. JAMA 273:402, 1995.

Pawlak, L: Life Without Diets. Communications Marketing Incorporated, Palm Springs, CA 1989.

Petersmark, KA: Toward Safe Weight Loss. Michigan Health Council, East Lansing, MI, 1989.

Polivy, J: Psychological consequences of food restriction. J Am Diete Assoc 96:589, 1996.

Pyle, RL, Mitchell, JE, and Eckert, ED: Bulimia: A report of 34 cases. J Clin Psychiatry 42:60, 1981.

Rock, CL, and Coulson, AC: Evaluation of weight loss programs. Nutrition and the MD 15:2, 1989.

Roe, DA, and Eickwork, KR: Relationships between obesity and associated health factors with unemployment among low income women. J Am Med Wom Assoc 31:193, 1976.

Rohner-Jeanrenaud, F, and Jeanrenaud, B: Obesity, leptin, and the brain. N Engl J Med 334:324, 1996.

Romsos, DR: Efficiency of energy retention in genetically obese animals and in dietary-induced thermogenesis. Fed Proc 40:2524, 1981.

Romsos, D: "Gene-Whiz" The Obesity/Gene Connection. (Unpublished lecture) 23rd Annual Nutrition Conference. Michigan State University, East Lansing, MI, March 6, 1996.

Russell, RM: Nutrition. JAMA 273:1699, 1995.

Scheingart, DE: Unpublished material, 1989.

Sims, EA: Why, oh why can't they lose weight? Nutrition and the MD 11:1, 1985.

Stern, JS, and Lowney, P: Obesity: The role of physical activity. In Brownell, KD and Foreyt, JP (eds): Handbook of Eating Disorders: Physiology, Psychology, and Treatment of Obesity, Anorexia, and Bulimia. Basic Books, New York, 1986.

Strand, G: Some Basic Facts About Losing Weight. Insights, March 1990.

Stunkard, AJ: A History of Binge Eating. In Fairburn, CG, Wilson, GT (eds): Binge Eating: Nature, Assessment and Treatment. Guilford Press, New York, 1993.

Stunkard, AJ, and Burt, V: Obesity and body image II. Age on onset of disturbances in the body image. Am J Psych 123:1443, 1967.

Stunkard, AJ, and Mendelson, M: Disturbances in body image of some obese persons. J Am Diet Assoc 38:328, 1961.

Van Itallie, TB: Fiber and obesity. Am J Clin Nutr 31:S252, 1978.

Van Itallie, T, and Yang, M: Cardiac dysfunction in obese dieters: A potential complication of rapid weight loss. Am J Clin Nutr 39:695, 1984.

Van Itallie, TB: Obesity. In Jeejeebhoy, KN (ed): Current Therapy in Nutrition. BC Decker, Toronto, Canada, 1988.

Wadden, T, and Stunkard, A: Social and psychological consequences of obesity. Ann Int Med 103:1062, 1985.

Weigley, ES: Average? Ideal? Desirable? A brief overview of height-weight tables in the United States. J Am Diet Assoc 4:84.

CHAPTER 18

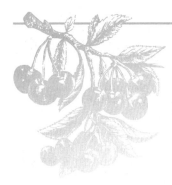

Diet in Diabetes Mellitus and Hypoglycemia

LEARNING OBJECTIVES

After completing this chapter, the student should be able to:

1   Define and classify diabetes mellitus and describe the treatment for each type.
2   Discuss the goals of nutritional care for persons with diabetes mellitus.
3   List nutritional guidelines for illness, exercise, delayed meals, alcohol, hypo-glycemic episodes, vitamin/mineral supplementation, and eating out for people with diabetes.
4   Describe dietary treatment for reactive hypoglycemia as compared to dia-betes mellitus.

This chapter discusses two diseases associated with insulin secretion and/or resistance to insulin accompanied by characteristic long-term complications. Diabetes mellitus is caused by the low secretion and/or use of insulin. Hypoglycemia is caused by excessive secretion of insulin. Diabetes mellitus has been diagnosed in approximately 6 million people in the United States, and an additional 4 to 5 million individuals are believed to have undiagnosed diabetes. Each year about 500,000 new cases are diagnosed (National Research Council, 1989). Nationally, diabetes is the seventh leading cause of death. Hypoglycemia is much rarer than diabetes mellitus. Nutrition is integral to the management of diabetes. This chapter provides an introduction to the importance of nutrition in diabetes and hypoglycemia.

Definition and Classification

Diabetes mellitus is a disorder characterized by the passage of sweet urine, excessive urine production, thirst, excessive hunger, and in some cases, weight loss. Records from the ancient Greeks described this condition as early as the first century AD. Diabetes mellitus can be defined as a group of disorders with a common characteristic of hyperglycemia. **Hyperglycemia** means an elevated level of glucose in the blood. Definitions and classifications for the various subclasses of diabetes mellitus have been standardized. The following sections define and classify the major types of diabetes.

Definition

Diabetes is diagnosed and defined by laboratory analysis. Multiple tests of a client's blood sugar level are necessary before the diagnosis can be established. Fasting glucose levels of at least 140 milligrams per deciliter on more than one occasion are required for diagnosis in nonpregnant adults. Refer to Clinical Application 18–1 for an explanation of other tests used for diabetes.

Classification

There are two major forms of diabetes: **insulin-dependent diabetes mellitus** (IDDM) and **noninsulin-dependent diabetes mellitus** (NIDDM). The World Health Organization (WHO) has further classified diabetes into three additional categories: secondary diabetes, impaired glucose tolerance (IGT), and gestational diabetes.

Insulin-Dependent Diabetes Mellitus

IDDM is also called type I diabetes. Patients with this disorder cannot survive without daily doses of insulin because their blood glucose levels vary significantly from the norm. These variations in blood glucose levels make these patients prone to two conditions. The first condition is **ketoacidosis.** The signs of ketoacidosis are hyperglycemia and excessive ketones. More is said about ketoacidosis later in this chapter. The second condition is **hypoglycemia** or a low blood glucose level. IDDM can occur at any age, although its usual onset is during childhood. Five to ten percent of the people with diabetes have IDDM. The onset of this disorder is usually abrupt, and the condition is difficult to control.

Noninsulin-Dependent Diabetes Mellitus (NIDDM)

NIDDM is also called type II diabetes. Persons with NIDDM are not insulin dependent or prone to ketoacidosis. However, some of them do use insulin because of persistent hyperglycemia. Clients with this condition can manufacture some insulin but do not make a sufficient amount or cannot use insulin efficiently. Typically, the noninsulin-dependent diabetic client develops his or her condition after age 45. Most of these clients are obese, and weight reduction usually improves their ability to process glucose. About 90 to 95 percent of all people with diabetes in the United States have NIDDM. The prevalence of NIDDM is markedly increased among Native Americans, African Americans, and Latinos. The cultural implications of these statistics were discussed in the chapter on individualized care. The

---

Hyperglycemia—An elevated level of glucose in the blood; fasting value above 110 or 120 milligrams per deciliter, depending on technique used.

Insulin-dependent diabetes mellitus (IDDM)—Type I diabetes; persons with this disorder must take insulin to survive.

Noninsulin-dependent diabetes mellitus (NIDDM)—Type II diabetes; although some persons with this disorder take insulin, it is not necessary for their survival.

Ketoacidosis—Acidosis due to an excess of ketone bodies.

Hypoglycemia—An abnormally low level of glucose in the blood.

Laboratory Tests for Diabetes

Several types of biochemical tests are discussed below: fasting blood sugar, glucose tolerance test, urine tests, and glycolated hemoglobin.

Fasting Blood Sugar

A measurement of a fasting blood sugar (FBS) is performed routinely on most diabetic clients. In preparation, the client should be instructed not to eat or drink for 12 hours before the test. Water is the exception, as it will not interfere with test results. If the client usually takes insulin or a hypoglycemic agent, the medication should not be taken or given until the blood test is done. Normal FBS should be 70 to 110 mg/dL. A finding of 140 mg/dL on two occasions is diagnostic of diabetes mellitus.

Glucose Tolerance Test

In the glucose tolerance test, a measured amount of glucose is given orally or intravenously after a fasting blood sugar sample has been drawn. Blood samples are then drawn at specified intervals. The client's ability to process glucose can be evaluated by this means. A blood glucose value above or equal to 200 mg/dL at 2 hours and at least one other sample at less than 2 hours are required for the diagnosis in nonpregnant adults. A normal 2-hour blood sample would have an upper level of 140 mg/dL. Values between 140 and 200 mg/dL are indicative of impaired glucose tolerance.

Clients may need to discontinue certain drugs for 3 days prior to the test. Also, a high-carbohydrate diet of 300 g of carbohydrate per day should be followed for the same period. The client should be given written instructions explaining the pretest dietary requirements. An inadequate diet prior to the glucose tolerance test may diminish carbohydrate tolerance and cause high glucose levels, creating a false-positive result. During the test, the client should not be permitted to have anything by mouth except water. Tobacco, coffee, and tea can alter the test results.

Urine Tests

For most people, when blood glucose reaches 180 to 200 mg/100 mL, the kidneys begin to spill glucose into the urine. This point of spillage is called the **renal threshold.** At one time, this test was assumed to reflect the glucose content of the blood, but the renal threshold varies from individual to individual. The renal threshold may also change in a given individual with decreasing kidney function. Although urine tests are used as screening tests, they are less reliable than the blood glucose tests available for home use.

Urine Acetone

As a consequence of the body's inability to metabolize glucose, fat is partially broken down for energy. The intermediate products of fat breakdown are ketone bodies. These ketone bodies build up in the blood because the quantity of fat being catabolized exceeds the body's capacity to process these intermediate products effectively. As this occurs, ketone bodies begin to spill into the urine. One of the ketone bodies is acetone, which can be measured in the urine. The presence of acetone in the urine is called **ketonuria.** Ketonuria is a sign that the diabetes is out of control. Clients are often taught to test for urinary ketones if their blood glucose level exceeds 240 mg/dL. When a client exhibits ketonuria, the physician should be consulted for changes in the diet prescription or insulin dosage.

Glycosylated Hemoglobin

Glucose attaches to the hemoglobin molecule in a one-way reaction throughout the 120-day life of the red blood cell. In a high-glucose environment, a greater percentage of the hemoglobin is glycosylated. This blood test is performed on a random blood sample; the client does not have to fast. The result is not influenced by exercise or diabetic drugs.

Because the **glycosylated hemoglobin** value reflects the average blood glucose level for the preceding 2 to 3 months, it is a good test of the effectiveness of long-term therapy. A client cannot follow the prescribed regimen for just a few days prior to a doctor's visit and claim otherwise. Glycosylated hemoglobin will be 4 to 8 percent of the total hemoglobin in adults without diabetes. In clients with diabetes, a value of 7 percent indicates good control of the disease, 10 percent fair control, and 13 to 20 percent poor control (Pagana, and Pagana, 1995).

TABLE 18–1 Insulin-Dependent and Noninsulin-Dependent Diabetes Mellitus

	IDDM	*NIDDM*
Cause	Beta cells damaged	Tissues resist insulin
Most common age at onset	Under 20 years	Over 45 years
Medication	1. Insulin injections OR 2. Insulin injections and oral agents	1. None OR 2. Oral agents OR 3. Some individuals may require insulin injections to attain optimal blood glucose levels.
Usual body build	Thin, underweight	Obese
Nutrition therapy	Integration of insulin therapy, activity, and food intake Consistent timing of food intake	Achievement of near normal glucose, lipid, and blood pressure goals. Weight loss is desirable and possible with some clients.

onset of this disorder is gradual. The condition is usually easier to control than IDDM. Table 18–1 summarizes the differences between IDDM and NIDDM.

Secondary Diabetes

Most diabetes results from a primary failure of insulin production and/or use, but diabetes can occur as a result of a variety of disorders including pancreatitis, surgical removal of the pancreas, Cushing's disease, pharmacologic doses of glucocorticoids (e.g., prednisone) or other hormones or drugs. The term **secondary diabetes** is used when one of these disorders is responsible for the hyperglycemia. The diabetes may be resolved if the cause is alleviated. If the cause is not correctable, secondary diabetes is treated similarly to other forms of diabetes.

Impaired Glucose Tolerance

Impaired glucose tolerance (IGT) is the term used for clients who do not meet the criteria for diabetes as defined by the WHO. These clients have fasting plasma glucose levels of less than 140 milligrams per deciliter or 2-hour tolerance plasma glucose values between 140 and 200 milligrams per deciliter, and intervening oral tolerance test plasma glucose values greater than 200 milligrams per **deciliter.** IGT may represent a step in the development of IDDM or NIDDM. In fact, 25 percent of the clients with IGT later develop diabetes mellitus.

Gestational Diabetes

Gestational diabetes (GDM) is the term for glucose intolerance in pregnancy. Women who are diag-

nosed as diabetic before pregnancy are not classified as having gestational diabetes. Clinical Application 18–2 discusses diabetes mellitus in pregnancy. Gestational diabetes is diagnosed slightly differently than other forms of diabetes. After an oral glucose load, diagnosis of gestational diabetes is made if two plasma values equal or exceed the following (Pastors, 1992).

Fasting: 105 milligrams per deciliter
1 hour: 190 milligrams per deciliter
2 hours: 165 milligrams per deciliter
3 hours: 145 milligrams per deciliter

Women who have had gestational diabetes are at an increased risk for developing NIDDM as they mature.

Normal Nutrient Metabolism

An understanding of diabetes mellitus is based on knowledge of the pancreas, the organ that produces

---

Secondary diabetes—A World Health Organization (WHO) classification for diabetes when the hyperglycemia occurs as a result of another disorder.

Impaired glucose tolerance (IGT)—A type of classification for hyperglycemia; for persons who have a glucose intolerance but do not meet the criteria for diabetes.

Deciliter—100 milliliters or 100 cubic centimeters.

Gestational diabetes (GDM)—Hyperglycemia related to the increased metabolic demands of pregnancy.

Diabetes in Pregnancy

Pregnancy raises blood insulin levels in all women. It is an adaptive mechanism. Early in pregnancy, the woman's body cells store energy. Later, the woman's tissues become insulin resistant so that the fetus can draw on energy stores when the woman is fasting.

When the pregnant woman has or develops hyperglycemia, the mother's blood glucose crosses the placenta but her insulin does not. Then the fetus produces more insulin, which increases his/her fat deposition. Women with diabetes have large babies for this reason.

Perinatal mortality of infants born to women with diabetes is higher than that of infants of women who do not have diabetes. Ketosis in early pregnancy can produce congenital malformations, central nervous system disorders, and low intelligence. With strict control of the diabetes, however, 97 percent of the fetuses survive, compared with 98 to 99 percent born to women without diabetes.

Insulin resistance is greater in the morning in pregnant women. For this reason, usually only 10 to 15 percent of the total kilocalories from carbohydrate are usually planned into the breakfast meal plan. There is a heightened tendency for maternal ketosis during fasting, and the possible adverse effects of ketones on the fetus suggest that periods of fasting during pregnancy should be avoided. A bedtime snack that contains at least 15 percent of the total kilocalories from carbohydrate is recommended to minimize an accelerated production of ketones, which has been known to occur during sleeping. Clients should also be reminded not to skip meals.

Pregnant Women with Diabetes Mellitus

Nutritional regulation is central to management of diabetes in pregnant women. During pregnancy the most commonly recommended kilocaloric distribution is: 40 to 45 percent carbohydrate, 20 to 25 percent protein, and 30 to 40 percent fat. This is not the same kilocaloric distribution commonly used in nonpregnant diabetic individuals.

The treatment goal is to prevent hypoglycemia, defined as fasting plasma concentrations of 70 to 90 mg/dL and 2-hour postprandial plasma glucose levels of less than 140 mg/dL. Some medical experts believe that this goal is too rigid because hypoglycemia during early pregnancy may be teratogenic. Hypoglycemic agents have been shown to cause significant risk to the fetus. In most instances, women are advised to discontinue use of hypoglycemic agents before conception. If medication is necessary to control hyperglycemia, insulin is safer for the fetus.

Preconception Care

Early pregnancy loss and congenital malformations can be minimized by optimal medical care and client education before conception in women with diabetes. Contraception, timing of conception, control of metabolic state, self-management techniques, assessment of diabetic complications, and other medical complications should be discussed with the female client of child-bearing age. The desired outcome of glycemic control in the preconception phase of care is to lower glycohemoglobin so as to achieve maximum fertility and optimal embryo and fetal development (American Diabetes Association, 1996). Preconception counseling is best accomplished by a multidisciplinary team approach including a diabetologist; internist or family practice physician; obstetrician; and diabetes educators, including nurses, registered dietitians, social workers, and other specialists as necessary. Self-management skills essential for control during pregnancy include (Position Paper of the American Dietetic Association, 1996a):

- Using an appropriate meal plan
- Timing of meals and snacks
- Planning physical activity
- Choosing time and site of insulin injections
- Using carbohydrate and glucagon for hypoglycemia
- Reducing stress, coping with denial
- Testing capillary blood glucose
- Self-adjusting insulin doses

insulin. It is also important to know the cellular sources of glucose, the normal blood glucose curve, and the functions of insulin and other hormones. All of these are discussed in the following sections of this chapter.

Anatomy of the Pancreas

The pancreas is a gland that lies behind the stomach. It has both exocrine and endocrine secretions. The exocrine functions of the pancreas include the flow of enzymes into the intestine via ducts. Endocrine secretions (hormones) flow directly into the bloodstream.

Clusters of cells in the pancreas called the **islets of Langerhans** produce three hormones. These islets contain three types of cells: alpha, beta, and delta. The alpha cells produce **glucagon,** the beta cells produce insulin, and the delta cells produce **somatostatin** (Fig. 18–1). Special sensors at junctions of the three types of cells monitor levels of blood glucose and stimulate the release of the appropriate hormone.

Functions of Insulin

Insulin is the only hormone that lowers blood glucose. A person normally secretes insulin in response to an elevated blood glucose level. Insulin decreases blood glucose by accelerating its movement from the blood into cells. As glucose enters the cells, it may be metabolized to yield energy, may be stored as glycogen, or may be converted to fat (Table 18–2).

TABLE 18–2   Metabolic Activities Promoted by Insulin

Activity	Name of Metabolic Pathway
Movement of glucose into cells	None
Energy production from glucose	Glycolysis
Manufacture of glycogen	Glycogenesis
Fat formation from carbohydrate and protein	Lipogenesis

Note: "Genesis" means building up.

The ultimate fate of glucose once inside the cell depends on body need and the amount of glucose that enters the cell. The cells' energy needs will be met first. If cells have available glucose over and above immediate energy needs, the excess glucose is stored as glycogen. Insulin stimulates the storage of glucose as glycogen. Once the glycogen stores are filled to capacity, any remaining glucose is converted to fat.

Insulin influences the metabolism of protein and fat. Insulin stimulates entry of amino acids into cells and enhances protein formation. It also enhances fat storage in adipose tissue and indirectly inhibits the breakdown of fat for energy. If the body has ample glucose available for energy, protein and fat need not be broken down to meet energy needs.

Insulin levels fluctuate in the blood. Normally, blood insulin levels increase as the blood glucose level increases. A high level of insulin in the blood signals the cells not to break down stores for energy (Table 18–3). An anabolic or building state exists when metabolism is normal and glucose and insulin levels are high. Insulin levels decrease as the blood sugar level decreases. A low level of insulin in the blood indirectly signals the body to begin to break down body stores for glucose. A catabolic or breaking-down state exists when metabolism is normal and glucose and insulin levels are low. Figure 18–2 illustrates glucose use by the cells.

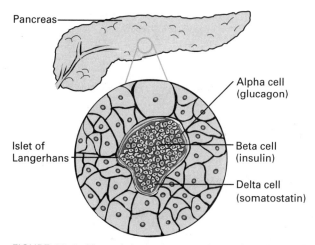

Pancreas

Islet of Langerhans

Alpha cell (glucagon)

Beta cell (insulin)

Delta cell (somatostatin)

FIGURE 18–1 View of the pancreas and an enlarged islet of Langerhans. Alpha cells secrete glucagon, beta cells secrete insulin, and delta cells secrete somatostatin.

Glucagon—A hormone secreted by the alpha cells of the islets of Langerhans; it increases the concentration of glucose in the blood.

Somatostatin—A hormone produced by the delta cells of the islets of Langerhans; it inhibits both the release of insulin and glucagon production.

TABLE 18–3 Metabolic Activities Inhibited by a High Level of Insulin

Activity	Name of Metabolic Pathway
Manufacture of glucose from noncarbohydrate sources, e.g., glycerol and amino acids	Gluconeogenesis
Release of glucose from glycogen	Glycogenolysis
Breakdown of fat from adipose tissue	Lipolysis

Note: "Lysis" means breaking down.

Other Hormones

Glucagon and somatostatin assist in coordinating the storage and mobilization of the energy nutrients. Glucagon increases blood glucose levels and stimulates the breakdown of body protein and fat stores. Somatostatin acts locally within the islets of Langerhans to depress the secretion of both insulin and glucagon. Evidence has shown these hormones may not be at optimal levels in some clients with diabetes.

Cellular Sources of Glucose

The cells obtain glucose from food eaten and internal glucose stores. All of the carbohydrate eaten, about 50 percent of the protein eaten, and about 10 percent of the fat eaten will enter the blood as glucose. The internal body stores that can be converted to glucose are glycogen, some protein, and the glyc-

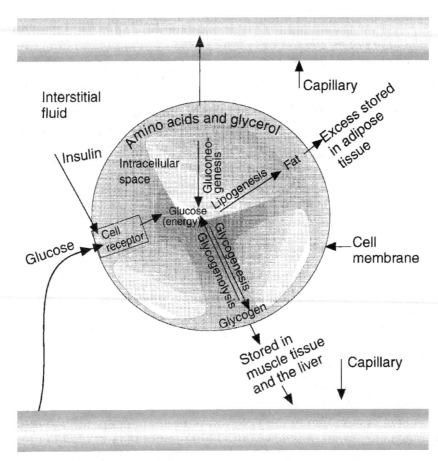

FIGURE 18–2   Insulin is necessary for glucose to gain entry into a cell. Once inside the cell, glucose can meet several fates. Glucose can be burned as energy, stored as glycogen, or stored as fat. In the event that the cell lacks sufficient glucose for energy needs, glycogen, or the glycerol portion of a fat molecule, or some amino acids can be broken down into glucose.

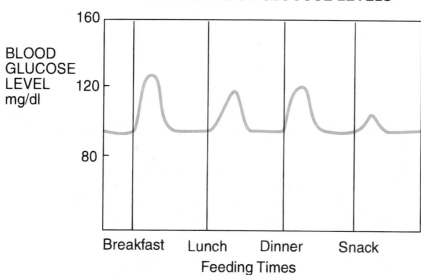

NORMAL BLOOD GLUCOSE LEVELS

FIGURE 18–3 A person's blood glucose level normally goes up after food consumption and then down between feedings.

erol portion of triglycerides. Body fat is stored as triglycerides in adipose tissue. To understand diabetes it is necessary to know how the body coordinates all internal and external sources of glucose to maintain a normal blood glucose range.

Blood Glucose Curve

Given the vital need for every cell to have an uninterrupted supply of energy, the human body has evolved to allow an uninterrupted energy supply to reach cells without continuous eating. A normal blood glucose range is usually about 70 to 110 milligrams per deciliter. (Some laboratories assign a normal blood glucose range of 80 to 120 milligrams per deciliter. The difference is due to the type of equipment the laboratory uses, not the glucose content of the blood.) The blood glucose level increases in the fed state and decreases in the fasting state. Figure 18–3 illustrates the normal blood glucose curve.

Causes of Diabetes

The causes of diabetes include genetic factors, lifestyle, and viral infections. Although these causes are explained separately for the sake of clarity, in reality they are often interconnected.

Genetic Factors

Some of the susceptibility to diabetes is genetic. Researchers have discovered that people with IDDM

have certain genes associated with their immune response. These particular genes are often found in children with IDDM. However, not everyone with these genes displays clinical diabetes. Before diabetes becomes apparent, this genetic susceptibility is often triggered by the individual's lifestyle or other environmental factors. These factors cause a series of events that result in damage to or destruction of the pancreatic beta cells. Inheritance is even more prominent in the development of NIDDM than in IDDM, as the next section describes.

Insulin Resistance

A person may be genetically susceptible to **insulin resistance.** Insulin resistance occurs when both the client's glucose and blood insulin levels are elevated. Insulin may not be released at the right times and/or be unable to assist the movement of glucose into the cells because of a lack of receptor sites. Before glucose can enter the cells, the insulin must first attach itself to specific receptor sites on the cells' outer surfaces. Persons with type II diabetes may lack enough receptor sites, have faulty receptor sites, or have postreceptor defects. Excess body fat seems to be related to a decrease in the number of receptor sites

Insulin resistance—A disorder characterized by elevated glucose and insulin levels; thought to be related to a lack of insulin receptors.

(Pastors, 1992). NIDDM is often associated with insulin resistance.

Lifestyle

A healthy lifestyle is particularly important for the prevention of diabetes in genetically susceptible clients. Excessive body fat, inactivity, and stress are risk factors for diabetes. Up to 90 percent of noninsulin-dependent diabetic clients are overly fat. A loss of body fat alone is sometimes sufficient to balance the insulin produced with a modified food intake. Inactivity is a risk factor that predisposes one to diabetes. Sometimes emotional or physical stress is the stimulus that causes the hyperglycemia. The body's stress response involves the release of epinephrine from the adrenal glands. One action of epinephrine is to raise the blood sugar level so the person has energy for "fight or flight."

Viral Infections

Links have been noted between viral epidemics and the onset of diabetes. During the late fall and winter months, a disproportionate number of cases of IDDM diabetes are diagnosed. Because these seasons are also associated with peak occurrence of childhood viral diseases, it is possible there is a causal connection between viral epidemics and the onset of IDDM.

Antibodies to islet cells have been found in some people with diabetes. This lends credence to the concept of IDDM as an autoimmune process, in which the body destroys its own beta cells. In **autoimmune diseases,** the body cannot recognize its own cells but rather treats them as foreign invaders. The event that provokes this process usually is a viral infection. Both islet cell antibodies (ICAs) and anti-insulin antibodies (AIAs) have been found to be elevated in clients with IDDM. These elevated antibodies may be detected in about 90 percent of clients prior to the diagnosis of diabetes.

Signs and Symptoms of Diabetes

The classic triad of signs and symptoms includes **polyuria,** increased urination; **polydipsia,** increased thirst; and **polyphagia,** increased appetite. The triad is most commonly seen in IDDM. The following section describes these and other signs and symptoms commonly seen in persons with diabetes.

Classic Triad

In diabetes, glucose cannot optimally move from the intravascular space across a cell membrane into the intracellular space. This is why the diabetic person's blood glucose level remains elevated after eating. Under normal circumstances, the blood glucose level does not increase excessively because excess glucose undergoes glycolysis and is readily converted to adipose tissue or stored as glycogen inside the cell. As the glucose-rich blood circulates through the kidneys, these organs reabsorb all of the glucose of which they are capable. After this point is reached, glucose enters the urine. **Glycosuria** means an abnormally high amount of glucose in the urine. As the glucose exits the body in the urine, water is pulled out also as a result of the osmotic effect of glucose. This results in polyuria, or a large urine output. The large loss of water causes excessive thirst, polydipsia, and prompts the person to drink fluids.

When glucose is not available for energy inside the cells, the body will begin to break down protein and fat for energy. In untreated IDDM, the body's cells are starving. These starving cells send a message to the brain to turn on the person's appetite. The person responds by eating to satisfy the craving for food. The third symptom or sign of diabetes is polyphagia, an abnormal increase in appetite. Polyphagia, polyuria, and polydipsia are the three classic signs or symptoms reported or seen in clients with diabetes.

Other Signs and Symptoms

The abnormal carbohydrate metabolism of diabetes and its effects on the body's tissues cause other problems. Weight loss is more commonly seen in clients with IDDM than in clients with NIDDM. Blurred vision is common in both types. Fatigue is frequently seen in these clients. High glucose levels impair white blood cell functioning, thus increasing the client's susceptibility to infection. Commonly involved agents are *Staphylococcus aureus* and *Candida albicans* involving the skin and mucous membranes. Recurrent boils, **vaginitis,** or bladder infections in a client may stimulate testing for diabetes. Poor wound healing is related to decreased circulation. Circulatory problems in men may be manifested as *impotence*.

Complications

The complications of diabetes mellitus are both acute and chronic. Acute complications require immediate care. Chronic complications include diseases of the eye, kidneys, heart, and nervous system. Chronic complications are responsible for the increased death rate among individuals with diabetes and the diminished quality of life that many of these clients experience.

Acute Clinical Situations

Three acute complications are seen in clients with diabetes: ketoacidosis, hyperglycemic hyperosmolar nonketotic syndrome, and hypoglycemia.

Ketoacidosis

Individuals with IDDM who experience a profound insulin deficiency may progress to the condition of ketoacidosis. The three main precipitating factors in ketoacidosis are: a decreased or missed dose of insulin, an illness or infection, or uncontrolled disease in a previously undiagnosed person. Ketoacidosis is a complex life-threatening condition demanding emergency treatment. The predominant clinical manifestations of dehydration, acidosis, and electrolyte imbalances and general principles of treatment will be discussed.

DEHYDRATION   Without insulin, glucose cannot be transferred across the cell membranes into the cells. A greatly increased number of glucose molecules (300 to 800 milligrams per deciliter) in the blood exert an osmotic effect, causing water to move from within the cells to the intravascular space, producing cellular dehydration. The body excretes the water and the glucose in the urine, along with electrolytes, producing polyuria.

ACIDOSIS   Unaware that the problem is not lack of glucose, but lack of insulin, the body proceeds to increase blood glucose by mobilizing protein and fat from the tissues to be converted to glucose by the liver. As the human body can use only the glycerol portion of the triglyceride molecule for glucose, the fatty acid portion is processed into ketones. Normally the ketones are metabolized and excreted as carbon dioxide and water. Under conditions of ketoacidosis, however, the body cannot metabolize this overload of ketones rapidly enough to maintain homeostasis, thus the client displays excessive ketones in the blood (ketonemia) and spills ketones in the urine (ketonuria). Acetone is one of the ketone bodies for which urine is tested. The ketone bodies are acid, thus the term, ketoacidosis.

Several homeostatic mechanisms can be initiated by the body as it attempts to correct the acidosis. It decreases the level of carbonic acid in the blood by increasing the excretion of carbon dioxide through involuntary deep, rapid breaths called **Kussmaul respirations.** The client's breath has a fruity odor from the ketonemia. The kidney increases the hydrogen ion content or acidity of the urine it excretes. Buffering of hydrogen can occur in the cells, also, where it displaces potassium to the extracellular fluid.

ELECTROLYTE IMBALANCES   Clients with severe ketoacidosis may excrete 6.5 liters of fluid and 400 to 500 milliequivalents of sodium, potassium, and chloride in 24 hours. A fluid loss of 15 percent of body weight is not unusual. Most critical in the treatment of electrolyte imbalances in diabetic ketoacidosis is the body's level of potassium. As the cells are being catabolized for fuel, the intracellular potassium is transferred to the intravascular space. Serum potassium levels can be low, normal, or elevated in the person with ketoacidosis, depending upon the body's current coping mechanism. Regardless of the serum concentrations of potassium and sodium, the pathological process of diabetic ketoacidosis depletes these electrolytes. Either hypokalemia or hyperkalemia can lead to cardiac arrhythmias and must be carefully managed in the client with ketoacidosis.

TREATMENT   Clients with severe diabetic ketoacidosis are critically ill. Serum electrolyte levels change dramatically once treatment commences. Intensive care is necessary to provide the careful monitoring and frequent adjustments in therapy required as the fluids and electrolytes are being replaced. Intravenous regular insulin will permit the use of carbohydrate for energy and will halt the body's excessive use of fat, which has produced the ketone bodies. Insulin drives glucose back into the cells. Potassium, too, moves from the intravascular space to the intracellular space, necessitating frequent measurement

---

Autoimmune disease—A disorder in which the body produces an immunological response against itself.

Polyuria—Excessive urination.

Polydipsia—Excessive thirst.

Polyphagia—Excessive hunger.

Glycosuria—abnormally high amount of glucose in the urine.

of the serum levels of both glucose and potassium. When the client recovers, identification of the precipitating factor for the ketoacidosis and education focused on preventing additional occurrences is essential.

Hyperglycemic Hyperosmolar Nonketotic Syndrome

The four signs of **hyperglycemic hyperosmolar nonketotic syndrome** (HHNS) are blood glucose level greater than 600 milligrams per deciliter, absence of or slight ketosis, plasma hyperosmolality, and profound dehydration. This life-threatening emergency is usually seen in the elderly or undiagnosed people with NIDDM. HHNS is like DKA except that the insulin deficiency is not as severe, so increased **lipolysis** does not occur. Because these clients do not have symptoms of vomiting, nausea, and acidosis brought on by severe ketosis as do clients with type I diabetes, they often do not seek prompt medical help. Their blood sugar levels are higher and their dehydration more severe than is seen in ketoacidosis.

In these clients, prolonged osmotic diuresis and dehydration secondary to hyperglycemia lead to decreased renal blood flow and allow the blood glucose to reach very high levels. Medications that cause an increase in blood glucose levels, chronic disease, and infection may contribute to this condition. Treatment includes correction of the electrolyte imbalance, hyperglycemia, and dehydration.

Hypoglycemia

In both IDDM and NIDDM (treated with medications) the person can develop hypoglycemia. Hypoglycemia may be caused by too much insulin (accidental or deliberate); too little food intake; a delayed meal; excessive exercise; alcohol (especially in the fasting state); and/or medications such as oral hypoglycemic agents. Symptoms may include confusion, headache, double vision, rapid heartbeat, sweating, hunger, seizure, and coma. The treatment of hypoglycemia is discussed later in the chapter.

Chronic Complications

Clients with both IDDM and NIDDM of sufficient duration are vulnerable to serious complications involving the eyes, kidneys, and nervous system. Diabetic **retinopathy** is a disorder that involves the retina. Diabetes is a leading cause of blindness and of visual loss in the adult US population. The blurred vision reported by these clients is related to retinopathy. These clients are also at a higher risk for cataracts.

Diabetic neuropathy is a chronic complication of diabetes mellitus. Clients may complain of a lack of sensation in their extremities. They may puncture, cut, or burn their feet and not feel any pain. A wound may become infected and heal poorly. Gangrene, or tissue death, may follow. The treatment for gangrene is amputation. Neuropathy can affect gastric or intestinal motility, erectile function, bladder function, cardiac function, and vascular tone (Nathan, 1993). **Gastroparesis** may occur and alter the absorption of meals, which makes glycemic control problematic. Heart disease is more common in these clients.

Diabetic **nephropathy,** or kidney disease, is another common complication in diabetic clients. Tragically, some clients with diabetes do not take the threat of chronic complications seriously until much damage has occurred.

Treatment

The current medical goal is to *normalize* the blood glucose throughout the day, which goes far beyond what has been clinical practice in the past. A normal blood glucose level is 60 to 120 milligrams per deciliter before a meal and less than 140 milligrams per deciliter 2 hours after a meal. Realistic target levels for individuals with diabetes treated intensively are 70 to 140 milligrams per deciliter before meals; less than 180 milligrams per deciliter 2 hours after meals; and glycosylated hemoglobin within 1 percent of normal. A landmark study known as the Diabetes Control and Complications Trial (DCCT) in individuals with IDDM demonstrated that intensive control of blood glucose levels delays the onset and slows the progression of diabetic retinopathy, nephropathy, and neuropathy (Diabetic Control and Complications Trial Research Group, 1993).

According to this study's results, people with type I diabetes who followed a tightly controlled regimen, compared with those who followed a standard regimen, showed reductions of about:

- 76 percent in progression of diabetic retinopathy
- 54 percent in albuminuria
- 36 percent in microalbuminuria
- 60 percent in rates of neuropathy

A tightly controlled regimen is not without problems, however. Among these are an increased inci-

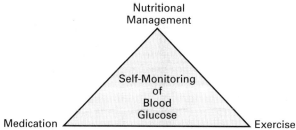

FIGURE 18–4 Nutritional management, medication, and exercise are the three cornerstones of treatment for diabetes. Each of these cornerstones has an influence on blood glucose levels. An individual can identify how each of these cornerstones impacts his or her blood glucose level by self-monitoring of blood glucose.

dence of insulin-induced hypoglycemic episodes. A recent study showed clients undergoing intensive diabetes treatment do not face deterioration in the quality of their lives, even while the rigor of their diabetes care is increased (The Diabetes Control and Complication Trial Research Group, 1996).

All health care workers should assist the general population in the early detection of diabetes and prevention of complications. As Figure 18–4 emphasizes, the three cornerstones of the management of diabetes after diagnosis are physical activity, medication, and nutritional management. Self-monitoring of blood glucose levels enables the client to assess how each of these factors interact. Blood glucose monitoring, physical activity, medication, and diet are discussed next.

Self-Monitoring of Blood Glucose

Many individuals monitor their own blood glucose levels with a device called a blood glucose meter. This procedure is called **self-monitoring of blood glucose** (SMBG). Individual response to medication, diet, and exercise can be determined with this advanced technology. SMBG can be performed using a single drop of blood. The client obtains the drop of blood from a finger with either a lancet or a spring-loaded device. The blood sample is placed in the meter, and the test results are available in 1 minute. The client can then adjust insulin dose and food and exercise behaviors accordingly. Many experts consider SMBG to be the most important development in diabetes management since the discovery of insulin.

SMBG has allowed clients to try to normalize their blood glucose levels throughout the day. Health care workers need to carefully teach clients how to interpret the results of SMBG. Continual reassessment of the client's technique and blood glucose

records are necessary to guide treatment decisions. To evaluate the need for changes in diet or medications, monitoring should be done at least twice a day. Four times a day for 3 days each week is preferable for clients who are stable. If near-normalization of blood glucose is the treatment goal, SMBG must be done four to eight times daily (before and 2 hours after each meal and/or snack). During acute illness, more frequent self-monitoring is indicated.

Physical Activity

Exercise plays a key role in the management of diabetes. All individuals with diabetes who exercise should be encouraged to follow these guidelines:

1. Use proper footwear, and other protective equipment if necessary.
2. Avoid exercise in extremely hot and cold environments.
3. Inspect feet daily and after exercise for open areas, blisters, punctures, swelling, and redness; report any of these signs to the physician immediately.
4. Avoid exercise during periods of poor metabolic control (blood glucose levels which are <60 or >240 milligram per deciliter levels).
5. Wear a diabetes ID badge or bracelet during exercise.

Exercise and Noninsulin-Dependent Diabetes Mellitus

Physical activity is widely endorsed for persons with type II diabetes. Physical activity increases the number and binding capacity of insulin receptors, assists in lowering blood glucose levels, and reduces insulin requirements in persons who use insulin. Improved blood lipid levels occur in some clients who engage in regular exercise. This helps delay or prevent the heart disease complications often seen in these clients. Exercise also assists in weight control and improves muscle strength and flexibility.

Lipolysis—Catabolism of adipose tissue.

Retinopathy—Any disorder of the retina; diabetes is a leading cause of both visual loss and blindness in the adult population in the United States.

Neuropathy—Any disease of the nerves.

Gastroparesis—Partial paralysis of the stomach.

Nephropathy—A kidney disease characterized by inflammation and degenerative lesions.

Aerobic exercise should be encouraged at 50 to 70 percent maximum heart rate and at least 40 minutes duration to promote breakdown of body fat. Daily exercise is recommended, but three times a week is considered the minimum required to aid blood glucose management.

Exercise and Insulin-Dependent Diabetes Mellitus

The American Diabetes Association strongly endorses an exercise program for people with IDDM because of the potential to improve cardiovascular fitness and psychological well-being. Exercise involves some risk for individuals with IDDM because it changes insulin requirements in sometimes unpredictable ways more than 24 hours after the exercise. Retinopathy, neuropathy, and renal disease may worsen in some clients with IDDM who exercise. Blood pressure may also become elevated. For this type of client, self-monitoring of blood glucose should be incorporated into a modified exercise program tailored to individual client needs and limitations. The client should demonstrate the ability to self-treat a hypoglycemic episode.

Exercise, SMBG, and Food Intake

Type I clients with diabetes who do exercise and all type II clients who engage in nonroutine exercise should monitor their blood glucose levels before, during, and after exercise. If the blood glucose level is greater than 100 milligrams per deciliter before exercise, there is usually no need for additional food if the planned exercise is of short duration and low intensity. Exercise of long duration and high intensity will generally require more kilocalories. Snack food containing an additional 15 to 30 grams of carbohydrate-containing food should be ingested for every 30 to 60 minutes of exercise (Franz, 1987). Good choices for snack foods include fruit, starch, and milk exchanges. Exercise is best done 60 to 90 minutes after meals when the blood glucose level is highest.

Medications

Two types of medications are used with diabetic clients: insulin and oral hypoglycemic agents. Clients with IDDM (type I) require insulin. Clients with NIDDM (type II) may not require any medication or may need to have an oral hypoglycemic agent or insulin prescribed. Frequently, clients with type II diabetes are able to discontinue the medication after a loss of body fat.

Insulin

The four sources of insulin are beef, pork, biosynthetic human, and semisynthetic human. Human insulin is made by converting pork insulin to the human amino-acid sequence (semisynthetic) or manufactured by recombinant-DNA technology (biosynthetic). Human insulin (Humulin) produces fewer allergic reactions. Human insulin is also the drug of choice by vegetarians. Insulin cannot be taken orally because the gastrointestinal tract enzymes would digest it before absorption. Insulin must be administered by needle either **subcutaneously** (beneath the skin) or intravenously (IV). Only regular insulin is given IV. The substances used to delay absorption of intermediate- and long-acting insulins are not designed for IV administration. Regular insulin is usually administered IV only for the severely hyperglycemic client.

Insulin can also be administered with an insulin pump. These pumps are designed to provide a small inflow of insulin continuously and large inflows before eating, thus mimicking normal insulin secretion.

Medications are described according to the onset, peak, and duration of action. Insulin is categorized as rapid-acting, intermediate-acting, or long-acting. Table 18–4 lists the times of onset, peak, and duration of insulin. Variation in duration makes it possible to inject insulin in a pattern that is as close as possible to normal insulin activity. Ideally, the medication is planned around the diet, not vice-versa. Most experts know that it is far easier to change a medication than a food behavior.

Oral Hypoglycemic Agents

Oral hypoglycemic agents lower blood glucose levels in noninsulin-dependent diabetics. These drugs stimulate insulin release from the pancreatic beta cells and reduce glucose output from the liver. Recently, oral agents and insulin administered simultaneously have been used successfully to treat type I diabetes. Commonly prescribed oral hypoglycemic agents include glipizide, glyburide, and tolazamide.

Medical Nutritional Management

Diabetes is directly related to how the body uses food. Nutrition is thus an essential component of management for all persons with diabetes. Clients report improved health, better control of body weight, improved control of blood glucose and lipid levels, and improved use of insulin when they adhere to dietary recommendations. The goals of nutritional care for the person with diabetes are the control and prevention of complications. This in-

TABLE 18–4 Times of Onset, Peak, and Duration of Action for Rapid-Acting, Intermediate-Acting, and Long-Acting Insulin*

Insulin	Time in Hours		
	Onset	Peak	Duration
Rapid-acting			
Regular intravenously	0.17–0.5	0.25–0.5	0.5–1
Regular subcutaneously	0.5–1	2–4	5–7
Intermediate-acting			
Lente subcutaneously	1–3	8–12	18–28
NPH subcutaneously	1–4	6–12	18–28
Long-acting			
Ultralente subcutaneously	4–6	18–24	36

* References differ. Deglin, and Vallerand, 1995.

volves the promotion of normal nutrition and dietary manipulation to control blood glucose and lipid levels. Each client's nutritional goals need to be determined individually. There is no "diabetic diet" or "ADA diet," however, several meal planning approaches are widely endorsed by the American Diabetes and the American Dietetic Associations. The next sections of the chapter describe: the overall goals of nutritional care, the need to individualize nutritional care to meet each client's goals, assessment of client readiness to change negative eating behaviors, survival skills needed by all clients with diabetes, and various meal planning approaches widely used for these clients.

Nutritional Goals

The goal of medical nutritional therapy is to educate the person with diabetes to make changes in food and exercise habits that lead to improved metabolic control. Specifically, the client needs assistance with:

1. The attainment and maintenance of near-normal blood glucose levels as feasible by the coordination of food intake, endogenous and exogenous insulin and/or hypoglycemic agents, and with physical activity
2. The attainment and maintenance of optimal serum lipid levels
3. Provision of adequate kilocalories to attain and maintain: a healthy body weight for adults, normal growth and development for children, and recovery from catabolic illnesses and to meet the metabolic needs of pregnancy and lactation
4. The prevention and treatment of the acute and chronic complications of diabetes such as renal

disease, autonomic neuropathy, hypertension, and cardiovascular disease
5. Improvement of overall health through good nutrition. *The Food Guide Pyramid* and *Dietary Guidelines for Americans* illustrate and summarize nutritional guidelines for all Americans including people with diabetes.

Goal Priority

The medications prescribed, the type of diabetes the individual has, and the client's desire to change behavior determine goal priority. A high priority for the person taking insulin is to facilitate consistency in the timing of meals and snacks to prevent wide swings in blood glucose. This requires coordination among exercise, insulin, and food intake. A high priority for the individual with type II diabetes is achieving glucose, blood pressure, and lipid goals. Although weight reduction for these clients usually improves short-term glycemic levels and long-term metabolic control, traditional weight loss strategies have not been effective in achieving long-term weight loss. The client's motivation to lose weight needs to be carefully assessed by the health care educator.

Meal Frequency

Meal spacing is more crucial in IDDM than in NIDDM. Consistent timing and meal size assist in stabilization of blood glucose levels in IDDM.

Client Readiness to Change Behavior

Food behaviors are difficult to change. Although some clients with diabetes do successfully change or alter food behaviors to enhance their outcomes, many clients do not, will not, or cannot change negative food behaviors. Modification of addictive behaviors involves progression through five stages: precontemplation, contemplation, preparation, action, and maintenance (Prochaska, DiClemente, and Norcross, 1993). Individuals typically recycle through these stages several times before terminating negative behaviors. Following is a brief description of each of these stages:

1. *Precontemplation:* individuals exhibit no intention to change behavior in the foreseeable future.
2. *Contemplation:* individuals know they have a problem and they are seriously thinking about overcoming the negative behavior but are not ready to take action.
3. *Preparation:* individuals plan to take action in the near future, have taken action unsuccessfully in the past, and may report small behavioral changes.
4. *Action:* individuals modify their behavior, experiences, and/or environment to overcome the negative behavior. This stage requires considerable commitment of time and energy.
5. *Maintenance:* individuals continue to work to prevent relapse and to consolidate gains.

Health care workers can assist clients in the precontemplation and contemplation stages by attempting to raise patients' consciousness about the benefits of behavioral change. Stimulus control and reinforcement (Weight Control Chapter) also help patients become more aware of the need to alter behaviors. The most difficult problems posed by clients for the health educator are at the precontemplation phase (Jacobson, 1993).

The health care educator needs to carefully consider how much information the client desires and how ready he or she is to change food behaviors. An educational tool that takes three to four hours to review with a client is inappropriate for the client who is willing to devote just a few minutes to learning about his or her diet. In contrast, the client who wants to learn everything he or she can about self-care will not be satisfied with an elementary meal plan.

Survival Skills

Initially the newly diagnosed client needs to learn basic survival skills. See Box 18–1 for information the client needs to know immediately. Once the client has demonstrated an understanding of this basic knowledge, a firm foundation has been set for the acquisition of additional information.

Meal-Planning Approaches

There are about a dozen appropriate meal-planning approaches. The most elementary approaches include: *The Food Guide Pyramid, Dietary Guidelines for Americans,* and *The First Step in Diabetes Meal Panning* (Figure 18–5). Any one of these meal-planning approaches is considered survival skill level information. After the client has demonstrated an understanding of the meal-planning approach initially used by the health educator, the use of a more advanced approach should be considered. The client will achieve optimal blood glucose and lipid control with a more sophisticated meal-planning approach. Two of the more widely used, more advanced meal-planning systems are discussed in the next sections. Various meal-planning approaches are discussed in Box 18–2.

THE EXCHANGE LISTS OF THE AMERICAN DIETETIC AND THE AMERICAN DIABETES ASSOCIATIONS   This approach to meal planning introduced in Chapter 2, "Individualized Nutritional Care," allows the learner to acquire some knowledge about food composition. Usually the registered dietitian reviews this approach with the client and then the nurse reinforces the dietitian's teaching. The educator needs to anticipate spending a total of one to two hours to thoroughly explain this approach to a client. This can best be accomplished in two or more sessions. *The Exchange Lists of the American Dietetic and American Diabetes Associations* is used to calculate energy nutrient distribution.

Energy Nutrient Distribution. Total energy requirements for the individual with diabetes do not differ from the individual without diabetes. Therefore, please refer to the chapter on Energy Balance to determine the total kilocalorie requirement for a person. The distribution of energy nutrients refers to the percentage of total kilocalories that should be derived from each of carbohydrate, fat, and protein. Distribution also refers to the division of carbohydrate, fat, and protein among the day's meals/feedings. Clinical Calculation 18–1 shows how the percentage of energy nutrients is converted to grams of carbohydrate, fat, and protein and distributed throughout the day's meals/feedings. The next three parts of this chapter elaborate on energy nutrient distribution.

Carbohydrate. Complex carbohydrate should ideally provide the majority of kilocalories in the diet or about 55 to 60 percent of the total kilocalories. Many complex carbohydrates are also excellent sources of dietary fiber. Water-soluble fibers found in fruits, oats, barley, and legumes can influence glu-

BOX 18–1 SURVIVAL INFORMATION FOR THE CLIENT WITH DIABETES

Initial education for the client with diabetes should include basic knowledge that will facilitate the maintenance of acceptable (safe) blood glucose levels. Individuals with diabetes must come to accept responsibility for self-management and the need for ongoing education. Survival skills are typically reviewed with these clients during the first educational session.

1. Diabetes is caused by a lack of insulin and/or an inability to use the insulin the body produces. There is no cure for diabetes, but it can be controlled through diet, exercise, and medications.

2. An acceptable blood glucose is 80 to 120 mg/dL before meals and less than 200 mg/dL two hours after meals. The client is said to be adequately controlled if the blood glucose level is between these numbers relative to the time meals are eaten. Better control can be possible with more finely controlled blood glucose levels.

3. Monitoring and recording blood glucose levels can be done with a blood glucose monitor. All individuals with diabetes are encouraged to monitor their blood glucose levels. Hospital nurses and dietitians, home health care agencies, and health care workers in physicians' offices can teach the client how to monitor blood glucose levels.

4. Nutrition is an important part of blood glucose control. The Food Pyramid provides an initial acceptable dietary guide of what foods should be eaten. Foods chosen from the Food Pyramid guide should be divided into three or more equal feedings. It is important to eat at regular times each day, to avoid skipping meals, and to eat about the same amount each day. Try to limit fat, salt, sugar, and alcohol intake. Alcohol consumption on an empty stomach may cause a low blood glucose reaction. Try to increase intake of fruits, vegetables, and whole grains.

5. Exercise is beneficial for most people with diabetes, however, before beginning any exercise program, consult the doctor. Exercise is the most beneficial when the blood glucose is below 200 mg/dL. Regular exercise is more beneficial than sporadic exercise and best done 60 to 90 minutes after eating.

6. An understanding of the peak, onset, and duration of any medication used to treat a high blood glucose is important. Good insulin injection technique (if applicable) is essential.

7. A high blood glucose (greater than 240 mg/dL) is potentially dangerous, especially if untreated. Always check the urine for ketones if the blood glucose is more than 240 mg/dL. Contact the physician if the blood glucose is greater than 240 mg/dL and the urine is positive for ketones.

8. A blood glucose of less than 60 mg/dL is dangerous and may lead to confusion, disorientation, and coma. Signs of a low blood glucose include: sweating, slurred speech, headache, weakness, tremors, hunger, nervousness, tingling of the lips, and rapid heart beat. In the event these signs are noted, immediately:

    1. Check the blood glucose, if low proceed to step 2
    2. Take 1/2 cup of fruit juice OR 1/2 cup of milk OR 6 hard candies
    3. Wait 15 minutes and then recheck the blood glucose

    Repeat the process if the blood glucose is less than 100 mg/dL.

9. Over the long term, diabetes can lead to foot problems, including infection and amputation. Check the feet (and legs) daily. Look for sores, redness, infection, drainage, swelling, or bruises. Report problems to the doctor early. Keep the feet clean and dry. Never go barefoot. Protect any area where sensation is lost.

10. Have an annual examination with a board certified ophthalmologist (a doctor specializing in eye care).

11. The person with diabetes should wear a personal identification bracelet or necklace.

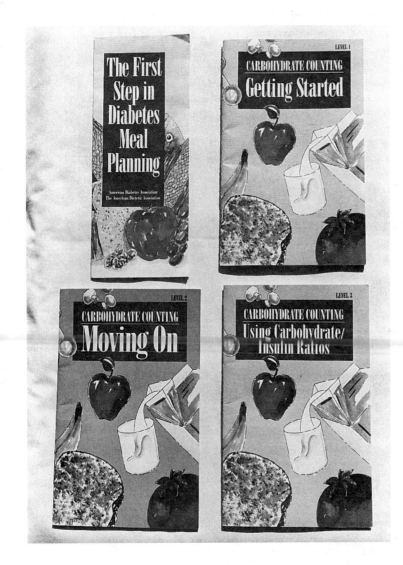

FIGURE 18–5 Teaching materials available from the American Diabetes and the American Dietetic Associations. (American Diabetes Association and The American Dietetic Association.© 1995. *Carbohydrate Counting: Getting Started*, with permission.)

cose and insulin levels by smoothing out the postprandial glucose curve, thereby helping to lower plasma lipid levels. Complex carbohydrates also provide many needed vitamins. A limited amount of carbohydrate or about 5 percent of the total carbohydrate may be derived from simple carbohydrates (single or double sugars found in simple sugars, fruits, some starches, and milk).

Clinical Application 18–3 discusses the glycemic index of foods. Note that while glucose has a high glycemic index, honey has a low glycemic index, and sucrose falls somewhere between them. White bread, potatoes, and cornflakes all have a higher glycemic index than sucrose. Thus, it is incorrect to tell a client that sucrose and honey cause the blood glucose level to increase faster or higher than an equal amount of carbohydrate from some complex carbohydrates.

The Food Guide Pyramid and *Dietary Guidelines for Americans* also recommend that the bulk of kilocalories be derived from complex carbohydrate and only minimal amounts of simple sugars be consumed. Simple sugars are empty kilocalories that contain almost no vitamins, minerals, and fiber.

Protein. The need for protein in the diabetic population is the same as in the general population. For example, the adult RDA of 0.8 grams per kilogram of protein or approximately 12 to 20 percent of total kilocalories is indicated. Excessive amounts of dietary protein should be avoided in people with diabetes just as it should be avoided by members of the general population.

BOX 18–2   MEAL-PLANNING APPROACHES

Approach	Comments	Availability
Food Pyramid	Initial phase of teaching Provides a basic foundation in normal nutrition. Does not emphasize meal consistency.	A colorful version is available from the National Dairy Council, 10255 West Higgins Road, Suite 900, Rosemont, IL 60018-4233 1-708-803-2000
Dietary Guidelines	Initial phase of teaching Provides a basic foundation in normal nutrition, 40 pages in length. Does not emphasize meal consistency.	United States Department of Agriculture Home & Garden Bulletin #232, Local Cooperative Extension Office
The First Step in Diabetes Meal Planning	Initial phase in teaching Combines Food Pyramid and Dietary Guidelines, and provides information on meal consistency in a simplified format.	The American Dietetic Association, 216 West Jackson Boulevard, Suite 800 Chicago, IL 60606-6995 1-800-366-1655
CHO Counting Level I Level II Level III	Progressive teaching tool that leads to maximum control of blood glucose and lipid levels. Decreased emphasis on balance and variety.	The American Dietetic Association, 216 West Jackson Boulevard, Suite 800 Chicago, IL 60606-6995 1-800-366-1655
Month-O-Meals	Each book contains 28 complete and interchangeable menus for breakfast, lunch, dinner, and snacks. Excellent approach for the client who "just wants to be told what and when to eat."	The American Dietetic Association, 216 West Jackson Boulevard, Suite 800 Chicago, IL 60606-6995 1-800-366-1655
Exchange Lists of the American Dietetic and the American Diabetes Associations	Allows the health care educator to distribute all of the energy nutrients. More emphasis on the importance of eating a balanced diet than the CHO counting approach. Time consuming to learn and teach	The American Dietetic Association, 216 West Jackson Boulevard, Suite 800 Chicago, IL 60606-6995 1-800-366-1655
Healthy Dividends: A Plan for Balancing Your Fat Budget	This approach is based on kcaloric density alone. Ignores glycemic effect, nutrient or fiber content Clients make food choices.	National Dairy Council 10255 West Higgins Road Suite 900 Rosemont, IL 60018-4233 1-708-803-2000

How to Distribute the Energy Nutrients and Calculate a Diet Using the Exchange System

In the following example, an 1800-kcal diet is being converted to 55 percent carbohydrate, 20 percent protein, and 25 percent fat.

$$1800 \text{ kcal} \times 0.55 = 990 \text{ kcal} \div 4 \text{ kcal/g} = 248 \text{ g carbohydrate}$$

$$1800 \text{ kcal} \times 0.20 = 360 \text{ kcal} \div 4 \text{ kcal/g} = 90 \text{ g protein}$$

$$1800 \text{ kcal} \times 0.25 = 450 \text{ kcal} \div 9 \text{ kcal/g} = 50 \text{ g fat}$$

In the following example, 248 g of carbohydrate, 90 g of protein, and 50 g of fat are converted to a 1/5, 2/5, 1/5, and 1/5 distribution. Each fraction represents one meal: thus 1/5 of the energy nutrients are to be provided each at breakfast, supper, and the evening snack; 2/5 of the energy nutrients are to be provided at the noon meal. Please note: 1/5 equals 20 percent and 2/5 represents 40 percent.

$$248 \text{ g of carbohydrate} \times 0.20 = 50 \text{ g} \times 3 \text{ meals} = 150$$

$$248 \text{ g of carbohydrate} \times 0.20 = 99 \text{ g} \times 1 \text{ meals} = \frac{99}{249}$$

$$90 \text{ g of protein} \times 0.20 = 18 \text{ g} \times 3 \text{ meals} = 54$$

$$90 \text{ g of carbohydrate} \times 0.40 = 36 \text{ g} \times 1 \text{ meal} = \frac{36}{90}$$

Because only a small percentage of dietary fat enters the bloodstream as glucose, normally fat is not calculated into the distribution. Lunch (2/5 distribution) would contain about 99 g of carbohydrate and 36 g of protein. Each of the other meals (1/5 distribution) would contain about 50 g of carbohydrate and 18 g of protein.

The next step is to determine the number of exchanges to be provided from each of the six exchange groups. There is no exact method used to determine this step. Usually the client is consulted to determine the amount of nonfat milk, fruits, vegetables, and so forth that he or she would be willing to consume. An effort should be made to calculate the diet with at least the recommended servings given in the Food Pyramid guide. Many health care workers determine the amount of nonfat milk, fruits, and vegetables to be provided first. This is followed by the grams of carbohydrate to be contributed by these groups. The remaining carbohydrate is then allocated to the starch group.

The protein is determined by first calculating the amount previously provided by nonfat milk, vegetables, and starches; the remaining protein is then allocated to meat exchanges. The fat is determined by first calculating the amount previously provided by the meat exchanges; the remaining fat is then allocated to fat exchanges. The calculations and meal plan for our sample 1800 kcal with 55 percent carbohydrate, 20 percent protein, and 25 percent fat with a 1/5, 2/5, 1/5, and 1/5 distribution appear in Table 18–5.

Fat. The American Diabetes Association recommends that total fat be less than 30 percent of total kilocalories. Note again this is similar to the *Dietary Guidelines for Americans.* Ten percent of fat should come from polyunsaturated fat, 10 percent from saturated fat, and 10 percent from monounsaturated fat. In addition, cholesterol should ideally be kept under 300 milligrams per day.

CARBOHYDRATE COUNTING   In 1995, the American Diabetes and Dietetic Associations introduced carbohydrate counting, a new menu planning concept. Carbohydrate counting refers to a teaching tool that includes three progressive levels of difficulty, sophistication, achievement, and self-care to be mastered by the client. These 3 progressive levels are designated Level I, Level II, and Level III. They are summarized in Box 18–3. Because carbohydrate is assumed to be the main factor affecting postprandial blood glucose elevation, priority is given to counting the total amount of carbohydrate consumed at one meal and/or snack. Diabetes educators

TABLE 18–5   Sample 1800-Kilocalorie Diabetic Diet*

				DIVISION OF ENERGY NUTRIENTS AND EXCHANGES				
Exchange List	*Number of Daily Exchanges*	*Protein (90 g)*	*Fat (50 g)*	*Carbohydrate (218 g)*	*Breakfast*	*Lunch*	*Dinner*	*HS*
Skim milk	2	16	0	24	1/2	1		1/2
Starch	11	33	0	165	2	4	3	2
Fruit	3	0	0	45	1	1	0	1
Vegetable	3	6	0	15	0	2	1	0
Meat	5	35	25	0	1	2	1	1
Fat	5	0	25	0	1	1	2	1

	MEAL PLAN AND SAMPLE MENUS	
Meal Plan	*Sample Menu 1*	*Sample Menu 2*
Breakfast		
1/2 skim milk	1/2 cup skim milk	1/2 cup skim milk
2 starch	2 slices of toast	1 cup of oatmeal
1 fruit	1/2 cup orange juice	1/2 banana
1 meat	1/4 cup low-cholesterol egg substitute	1 low-fat sausage link
1 fat	1 tsp margarine	2 pecans
Lunch		
1 skim milk	1 cup skim milk	1 cup skim milk
4 starch	1 1/3 cup brown rice	2 slices of bread†
		1 cup broth-type vegetable soup and 3 ginger snaps
1 fruit	1 apple	1/2 cup pineapple juice
2 vegetables	1 cup green beans	1/2 cup asparagus and 1 cup raw carrots
2 meat	2 oz stir-fried chicken	2 slices low-fat cheese†
1 fat	1 tsp oil	1 tsp margarine†
Dinner		
3 starch	1 lg baked potato	1/4 10-in pizza, thin crust and 2 bread sticks (4 × 1/2 in)
1 vegetable	1/2 cup broccoli‡	Sliced tomato
Free vegetable	Lettuce salad	Lettuce salad
1 meat	1 oz ground beef‡	(on pizza)
2 fat	2 tbsp sour cream‡	(on pizza)
	1 tbsp French dressing	1 tbsp Italian dressing
Free	Coffee	Diet soft drink
HS		
1/2 skim milk	1/2 cup skim milk	1/2 cup skim milk
2 starch	1 1/2 oz pretzels	6 cups hot-air popped popcorn
1 fruit	15 grapes	1 peach
1 meat	1 oz low-fat cheese stick	1 tbsp Parmesan cheese
1 fat	2 walnuts	1 tbsp diet margarine

* The calculations and meal plan based on 55 percent carbohydrate, 20 percent protein, and 25 percent fat with a 1/5, 2/5, 1/5, and 1/5 distribution.
† Cheese sandwich.
‡ Potato toppings.

CLINICAL APPLICATION 18–3

Glycemic Index

Different food sources that contain equal amounts of carbohydrate have been found not to have an equal impact on blood glucose levels. The **glycemic index** of food attempts to classify foods according to their impact on blood glucose. The higher the glycemic index value, the higher the blood glucose would be expected to rise after ingestion of the food.

Foods high in water-soluble fiber, in the raw state, high in binders, and eaten as part of a mixed meal reduce the glycemic response. Dairy products, pasta, dried peas, and legumes are examples of foods with a low glycemic index. Potatoes, some cereals, and bread are examples of foods with a high glycemic index.

Food is usually eaten as mixed nutrient sources. For example, spaghetti is usually eaten with tomato sauce or as part of a meal. Because a mixed meal tends to dilute the glycemic index of any one of the meal's constituents, the glycemic index is rarely taught in clinical practice. However, some highly motivated and well-educated people with diabetes are beginning to use information about the glycemic index of foods to assist in meal planning. Thus it is important to understand this concept. The following table compares effects of foods based on equal amounts of carbohydrate, not serving sizes or energy content. By convention, white bread is assigned a value of 100.

Food	*Glycemic index*
Glucose	138
Potato, russet, baked	135
Cornflakes	119
White bread	100
White table sugar (sucrose)	86
Rice	83
Banana	79
All-bran cereal	73
Spaghetti	66
Dried peas	56
Apple	53
Ice cream	52
Milk	49
Honey (fructose)	30

use Level I, then Level II, and possibly Level III as a client masters the previously taught level. The advantages of the Carbohydrate Counting meal plan concept include: single-nutrient focused, more precise matching of food and insulin, flexible food choices, a potential for improved blood glucose, and a feeling of controlling his or her own treatment. Challenges for the client who uses this system include: the need to weigh and measure food, maintenance of extensive food records, monitoring of the blood glucose before and after eating, the need to calculate grams of carbohydrate consumed, the need to maintain healthful eating, and weight management.

The rationale for Carbohydrate Counting is: a carbohydrate equals a carbohydrate equals a carbohydrate or one starch exchange equals one fruit exchange equals one milk exchange. One carbohydrate unit is about 15 grams of carbohydrate with an acceptable range of 8 to 22 grams per carbohydrate choice. Food labels, tables of food composition, and *Exchange Lists for Meal Planning* are some of the tools clients can use to determine the carbohydrate content of a particular food. Following is a typical meal plan for a client who has been taught to count carbohydrates:

Breakfast: 3 carbohydrates (range 38 to 52 grams)
 Example: 1 whole bagel and 1 cup skim milk
Lunch: 3 carbohydrates (range 38 to 52 grams)
 Example: 1 cup regular cola and 1 fresh orange and 1 slice whole wheat bread
Dinner: 3 carbohydrates (range 38 to 52 grams)
 Example: 1 1/2 cups pasta
Snack: 1 carbohydrate (8 to 22 grams)
 Example: 1 cup skim milk

The amount of time a client must be willing to spend to learn the carbohydrate counting method is underestimated by most health care workers (including students). The American Diabetes and the American Dietetic Associations estimate that clients need between 90 to 180 minutes to master one Level of this menu-planning system (The American Diabetes and the American Dietetic Associations, 1995). Client visits (usually three) should be spread over several months.

Special Considerations

Persons with diabetes frequently ask questions about nutritional problems related to vitamin mineral supplementation, alcohol, acute illness, eating out, and delayed meals. The following sections of this chapter discuss these nutrition-related problems.

Vitamin and Mineral Supplementation

There is no evidence to support the need for vitamin and mineral supplementation in persons with diabetes. Individuals on very low-calorie diets (less than

---

BOX 18–3   CARBOHYDRATE COUNTING

Title	Level I	Level II	Level III
Food Pyramid	Getting Started	Moving On	Intensive Diabetes Management Using Carbohydrate/ Insulin Ratios
Educational concepts	Foods that should be eaten Importance of eating on time Use of foods to counteract hypo- glycemia	Rationale for meal plan Expands on the selection of healthy foods Provides additional tips for meal planning	Sets the stage for self-management skills that provide flexibility and best control of diabetes The nutrient con- tent of food Interpretation of food labels Use of dietetic foods and sweeteners Advice for dealing with fast food, eating out, and parties
Client goals	Carbohydrate die- tary consistency Flexible food choices	Adjust food, medi- cation, and activ- ities based on patterns from cli- ent daily records.	Adjust insulin dose using ratio of carbohydrate/ insulin dosage
Intended audiences	IDDM NIDDM GDM	Person on diet only, oral agents, or insulin who has mastered basics of carbohydrate counting	People on intensive therapy People who have mastered insulin adjustment and supplementation
Primary distribu- tion channels	Physician's offices Hospitals HMOs Clinics with regis- tered dietitians on staff	Settings with a reg- istered dietitian or certified diabetes educator who has diabetes training and experience	Settings with health care team trained in intensive insulin therapy

---

800 kilocalories) or pregnant women may need a vitamin and mineral supplement. Any disease condition that normally affects the ingestion, digestion,
absorption, metabolism, and excretion of nutrients
may require a supplement as it would for the person
without diabetes.

Alcohol

The moderate use of alcohol will not adversely affect
diabetes in the well-controlled client. Recommendations follow (The American Diabetes Association,
1994):

For insulin users:

- Limit to 2 drinks per day.
- Drink only with food.
- Do not cut back on food.
- If history of alcohol abuse, abstain.
- Abstain during pregnancy.

For noninsulin users:

- Substitute for fat kilocalories.
- Limit to promote weight loss or maintenance.
- Limit with elevated triglycerides.
- If there is a history of alcohol abuse, abstain.
- Abstain during pregnancy.

Nutrition During Acute Illness Episodes

Acute illness affects everyone, including the diabetic person. Colds and flu-like symptoms can be fatal for some people with diabetes unless precautions are taken. Secretion of both glucagon and epinephrine increases during illness and contributes to an increase in blood glucose levels. This may lead to a loss of glucose, fluid, and electrolytes. Dehydration, electrolyte depletion, and a loss of nutrients may follow. Acute illnesses can lead to DKA in IDDM and to HHNS in NIDDM.

Dehydration is more rapid if the electrolytes and fluids are not replaced. Vomiting, diarrhea, and fever all represent fluid loss. During acute illness the individual should be instructed to monitor his or her blood glucose level every 4 to 6 hours until the symptoms subside. Urine ketone levels should be checked if the blood glucose level is above 240 milligrams per deciliter. Generally, if the blood glucose level exceeds 240 milligrams per deciliter for longer than 24 hours, the physician should be informed immediately. Some physicians may provide their clients with slightly different instructions. Care must be taken not to confuse the client.

The risk of dehydration is reduced by increased fluids. Clients who are vomiting or nauseated and are unable to tolerate regular food should drink liquids that contain carbohydrate and/or electrolytes (Table 18–6). A general guideline is that approximately 15 grams of carbohydrate should be consumed every 1 to 2 hours. Some clients have an individually calculated sick-day menu based on the carbohydrate content of their regular diet.

Other meal-planning tips that may prove helpful during periods of acute illness include (1) increasing water intake even for clients who can eat regular food; (2) eating smaller, more frequent feedings; and (3) eating soft, easily digested foods.

Eating Out and Fast Foods

The best advice for persons with diabetes who enjoy eating out is that they know their meal-planning system and order small. For example, a small hamburger at McDonald's with a side salad, diet dressing, and a glass of skim milk are equal to:

	Grams of CHO
3 carbohydrates	
2 starches (hamburger bun)	30
1 milk	12
	42

The individual can always mix 4 ounces of orange juice with diet soft drinks for a fruit punch drink if he or she needs an additional 15 grams of carbohydrate.

Hypoglycemia in Diabetes Mellitus

The immediate treatment goal for a glucose level of less than 60 milligrams per deciliter is to increase blood glucose to within a normal level as rapidly as possible. Take care not to over-treat hypoglycemia. If the client is monitoring his or her blood glucose level, at the first sign or symptom of hypoglycemia he or she should measure the blood glucose level. If the blood glucose level is less than 60 milligrams per deciliter, 15 grams of carbohydrate should be consumed. Fifteen grams of carbohydrate is equal to 2 to 3 glucose tablets, 6 to 10 Lifesavers candy, or 4 to 6 ounces of juice. Fifteen minutes later, he or she should measure the blood glucose a second time. This is called the 15–15. The process may need to be repeated a second time to achieve a blood glucose

TABLE 18–6 Easily Consumed Carbohydrate-Containing Foods for "Sick Days"

Food	Amount	Grams of Carbohydrate
Regular cola	1/2 cup	13
Ginger ale	3/4 cup	16
Milk	1 cup	12
Apple juice	1/2 cup	15
Grape juice	1/3 cup	15
Orange juice	1/2 cup	15
Pineapple juice	1/2 cup	15
Prune juice	1/3 cup	15
Regular gelatin	1/2 cup	20
Sherbet	1/2 cup	30
Tomato juice*	1/2 cup	5

* High in sodium.

Children with Diabetes

Kilocalorie allowances are based on a person's weight. As a rough estimate, a 1-year-old child needs 1000 kcal per day. For older children, 100 kcal per year of age are added to the daily intake. For a 9-year-old child, this would equal 1900 kcal. Typically, 55 percent of the total kilocalories should be consumed as carbohydrate. 1900 kcal multiplied by 55 percent equals 1045 kcal. To convert kilocalories from carbohydrate to grams of carbohydrate divide by 4. 1045 kcal divided by 4 kcal/g equals 260 g of carbohydrate.

How these grams of carbohydrate are divided among the day depends on the child's prescribed medications and lifestyle. Let's assume the child eats three meals and two snacks (at mid-afternoon and bedtime) and takes one dose of basal insulin in the morning and three doses of regular insulin, one before each meal.

The diet could be planned to provide 20 percent of the carbohydrate at each feeding. Twenty percent of 260 g of carbohydrate equals 52 g or 3 1/2 carbohydrate choices. The child and the child's parents would be instructed to provide about 52 g of carbohydrate at each feeding.

As long as the child eats balanced meals that provide all the essential nutrients, the source of the carbohydrate is not important. Scientific evidence has shown that the use of sucrose as part of the meal plan does not impair blood glucose control in individuals with type I and type II diabetes (American Dietetic Association, 1994). A typical menu for the child follows:

Breakfast	Grams of Carbohydrate Acceptable range 46 to 60
1/2 cup of Honey Nut Cheerios	12 (package label)
3/4 cup skim milk	9 (exchange value)
1/2 cup orange juice	15 (exchange value)
1 slice toast	15 (exchange value)
1 tsp peanut butter	0
Total carbohydrates	51

Lunch	
Ham and cheese sandwich with 2 slices of bread	30 (exchange value)
1 apple	15 (exchange value)
3/4 cup skim milk	9 (exchange value)
Carrot sticks	0 (free with this system)
Total carbohydrates	54

Mid-Afternoon Snack	
3/4 cup apple juice	23 (exchange value)
13 animal crackers	25 (exchange value)
Total carbohydrates	48

Dinner	
1/8 15-in cheese pizza	39 (table of food composition)
6 oz regular cola	20 (table of food composition)
Total	59

Bedtime Snack	
1/2 cup skim milk	6 (exchange value)
Raw broccoli with dip	0 (free with this system)
10 (1 1/2 oz) whole-wheat crackers (no added fat)	30 (exchange value)
1/2 oz jelly beans	14 (table of food composition)
Total carbohydrates	50
Total carbohydrates for the day	262

level between 80 to 120 milligrams per deciliter (or 70 to 110 milligrams per deciliter; check laboratory's normal range). Treat with 15 grams of carbohydrate, wait 15 minutes, and retest. If the reaction is not resolved, treat again. Overtreatment can be avoided by adherence to the 15–15 rule. Those clients who do not test their blood glucose levels should be taught to do so.

Clients should be advised to carry a source of carbohydrate with them at all times. In the event that a meal or snack is delayed (preplanned or not preplanned) by 1/2 hour or more, a snack should be consumed. At least one other significant other should be instructed about hypoglycemia and the 15–15 rule.

Teaching Self-Care

Persons with diabetes ultimately treat themselves. The better educated the individual is about diabetes, the better the likelihood of his or her avoiding the acute and chronic complications of this disease. Many public health departments, hospitals, and clinics hold classes for clients with diabetes. Initially, these persons need to learn survival skills. The health care worker often has to repeat instructions several times before the client understands the survival skills being taught. Because of the genetic predisposition toward diabetes, many newly diagnosed clients have relatives who have suffered from the acute and chronic complications of diabetes. Hearing about such complications firsthand often creates fear in newly diagnosed clients. They need time to accept their condition. Occasionally, it may take as long as a full year before clients can grasp the principles of self-care. This is especially difficult for children (see Clinical Application 18–4).

Hypoglycemia

Hypoglycemia, caused by increased endogenous insulin production (hyperinsulinism), is rarer than diabetes mellitus. Hyperinsulinism is most likely caused by islet cell tumors or, less often, by reactive hypoglycemia. Hypoglycemia that occurs 1 to 3 hours after a meal and resolves spontaneously with the ingestion of carbohydrate is often termed "reactive hypoglycemia."

The dietary management of reactive hypoglycemia consists of avoiding simple carbohydrates and sometimes taking small, frequent feedings. The meal plans for diabetes offer a reasonable guide to meal planning. Table 18–7 is a 1-day meal plan for this type of diet.

The dietary treatment for hypoglycemia caused by an islet cell tumor is food given at frequent intervals in amounts necessary to prevent symptoms. Sugar is not avoided in these clients, as it may be particularly useful for the rapid correction of symptoms. In fact, some reports have indicated as much as 1000 grams of glucose administered each 24 hours are occasionally indicated to counteract a tremendous production of insulin (Guyton, 1986).

TABLE 18–7   Sample Meal Plan for Hypoglycemic Diet

Exchange Group	Sample Menu
Morning	
1 fruit	1/2 cup unsweetened orange juice
1 starch	3/4 cup whole-grain cereal
1 meat	1 low-fat cheese or
1/2 skim milk	1/2 cup skim milk
Free	Decaffeinated coffee
Mid-morning	
1 meat	1 tbsp peanut butter
1 starch	4 whole-grain crackers
Noon	
Chef's salad	
2–4 meat	2–4 oz lean meat
1 vegetable	Lettuce, tomatoes, and
1 fat	Dressing
1 fruit	1 small piece fresh fruit
1 skim milk	1 cup skim milk
1 starch	2 breadsticks (4 × 1/2 in)
Mid-afternoon	
1 meat	1 oz low-fat cheese
1 starch	4 whole-grain crackers
Evening	
2–4 meat	2–4 oz lean meat
1 starch	1/2 cup potato or pasta
1 vegetable	1/2 cup vegetable
1 fat	Lettuce salad with dressing
1 fruit	1 pce fresh fruit
Free	Decaffeinated coffee or tea
Bedtime	
1 starch and 1 meat	1/2 sandwich (1 slice whole-grain bread and 1 oz lean meat)
1 vegetable	Fresh vegetables
Free	Decaffeinated beverage

Summary

Diabetes mellitus is caused by an undersecretion of insulin and/or receptor defects. Diabetes is actually a group of disorders with a common sign of hyperglycemia. There are two major types of diabetes: insulin-dependent diabetes mellitus (IDDM) and non-insulin-dependent diabetes mellitus (NIDDM). Impaired glucose tolerance, secondary diabetes, and gestational diabetes are recently named new categories of this disease. Persons with diabetes suffer from acute and chronic complications. Treatment involves medication, nutrition management, and exercise. Nutrition is a fundamental part of treatment. Hypoglycemia, a rarer condition than diabetes, is caused by oversecretion of insulin, and is also treated with dietary manipulation.

Case Study 18–1

Mrs. S, a 45-year-old black woman, admitted to the hospital with medical diagnoses of NIDDM and cellulitis of the left leg. Her admitting height was 5 ft, 5 in and weight 200 lb. Wrist measurement shows Mrs. S has a large frame. Vital signs were temperature 98.6°F, pulse 70 beats per minute, respirations 16 per minute, and blood pressure 160/95.

Mrs. S reported a gradual increase in her weight since her third child was born 20 years ago. That baby weighed 12 lb. Two previous pregnancies produced infants weighing 10 and 11 lb. She has no known allergies.

None of the children live at home. Mrs. S lives with her husband, who works fairly regularly as a construction laborer. She has been seasonally employed as a hotel maid at a nearby resort. Health insurance coverage is sporadic. They have a new insurance policy now.

Mrs. S is the oldest of six children. Her father died of a heart attack at age 60. Her mother died of a stroke at age 62 following 15 years of treatment for diabetes mellitus. The sister who is closest to Mrs. S in age developed diabetes mellitus 3 years ago and is being treated with oral medication. Their youngest sister was diagnosed as an insulin-dependent diabetic at age 18 following an episode of mumps.

Mrs. S reports a good appetite and a fluid intake of about 3 quarts per day. Her favorite beverage is iced tea with sugar and lemon. She does most of the grocery shopping and cooking.

Mrs. S hit her left ankle with the screen door about 2 months ago. The resulting sore has not healed but has gotten worse. Mrs. S knows that a sore that does not heal is a sign of cancer, which is why she sought medical attention. The ankle now has an open lesion 5 cm in diameter over the lateral ankle bone. The entire foot is swollen to twice the size of the right foot. The bandage over the sore had greenish-yellow drainage on it.

A random blood glucose test in the doctor's office 3 hours after her last meal was 400 mg/dL. Her urine glucose was negative for ketones. Before she left the office, the physician told Mrs. S she has noninsulin-dependent diabetes mellitus.

The physician prescribed the following care for Mrs. S:

- Bed rest with left leg elevated
- Bedside commode
- Diet assessment and teaching
- Multivitamin, 1 capsule, daily
- Culture and sensitivity of drainage from left leg
- Cefuroxime, 250 mg, orally every 12 h
- Warm, moist dressing to left leg ulcer four times per day
- Fasting blood sugar (FBS), electrolytes in AM

The admitting nurse constructed the following Nursing Care Plan for Mrs. S.

Assessment

Subjective Data Family history of diabetes mellitus

Large appetite

Large fluid intake

Delay in seeking medical attention

Objective Data Obesity (HBW 134 percent)

Newly diagnosed NIDDM

Possible hypertension (only one reading given)

Open lesion 5 cm diameter over left lateral ankle; purulent discharge

Nursing Diagnosis Health maintenance, altered: related to inappropriate self-care as evidenced by delay in seeking medical attention.

Desired Outcome/ Evaluation Criteria	Nursing Actions	Rationale
Client will verbalize self-care measures related to NIDDM by hospital discharge.	Refer to dietitian for nutritional assessment and education.	The cornerstone of treatment of NIDDM is weight loss. Although any weight loss will help, to reach a healthy weight, Mrs. S needs to lose 51 lb. A dietitian's expertise is needed.
Client will verbalize willingness to continue nursing/medical regimen after discharge.	Refer to social worker for sources of medical attention when uninsured.	Social workers are most familiar with community resources.
	Teach principles of wound care, including effect of high blood sugar on infection.	If Mrs. S understands that high blood sugar feeds the bacteria causing the infection, she may be more willing to work hard to control the diabetes.
	Reinforce dietitian's instruction. Have Mrs. S state the Dietary Guidelines and the reason why they are important.	Knowledge usually precedes behavior change.
	Have Mrs. S describe the meal plan she follows.	Short periods of instruction are most effective; frequent review of the material will help the client master it.
	Remind physician to discuss exercise regimen when the blood sugar is under control.	Mrs. S needs a prescribed exercise program suited to her level of conditioning.

Study Aids

Chapter Review

1. If a client has a history of ketoacidosis, he or she most likely has _____ diabetes.
   a. Type I
   b. Type II
   c. Pituitary
   d. Gestational

2. The following statement is true:
   a. Acute illness lowers blood glucose levels.
   b. Fluid and electrolyte replacement is essential during episodes of acute illness in all persons with diabetes.
   c. Persons with diabetes who have an acute illness require a vitamin and mineral supplement.
   d. Persons with diabetes should never eat forms of simple sugar.

3. Dietary guidelines for people with diabetes include:
   a. Drink alcohol in moderation.
   b. Consume no more than 2000 milligrams of sodium each day.
   c. Restrict fat intake to less than 30 percent of total kilocalories.
   d. Consume at least 50 grams of fiber each day.

4. For most clients, the cornerstone of treatment of NIDDM is:
   a. Stress management
   b. Weight loss
   c. Strict adherence to five planned meals per day
   d. Hypoglycemic drugs

5. The diet for reactive hypoglycemia includes the following features:
   a. Small, frequent meals with restricted simple sugar
   b. Three meals with ample simple sugars and high in complex carbohydrate
   c. Four to six small meals that are high in fat
   d. Three high-carbohydrate meals that are moderate in fat

Clinical Analysis

Ms. N, a 14-year-old white girl, has been an insulin-dependent diabetic for 1 year. Her blood sugar levels have been stable on an intermediate-acting insulin and a 370 gram CHO diet. She is now being seen in the doctor's office for routine follow-up. The nurse is reviewing Ms. N's knowledge of self-care.

1. To assess Ms. N's knowledge, the nurse asks Ms. N how she would handle a day when she could not eat solid foods. Which of the following answers would show Ms. N's understanding of the usual procedure?
   a. She would skip her insulin that day.
   b. She would call the doctor after missing one meal.
   c. She would replace the carbohydrates in the meal plan with liquids containing equal amounts of carbohydrate.
   d. She would take half her usual insulin dose and double her usual fluid intake.

2. Ms. N plays volleyball for her high-school team. She usually is moderately active during practices and games. SMBG records indicate a daily glucose level of between 120 and 140 milligrams per deciliter prior to the time she usually plays volleyball. Which of the following behaviors are appropriate for her before playing?
   a. No additional food is indicated.
   b. Increase her intake by 15 grams of carbohydrate.
   c. Decrease her intake by 15 grams of carbohydrate.
   d. Increase her intake by one vegetable exchange and fat exchange.

3. Ms. N says she is getting tired of pricking her finger several times a day. She asks the nurse why she cannot manage her diabetes using urine testing as her grandmother does. Which of the following responses by the nurse would be most appropriate?
   a. "The urine test is more accurate in older people."
   b. "The point at which sugar is spilled in the urine varies even for one individual. Therefore, the blood test is more accurate."
   c. "Urine tests are more costly."
   d. "The blood test is the newest thing. Your grandmother's doctor must be old-fashioned."

Bibliography

American Diabetes Association: Maximizing the Role of Nutrition in Diabetes Management. American Diabetes Association, Alexandria, VA, 1994.

American Diabetes Association: Position statement American Diabetes Association: Diabetes mellitus and exercise. Diabetes Spectrum 19:530, 1996a.

American Diabetes Association: Position statement American Diabetes Association: Nutrition recommendation and principles for people with diabetes mellitus. Diabetes Care (Suppl 1) 19:516, 1996b.

American Dietetic Association: Manual of Clinical Dietetics, ed 4. American Dietetic Association, Chicago, 1992.

Black, JM, and Matassarin-Jacobs: Luckmann and Sorenson's Medical-Surgical Nursing, ed 4. WB Saunders, Philadelphia, 1993.

Committee on Diet and Health Food and Nutrition Board Commission on Life Sciences National Research Council: Diet and Health. National Academy Press, Washington, DC, 1989.

Deglin, JH, and Vallerand, AH: Davis's Drug Guide for Nurses, ed 4. FA Davis, Philadelphia, 1995.

Diabetes Control and Complication Trial Group: Influence of intensive treatment on quality-of-life outcomes in the diabetes control and complications trial. Diabetes Care 19:195, 1996.

Diabetes Control and Complication Trial Group: The effect of intensive treatment of diabetes on the development and progression of long-term complications in insulin-dependent diabetes mellitus. New Engl J Med 329:977–986, 1993.

Franz, MJ: Exercise and the management of diabetes mellitus. J Am Diet Assoc 87:872, 1987.

Franz, MJ, et al: Nutrition principles for the management of diabetes and related complications. Diabetes Care 17:490, 1994.

Guthrie, AW, Hinnen, D, and De Shelter, E (eds): Diabetes Education: A Core Curriculum for Health Professionals. American Association of Diabetes Educators, Alexandria, VA, 1988.

Guyton, AC: Textbook of Medical Physiology, ed 7. WB Saunders, Philadelphia, 1986, p. 932.

Jacobson, AM: Commentary. Diabetes Spectrum 6:36–37, 1993.

Nathan, DM: Long-term complications of diabetes mellitus: New Engl J Med 328:1676, 1993.

Pagana, KD, and Pagana, TJ: Mosby's Diagnostic and Laboratory Test Reference, ed 2. Mosby, St. Louis, 1995.

Pastors, JG: Nutritional Care of Diabetes. Nutrition Dimension Inc., San Marcos, FL, 1992.

Pemberton, CM, et al: Mayo Clinic Diet Manual: 6th ed. BC Decker, Philadelphia, 1988.

Position paper of the American Dietetic Association. Nutrition recommendations and principles for people with diabetes mellitus. J Am Diet Assoc 94:504, 1994.

Position paper of the American Diabetes Association: Preconception care of women with diabetes. Diabetes Care (suppl) 19: 525, 1996a.

Prochaska, JO, DiClemente, Norcross: In search of how people change: Application to addictive behavior. Diabetes Spectrum 6:25–33, 1993.

CHAPTER 19

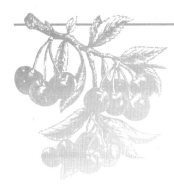

Diet in Cardiovascular Disease

LEARNING OBJECTIVES

After completing this chapter, the student should be able to:

1 Discuss the relationship of diet to the development of cardiovascular disease.
2 Distinguish between type II and type IV hyperlipoproteinemias as to aggravating factors and dietary modifications.
3 Identify strategies likely to reduce the risk of cardiovascular disease.
4 Describe the traditional 2-gram sodium diet.
5 List several flavorings and seasonings that can be substituted for salt on a sodium-restricted diet.

The cardiovascular system includes not only the heart and blood vessels but the blood-forming organs as well. This chapter discusses common diseases of the heart and blood vessels that can be influenced by diet modification. Conditions resulting from faulty blood forming are included in other chapters. Iron-deficiency anemia was discussed with minerals; pernicious anemia with vitamins and pregnancy. Nutritional care of the leukemia patient is included in Chapter 22, "Diet in Cancer."

Occurrence of Cardiovascular Disease

Diseases of the cardiovascular system are 2 of the 10 most common causes of death in the United States. Coronary heart disease is number one and cerebrovascular disease is third. Coronary heart disease causes one-third of all deaths, both of men and women. This is true despite the fact that coronary heart disease mortality in the United States declined by 54 percent between 1963 and 1990 (Johnson, et al, 1993). Coronary heart disease costs this country between $50 billion and $100 billion per year in medical treatment and lost wages (Expert Panel, 1993).

Cerebrovascular disease includes **cerebral vascular accident** (CVA) or stroke. Every year one-half million people in the United States suffer strokes. There is no gender preference but incidence increases sharply with age.

Underlying Pathology

Two major pathological conditions contribute to cardiovascular disease. One is atherosclerosis, the most common form of **arteriosclerosis.** The second is hypertension.

Atherosclerosis

Atherosclerosis is more common in older persons, but the process begins early in life. It is also becoming less widespread. On autopsy, 45 percent of young soldiers killed in Vietnam displayed atherosclerotic changes compared to 77 percent in Korea.

In **atherosclerosis** fatty deposits of cholesterol, fat, or other substances accumulate inside the artery. Initially, the deposited material, or plaque, is soft, but later it becomes fibrosed or hard. This disease process interferes with the pumping of blood through the artery in two ways: (1) the deposits gradually make the opening smaller and smaller, and (2) the fibrosis makes it progressively harder for the artery to constrict or dilate in response to the tissues' needs for oxygenated blood (Fig. 19–1). When the lumen, or opening through the artery, is 70 percent blocked by atherosclerotic plaque, the person is likely to show symptoms. Atherosclerosis is a major causative factor of peripheral vascular disease (PVD) affecting an estimated 2.4 million Americans (Grace, Crosby, and Ventura, 1995).

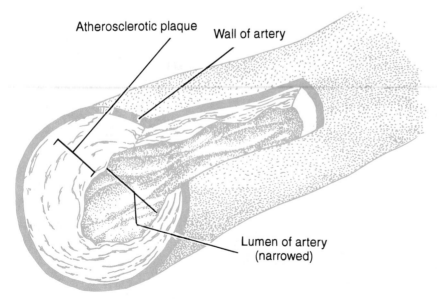

Atherosclerotic plaque   Wall of artery

Lumen of artery
(narrowed)

FIGURE 19–1 Buildup of atherosclerotic plaque within an artery. Note both the narrowed diameter and the roughness within the lumen. (From Scanlon and Sanders, p 284, with permission.)

Hypertension

Blood pressure is the force exerted against the walls of the arteries by the pumping action of the heart. It is reported in two numbers, such as 120/80. The top number, **systolic pressure,** is the pressure during a heartbeat. The bottom number, **diastolic pressure,** is the pressure between beats. Both numbers are reported in millimeters of mercury (mm Hg).

Diagnosis of Hypertension

Approximately 30 to 40 million adults in the US have high blood pressure and 2 million new cases are diagnosed annually. The prevalence steadily increases with age, from 4 percent in those 18 to 29 years old to 65 percent in individuals 80 and older (National High Blood Pressure Education Program, 1993). A measurement of 140/90 or higher on several occasions is diagnosed as hypertension. Several readings are taken on different days to eliminate the possibility of excitement or nervousness causing a transient hypertension. **Hypertension** is classified as mild, moderate, severe, or very severe. (See Table 19–1.) A person with hypertension may not feel sick, so blood pressure screening is often offered as a community service (Figure 19–2).

Types of Hypertension

Depending on the cause of the hypertension, it is labeled primary or secondary. About 90 percent of hypertensive patients have primary or **essential hypertension.** There is no single, clear-cut cause for this high blood pressure.

    Secondary hypertension occurs in response to another event or disease process in the body, such as pregnancy induced hypertension. Birth control pills that contain progesterone stimulate the production of renin, which results in an elevation in blood pressure. The combined intake of **monoamine oxidase (MAO) inhibitors** and tyramine-rich foods or beverages can cause hypertension. Secondary hypertension can result from diseases of the kidney, adrenal glands, or nervous system.

Positive Feedback Cycle

Many cardiovascular conditions have interlocking causative factors. The interaction between atherosclerosis and hypertension is a **positive feedback cycle.** The presence of the second condition worsens the first. Atherosclerosis narrows the lumen of the arteries, and the smaller opening increases the blood pressure. High blood pressure forces more lipids into the arterial wall.

End Result of Pathology

Most people do not have atherosclerosis or hypertension. They probably have both conditions. Although many organs are likely to be damaged by atherosclerosis and hypertension, here the concern is the effects on the heart and brain.

TABLE 19–1   Classification of Hypertension

Category	Systolic mm Hg	Diastolic mm Hg
Normal	<130	<85
High normal	130–139	85–89
Hypertension		
Stage 1 (mild)	140–159	90–99
Stage 2 (moderate)	160–179	100–109
Stage 3 (severe)	180–209	110–119
Stage 4 (very severe)	≥210	≥120

Cerebrovascular accident (CVA)—An abnormal condition in which the brain's blood supply is interrupted, resulting in damaged brain tissue.

Arteriosclerosis—A group of cardiovascular diseases characterized by the thickening, hardening, and loss of elasticity of the arterial walls.

Atherosclerosis—A form of arteriosclerosis characterized by the deposit of fatty material inside the arteries; major factor contributing to heart disease.

Blood pressure—Force exerted against the walls of blood vessels by the pumping action of the heart.

Systolic pressure—Pressure exerted against the arteries when the heart contracts; the upper number of the blood pressure reading.

Diastolic pressure—Pressure exerted against the arteries between heartbeats, the lower number of a blood pressure reading.

Hypertension—Blood pressure above normal, usually more than 140/90 on three successive occasions.

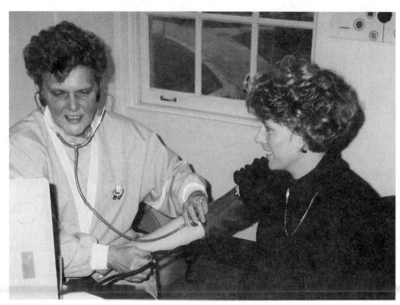

FIGURE 19–2   Hypertension is a silent killer. Even children are occasionally hypertensive. Many clinics routinely monitor blood pressure.

Coronary Heart Disease

Coronary heart disease (CHD) results when the coronary arteries that supply the heart muscle with blood become blocked. If the blockage is temporary, owing to increased activity and increased demand for oxygen, the person may display **angina pectoris,** or severe pain and a sense of constriction about the heart. Rest and the administration of vasodilating medications may stave off heart damage. However, if the vessel is blocked by a **thrombus,** a blood clot that develops at the site, or an **embolus,** a circulating mass of undissolved matter, the heart tissues beyond the point of obstruction receive no oxygen or nutrients. When this happens, the person has a **coronary occlusion,** or a heart attack. When the blood supply cannot be restored quickly, part of the heart dies. The medical diagnosis then becomes **myocardial infarction** (MI).

Congestive Heart Failure

Congestive heart failure affects an estimated 4 million Americans. Each year 200,000 clients die of CHF (Brady, Rock, and Horneffer, 1995). **Congestive heart failure** (CHF) occurs when the heart fails to maintain adequate circulation of the blood. CHF results from an injury or a reduction in function of the heart muscle. Causes may be atherosclerosis, hy-

pertension, myocardial infarction, rheumatic fever, or a birth defect. When the heart cannot keep up with the demands on it, a sequence of events sets up another positive feedback cycle.

The right side of the heart collects the blood returning from the body and pumps it to the lungs to be cleared of carbon dioxide and refilled with oxygen. If the right ventricle is failing, usually owing to lung disease, the blood backs up into the veins that empty into the right atrium, and the client will display the signs of peripheral edema. The elevated venous pressure also produces changes in the small bowel, which impacts the client's appetite (Brady, Rock, and Horneffer, 1995).

The left side of the heart receives the oxygenated blood from the lungs and pumps it out to the body. If the left ventricle is failing, usually following a myocardial infarction, the blood will back up into the lungs. The client will display shortness of breath and moist lung sounds and will expectorate a frothy pink sputum.

In addition, if the heart cannot pump enough to maintain blood pressure, the body will implement the renin-angiotensin response. Angiotensin II constricts the blood vessels, raising blood pressure. Aldosterone prompts the kidney to conserve sodium, and with it, water. More fluid fills the blood vessels. The higher blood pressure pushes this fluid out into the interstitial spaces, causing edema.

Obviously, one side of the heart cannot function indefinitely while the other side is failing. Nevertheless, the health care worker learns to look for signs of early heart failure in the extremities in right-sided failure or in the lungs in left-sided failure.

Cerebrovascular Accident

When a blood vessel in the brain becomes blocked by atherosclerosis, the tissue supplied by that artery dies. This is the most common cause of cerebrovascular accidents, or strokes. Strokes also can be caused by an embolus or a ruptured blood vessel. Cerebrovascular accidents are usually secondary to atherosclerosis, hypertension, or a combination of both.

Risk Factors in Cardiovascular Disease

The occurrence of cardiovascular disease in a person cannot be predicted with certainty. Many attributes and behaviors interact to produce the illness.

Unchangeable Risk Factors

Age, sex, race, and family history can be predictive of atherosclerosis and hypertension in some people.

Age, Sex, and Race

Coronary atherosclerosis is seen more frequently in individuals over the age of 40. Hypertension usually develops at about age 50 or 60. Prevalence is higher in men until middle age, but in women after middle age. Coronary heart disease risk increases in males after age 45 and females after age 55.

Until menopause, females have less atherosclerosis and coronary heart disease than males. Females past menopause and younger diabetic women are stricken just as often as men.

Hypertension is twice as common in blacks as in whites. Blood pressure shows steeper increases with advancing age in blacks than in whites (Melby, Toohey, and Cebrick, 1994).

Family History

A family history of premature coronary heart disease in a parent or sibling increases a person's risk of the disease. Premature coronary heart disease has been defined as occurring in a male under the age of 50

or a female under age 60 (Williams, and Bollella, 1995).

Of special concern are the **hyperlipoproteinemias,** or increased lipoproteins and lipids in the bloodstream (Table 19–2). One of these hyperlipoproteinemias, type IV, is very common and is often associated with **noninsulin-dependent diabetes mellitus** (NIDDM). Some of the other types are seen less often. All six types have a connection to food intake of fats, carbohydrates, or both. Blood plasma values vary in each condition. For example, type I hyperlipoproteinemia is aggravated by fat, and the chylomicrons are elevated because they carry exogenous triglycerides that cannot be broken down. Thus, plasma triglyceride levels are elevated as well.

Type II hyperlipoproteinemia results from a single gene defect in the cell receptor that binds circulating low-density lipoproteins. It is an autosomal dominant characteristic. Individuals with this defect manifest a rate of coronary heart disease 25 times that of the normal population. In addition, clients with type IIA hyperlipoproteinemia generally develop heart disease 15 years earlier than the rest of the population. Some even suffer heart attacks in infancy and childhood.

Coronary heart disease (CHD)—Disease resulting from the decreased flow of blood through the coronary arteries to the heart muscle.

Angina pectoris—Severe pain and sense of constriction about the heart caused by relative lack of oxygen.

Thrombus—A blood clot that obstructs a blood vessel.

Embolus—A circulating mass of undissolved matter in a blood or lymphatic vessel; may be composed of cells, tissues, fat globules, air bubbles, clumps of bacteria, or foreign bodies including pieces of medical devices.

Coronary occlusion—Blockage of one or more branches of the coronary arteries, which supply the heart muscle with oxygen and nutrients.

Myocardial Infarction—Area of dead heart muscle; usually the result of coronary occlusion.

Congestive heart failure (CHF)—Condition resulting from failure of the heart to maintain adequate blood circulation; due to complex reactive mechanisms, fluid is retained in the body's tissues.

Hyperlipoproteinemias—Increased lipoproteins and lipids in the blood.

TABLE 19–2 Hyperlipoproteinemias

Type	Frequency	Aggravated	Increased Plasma Values				
			Lipoprotein			Lipid	
			Chylomicrons	VLDL	LDL	Cholesterol	Triglycerides
I	Very rare	Fat	X				X
IIA	Common	Fat			X	X	
IIB	Common	Fat		X	X	X	X
III	Uncommon	Carbohydrate	Remnants			X	X
IV	Very common	Carbohydrate		X			X
V	Rare	Fat and carbohydrate	X	X		X	X

Changeable Risk Factors

Unlike age, sex, race, and family history, some risk factors for cardiovascular disease can be modified. For hypertension the modifiable risk factors are weight, high salt intake, physical inactivity, and excessive alcohol consumption. For coronary heart disease modifiable risk factors are cigarette smoking, hypertension, elevated LDL, or low HDL cholesterol, and diabetes mellitus.

Hypertension

A person who has blood pressure greater than 140/90 millimeters of mercury or is taking antihypertensive medication is classified as hypertensive. A 2 millimeters of mercury decrease in systolic pressure is estimated to have the potential to reduce annual mortality from stroke by 6 percent and from coronary heart disease by 4 percent.

OVERWEIGHT People who are overweight have 2 to 6 times the risk of developing hypertension as people with a healthy body weight. An estimated 50 percent of hypertension could be prevented by weight control. The location of the body fat is significant: abdominal fatness is related to cardiovascular disease and diabetes mellitus more than is gluteal-femoral fatness. Even a ten pound weight loss has been effective in lowering blood pressure.

Excess body fat is a cause of hypertension and coronary heart disease. The Nurses Health Study showed the risk of coronary heart disease in middle age increased by 2.6 to 3.6 percent in these women for every kilogram of weight gain after age 18. Using the BMI as the criterion, the risk of coronary heart disease was 20 to 77 percent greater for women with BMIs between 23 and 24.9 compared to women with BMIs of less than 21. For women with BMIs of 29 or more, the risk was 3.5 times that of the women with BMIs of 21 (Willett, et al, 1995).

HIGH-SALT INTAKE Increased blood pressure values with age are significantly related to sodium intake (Elliott, et al, 1996). A large study showed a 100 millimole (2.5 grams) difference in sodium intake was associated with differences in systolic pressure ranging from 5 millimeters of mercury in those aged 15 to 19 years, to 10 millimeters of mercury in ages 60 to 69. Clinical trials showed greater effectiveness of sodium restriction in hypertensive subjects than in normotensive subjects. Decreases in systolic and diastolic pressures averaged 5 and 3 millimeters of mercury in the former but 2 and 1 millimeters of mercury in the latter (National High Blood Pressure Education Program, 1993).

PHYSICAL INACTIVITY Activity is inversely related to blood pressure independent of being overweight in both sexes and across all ages. Hypertension is less prevalent in active adults than in age-matched subjects for whites and blacks, for both sexes, and for younger and older persons. Increasing physical activity has been shown to decrease both systolic and diastolic pressures by 6 to 7 millimeters of mercury (National High Blood Pressure Education Program, 1993).

ALCOHOL CONSUMPTION An estimated 30 to 60 percent of alcoholics have hypertension. When hospitalized for detoxification, the average alcoholic's systolic blood pressure decreases by 20 millimeters of mercury. Alcohol has been found to induce strokes, even in normotensive clients. A high intake of alcohol also increases serum triglyceride levels.

Blood pressure is positively correlated with an alcohol intake of three or more drinks per day, independent of age, BMI, and cigarette smoking. An estimated 5 to 7 percent of hypertension is attributed to an alcohol intake of three or more drinks per day (National High Blood Pressure Education Program, 1993). Generally, a **drink** is 12 ounces of beer, 4 ounces of wine, or 1.5 ounces of liquor.

UNPROVEN FACTORS RELATING TO HYPERTENSION
Other dietary components have been associated with hypertension, but inconsistently. Low potassium, especially the sodium/potassium ratio, is implicated in hypertension. Potassium supplementation is judged less important than controlling weight and sodium intake. Other factors, omega-3 fatty acids, calcium, magnesium, protein, and fiber have been studied as impacting hypertension but with inconclusive or clinically minimal results (Allender, et al, 1996; National High Blood Pressure Education Program, 1993).

Cigarette Smoking

Nicotine is a vasoconstrictor that raises blood pressure. Smokers also have lower levels of HDL even when weight is held constant. Lower HDL levels increase the risk of coronary heart disease.

Elevated Blood Cholesterol

The segment of the public who have had their blood cholesterol checked rose from 35 percent in 1983 to 65 percent in 1990 (10th Anniversary of NCEP, 1995). The recommended frequency is every five years in healthy people (Expert Panel, 1995). Concern has been raised that mass screenings increase health care costs through repetitive testing of known cases (Strychar, 1994).

Mean total cholesterol increases through age 54 and then declines (Johnson, et al, 1993). Between 1976 and 1991 the proportion of adults with blood cholesterol levels of 240 milligrams per deciliter or higher declined from 26 to 20 percent while those with levels of 199 milligrams per deciliter or lower rose from 44 to 49 percent (Sempos, et al, 1993). These changes occurred across all age and sex groups (Johnson, et al, 1993).

Among 2- to 11-year-old children, 25 percent are reported to have borderline high cholesterol. Table 19–3 compares desirable serum cholesterol levels in children and adults. It is recommended that a child's risk of CHD be evaluated by family history between the ages of 2 and 6 and updated regularly (Williams and Bollella, 1995). Children who are determined to have elevated serum cholesterol levels have to be managed carefully so that sufficient food is provided to support growth. Universal screening of children for hypercholesterolemia is not recommended (Committee on Nutrition, 1992).

RELATIONSHIP TO PATHOLOGICAL CHANGES Serum cholesterol levels are directly associated with CHD mortality in the United States and Northern Europe

TABLE 19–3 Desirable Serum Cholesterol Levels (mg/dL) in Children and Adults

	Ages 2 to 19 years*	Ages >20 years
Total cholesterol	<170	<200
Low-density lipoprotein	<110	<130
High-density lipoprotein	>45	>35

* Recommended by Williams and Bollella, 1995.

(Verschuren, et al, 1995) and with atherosclerosis and CHD risk. There is no threshold level below which there is no risk (Montague, et al, 1994). The importance of cholesterol levels on risk of CHD in persons older than 70 years is controversial. One study of 997 men and women found no relationship between **hypercholesterolemia** or low HDL cholesterol and CHD morbidity, CHD mortality, and all cause mortality (Krumholz, et al, 1994) while another of 4099 men and women related low HDL cholesterol to CHD mortality and new CHD events (Corti, et al, 1995). All cholesterol-lowering clinical trials show angiographic improvement in coronary perfusion. For every 1 percent reduction in serum cholesterol, a person decreases his risk of CHD by 2 percent. Even so, cholesterol-lowering alone is unlikely to reduce CHD mortality in the United States and Northern Europe to the level of Mediterranean and Japanese people (Verschuren, et al, 1995).

RELATIONSHIP TO DIET Cholesterol is produced by the liver, but diet also influences serum cholesterol levels. Only foods of animal origin contain cholesterol. Limiting their intake impacts cardiovascular risks. Only 16 percent of African Americans consuming vegetarian diets were hypertensive compared to 31 percent of nonvegetarians (Melby, Toohey, and Cebrick, 1994).

LIPOPROTEINS AS RISK FACTORS Fats cannot dissolve in water but are bound to proteins for transportation in the bloodstream. These fat-carrying complexes are called lipoproteins. There are four main classes of lipoproteins: **chylomicrons, very low-density lipoproteins** (VLDL), **low-density**

Chylomicron—A lipoprotein that carries triglycerides after meals.

Very low-density lipoprotein (VLDL)—A plasma protein containing mostly triglycerides with small amounts of cholesterol, phospholipid, and protein; transports triglycerides from the liver to the tissues.

lipoproteins (LDL), and **high-density lipoproteins** (HDL). Table 19–4 summarizes the functions, significance, and normal laboratory values of these four lipoproteins:

The higher the LDL, the greater the risk of CHD. Therefore, the primary target of cholesterol-lowering regimens is the LDL cholesterol. The goals of therapy are to lower the LDL value to (1) below 160 milligrams per deciliter if fewer than two other risk factors are present or (2) below 130 milligrams per deciliter if two or more other risk factors are present (Expert Panel, 1993). LDL cholesterol is deposited as part of the atherosclerotic plaque. Because LDL has to be oxidized before it becomes atherogenic, much current research involves antioxidants. Box 19–1 summarizes some of the findings.

Conversely, the higher a person's HDL levels, the less the risk of coronary heart disease. A high HDL level (60 mg/dL or more) negates one other risk factor in tallying a person's risk. A low HDL value of less than 35 milligrams per deciliter is added as a risk factor. Increased HDL levels related to exercise have been clearly demonstrated in men, but the findings are controversial in women (Hartung, 1995).

Adding to this complex issue is a nutrient-drug interaction. Beta-adrenergic blocking agents, given for hypertension and angina, increase serum triglyceride and VLDL levels (Lamont, 1995).

Diabetes Mellitus

At any given cholesterol level, diabetic persons have two to three times the risk of atherosclerosis as other people. Diabetic women lose the preventive advantages usually associated with women regarding cardiovascular risk.

Insulin is required to maintain adequate levels of **lipoprotein lipase,** an enzyme that breaks down chylomicrons. When lipoprotein lipase is inadequate, chylomicrons and VLDL particles accumulate in the blood. After the diabetes is controlled, serum lipid levels decrease. Lipoprotein lipase is more active in physically active subjects and increases with exercise. Another example of altered physiology is described in Box 19–2, relating undernutrition in utero to increased risk for diabetes mellitus and cardiovascular disease in adulthood.

Prevention of Cardiovascular Disease

Prevention of cardiovascular disease depends on minimizing a person's changeable risk factors. Focused on hypertension, these are: weight control, decreased sodium intake, regular exercise, and moderation in alcohol consumption. Modifying the changeable risk factors for CHD would entail: smoking cessation, decreased saturated fat intake, and control of diabetes mellitus.

People in the United States have changed their sources of animal protein between 1977 and 1987. Red meat consumption decreased from 91 to 73 pounds per person per year. Chicken consumption increased from 30 to 43 pounds and seafood from 13 to 15 pounds in the same period (Denke, 1994).

TABLE 19–4 Functions and Significance of Various Lipoproteins

Lipoprotein	Normal Value in 12- to 14-Hour Fasting Specimen	Function	Clinical Significance
Chylomicrons	0	Transport exogenous triglycerides from intestines to blood stream	Present in blood only after a meal
VLDL	13–32 mg/dL	Main transporter of endogenous triglyceride	Synthesized by liver and small intestine from free fatty acids, glycerol, and carbohydrate
LDL	38–40 mg/dL	Transports cholesterol to body cells	Major form of lipoprotein in atherosclerotic lesions. The higher the LDL level, the greater the risk of CHD
HDL	20–48 mg/dL	Transports cholesterol from body cells to liver to be excreted	Synthesized by liver and intestines. The higher the HDL level, the lower the risk of CHD; aerobic exercise increases HDL level in men but only slightly in women

BOX 19–1   RESEARCH ON ANTIOXIDANTS IN CARDIOVASCULAR DISEASE

Animal subjects fed antioxidants showed regression in their atherosclerotic lesions (Fuller and Jialal, 1994). In laboratory experiments, the antioxidant vitamins are expended in a particular order: C, E, and beta-carotene (Frei, B, 1994). High dietary intake of these vitamins was inversely correlated with coronary heart disease in 5133 Finnish men and women (Abbey, Noakes, and Nestel, 1995).

Higher vitamin E intake was associated with a lower incidence of CHD (Rimm, et al, 1993; Stampfer, et al, 1993) and with lower coronary mortality (Knekt, et al, 1994; Kushi, et al, 1996). The vitamin E reciprocally-sparing-mineral, selenium, was lower in the blood of acute MI clients than in healthy controls.

Beta-carotene intake through vegetables and fruit was inversely related to cardiovascular mortality and to incidence of myocardial infarction. Men in the placebo group of a hyperlipidemia study with the highest total serum **carotenoid** levels (of which beta carotene is only 25 percent) had a **relative risk** of CHD events of 0.64 compared to men with the lowest serum carotenoid levels (Morris, Kritchevsky, and Davis, 1994). Supplements of beta carotene were not effective in reducing cardiovascular disease (Hennekens, et al, 1996).

Antioxidant flavonoids, found in vegetables, fruits, tea and wine, inhibit oxidation of LDL and reduce thrombotic tendency in laboratory experiments. A high flavonoid intake in elderly men, mainly from tea, onions, and apples, was associated with lower mortality from CHD (Hertog, et al, 1993). A similar association was found for women, but not men, in Finland (Knekt, et al, 1996). After 25 years of follow-up in a cross-cultural study, intake of flavonoids was inversely associated with CHD mortality and explained about 25 percent of the variance in CHD rates in 7 countries (Hertoz, et al, 1995).

The declining heart disease rate has been correlated with increased fruit and vegetable consumption in the United States. In large prospective studies women with the highest intakes of beta-carotene and vitamin E had a 22 percent and 34 percent reduction in the risk of coronary events; men showed a 25 percent and 39 percent reduction (Gaziano, 1994). The evidence is not conclusive, but reinforces the importance of ample fruits and vegetables in the diet.

To implement the Food Pyramid recommendations, meats, fish, and poultry should be baked, broiled, or grilled, not fried. Legumes are an excellent meat substitute and contribute soluble fiber.

Not all animal fat is equally threatening to one's heart and blood vessels. Eskimos following their traditional diet eat a lot of animal fat; they also have a low rate of CHD. Many researchers attribute this to the high omega-3 fatty acid content of the fish Eskimos eat. Cold water ocean fish, some cold water inland fish, and some other foods contain this substance in varying amounts. It helps to decrease serum triglycerides, while lowering total cholesterol and blood pressure. Fish that contain omega-3 fatty acids include herring, mackerel, rainbow trout, salmon, swordfish, and tuna. Risk of death from CHD was 25 percent less in health professionals eating some fish versus those eating none at all. One or two servings a week seems to achieve maximum results (Katon, 1995). Fish intake was not related to coronary disease risk (Ascherio, et al, 1995) but was inversely related to the risk of primary cardiac arrest possibly because of changes in the cell membrane fatty acid composition (Siscovick, et al, 1995). Not all research is easily interpreted. Clinical Application 19–1 describes apparent paradoxes in diet and disease in different countries. Other food sources of omega-3 fatty acids are butternuts, soybeans, and walnuts.

Low-density lipoprotein (LDL)—A plasma protein containing more cholesterol and triglycerides than protein; elevated blood levels are associated with increased risk of heart disease.

High-density lipoproteins (HDL)—A plasma protein which carries fat in the bloodstream to the tissues or to the liver to be excreted; elevated blood levels are associated with a decreased risk of heart disease.

BOX 19–2 FETAL NUTRITION AND CARDIOVASCULAR DISEASE IN ADULTHOOD

Studies have connected low growth rates in utero and in infancy with high death rates from cardiovascular disease. The associations are seen in small for gestational age (SGA) babies rather than premature infants, and are independent of social class or lifestyle. Babies who are thin at birth tend to be insulin resistant as adults and have a high prevalence of diabetes mellitus, hypertension, and hyperlipidemia as adults. It is suggested that undernutrition during gestation alters the relationships between glucose and insulin and between growth hormone and insulin-like growth factors. In this way, the fetus adapts to its environment to permit survival, but its changed physiology makes it susceptible to cardiovascular disease in later life (Barker, et al, 1993).

CLINICAL APPLICATION 19–1

The Limits of Population Studies

In the 1960s, the lowest rates of heart disease reported among 7 countries were in Japan and Greece. People in those two countries were poles apart in fat consumption: 10 percent of kilocalories in Japan; 40 percent on the island of Crete. The Greeks derived 33 percent of their kilocalories from olive oil, which is 82 percent monounsaturated, and less than 10 percent of kilocalories from animal protein. A high monounsaturated fat intake was inversely correlated with cardiovascular disease. Diets high in monounsaturates enhance the resistance of LDL cholesterol to oxidation, whereas polyunsaturates are more susceptible to oxidation (Hiser, E, 1995).

Since 1976, a decrease in cardiovascular mortality in men and women was experienced in Spain despite increased intakes of dairy products and meat, particularly pork and poultry. If attention focused only on those foods, the rationale for the decreased mortality would be missed. Spanish intakes of fish and fruit also increased but consumption of olive oil, sugar, carbohydrates, and wine decreased. Most of the decrease in cardiovascular mortality was due to a decline in stroke mortality. Improved hypertension control, including decreased intake of salt and salt-cured foods, is thought to have influenced this trend. Other contributing factors are increased consumption of fruit and fish, reduction in cigarette smoking, and expanded access to clinical care, including a major increase in aspirin as a platelet inhibitor (Serra-Majem, L, et al, 1995).

Among 21 countries, The highest alcohol intake, the highest wine intake, and the second lowest coronary heart disease mortality rate was in France. Between 1965 and 1988, annual wine **ethanol** intake decreased from 13.3 to 9.1 L per person. If the wine were preventing deaths from heart disease, the mortality rate from CHD should have risen. Instead it fell from 94.9/100,000 to 71.3/100,000. Other studies showed a maximum protective effect of alcohol against CHD at one to two drinks per day. Higher alcohol intake is progressively associated with higher risks of cardiovascular disease and other causes of mortality. Simultaneously with the decrease in CHD deaths, French mortality from cirrhosis of the liver fell precipitously, from 68.5/100,000 to 37.9/100,000 (Criqui and Ringel, 1994). In Spain, too, a decline in alcohol consumption was reflected in a decrease in mortality from cirrhosis of the liver. It is suggested that antioxidant flavonoids in red wine, not alcohol, contributes to wine's protective effect against heart disease (Hertog, et al, 1993; van Poppel, et al, 1994) by inhibiting the copper-catalysed oxidation of LDL (Frankel, et al, 1993). Given the potential for abuse, no one should propose alcohol as a preventive measure against heart disease. The dietary guideline is "If you drink alcoholic beverages, do so in moderation."

Men in eastern Finland have one the highest recorded incidence of an mortality from CHD. An early study reported an association between high levels of stored iron (as assessed by serum ferritin levels) and increased risk for acute myocardial infarction (Salonen, et al, 1992). Iron overload was hypothesized to cause the higher occurrence of CHD in men compared to women. Subsequent studies on other populations did not support the relationship between iron and coronary heart disease (Cooper and Liao, 1993; Rimm, et al, 1993), between iron and carotid atherosclerosis (Rauramaa, et al, 1993; Rauramaa, et al, 1994), or between iron and myocardial infarction (Stampfer, et al, 1993). Another investigation on the same Finnish men correlated a high intake of mercury from nonfatty freshwater fish with an excess risk of acute myocardial infarction possibly due to promotion of lipid peroxidation by mercury (Salonen, et al, 1995).

Thus evidence accumulates slowly and must be interpreted cautiously. Many correlations are found in large studies but do not prove causation and may not be clinically useful. In human beings, multiple factors may be interacting to produce the result.

Dietary Modifications in Cardiovascular Disease

The major diet modifications for clients with cardiovascular disease involve cholesterol and sodium. In addition to weight control, sodium restriction may be effective for some clients with hypertension. Dietary intervention is recommended for six weeks in cases of mild hypertension before other treatments are instituted. Although clinical trials often isolate specific nutrients or foods to test, a diet prescription most likely will use a multipronged approach.

Cholesterol-lowering Diets

Based on large studies of blood cholesterol, 32 percent of men and 27 percent of women would be candidates for dietary intervention (Sempos, et al, 1993). A cardiovascular screening program in Canada identified only 14 percent of 3432 participants with high blood cholesterol. Of these, only 203 or 6 percent of those screened, were newly identified (Strychar, et al, 1994).

The Step 1 and Step 2 Diets

Dietary modification for hyperlipoproteinemia is well structured. The Step 1 diet is usually reviewed with the client in the physician's or clinic office, often by the nurse. A reduction of total and LDL cholesterol of 10 to 20 percent is the expected outcome (Sempos, et al, 1993; Williams and Bollella, 1995). If, after 3 months, no significant change is seen in serum cholesterol levels, the client is referred to a registered dietitian for instruction in the Step 2 diet. Only after 6 months of intensive dietary therapy and counseling should drug therapy be considered. Of 606 clients of cardiologists, 92 percent had received dietary literature, but only 31 percent reported completely understanding of it. A minimum of four nutrition counseling sessions is recommended (Plous, Chesne, and McDowell, 1995). If used, drug therapy is added to dietary therapy, not substituted for it. Clients with established CHD or atherosclerotic disease should begin immediately on the Step 2 diet (Expert Panel, 1993). The standards for the Step 1 and Step 2 diets are shown in Table 19–5. The diets are profiled in Table 19–6.

Rationale for Selection of Foods

Clients should be taught healthy choices and portion control, not that any foods are good or bad.

Some of the reasons certain foods should be limited are given below.

FAT   Monounsaturated fats may significantly lower LDL and cholesterol as well as protect against blood clots. Any oil contributes substantial kilocalories. See Figure 19–3.

Reducing saturated fat intake decreases blood cholesterol more than reducing dietary cholesterol. Two saturated fatty acids, palmitic acid in whole milk and stearic acid in red meat, increase cholesterol levels. Using nonfat or low-fat dairy products rather than higher fat ones can reduce fat intake by as much as 90 percent. Warm water rinsing of crumbled ground beef containing 30 percent fat reduced its fat content by 33 to 52 percent (Love and Prusa, 1992). Other techniques to reduce fat in meat are shown in Figure 19–4.

A dietary trial of survivors of myocardial infarction was stopped after an average of 27 months because the experimental group had a 73 percent reduction in risk of re-infarction or death compared to the control group (de Lorgeril, et al, 1994). The diet used more bread, more vegetables, more fish, less red meat replaced by poultry, and fruit every day. Olive or canola oils and canola margarine were the only fats used for salad and food preparation. Despite the significant differences in outcomes, no difference between groups was shown in serum cholesterol, triglycerides, or HDLs.

Sometimes a dietary change to improve health has unexpected consequences, as happened when hydrogenated vegetable oils were substituted for saturated fats. Hydrogenation increases the amount of trans fatty acids in the product (see illustration of trans fatty acid in Chapter 4, "Fats"). Intake of trans fatty acids was directly related to the risk of CHD in

TABLE 19–5   Standards for the Step 1 and Step 2 Diets

	Step 1 Diet Percent Total Kilocalories	Step 2 Diet Percent Total Kilocalories
Total fat	<30	<30
Saturated	<10	<7
Polyunsaturated	<10	<10
Monosaturated	10–15	10–15
Carbohydrate	50–60	50–60
Protein	10–20	10–20
Cholesterol	<300 mg/day	<200 mg/day

Kilocalories sufficient to achieve and maintain healthy body weight.

TABLE 19–6   Cholesterol-Lowering Diets

Description	Indication	Adequacy
These diets limit lipids. The Step 1 diet is strict interpretation of the Food Pyramid. The Step 2 diet is more restrictive.	These diets are prescribed when clients have elevated serum cholesterol.	The diets are adequate in all nutrients with the possible exception of iron because of the restriction on red meat. If the client is also on a sodium restricted diet, imitation cheese, bacon, and eggs may exceed the prescription. Clients must be encouraged to consume enough energy to maintain a healthy body weight.

Food Group	Allowed	Avoided

Milk
  Step 1:
    3 servings/day
  Step 2:
    2 servings/day
	Skim milk, 1 percent milk, cultured buttermilk, evaporated skim or nonfat milk
	Nonfat or low-fat yogurt and frozen yogurt
	Low-fat soft cheese
	  Farmer and pot labeled no more than 2 to 6 g of fat/oz
	1 percent or 2 percent fat cottage cheese
		Whole milk, regular, evaporated, condensed
		Cream: half-and-half, most nondairy creamers
		Real or nondairy whipped cream
		High fat cheeses: Neufchatel, Brie, American, feta, mozzarella, cheddar, muenster
		Cream cheese
		Ice cream
		Sour cream
		Custard-style yogurt
		Whole-milk ricotta

Breads and Cereals
  Step 1:
    4–7 servings/day
  Step 2:
    5–8 servings/day
	Breads: whole wheat, rye, pumpernickel, pita, white, bagels, English muffins, sandwich buns, dinner rolls, rice cakes made without whole milk, eggs, or butter
	Low-fat crackers: sticks, rye crisp, saltines, zwieback
	Hot cereals, most dry cold cereals
	Pasta: noodles, macaroni, spaghetti
	Rice
	Dried peas and beans, split peas, black-eyed peas, chick peas, kidney beans, navy beans, lentils, soybeans, low-fat tofu
		Croissants, butter rolls, sweet rolls, Danish pastry, doughnuts
		Most snack crackers: cheese crackers, butter crackers, crackers containing saturated fat
		Granola-type cereal containing saturated fat
		Egg noodles
		Pasta and rice made with cream, butter, or cheese sauce

Fruits & Vegetables
  Steps 1 and 2:
    3 fruit servings/day
    4 vegetable servings/day
	Fresh, frozen, canned, or dried	Those prepared with butter, cream, or cheese sauce

TABLE 19–6   Cholesterol-Lowering Diets (Continued)

Food Group	Allowed	Avoided
Meat, Poultry, Fish, Shellfish *Steps 1 and 2:* 6 oz/day	Lean meat with fat trimmed: Beef-round, sirloin, chuck, loin Lamb—leg, arm, loin, rib Pork-tenderloin, leg, shoulder Veal—all except ground Poultry without skin Fish, shellfish Refer to very lean meat and substitutes list	Prime grade Fatty meat: Beef-corned, brisket, short ribs, regular ground Pork-spare ribs Goose, domestic duck Organ meats: liver, sweetbread brain, kidney Sausage, bacon Regular luncheon meats Frankfurters Caviar, roe
Eggs *Step 1:* 3 yolks/week *Step 2:* 2 yolks/week	Egg whites Cholesterol-free egg substitutes	Egg yolks except as specified
Fats and Oils *Step 1:* 4–6 servings/day *Step 2:* 5–7 servings/day	Polyunsaturated: Corn, safflower, sunflower, sesame, soybean Monounsaturated: Peanut, olive, canola (rapeseed) Margarine or shortening high in unsaturated fatty acids: tub, diet, liquid, stick with <2 g of saturated fat/tbsp Mayo, salad dressing high in unsaturated fats Low-fat dressings	Saturated oils and fat: butter, lard, bacon fat, coconut, palm, and palm kernel oils Margarine or shortening high in saturated fatty acid Dressings made with egg yolk
Desserts and Miscellaneous *Step 1 and 2:* 2 servings/day	Low-fat frozen desserts: sorbet, sherbet, Italian ice, frozen yogurt, popsicles Angel food cake Low-fat cookies: fig bars, gingersnaps Low-fat candy: hard candy, jelly beans Low-fat snacks: pretzels, plain popcorn Nonfat beverages: carbonated drinks, juices, tea, coffee	High-fat frozen desserts: ice cream, frozen tofu High-fat cakes: most store-bought, pound, frosted cakes Store-bought pie Most store-bought cookies Most candy Chips made with saturated fat Buttered popcorn High-fat beverages: frappes, milkshakes, floats, eggnogs

Sample Menus, Step 1

Breakfast	Lunch and Dinner
1/2 grapefruit 1/2 cup oatmeal 1 bagel 2 tsp. reduced fat margarine 1/2 cup skim milk Coffee	3 oz chicken or fish, baked without skin Wild rice Three bean salad with olive oil and vinegar Dinner roll with honey 1/2 cup steamed asparagus Angel food cake with strawberries 1 cup skim milk Herb tea

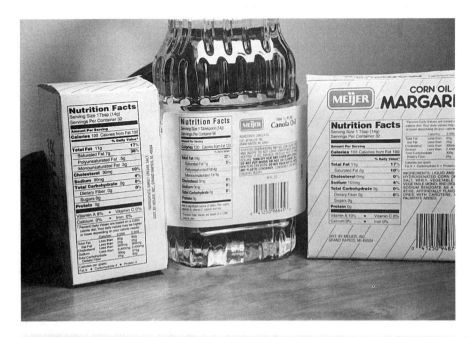

FIGURE 19–3 These labels clearly list the saturated fat in 1 tbsp of the product. Butter has 11 g; canola oil, 1 g; and corn oil margarine, 2 g.

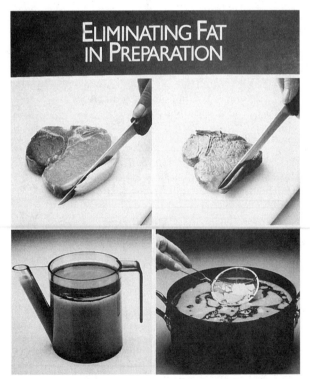

FIGURE 19–4 Selecting lean meat, trimming off visible fat, and skimming fat from meat juices reduce the amount of fat consumed. (From National Live Stock and Meat Board, Chicago, 1990, with permission.)

women (Willett, et al, 1993) and to risk of myocardial infarction in both men and women (Ascherio, et al, 1994). The latter increased risk was significant only for clients consuming more than 2 1/2 pats of margarine per day compared to those consuming less than 1 pat per day. Liquid or soft (tub) margarines generally have lower trans fatty acid content than hard (stick) margarines but even hard margarines have less cholesterol-raising potential than butter (Expert Panel, 1994).

FIBER Soluble fiber lowers serum cholesterol by binding with it, promoting fecal elimination. Examples of foods high in soluble fiber are: legumes, oats, barley, broccoli, apples, and citrus fruits. A diet supplemented with oat bran reduced the LDL levels by an additional 6 percent in children with hypercholesterolemia (Williams, 1995). After adjusting for other risk factors, a 10 gram increase in dietary fiber was associated with a 44 percent decrease in MI. Further analysis indicated cereal fiber, rather than vegetable or fruit fiber, was the main reason for the reduction (Rimm, et al, 1996).

The soybean diet, the most potent dietary tool to treat hypercholesterolemia, has given a 20 percent reduction in LDL levels. It is not effective in individuals with normal cholesterol values, suggesting that soy protein stimulates LDL receptors, which are chronically depressed in hypercholesterolemia

(Sirtori, et al, 1995). The search for more palatable soy products is ongoing (Klein, Perry, and Adair, 1995).

SUGAR   In persons with elevated serum triglycerides, a high-sucrose intake further increases triglyceride levels. Almost any recipe can be satisfactorily made with two-thirds to three-fourths the usual sugar. Increasing the amounts of vanilla extract and cinnamon will give the impression of sweetness.

Diet Tailored to Types of Hyperlipoproteinemia

Because of altered physiology, clients with the different types of hyperlipoproteinemia may need modification of the cholesterol-lowering diets. The dietitian will work with clients to maximize compliance.

Beyond the general recommendations to lower saturated fat consumption, clients with hyperlipoproteinemia need more stringent diets. All of these clients who are overweight are urged to lose the excess weight. You may wish to refer again to Table 19–2 as you read about diet modifications for the different types of hyperlipoproteinemias.

TYPE 1   This person is deficient in the enzyme triglyceride lipase. The serum chylomicrons are elevated because they carry the exogenous triglyceride in the bloodstream after meals. To treat this condition, food sources of triglyceride are restricted. Usually a 20- to 30-gram fat diet is prescribed, which generally limits the person to 3 to 4 ounces of lean meat per day.

TYPE 2A   This diet contains less than 200 milligrams of cholesterol per day. LDL and cholesterol elevations characterize Type 2A hyperlipoproteinemia. Polyunsaturated and monounsaturated fats should outnumber saturated fats by a factor of 1.5 or 2 to 1.

TYPE 2B   This diet is the same as for Type 2A, plus limitation in alcohol and high-carbohydrate foods, especially simple sugars. In Type 2B hyperlipoproteinemia, triglyceride levels are elevated, whereas in Type 2A they are not. Alcohol and carbohydrate stimulate triglyceride production, and therefore are to be restricted. Usually the diet is calculated to provide only 40 percent of the kilocalories from carbohydrate.

TYPE 3   Carbohydrate aggravates Type 3 hyperlipoproteinemia. Here dietary carbohydrate is limited to 35 to 40 percent of kilocalories. Because triglycerides are elevated, alcohol and sugar should be restricted. If cholesterol levels continue to be high after weight loss, dietary cholesterol should be moderately reduced.

TYPE 4   This very common hyperlipoproteinemia also is aggravated by carbohydrate. Therefore only 35 to 40 percent of kilocalories come from carbohydrate. Triglycerides are elevated, so sugar intake should be limited. Alcohol should be consumed at a rate of 1 to 2 ounces per week, if at all.

TYPE 5   Type 5 hyperlipoproteinemia is treated the same as Type 4. In fact, excessive fat and kilocalorie intake can convert a severe Type 4 client into a Type 5.

Because all hyperlipoproteinemias are not the same, neither are the dietary treatments. For best results, the clinical dietitian should individualize the diet with the client.

Sodium-Controlled Diets

As many as one-third of mild hypertensive cases can be controlled with sodium restriction. Usually a 2 gram sodium diet is prescribed for mild hypertension. Up to 8 weeks may be necessary before results are seen. The preference for salty foods is learned and culturally transmitted even when heavy salting is no longer necessary for preservation of food. After 3 months on a sodium-restricted diet, most individuals lose their appetite for salt. Box 19–3 lists the legal definitions for sodium and salt descriptions on labels.

Unseen contributions to sodium intake may come from other beverages, over-the-counter medications, and drinking water. Table 19–7 lists sodium content of beverages. Many toothpastes and mouthwashes contain significant amounts of sodium and should not be swallowed. Over-the-counter medications that may contain significant amounts of sodium include: analgesics, antacids, antibiotics, antitussives, laxative, and sedatives.

The American Heart Association recommends a limit of 20 milligrams of sodium per liter of water as a standard for persons who require a restricted sodium diet. As much as 42 percent of the nation's water supply exceeds this amount (Korch, 1986). Many municipal water supplies are softened, which can increase the water's sodium content excessively. City water supplies vary from 1.2 milligrams per liter in Seattle to 100 milligrams per liter in Phoenix.

Many households have water softeners in their homes that increase the water's sodium content. Clients who require a diet containing less than 2 grams of sodium may have to use bottled, distilled,

BOX 19–3 LABELING REGULATIONS FOR SODIUM CONTENT DESCRIPTORS

Term	Legal Definition
Free	Less than 5 mg of sodium per serving.
Salt Free	Must meet the criteria for free.
Very Low* Sodium	Less than 35 mg of sodium per serving. For meals and main dishes: 35 mg or less per 100 g.
Low* Sodium	Less than 140 mg of sodium per serving. Meals and main dishes: 140 mg or less per 100 g.
Reduced or Less	This term means that a nutritionally altered product contains 25 percent less sodium than the regular, or reference, product. However, a reduced claim can't be made on a product if its reference food already meets the requirement for a "low" claim.
Light in sodium or Lightly salted	May be used on food in which the sodium content has been reduced by at least 50 percent compared to an appropriate reference food.
Unsalted or No Added Salt	Must declare "This is not a sodium free food" on information panel if the food is not sodium free.

* Synonyms for low include "little," "few," and "low source of".

deionized, or demineralized water for drinking and cooking.

Consideration should be given to the sodium content of specialty bottled waters also. "Mineral waters" contain from 8 to 172 milligrams of sodium per liter. "Read the label" is appropriate advice here.

The amount of sodium in foods can be calculated.

Many dietitians will work with a client to develop individualized diet plans. Some clients prefer a daily allotment of salt in a shaker to be used as desired. If this strategy is adopted, the foods high in sodium must be limited to a greater extent than used on a standardized sodium-controlled diet.

A number of salt substitutes are available. Many of

TABLE 19–7 Sodium Content of Beverages*

Beverage†	Regular Sodium (mg)	Regular Kilocalories	Diet Sodium (mg)	Diet Kilocalories
Club soda			75	0
Cola	15	151		
With aspartame			21	2
With saccharin			75	2
Gatorade	39	123		
Ginger ale	25	125	130	4
Kool-Aid	0	150		
With aspartame			0	6
Lemonade	12	150		
Lemon-lime soda	41	149	70	4
Pepper-type	38	151	70	0
Root beer	49	152	170	4

* Serving size is 12 fluid ounces.
† Sodium content may vary, depending on the source of water.

TABLE 19–8   Sodium-Controlled Diets

Description	Indication	Adequacy
These diets control sodium intake to prescribed levels.	Clients with hypertension, congestive heart failure, fluid-retaining kidney or endocrine disease, or other edematous conditions.	The 500 mg and 250 mg diets may be deficient in some nutrients.

Meal Plans for Restricted-Sodium Meal Plan				
Food/Item or Group	2 Grams	1 Gram	500 Milligrams	250 Milligrams
Soups	LS*	LS	LS	LS
Milk	2 cups	2 cups	1 cup	LS
Bread	3 slices	3 slices	LS	LS
Cereal	1 serving	LS	LS	LS
Fruits	Free	Free	Free	Free
Egg	1	1	1	1
Meat/substitutes	6 oz	5 oz	4 oz	4 oz
Vegetables	LS	LS	LS	LS
Desserts	1 serving	LS	LS	LS
Margarine	5 tsp	3 tsp	3 tsp	LS
Condiments	LS	LS	LS	LS

Food Group	Lower in Sodium (LS)	Higher in Sodium
Milk	Commercially made low-sodium milk Low-sodium cheese	All milk from animals Yogurt Regular cheese Commercial milk products
Breads and cereals	Bread and crackers prepared without salt Rice, barley, and pasta without added salt Baked goods made without salt, baking soda, or baking powder Unsalted cooked cereal Puffed rice, puffed wheat, shredded wheat Cornmeal, cornstarch	Commercial mixes Frozen bread dough Regular crackers Instant rice and pasta mixes Instant and quick cooking cereals Commercial stuffing and casserole mixes Self-rising flour and cornmeal Baked goods and quick breads made with salt, baking soda, baking powder, or egg white
Fruits	Fresh, frozen, dried, or canned fruit without added sodium All fruit juices	Crystallized or glazed fruit Maraschino cherries Dried fruit with sodium preservatives
Vegetables	Fresh, frozen without salt, low-sodium canned vegetables except those listed at right	Canned and frozen vegetables and juices Sauerkraut

Table continued on following page

them use potassium instead of sodium. These may be unsuitable for clients with kidney disease or those taking potassium-sparing diuretics. Salt substitutes are not useful for cooking because they turn bitter.

In clinical practice, diet orders such as "no-added-salt diet" or "low-sodium diet" require clarification. Usually, a facility's diet manual defines the terms. A "no-added-salt diet" may be calculated as 4 grams of sodium and a "low-sodium diet" as 2 grams in one facility and at different levels in another. Table 19–8 describes diets with various levels of sodium control.

Other Modifications

Clients on potassium-wasting diuretics may require dietary or supplemental potassium. The choices become more complex when the client also receives a sodium-controlled diet. In general, fruits are high in potassium and low in sodium. Another adjunct source of supplemental potassium is a salt substitute.

After a heart attack, the client is in shock. One adaptive response of the body is to slow gastrointestinal function. Thus the client should receive

TABLE 19–8   Sodium-Controlled Diets (Continued)

Food Group	Lower in Sodium (LS)	Higher in Sodium
Meat, poultry, fish, shellfish	Fresh, frozen, or canned low-sodium meat and poultry Low sodium luncheon meats Eggs Low-sodium peanut butter Fresh fish Canned low-sodium tuna and salmon	Real and imitation bacon Luncheon meat Chipped or corned beef Smoked or salted meat or fish Kosher meat Frozen and powdered egg substitutes Regular peanut butter Brain, kidney, clams, lobster, crab, oysters, scallops, shrimp, and other shellfish
Fats and oils	Cooking oil Unsalted butter, margarine, salad dressings, and shortening	Salted butter and margarine Commercial salad dressings
Desserts and miscellaneous	Alcohol Coffee, coffee substitutes Lemonade Tea Low-sodium candy Unflavored gelatin Jam, jelly, maple syrup, honey Unsalted nuts and popcorn	Regular canned or frozen soups Soup mixes Salted popcorn, nuts, potato chips, snacks Instant cocoa or powdered drink mixes Canned fruit drinks Commercial pastry, candy, cakes, cookies, gelatin desserts
Condiments and seasonings	Sweet: Allspice, Almond extract, Anise seed, Apricot nectar, Baking chocolate, Cardamon, Cinnamon, Coriander, Ginger, Lemon extract, Lemon juice, Mace, Maple extract, Mint, Nutmeg, Orange extract, Orange juice, Peppermint extract, Pineapple, Pineapple juice, Unsalted pecans, Vanilla extract, Unsalted walnuts, Walnut extract Tangy: Basil, Bay leaves, Caraway seeds, Cayenne pepper, Chili powder, Chives, Cloves, Curry powder, Dill weed, Garlic, Garlic powder (not salt), Green pepper, Horseradish without salt, Marjoram, Mustard powder (not prepared), Mustard seed, Onion powder (not salt) Onions, Oregano, Paprika, Parsley, Pepper, Poppy seed, Rosemary, Sage, Savory, Sesame seeds, Tarragon, Thyme, Turmeric	Any salt Barbecue sauce Bouillon cubes or granules Catsup Chili sauce Tartar sauce Horseradish sauce Meat extracts, sauces, and tenderizers Kitchen Bouquet Gravy and sauce mixes Monosodium glutamate Prepared mustard Olives Pickles Saccharin, other sugar substitutes containing sodium Soy sauce Teriyaki sauce Worcestershire sauce

Sample Menus for 2-g Sodium Diet	
Breakfast	**Lunch and Dinner**
1/2 cup orange juice 1/2 cup shredded wheat 2 slices toast 2 tsp margarine 1 tbsp strawberry jam 1 cup 1 percent milk Sugar Coffee	3 oz chicken breast, turkey, or fish baked in lemon juice Baked potato 2 tsp margarine 1/2 cup broccoli Tossed salad with homemade oil and vinegar dressing 1 dinner roll 1/2 cup sherbet 1 cup 1 percent milk (one meal only) Tea

* LS any food on the following lower in sodium list.

nothing by mouth while shock persists. Fluid is given intravenously to maintain fluid balance and to keep an access site open for intravenous medications. As the client recovers, the diet usually progresses from a 1000- to 1200-kilocalorie liquid diet to a soft, "cardiac" diet of small, frequent meals. Large meals can increase the workload of the heart. Food is served at a moderate temperature. Very hot or very cold foods are thought to produce irregular heart rhythms.

Caffeine should be avoided by clients after heart attacks. Normal people have been observed to have serious **arrhythmias** after 9 or more cups of coffee or tea. Persons with histories of abnormal rhythms showed the same effects after 2 cups. The hypertensive client should use caffeine in moderation because it increases blood pressure.

For the person in congestive heart failure, the diet order may read "as tolerated." Food should be easily eaten and easily digested. An hour's rest before meals conserves energy. Large meals, which would exert upward pressure on the chest, are undesirable. Liquid formulas can be used to provide nutrients without fullness.

The person who has had a stroke may have chewing or swallowing problems. Often, thicker rather than thinner liquids are easier for a person with swallowing difficulty to manage. The nurse feeding a client with hemiplegia should place the food on the unaffected side of the tongue. Turning the client's head toward the weak side while sitting upright may help with swallowing. In addition, stroke clients may be aphasic and unable to communicate their needs or desires. A speech therapist is skilled in adaptive devices and restorative therapy for clients with dysphagia and aphasia.

Summary

Cardiovascular diseases are responsible for more deaths in the United States than are diseases of any other body system. Some of the causative factors such as age, sex, race, and heredity are beyond a person's control. Other risk factors can be modified by a motivated person.

Underlying pathology in cardiovascular diseases involves both atherosclerosis and hypertension. Each reinforces the other in a vicious circle, often leading to coronary heart disease, congestive heart failure, or stroke.

The most important risk factors for coronary heart disease are cigarette smoking, hypertension, and elevated blood cholesterol. The most important risk factors for hypertension are obesity, excessive salt intake, inactivity, and alcohol consumption.

Closely linked to cardiovascular diseases are specific elevations of blood lipids and lipoproteins. The most common hyperlipoproteinemia is type 4. It is aggravated by carbohydrate intake, which must be limited as part of the treatment.

Dietary modifications in cardiovascular disease most often involve cholesterol-lowering or sodium-controlling measures. Other qualities of the diet may require adjustment, such as potassium intake, amount, timing, and texture of meals.

Arrhythmia—Irregular heartbeat.

Case Study 19–1 Mr. Z is a 59-year-old white man who was admitted to the acute care hospital with a diagnosis of possible myocardial infarction. Subsequent testing proved Mr. Z did not have an infarction. His medical diagnoses are myocardial ischemia and type 4 hyperlipoproteinemia. He is being readied for discharge to home.

Mr. Z is vice president for sales of a large manufacturing company. His business activities involve luncheon and dinner meetings at which alcohol consumption is common. He stated he has "at least one cocktail, usually two" with lunch and with dinner.

The clinical dietitian visited Mr. Z to instruct him on the diet prescribed by the physician. After the dietitian left, Mr. Z said to the nurse, "That diet is impossible for my situation. She just doesn't understand the business world. I don't believe there's anything wrong with my heart, anyway. It was just indigestion."

Providing client care is a dynamic process. Based on the above information, the nurse added the following modifications to Mr. Z's nursing care plan.

NURSING CARE PLAN

Assessment

Subjective Data	Reported alcohol intake of 2 to 4 oz per day
	Perceived incompatibility of prescribed diet with lifestyle
	Stated disbelief in medical diagnosis
Objective Data	Elevated blood VLDL and triglyceride

Nursing Diagnosis   Noncompliance: related to denial of illness and negative perception of treatment regimen as evidenced by statements to nurse.

Desired Outcome/ Evaluation Criteria	Nursing Actions	Rationale
Client will acknowledge consequences of noncompliant behavior by time of hospital discharge.	Review pathophysiology of hyperlioproteinemia and atherosclerosis with client.	Mr. Z is a competent adult. He is able to make his own choices. Repeating the information on atherosclerosis is an attempt to be sure his choice to reject the treatment regimen is informed.
	Analyze with the client the possibility of partial compliance.	Perhaps the many changes required are overwhelming Mr. Z. One or two alterations might be acceptable as a starting point.
	Obtain client's permission to discuss discharge instructions with significant other.	Enlisting a support person might, over time, give Mr. Z reason to reconsider his decision.
	Inform physician of extent of intended noncompliance.	This is a change in the client's mental condition. It is appropriate to notify the physician and record it on the client's medical record.

Study Aids

Chapter Review

1. The underlying pathological processes in cardiovascular disease are:
   a. Atherosclerosis and hypertension
   b. Coronary occlusion and obesity
   c. Diabetes mellitus and cerebrovascular accidents
   d. Kidney failure and congestive heart failure

2. The first action a hypertensive client should take to lower blood pressure is to:
   a. Restrict fluid to 1500 milliliters per day
   b. Eliminate saturated fat from the diet
   c. Lose weight if necessary
   d. Limit sodium intake to 1 gram per day

3. Soluble fiber also helps to lower blood cholesterol levels. Which of the following are good sources of soluble fiber?
   a. Broccoli and prunes
   b. Whole-wheat bread and grapes

c. Green beans and raspberries

d. Oats and legumes

4. Which of the following seasonings are permitted on a sodium controlled diet?

a. Catsup, horseradish mustard, and tartar sauce

b. Chili powder, green pepper, and poppy seeds

c. Celery seeds, seasoned meat tenderizer, and teriyaki sauce

d. Dry mustard, garlic, and Worcestershire sauce

5. A high sucrose intake is related to cardiovascular disease because:

a. Many cardiac clients have a genetic deficiency of sucrase.

b. A high-sugar diet causes hyperactivity and hypertension.

c. Excess sugar has to be excreted, causing premature aging of the kidney.

d. Sucrose is positively related to triglyceride levels in the body.

Clinical Analysis

Mr. T is a 55-year-old black man being seen in a health clinic for hypertension. His blood pressure was 150/102 three months ago when first diagnosed. It has remained below that level but has not returned to normal. Today his blood pressure is 146/100.

Mr. T is 5 feet 9 inches tall and weighs 173 pounds. He has a medium frame. When first diagnosed, he weighed 178 pounds. A weight-loss diet with no added salt was prescribed, but progress has been slow.

Now the physician is prescribing a 2-gram sodium diet and starting Mr. T on a mild potassium-wasting diuretic. The clinic nurse is responsible for instructing the client.

1. Before he or she instructs Mr. T, which of the following actions by the nurse would best assure his compliance with the diet?

a. Doing a financial analysis to see if Mr. T can afford the special foods on his new diet

b. Finding out which favorite foods Mr. T would have most difficulty giving up

c. Listing the possible consequences of hypertension if it is not controlled

d. Asking to see Mrs. T to instruct her on the preparation of foods for the new diet

2. Which of the following breakfasts would be best for Mr. T?

a. Applesauce, raisin bran, 1 percent milk, and a bagel with cream cheese

b. Canned pears, cornflakes, whole milk, and a cholesterol-free plain doughnut

c. Cooked prunes, instant oatmeal, 2 percent milk, and raisin toast with margarine

d. Orange juice, shredded wheat, skim milk, and whole-wheat toast with jelly

3. Mr. T has agreed to limit his alcohol intake to two drinks per week. He asks the nurse to recommend beverages compatible with his diet. Which of the following is the best choice?

a. Tomato juice

b. Buttermilk

c. Diet cola with aspartame

d. Gatorade

Bibliography

10th anniversary of the NCEP. National Institutes of Health Heart Memo Summer NCEP Suppl:1, 1995.

Abbey, M, Noakes, M, and Nestel, PJ: Dietary supplementation with orange and carrot juice in cigarette smokers lowers oxidation products in copper-oxidized low-density lipoproteins. J Am Diet Assoc 95:671, 1995.

Allender, PS, et al: Dietary calcium and blood pressure: A meta-analysis of randomized clinical trials. Ann Intern Med 124:825, 1996.

Archer, L, Grant, BF, and Dawson, DA: What if Americans drank less? The potential effect on the prevalence of alcohol abuse and dependence. Am J Public Health 85:61, 1995.

Ascherio, A, et al: Dietary intake of marine n-3 fatty acids, fish intake, and the risk of coronary disease among men. N Engl J Med 332:977, 1995.

Ascherio, A, et al: Trans-fatty acids intake and risk of myocardial infarction. Circulation 89:94, 1994.

Barker, DJ, et al: Fetal nutrition and cardiovascular disease in adult life. Lancet 341:938, 1993.

Beadle, L: The management of dysphagia in stroke. Nurs Stand 9:37, 1995.

Brady, JA, Rock, CL, and Horneffer, MR: Thiamin status, diuretic medications, and the management of congestive heart failure. J Am Diet Assoc 95:541, 1995.

Bulliyya, G, et al: Fatty acid profile and the atherogenic risk in fish consuming and non fish consuming people. Indian J Med Sci 48:256, 1994.

Committee on Nutrition, American Academy of Pediatrics: Statement on Cholesterol. Pediatrics 90:469, 1992.

Cooper, RS, and Liao, Y: Iron stores and coronary heart disease: Negative findings in the NHANES I epidemiologic follow-up study (abstract). Circulation 87:35, 1993.

Corti, M-C, et al: HDL cholesterol predicts coronary heart disease mortality in older persons. JAMA 274:539, 1995.

Criqui, MH, and Ringel, BL: Does diet or alcohol explain the French paradox? Lancet 344:1719, 1994.

de Lorgeril, M, et al: Mediterranean alpha-linolenic acid-rich diet in secondary prevention of coronary heart disease. Lancet 343:1454, 1994.

Denke, MA: Role of beef and beef tallow, an enriched source of stearic acid, in a cholesterol-lowering diet. Am J Clin Nutr (suppl)60:1044S, 1994.

Donahue, PA: When it's hard to swallow. Journal of Gerontological Nursing 16:6, 1990.

Elliott, P, et al: Intersalt revisited: Further analyses of 24-hour sodium excretion and blood pressure within and across populations. Br Med J 312:1249, 1996.

Expert Panel on Detection, Evaluation and Treatment of High Blood Cholesterol in Adults (Adult Treatment Panel II): Second report of the Expert Panel on detection, evaluation and treatment of high blood cholesterol in adults (Adult Treatment Panel II). Circulation 89:1329, 1994.

Expert Panel on Detection, Evaluation and Treatment of High Blood Cholesterol in Adults: Summary of the second report of the National Cholesterol Education Program (NCEP) Expert Panel on detection, evaluation and treatment of high blood cholesterol in adults (Adult Treatment Panel II). JAMA 269:3015, 1993.

Feldman, EB: Essentials of Clinical Nutrition. FA Davis, Philadelphia, 1988.

Flavell, CM: Women and coronary heart disease. Prog Cardiovasc Nurs 9:18, 1994.

Frankel, EN, et al: Inhibition of oxidation of human low-density lipoprotein by phenolic substances in red wine. Lancet 341:454, 1993.

Frei, B: Reactive oxygen species and antioxidant vitamins: Mechanisms of action. Am J Med (suppl 3A)97:3A–5S, 1994.

Fuller, CJ, and Jialal, I: Effects of antioxidants and fatty acids on low-density-lipoprotein oxidation. Am J Clin Nutr (suppl)60:1010S–3S, 1994.

Gaziano, JM: Antioxidant vitamins and coronary artery disease risk. The American Journal of Medicine (suppl 3A)97:3A–18S, 1994.

Grace, ML, Crosby, FE, and Ventura, MR: Nutritional education for patients with peripheral vascular disease. J Health Educ 25:142, 1995.

Hartung, GH: Physical activity and high density lipoprotein cholesterol. J Sports Med Phys Fitness 35:1, 1995.

Hennekens, CH, et al: Lack of effect of long-term supplementation with beta carotene on the incidence of malignant neoplasms and cardiovascular disease. N Engl J Med 334:1145, 1996.

Hertog, MGL, et al: Dietary antioxidant flavonoids and risk of coronary heart disease: The Zutphen Elderly Study. Lancet 342:1007, 1993.

Hertog, MGL, et al: Flavonoid intake and long-term risk of coronary heart disease and cancer in the Seven Countries Study. Arch Intern Med 155:381, 1995.

Hiser, E: The Mediterranean diet and cardiovascular disease. J Cardiopulm Rehabil 15:179, 1995.

Johnson, CL, et al: Declining serum total cholesterol levels among US adults. JAMA 269:3002, 1993.

Karp, RJ: Problem of changing food habits: How food habits are formed. In Karp, RJ (ed): Malnourished Children in the United States. Springer, New York, 1993.

Katan, MB: Fish and heart disease: What is the real story? Nutrition Reviews 53:228, 1995.

Kirchhoff, KT, et al: Electrocardiographic response to ice water ingestion. Heart Lung 19:41, 1990.

Klasky, AL, and Friedman, GD: Annotation: Alcohol and longevity. Am J Public Health 85:16, 1995.

Klein, BP, Perry, AK, and Adair, N: Incorporating soy protein into baked products for use in clinical studies. J Nutr 125:666S–74S, 1995.

Knekt, P, et al: Antioxidant vitamin intake and coronary mortality in a longitudinal population study. Am J Epidemiol 139:1180, 1994.

Knekt, P, et al: Flavonoid intake and coronary mortality in Finland: A cohort study. Br Med J 312:478, 1996.

Korch, GC: Sodium content of potable water: Dietary significance. J Am Diet Assoc 86:80, 1986.

Krumholz, HM, et al: Lack of association between cholesterol and coronary heart disease mortality and morbidity and all-cause mortality in persons older than 70 years. JAMA 272:1335, 1994.

Kuski, LH, et al: Dietary antioxidant vitamins and death from coronary heart disease in postmenopausal women. N Engl J Med 334:1156, 1996.

Lamont, LS: Beta-blockers and their effect on protein metabolism and resting energy expenditure. J Cardiopulm Rehabil 15:183, 1995.

Love, JA, and Prusa, KJ: Nutrient composition and sensory attributes of cooked ground beef: Effects of fat content, cooking method, and water rinsing. J Am Diet Assoc 92:1367, 1992.

Martinez, G: Hypertension and electrolyte therapy. Progress in Cardiovascular Nursing 9:32, 1994.

Melby, CL, Toohey, ML, and Cebrick, J: Blood pressure and blood lipids among vegetarian, semivegetarian, and nonvegetarian African Americans. Am J Clin Nutr 59:103, 1994.

Mensink, RP, and Katan, MB: Effect of dietary trans fatty acids on high-density and low-density lipoprotein cholesterol levels in healthy subjects. N Engl J Med 323:439, 1990.

Montague, T, et al: Prevention and regression of coronary atherosclerosis. Chest 105:718, 1994.

Morris, DL, Kritchevsky, SB, and Davis, CE: Serum carotenoids and coronary heart disease. JAMA 272:1439, 1994.

Murray, ND, Young, RJ, and Reimers, KJ: The role of nutrition in cardiovascular disease. J Home Health Care Prac 4:13, 1991.

National High Blood Pressure Education Program: Working Group Report on Primary Prevention of Hypertension. National Institutes of Health (No. 93-2669), Bethesda, MD, 1993.

Plous, S, Chesne, RB, and McDowell, AV: Nutrition knowledge and attitudes of cardiac patients. J Am Diet Assoc 95:442, 1995.

Rauramaa, R, et al: Association of risk factors and body iron status to carotid atherosclerosis in middle-aged Eastern Finnish men. Eur Heart J 15:1020, 1994.

Rauramaa, R, et al: Association of risk factors and iron to carotid atherosclerosis in middle-aged Eastern Finnish men (abstract). Circulation (suppl)88:I-71, 1993.

Rimm, EB, et al: Dietary iron intake and risk of coronary disease among men (abstract). Circulation 87:692, 1993.

Rimm, EB, et al: Vegetable, fruit, and cereal fiber intake and risk of coronary heart disease among men. JAMA 275:447, 1996.

Rimm, EB, et al: Vitamin E consumption and the risk of coronary heart disease in men. N Engl J Med 328:1450, 1993.

Salonen, JT, et al: High stored iron levels are associated with excess risk of myocardial infarction in Eastern Finnish men. Circulation 86:803, 1992.

Salonen, JT, et al: Intake of mercury from fish, lipid peroxidation, and the risk of myocardial infarction and coronary, cardiovascular, and any death in Eastern Finnish men. Circulation 91:645, 1995.

Scanlon, VC, and Sanders T: Essentials of Anatomy and Physiology, ed 2. FA Davis, Philadelphia, 1995.

Sempos, CT, et al: Prevalence of high blood cholesterol among US adults. JAMA 269:3009, 1993.

Serra-Majem, L, et al: How could changes in diet explain changes in coronary heart disease mortality in Spain? The Spanish paradox. Am J Clin Nutr (suppl)61:1351S–9S, 1995.

Sirtori, CR, et al: Soy and cholesterol reduction: Clinical experience. J Nutr 125:598S–605S, 1995.

Siscovick, DS, et al: Dietary intake and cell membrane levels of long-chain n-3 polyunsaturated fatty acids and the risk of primary cardiac arrest. JAMA 274:1363, 1995.

Stampfer, MJ, et al: A prospective study of plasma ferritin and risk of myocardial infarction in US physicians (abstract). Circulation 87:688, 1993.

Stampfer, MJ, et al: Vitamin E consumption and the risk of coronary disease in women. N Engl J Med 328:1444, 1993.

Steinberg, D, et al: Antioxidants in the prevention of human atherosclerosis. Circulation 85:2338, 1992.

Strychar, IM, et al: A supermarket cardiovascular screening program: Analysis of participants' solicitation of follow-up care. Am J Prev Med 10:283, 1994.

Suzukawa, M, et al: Effects of supplementing with vitamin E on the uptake of low density lipoprotein and the stimulation of cholesterol ester formation in macrophages. Atherosclerosis 110:77, 1994.

Taylor, PA, and Ward, A: Women, high-density lipoprotein cholesterol, and exercise. Arch Intern Med 153:1178, 1993.

Van Horn, L, et al: Effects on serum lipids of adding instant oats to usual American diets. Am J Public Health 81:183, 1991.

van Poppel, G, et al: Antioxidants and coronary heart disease. Ann Med 26:429, 1994.

Verschuren, WMM, et al: Serum total cholesterol and long-term coronary heart disease mortality in different cultures. JAMA 274:131, 1995.

Willett, WC, et al: Intake of trans fatty acids and risk of coronary heart disease among women. Lancet 341:581, 1993.

Willett, WC, et al: Weight, weight change, and coronary heart disease in women. JAMA 273:461, 1995.

Williams, CL: Importance of dietary fiber in childhood. J Am Diet Assoc 95:1140, 1149, 1995.

Williams, CL, and Bollella, M: Guidelines for screening, evaluating, and treating children with hypercholesterolemia. J Pediatr Health Care 9:153, 1995.

CHAPTER 20

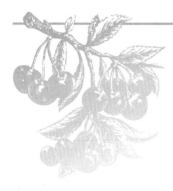

Diet in Renal Disease

LEARNING OBJECTIVES

After completing this chapter, the student should be able to:

1 Identify the major causes of acute and chronic kidney failure.
2 List the goals of nutritional care for a client with kidney disease.
3 List the nutrients commonly modified in the dietary treatment of kidney disease.
4 Discuss the relationship among kilocaloric intake, dietary protein utilization, and uremia.
5 Discuss the nutritional care of clients with kidney disease in relation to their medical treatment.

Before diet therapy can be used to treat kidney disease, the normal function of the kidneys and basic concepts of pathophysiology of renal diseases must be understood. (**Renal** means pertaining to the kidneys.) The nutritional care of clients with renal disease is complex. These clients must frequently learn not just one diet with one to seven nutrients controlled but several different diets as their medical condition changes, and along with it the treatment approach. Failure to follow through with necessary changes in dietary behavior can result in death. One aspect of working with these clients is that inattentiveness to dietary restrictions can be objectively measured in weight changes or changes in the blood chemistry.

This first part of chapter discusses the internal structure and functions of the kidneys. Common kidney diseases, major forms of treatment available for clients, and dietary treatment for renal disease are then presented. A brief discussion of urinary calculi and urinary tract infections concludes the chapter.

Anatomy and Physiology of the Kidneys

Internal Structure

The functioning unit of the kidney is the **nephron.** Each kidney contains about a million nephrons. Figure 20–1 shows an individual nephron. Each nephron has two main parts. The first part is **Bowman's capsule.** Bowman's capsule is the cup-shaped top of the nephron. Inside Bowman's capsule is a network of blood capillaries called the **glomerulus** (plural, *glomeruli*). The second part of the nephron is the **renal tubule.** (A **tubule** is a small tube or canal.) The renal tubule is the rope-like portion of the nephron. This rope-like structure ends at the **collecting tubule.** Several nephrons usually share a single collecting tubule.

Functions

The kidneys assist in the internal regulation of the body by performing the following functions:

1. *Filtration:* The kidneys remove the end products of metabolism and substances that have accumulated in the blood in undesirable amounts during the filtration process. Substances removed from the blood include urea, creatinine, uric acid, and urates. Undesirable amounts of chloride, potassium, sodium, and

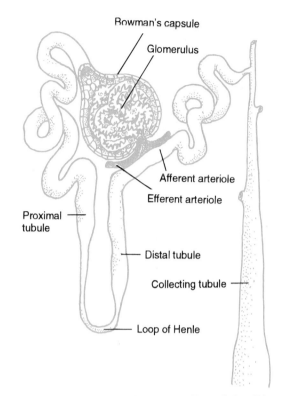

FIGURE 20–1 An individual nephron. (From Gylys, BA, and Wedding, ME: Medical Terminology: A Systems Approach, ed 3. FA Davis, Philadelphia, 1995, p 241, with permission.)

hydrogen ions are also filtered from the blood. The **glomerular filtration rate** (GFR) is the amount of fluid filtered each minute by all the glomeruli of both kidneys and is one index of kidney function. This is normally about 125 milliliters per minute.

2. *Reabsorption:* Previously filtered substances (e.g., water and sodium) needed by the body are reabsorbed into the blood in the tubules.

Nephron—The structural and functional unit of the kidney. There are approximately 1 million nephrons in each kidney.

Bowman's capsule—Part of the nephron that encloses the glomerulus; functions as a filter in the formation of urine.

Glomerulus—A cluster of capillaries through which blood is delivered for filtration; a part of the nephron.

Glomerular filtration rate (GFR)—Amount of fluid filtered each minute by all glumeruli; an index of kidney function.

3. *Secretion of Ions to Maintain Acid-Base Balance:* Secretion is the process of moving ions from the blood into the urine. Secretion allows for the amount of a particular substance to be excreted in the urine in concentrations greater than the concentration filtered from the plasma in the glomeruli. The kidneys regulate the balance between bicarbonate and carbonic acid by the secretion and exchange of hydrogen ions for sodium ions, which are used to form base.

4. *Excretion:* The kidneys eliminate unwanted substances from the body as urine.

5. *Renal Control of Cardiac Output and Systemic Blood Pressure:* The kidneys adapt to changing cardiac output by altering resistance to blood flow both at the beginning of the glomerulus and at the end.

6. *Calcium, Phosphorus, and Vitamin D:* The kidneys produce the active form of vitamin D, **calcitriol.** Activated vitamin D regulates the absorption of calcium **and** phosphorus from the intestinal tract and assists in the regulation of calcium and phosphorus levels in the blood.

7. *Erythropoietin:* The kidneys produce a hormone called **erythropoietin,** which stimulates maturation of red blood cells in bone marrow.

Kidney Disease

Because the kidneys perform so many different metabolic functions, kidney disease has serious consequences. This section of the text discusses the causes of kidney disease and describes several common kidney disorders.

Causes

Renal disease can be caused by many factors, including trauma, infections, birth defects, medications, chronic disease (e.g., artherosclerosis, diabetes, hypertension), and toxic metal consumption. A physiological stress such as a MI or an extensive burn can precipitate renal disease by decreasing the perfusion of the kidney or markedly increasing catabolism. Clinical Application 20–1, which describes the renal response after MI, illustrates the effect of reduced renal blood flow. Catabolism causes an increase in nitrogenous products and potassium; these must be excreted, thus overworking the kidneys. There is some evidence that a habitually high intake of dietary protein can cause kidney damage.

Renal disease is a feared complication of many pathologies and treatments.

Hypertensive Kidney Disease

High blood pressure can cause vascular or glomerular lesions. A **lesion** is an area of injured or diseased tissue.

Specific Tubular Abnormalities

A structural problem in the renal tubules may result in abnormal reabsorption or lack of reabsorption of certain substances by the tubules. The effect of a tubular abnormality is that the blood is not effectively cleansed.

Glomerulonephritis

A general term for an inflammation of the kidneys is **nephritis.** Inflammation of the glomeruli is called **glomerulonephritis,** which can be either acute or chronic. This condition often follows scarlet fever or a streptococcal infection of the respiratory tract. Young children and young adults are often victims. Symptoms include nausea; vomiting; fever; hypertension; blood in the urine, or **hematuria;** a decreased output of urine, or **oliguria;** protein in the urine, or **proteinuria;** and edema. Recovery is usually complete. However, in some clients the disease progresses and becomes chronic. This leads to a progressive loss of kidney function. Some clients de-

---

CLINICAL APPLICATION 20–1

Renal Response after a Myocardial Infarction

Immediately after a heart attack or MI, blood flow through the **systemic circulation** is diminished. Systemic circulation refers to the blood flow from the left part of the heart through the aorta and all branches (arteries) to the capillaries of the tissues. Systemic circulation also includes the blood's return to the heart through the veins. Following a heart attack, blood flow to the **myocardium,** or heart muscle, is decreased, and myocardial function is impaired. Less blood is thus delivered to the tissues. The kidneys sense the decreased cardiac output and try to compensate by reabsorption of additional water. This may lead to a fluid overload and edema. Most clients after a MI are on fluid restriction for this reason.

velop **anuria,** which is a total lack of urine output; without treatment, this condition is fatal.

Nephrotic Syndrome

The result of a variety of diseases that damage the glomeruli capillary walls is called **nephrotic syndrome.** Signs of nephrotic syndrome include proteinuria, severe edema, low serum protein levels, anemia, and hyperlipoproteinemia. Usually the higher the hyperlipoproteinemia, the greater the proteinuria. The disease is caused by the degenerative changes in the kidneys' capillary walls, which consequently permit the passage of albumin into the **glomerular filtrate.** Water and sodium are retained. Edema is sometimes so severe that it masks tissue wasting due to the breakdown of tissue protein stores. The degree of malnutrition is hidden until the excess fluid is removed.

Nephrosclerosis

A hardening of the renal arteries is known as **nephrosclerosis.** This condition is caused by arteriosclerosis and hypertension.

Progressive Nature of Kidney Failure

Kidney disease can be acute or chronic. In **acute renal failure,** the kidneys stop working entirely or almost entirely. Acute renal failure occurs suddenly and is usually temporary. It can last for a few days or weeks.

Chronic renal failure occurs when progressively more nephrons are destroyed until the kidneys simply cannot perform vital functions. Chronic renal failure occurs over time and is usually irreversible.

As individual nephrons are damaged, the remaining nephrons work harder to maintain metabolic homeostasis. As each functional nephron's workload is increased, the nephron becomes more susceptible to work overload and damage. The normal composition of the blood is altered when the remaining functional nephrons cannot assume any additional workload. Serum levels of **blood urea nitrogen** (BUN), creatinine, and uric acid become elevated. In some patients, even though the treatment of the underlying condition (e.g., diabetes mellitus or hypertension) is provided, chronic renal disease may lead to **end-stage renal failure.** During end-stage renal failure, most or all of the kidney's ability to produce urine and regulate blood chemistries is severely compromised.

Chronic renal failure often starts with sodium depletion. This occurs when the kidneys lose their ability to reabsorb sodium in the tubule. Symptoms associated with sodium depletion include a reduction of renal blood flow, dehydration, lethargy, decreased glomerular filtration rate, uremia (see next section), and client deterioration. The client's blood pressure and body weight drop. Urine volume may be increased initially in chronic renal failure. A loss of body fat and protein content is responsible for the weight loss. The client's serum albumin level may fall as protein is lost in the urine.

As kidney function further deteriorates, some of the above symptoms reverse. The kidneys lose the ability to excrete sodium. When this occurs, symptoms include sodium retention, overhydration, edema, hypertension, and CHF. The body can excrete little or no urine.

The GFR gradually declines in chronic renal failure. Most clients with a GFR below 25 milliliters per minute will eventually require either dialysis or transplantation, regardless of the original cause of failure.

If these measures were not implemented, uremia would develop. **Uremia** is the name given to the toxic condition associated with renal insufficiency. Uremia is produced by the retention in the blood of nitrogenous substances normally excreted by the kidneys. The uremic client manifests many symptoms in virtually every body system as toxic waste products build up in the blood. The client may com-

---

Glomerulonephritis—Inflammation (nephritis) of the glomeruli. May be acute or chronic.

Hematuria—Blood in the urine. Urine may be slightly smoky, reddish, or very red.

Oliguria—Diminished amount of urine formation.

Proteinuria—Protein in the urine. May be transient and benign or a symptom of severe renal disease.

Anuria—Absence of urine formation.

Nephrotic syndrome—The result of a variety of diseases that damage the glomeruli capillary wall.

End-stage renal failure—May occur as a result of chronic renal disease. Most or all of the kidney's ability to produce urine and regulate blood composition is severely compromised.

Uremia—Toxic condition associated with renal insufficiency produced by the retention in the blood of nitrogenous substances normally excreted in the kidneys.

plain of fatigue, weakness, and decreased mental ability. The client's muscles may twitch and cramp. Anorexia, nausea, vomiting, and **stomatitis** an inflammation of the mouth, may be present. Sometimes clients complain of an unpleasant taste in the mouth. To further complicate matters, gastrointestinal ulcers and bleeding are common. All of these symptoms have a direct effect on the client's willingness to eat.

Much research is under way to find a way to halt the progression of chronic renal failure. One study demonstrated that a low-protein diet produced a small benefit in clients with moderate renal impairment but did not significantly slow the progression of renal disease in clients with severe renal insufficiency (Klahr, et al, 1994). The idea is to decrease the work of the kidneys and thereby increase the kidneys' productive life span. Dietary intervention is now instituted simultaneously with initial diagnosis.

Treatment for Renal Disease

Renal functions cannot be assumed by another organ. There is no cure for chronic renal failure. However, many clients can be treated with dialysis (an artificial kidney) and/or a kidney transplant. Artificial kidneys have been used for about 40 years to treat clients with severe kidney failure.

Dialysis

Dialysis means the passage of solutes through a membrane. Two functions of the kidneys are (1) the removal of waste products and (2) the regulation of fluid and electrolyte balance. By removing waste products from the blood and assisting in the maintenance of fluid balance, dialysis reduces the symptoms of uremia, hypertension, edema, and the risk of CHF. Dialysis cannot restore the lost hormonal functions of the kidney. In addition, dialysis cannot correct the anemia, which occurs due to a lack of erythropoietin. Some dialysis clients still need treatment for hypertension.

Hemodialysis

During **hemodialysis,** blood is removed from the client's artery through a tube, forced to flow over a semipermeable membrane where waste is removed, and then rerouted back into the client's body through a vein. A solution called the **dialysate** is placed on one side of the semipermeable membrane while the client's blood flows on the other side. The dialysate is similar in composition to normal blood plasma. The client's blood has a higher concentration of urea and electrolytes than the dialysate, so these substances diffuse from the blood into the dialysate. The dialysate also contains glucose, and the more glucose the dialysate contains, the more fluid will move from the blood into the dialysate by osmosis. This process pulls extra fluid from the blood. The composition of the dialysate varies according to the requirements of each client.

Hemodialysis treatments usually last 4 to 8 hours and are administered three times per week. Some clients are taught to perform their own dialysis treatments at home. Dialysis is not as effective as normal kidney function because blood cleansing occurs only when clients are attached to artificial kidneys. Normal kidneys clear the blood 24 hours a day 7 days a week.

Peritoneal Dialysis

The **peritoneum** is the lining of the abdominal cavity. During **peritoneal dialysis,** the dialysate is placed directly into the client's abdomen. The dialysate enters the body through a permanent catheter placed in the abdominal cavity. The peritoneum thus functions as the semipermeable membrane.

INTERMITTENT PERITONEAL DIALYSIS Between 1 and 2 liters of fluid are introduced into the abdominal cavity during intermittent peritoneal dialysis. The fluid is allowed to remain in the abdomen for about 30 minutes and then drained from the body by gravity. One complete exchange takes about an hour. This process is repeated until the blood urea nitrogen level drops.

CONTINUOUS AMBULATORY PERITONEAL DIALYSIS **Continuous ambulatory peritoneal dialysis** (CAPD) is the dialysis method chosen by many clients. This is a form of self-dialysis. About 1 liter of dialysate is introduced into the abdominal cavity. The fluid remains in the cavity for 4 to 6 hours while the waste products diffuse into the dialysate. The dialysate is then replaced with a new solution. Clients can move about and pursue their activities of daily living during CAPD. The term "continuous" means that the client is dialyzing constantly. The advantage of CAPD is that the client's blood levels of sodium, potassium, creatinine, and nitrogen are kept within a much more stable range. Large shifts in fluid balance are also avoided.

Kidney Transplant

A kidney transplant can restore full renal function. Immunosuppressants to prevent rejection of the transplanted kidney are necessary. Some commonly used immunosuppressants are azathioprine, corticosteroids, and/or cyclosporine. These medications have many side effects, including diarrhea, nausea, and vomiting, which influence nutrient intake and absorption.

Nutritional Care of the Renal Client

The nutritional needs of clients with renal diseases are changing constantly. The reason for the change is that the disease state and treatment approach are not static. Clients with kidney disease require constant assessment, monitoring, and counseling. In addition, it is an ongoing challenge to provide quality nutritional care to these clients, who frequently must be coaxed to eat. Anorexia, nausea, and vomiting are frequent complaints. It is common for the dietitian to see these clients more than once per day for nutritional problems during hospitalization.

Malnutrition

The prevalence of malnutrition, especially in clients undergoing chronic dialysis treatment is high. One study found 8 percent of clients on CAPD were severely malnourished and 33 percent were moderately malnourished (Young, et al, 1991). Another study reported a 17 percent incidence of protein malnutrition in clients receiving hemodialysis (Oksa, et al, 1990). Among the reasons for the malnutrition are increased catabolism, metabolic derangement, decreased food intake, and low-economic status.

Goals of Nutrition Therapy

Well-planned nutritional management is a fundamental part of any treatment for renal disease. Every client with renal disease requires an individualized diet based on the following goals:

1. Attain and maintain optimal nutritional status
2. Prevent net protein catabolism
3. Minimize uremic toxicity
4. Maintain adequate hydration status
5. Maintain normal serum potassium levels
6. Control the progression of renal osteodystrophy (discussion follows)
7. Modify diet to meet other nutrition-related concerns such as diabetes, heart disease, gastrointestinal tract ulcers, and/or constipation
8. Retard the progression of renal failure and postpone the initiation of dialysis

No single diet is appropriate for all renal clients. Every client requires an individual assessment.

Dietary Components

Several basic components need to be monitored and, if possible, controlled in renal diets. These components are:

- Kilocalories
- Protein
- Sodium
- Potassium
- Phosphorus and calcium
- Fluid
- Saturated fat and cholesterol
- Iron, vitamins, and minerals

The need to restrict or encourage the consumption of any of the above nutrients changes according to the client's medical status and treatment approach. For example, it may not be necessary for a client to control his or her phosphorus intake at one time but vital at another time.

Kilocalories

Intake of kilocalories is often increased for clients with renal disease. Clients on high-kilocalorie diets are usually given all the simple carbohydrates and monounsaturated and polyunsaturated fats they will eat. The end products of fat and carbohydrate catabolism are carbon dioxide and water. Neither of

---

Dialysis—The passage of solute through a membrane; removes toxic materials and maintains fluid, electrolyte, and acid-base balance in cases of impaired kidney function or absence of kidneys.

Hemodialysis—A method of providing the function of the kidneys by circulating blood through a machine that contains synthetic semipermeable membranes.

Continuous ambulatory peritoneal dialysis (CAPD)—Method of self-dialysis chosen by many clients. The lining of the peritoneal cavity is used as the dialysis membrane.

these dietary constituents imposes a burden on the client's compromised excretory ability. Inadequate nonprotein kilocalories will, however, encourage tissue breakdown and aggravate the uremia. An adequate intake of kilocalories is crucial to the success of the dietary treatment.

Some individuals with diabetes mellitus and renal diseases still need to have their blood sugar levels controlled. For these clients, it may or may not be advisable to increase simple carbohydrates. The need to control the blood sugar is sometimes a secondary concern. In some situations, the primary nutritional goal is to decrease the uremia. Uremic diabetic clients may have relatively high amounts of sugar planned into their diets.

Some renal clients require an alternate feeding route to attain and maintain optimal nutritional status. Accordingly, some physicians order a peripheral intravenous infusion of lipids to supplement oral feedings. Total parenteral nutrition solutions for renal clients are commercially available.

Protein

A primary goal of nutritional therapy in renal clients is control of nitrogen intake. Control may mean an increase or decrease of dietary protein as the client's medical condition and treatment approach change. In addition, the kind of protein fed to the client may be important. High-biological-value protein is indicated for clients with an extremely high BUN level. Eggs, meat, and dairy products are examples of foods that contain protein of high biologic value. Protein restrictions are only effective if the client also consumes adequate kilocalories. Beginning renal insufficiency is usually referred to as a predialysis situation and requires a restriction of protein intake.

The treatment approach selected by the client and the physician influences protein requirements. Hemodialysis clients sometimes need increased protein because hemodialysis results in a loss of 1 to 2 grams of amino acids per hour of dialysis. A client on CAPD has an even higher protein need because he or she dialyzes continuously. During dialysis, protein passes out of the blood with the waste products and into the dialysate fluid. When the dialysate fluid is discarded, a significant amount of protein is lost from the body. A high-protein diet is necessary to replenish these losses.

Sodium

The desirable sodium intake of renal clients depends on individual circumstances and is usually determined by repeated measurements of sodium in the serum and in the urine (if any). The sodium intake of many clients with renal failure must be restricted to prevent sodium retention in the body with consequent generalized edema (Burton, and Hirschman, 1983).

The disease that precipitated the renal failure plays a role in determining the need for a sodium restriction. Because glomerulonephritis, for example, is more likely to produce hypertension and fluid retention, a sodium restriction is often necessary. Other renal diseases, such as pyelonephritis, are often characterized by low levels of sodium, absence of edema, and normal or low blood pressure. **Pyelonephritis** is an inflammation of the central portion of the kidney. In this situation, sodium intake should be higher than in the other groups of diseases but individualized to the client's needs.

Potassium

Dietary potassium, like sodium, needs to be evaluated on an individual basis. **Hypokalemia** (low blood potassium level) needs to be avoided because it introduces the danger of cardiac arrhythmias and eventually cardiac arrest. Tables 20–1 and 20–2 lists foods high and low in potassium. Salt substitutes are very high in potassium and should be avoided by most renal clients. Generally the need to restrict potassium increases with decreased urinary output.

The potassium content of fruits and vegetables varies according to the form eaten and the method of food preparation. For example, 1/2 cup of canned pears in heavy syrup has a potassium content of about 80 milligrams, while one fresh pear has a potassium content of about 200 milligrams. Potassium is water soluble. For this reason, some renal clients on very low potassium diets are taught to use large amounts of water when preparing vegetables and to discard the water after cooking. This decreases the potassium content of the vegetables. Unfortunately, it also decreases the water-soluble vitamins in the food. This is one reason why most renal clients need vitamin supplements. Clients should be taught to eat the fruits or vegetables in the form given on the list.

Phosphorus, Vitamin D, and Calcium

Phosphorus, vitamin D, and calcium are all normally balanced in the body. In clients with kidney disease, vitamin D cannot be activated. This leads to a low serum calcium level. At the same time, the kidneys cannot excrete phosphorus. This leads to an elevated serum phosphorus level. When the serum calcium level drops, calcium is released from the bones because of the increased secretion of **parathyroid hormone** (PTH). PTH is secreted in an effort to correct the calcium imbalance. This chain of events may lead to **renal osteodystrophy,** which is a complication of chronic renal disease. Renal osteodystrophy leads to faulty bone formation.

Control of the blood levels of calcium and phosphorus involve four treatment approaches. First, clients with hypocalcemia and hyperphosphatemia are currently given calcitriol, the activated form of vitamin D. Second, phosphate binders are frequently used if the phosphorus level of the blood is elevated. Phosphate binders work in the intestinal tract by binding dietary phosphorus and preventing its absorption into the blood. Phosphate binders are high in aluminum, which has been found to be elevated in the brains of clients receiving aluminum hydroxide or aluminum carbonate binders. Some researchers link the high levels of aluminum in the tissues of dialyzed clients to dialysis dementia. **Dialysis dementia** is a progressive loss of mental function seen in clients who have been on dialysis for a

TABLE 20–1 High-Potassium Foods to Avoid

Dairy products	(In excess of 2 cups per day)
Meats	(In excess of 6 oz per day)
Starches	Bran cereals and bran products
Fruits	Avocado
	Bananas
	Orange, fresh
	Mango, fresh
	Nectarines
	Papayas
	Dried prunes
	(All others if eaten in excess of allowance)
Vegetables	Bamboo shoots
	Beet greens
	Baked potato, with skin
	Sweet potato, fresh
	Spinach, cooked
	(All others if eaten in excess of allowance)
Others	Chocolate, cocoa
	Molasses
	Salt substitute
	Low-sodium broth
	Low-sodium baking powder
	Low-sodium baking soda
	Nuts

TABLE 20–2 Low-Potassium Foods and Beverages*

Gum drops
Hard, clear candy
Nondairy topping
Honey
Jams and jellies
Jelly beans
Lollipops
Marshmallows
Suckers
Sugar
Lifesavers
Chewing gum
"Poly-Rich" (nondairy creamer)
Cornstarch

Low-Potassium Beverages
Carbonated beverages
Lemonade
Limeade
Cranberry juice
Popsicles (1 stick = 60 mL of fluid)
Hawaiian punch
Kool-Aid

Low-Potassium Unsweetened Beverages
Diet carbonated beverages
Diet lemonade
Diet Kool-Aid

* *Note:* Foods with sugar should not be eaten freely by diabetics.

number of years. The third treatment approach is a dietary phosphorus restriction. Dietary phosphorus restriction is currently recommended over the use of phosphate binders; the intent is to minimize the problem of dialysis dementia. Fourth, calcium supplements and/or a high-calcium diet is frequently prescribed if the serum phosphorus is under control.

Phosphorus is found mainly in meat and dairy products. Clients on protein-restricted diets generally do not eat enough phosphorus to cause hyperphosphatemia. Clients on chronic renal dialysis with a more liberal protein intake may need to limit the intake of dairy products that are high in phosphorus.

> **Renal osteodystrophy**—Pathological changes in bone that often accompany renal failure in which calcium is lost from the bones.

Fluid

Predialysis (renal-insufficiency) and dialysis clients generally must restrict fluid intake because their kidneys can no longer excrete excess fluid. Fluids need to be allocated between meals and medications. Table 20–3 lists guidelines to follow for distributing fluids between meals and medications. Clients on hemodialysis are restricted to "500 to 1000 milliliters plus 24-hour urinary output." This allows for some fluid gain between dialysis treatments. For predialysis clients, fluid restrictions are usually "500 milliliters plus output." For clients on CAPD, fluid restriction is "as tolerated" according to their daily weight fluctuations and blood pressure.

Saturated Fat and Cholesterol

Clients with renal disease frequently have hyperlipoproteinemia. High serum lipid levels are thought to aid in the progression of renal disease, which contributes to an increased risk of cardiovascular disease. Total cholesterol levels may be increased tenfold (American Dietetic Association, 1992). This is believed to be especially a problem in clients with nephrotic syndrome, diabetes, and for an **LCAT deficiency.** LCAT is an enzyme that transports cholesterol from tissues to the liver for removal from the body. Most clients with an LCAT deficiency develop progressive glomerular injury.

Significant hypertriglyceridemia is often present in clients with a history of renal disease. The nutritional care of clients with elevated triglycerides (type 4 hyperlipoproteinemia) includes a modified fat diet and a modification of carbohydrate intake. Clients are usually counseled to avoid saturated fat and to increase their intake of polyunsaturated and monounsaturated fat. Thirty to 35 percent of the total kilocalories are provided as fat because excessive carbohydrate could worsen the hypertriglyceridemia (Moore, 1993). Simple sugars and alcohol are usually limited for the same reason.

Iron

The anemias seen in clients with renal disease may be due to a lack of erythropoietin; a decreased oral iron intake, which often occurs as a result of dietary restriction; or blood loss. *Epoetin alfa,* a pharmaceutical form of erythropoietin, may be used to increase red blood cell production and thereby correct the anemia. The treatment for iron-deficiency anemia is oral or parenteral iron products and an increase in dietary sources of iron. A diagnosis of iron-deficiency anemia can be made by a laboratory measure of ferritin. **Ferritin** is the storage form of iron found primarily in the liver. A small amount of ferritin circulates in the blood and reflects the amount of iron in body stores. A laboratory value of less than 12 micrograms per liter suggests iron deficiency.

Nutritional therapy with iron supplements consists of 200 milligrams of ferrous iron salts per day divided among three to four doses. Absorption is enhanced when iron supplements are taken on an empty stomach or with vitamin C.

TABLE 20–3   Guidelines for Fluid-Restricted Clients

If the Fluid Restriction Is:	Use This Amount of Fluids with Meals:	Use This Amount of Fluids with Medication:
1000 mL (4 cups)*	600 mL (2 1/2 cups)	400 mL (1 1/2 cups)
1200 mL (5 cups)	700 mL (3 cups)	500 mL (2 cups)
1500 mL (6 cups)	1000 mL (4 cups)	500 mL (2 cups)
2000 mL (8 cups)	1000 mL (4 cups)	1000 mL (4 cups)

All foods contain some fluids, but it is especially important to count the following as part of the fluid allowance:

Milliliters of Fluid per 1/2 Cup

Water	120	All juices	120	Watermelon	100
Coffee	120	soda-pop	120	Sherbet	65
Tea	120	Ice	60	Ice cream	40
Sanka	120	Gelatin	100	Ice milk	40
Milk	120	Soup	120	Popsicle	80

* Approximate

Vitamin and Mineral Supplementation

Deficiencies of water-soluble vitamins in clients with renal failure are caused by losses in the dialysate, metabolic alterations, and decreased intake (Panagis, 1995). Losses are most notable with pyridoxine, ascorbic acid, and folic acid (Wolfson, 1988). Supplementation of these nutrients is recommended for clients on dialysis. Fat-soluble vitamins are not lost in the dialysate and supplementation is not indicated except of vitamin D for another reason (see previous discussion). Because the body's ability to excrete excess fat-soluble vitamins is compromised, toxicity is a potential problem.

National Renal Diet

The American Dietetic Association and the National Kidney Foundation introduced the "National Renal Diet" in the fall of 1993. Because the dietary management of renal disease is tailored to the stage of disease and treatment approach, six meal-planning systems were developed. They are: renal insuffi-

ciency without diabetes; renal insufficiency with diabetes; hemodialysis without diabetes; hemodialysis with diabetes; peritoneal dialysis without diabetes; and peritoneal dialysis with diabetes. These national meal-planning systems offer standardized guidelines for nutrition intervention and client education.

Each system provides food lists and calculation figures (derived from the average nutrient content of foods included in each list). Although the food lists developed for the client booklets were patterned after the *ADA Exchange Lists,* the varied nutritional requirements of clients with renal disease at different stages of treatment necessitated creation of specific food lists for each treatment modality. Box 20–1 shows the General Dietary Recommendations for Renal Patients by treatment approach. In addition, separate calculation figures and food lists were devised for clients with diabetes receiving each treatment modality, because foods high in sugars were excluded from the food lists for clients with diabetes.

Box 20–2 is an example of the calculation of a diet for a client receiving hemodialysis without diabetes (one of the six meal-planning systems). A case study

---

BOX 20–1   GENERAL DIETARY RECOMMENDATIONS FOR RENAL PATIENTS

Dietary Component	Renal Insufficiency	Hemodialysis	Peritoneal Dialysis
Protein (g/kg HBW)*	0.6–0.8†	1.1–1.4	1.2–1.5
Energy (kcal/kg HBW)	35–40	30–35	25–35
Phosphorus (mg/kg HBW)	8–12‡	≤17§	≤17
Sodium (mg/day)	1000–3000	2000–3000	2000–4000
Potassium (mg/kg HBW)	Typically not restricted	40	Typically not restricted
Fluid (mL/day)	Typically not restricted	500–750 plus daily urine output or 1000 if anuric	≥2000
Calcium (mg/day)	1200–1600	Depends on serum level	Depends on serum level

*HBW = healthy body weight.

†The upper end of this range is preferred for patients with diabetes or malnutrition. Suggested protein intake for persons with nephrotic syndrome is 0.8 to 1.0 g/kg HBW.

‡Intake of 5 to 10 mg phosphorus per kilogram HBW is frequently quoted in the scientific literature, but 5 mg/kg HBW is practical only when used in conjunction with a very low-protein diet supplemented with specially formulated commercial feedings.

§It may not be possible to meet the optimum phosphorus prescription on a higher protein diet.

Source: Monsen, ER: Meeting the challenge of the renal diet. Copyright The American Dietetic Association. Reprinted by permission from Journal of the American Dietetic Association 93:638, 1993.

BOX 20–2 CALCULATING THE RENAL DIET: HEMODIALYSIS CASE STUDY

AVERAGE CALCULATION FIGURES FOR RENAL DIETS (NO DIABETES)*

Food Choices	Energy kcal	PRO g	CHO g	FAT g	Na mg	K mg	P mg
Milk	120	4	8	5	80	185	110
Nondairy milk substitute	140	0.5	12	10	40	80	30
Meat	65	7	...	4	25	100	65
Starch	90	2	18	1	80	35	35
Vegetable							
Low potassium	25	1	5	tr	15	70	20
Medium potassium	25	1	5	tr	15	150	20
High potassium	25	1	5	tr	15	270	20
Fruit							
Low potassium	70	0.5	17	...	tr	70	15
Medium potassium	70	0.5	17	...	tr	150	15
High potassium	70	0.5	17	...	tr	270	15
Fat	45	...	...	5	55	10	5
High-calorie	100	tr	25	...	15	20	5
Salt	...	...	...	...	250	...	...

CASE EXAMPLE

The client is a 55-year-old man who works full-time and has a sedentary lifestyle. He is 5 ft, 10 in tall, has a medium frame, and weighs 68 kg. His ideal and usual weight is 76 kg. During the past 6–9 months, he has been anorectic and has had intermittent nausea and episodes of vomiting. He receives 4 hours of hemodialysis 3 times per week. His predialysis blood chemistry values were blood urea nitrogen, 22.50 mmol/L (63 mg/dL); sodium, 135 mmol/L (135 mEq/L); potassium, 4.0 mmol/L (4.0 mEq/L); phosphorus, 2.0 mmol/L (6.2 mg/dL); calcium, 2.25 mmol/L (9.0 mg/dL); and albumin, 33 g/L (3.3 g/dL). His urine output ranges between 800 and 1000 mL per day.

DAILY RENAL DIET PLAN GOALS

Nutrient	Level	Rationale
Energy (kcal)	3000	40 kcal/kg HBW
Protein (g)	91	1.2 g/kg HBW
Sodium (mg)	2000	Control fluid weight gain
Potassium (mg)	3000 (75 mEq)	≤40 mg/kg HBW
Phosphorus (mg)	300	≤17 mg/kg HBW
Fluid (mL)	1500–1750	750 mL plus urine output